INTRODUCTION TO Splinting

A Clinical Reasoning and Problem-Solving Approach

Brenda M. Coppard, PhD, OTR/L
Associate Professor, Chair
Department of Occupational Therapy
Creighton University
Omaha, Nebraska

Helene Lohman, MA, OTD, OTR/L
Associate Professor
Department of Occupational Therapy
Creighton University
Omaha, Nebraska

3
THIRD EDITION

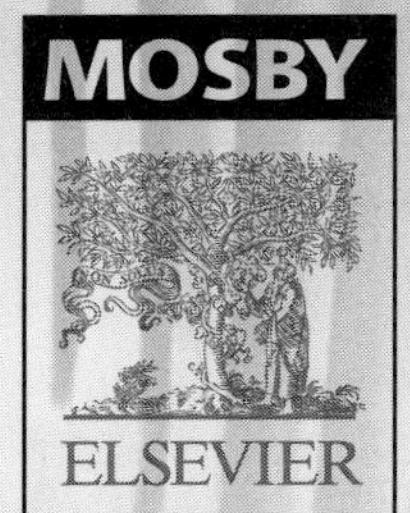
MOSBY
ELSEVIER

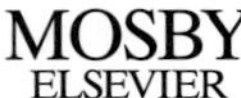

11830 Westline Industrial Drive
St. Louis, Missouri 63146

INTRODUCTION TO SPLINTING: A CLINICAL REASONING AND PROBLEM-SOLVING APPROACH, THIRD EDITION

ISBN: 978-0-323-03384-8

Library of Congress Control Number 2007932736

Publishing Director: Linda Duncan
Editor: Kathy Falk
Developmental Editor: Melissa Kuster Deutsch
Publishing Services Manager: Melissa Lastarria
Senior Project Manager: Joy Moore
Design Direction: Julia Dummitt
Text Designer: Julia Dummitt

Printed in the United States of America

Last digit is the print number: 9 8 7 6 5 4 3 2 1

This work is dedicated to the late Father Don Driscoll, SJ;
and Steve, Roman, and Margaret.

Brenda M. Coppard

With the writing of this book one can say that life happens.
Therefore, I appreciate the patience of everyone involved.
I specifically dedicate this book to my family, friends,
and students, who continue to inspire me.

Helene Lohman

CONTRIBUTORS

Debbie Amini, MEd, OTR/L, CHT
Director, Occupational Therapy Assistant Program
Cape Fear Community College
Wilmington, North Carolina

Omar Aragón, OTD, OTR/L
Assistant Clinical Professor
Department of Occupational Therapy
Creighton University
Director of Rehabilitative Science
Orthotics and Prosthetics
Lifestyles, Orthotics and Prosthetics
Omaha, Nebraska

Shirley Blanchard, PhD, OTR/L
Associate Professor
Department of Occupational Therapy
Creighton University
Omaha, Nebraska

Cynthia Cooper, MFA, MA, OTR/L, CHT
Director of Hand Therapy in Arizona
VibrantCare Rehabilitation
Phoenix, Arizona

Brenda M. Coppard, PhD, OTR/L
Associate Professor, Chair
Department of Occupational Therapy
Creighton University
Omaha, Nebraska

Lisa Deshaies, OTR/L, CHT
Adjunct Clinical Faculty
Department of Occupational Science & Occupational Therapy
University of Southern California
Los Angeles, California
Occupational Therapy Clinical Specialist
Occupational Therapy Department
Rancho Los Amigos National Rehabilitation Center
Downey, California

Deanna J. Fish, MS, CPO
Chief Clinical Officer
Clinical Operations
Linkia, LLC
Bethesda, Maryland

Linda S. Gabriel, PhD, OTR/L
Assistant Professor and Vice Chair
Department of Occupational Therapy
Creighton University
Omaha, Nebraska

Amy Marie Haddad, PhD
Director
Center for Health Policy and Ethics
Dr. C.C. and Mabel L. Criss Endowed Chair in the Health Sciences
Creighton University
Omaha, Nebraska

Karyn Kessler, OTR/L
Vice President
Clinical Operations
Linkia, LLC
Bethesda, Maryland

Dulcey G. Lima, OTR/L, CO
Clinical Education Manager
Orthomerica Products, Inc.
Orlando, Florida

Helene Lohman, MA, OTD, OTR/L
Associate Professor
Department of Occupational Therapy
Creighton University
Omaha, Nebraska

Michael Lohman, MEd, OTR/L, CO
Adjunct Clinical Professor
Department of Occupational Therapy
Creighton University
Director of Clinical Education Lifestyles Orthotics and Prosthetics
Omaha, Nebraska

Deborah A. Rider, OTR/L, CHT
Occupational Therapist, Fieldwork Coordinator
Therapy Department
Hand Surgery and Rehab
Marlton, New Jersey

Marlene A. Riley, MMS, OTR/L, CHT
Clinical Associate Professor
Department of Occupational Therapy
and Occupational Science
Towson University
Owner
Occupational Therapy Associates of Towson
Towson, Maryland

Linda S. Scheirton, PhD
Associate Dean for Academic Affairs
Associate Professor
Department of Occupational Therapy
Faculty Associate
Center for Health Policy and Ethics
Creighton University
Omaha, Nebraska

Kris M. Vacek, OTD, OTR/L
Chairperson, Associate Professor
Department of Occupational Therapy Education
Rockhurst University
Kansas City, Missouri

Jean Wilwerding-Peck, OTR/L, CHT
Clinical Coordinator
Creighton University Medical Center
Omaha, Nebraska

Aviva Wolff, OTR/L, CHT
Section Manager
Hand Therapy
Department of Rehabilitation
Hospital for Special Surgery
New York, New York

PREFACE

As instructors in a professional occupational therapy program who were unable to find an introductory splinting textbook that addressed the development of splinting theory and skills, we wrote the first edition and subsequently the second edition of *Introduction to Splinting: A Clinical Reasoning and Problem-Solving Approach*. Entry-level occupational therapy practitioners are expected to have fundamental skills in splinting theory, design, and fabrication. It is unrealistic to think that students gain these skills through observation and limited experience in didactic course work or fieldwork. With the growing emphasis in the health care environment on accountability, productivity, and efficacy, educators must consider what skills students need to apply theory to practice.

Several features are improved in this third edition. Evidence-based splinting practice is emphasized throughout the chapters both in narrative and chart formats. A focus on occupation-based splinting is present, including a chapter dedicated to the topic. The Occupational Therapy Practice Framework terminology is incorporated throughout the book.

The third edition of *Introduction to Splinting: A Clinical Reasoning and Problem-Solving Approach* was again designed with a pedagogy to facilitate the process of learning how to apply theory to practice in relationship to splinting. This text is primarily designed for entry-level occupational therapy students, occupational therapy practitioners and interdisciplinary practitioners who need to develop skills in splinting, therapists reentering the field, and students on fieldwork. In past editions, students found the book beneficial because it facilitated the mastery of basic theory and the principles and techniques of splinting that entry-level clinicians need for clinical competence. Instructors enthusiastically welcomed the text because the text was targeted for novice occupational therapy students. Novice practitioners also reported that the book was beneficial in developing their knowledge and skills related to splinting.

The pedagogy employed within the book facilitates learning. A unique aspect of this third edition is a **CD-ROM** that accompanies the book. The CD-ROM provides visual and auditory instructions on splint fabrication. There are additional **case studies** to stimulate clinical reasoning and problem-solving skills. **Self-quizzes** and **review questions** with answers provide the reader with excellent tools to test immediate recall of basic information. Readers are guided through splint fabrication in the laboratory with more illustrations and photographs than in the previous editions. The **forms** provided in the book present opportunities to promote reflection and to assist students' development of their self-assessment skills. Case studies, splint analyses, and documentation exercises are examples of learning activities designed to stimulate problem solving. The **learning exercises** and **laboratory experiences** provide opportunities to test clinical reasoning and the technical skills of splint pattern design and splint fabrication.

A cadre of expert contributors led to several new or expanded chapters that reflect current practice. This edition of *Introduction to Splinting* contains 19 chapters. The first five chapters consist of an introduction to splinting; occupation-based splinting; tools, processes, and techniques of splinting; a review of anatomic and biomechanical principles; and a review of the assessment process. These chapters provide fundamental information and are applied throughout the remaining chapters.

Chapter 6 addresses thorough clinical reasoning processes used in making decisions about practice involving splint design and construction. The material presented in this chapter helps answer questions in case studies presented in later chapters.

Chapters 7 through 13 present the theory, design, and fabrication process of common splints used in general clinical practice. The specific splints include wrist splints, hand immobilization splints, thumb immobilization splints, dynamic or mobilizing splints, and splints for the elbow and fingers.

The remaining six chapters in the book are geared toward more specialized topics and to intermediate-to-advanced splinting. Topics for these chapters include splinting for nerve injuries, antispasticity splinting, splinting on elders, splinting on children with congenital and developmental disabilities, splinting on the lower extremity, prosthetics, and ethical issues related to splinting.

A glossary of terms used throughout the book follows Chapter 19. This book also contains four appendixes. Appendix A provides answers to quizzes, laboratory exercises, and case studies. Appendix B contains updated copies of self-evaluation forms that appear in the chapters. Readers can complete these forms based on the splints they fabricate. Appendix C contains copies of classroom grading sheets that appear in the chapters. Appendixes B and C have perforated pages. Appendix D contains a list of web resources.

Although many therapists reviewed this book, each experienced therapist and physician may have a personal view on splinting and therapeutic approaches and techniques. This book represents the authors' perspectives and is not intended to present the only correct approach. Thus, therapists employ their clinical reasoning skills in practice.

We hope this third edition of the book complements your professional development!

Brenda M. Coppard, PhD, OTR/L
Helene Lohman, MA, OTD, OTR/L

ACKNOWLEDGMENTS

The completion of this third edition was made possible through the efforts of many individuals. We are grateful to Karen Schultz-Johnson, MS, OTR, CHT, FAOTA, for the peer-reviewing of the manuscripts. Additionally, we appreciate the talent and expertise of the following contributor authors to the current and previous editions: Debbie Amini, MEd, OTR/L, CHT; Omar Aragon, OTD, OTR/L; Serena M. Berger, MA, OTR; Shirley Blanchard, PhD, OTR/L; Maureen T. Cavanaugh, MS, OTR; Cynthia Cooper, MFA, MA, OTR/L, CHT; Lisa Deshaies, OTR/L, CHT; Beverly Duvall-Riley, MS, BSOT; Deanna J. Fish, MS, CPO; Linda Gabriel, PhD, OTR/L; Amy Marie Haddad, PhD; Karyn Kessler, OTR/L; Dulcey G. Lima, OTR/L, CO; Michael Lohman, MEd, OTR/L, CO; Peggy Lynn, OTR, CHT; Debra A. Monnin, OTR/L; Sally E. Poole, MA, OT, CHT; Debbie Rider, OTR/L, CHT; Marlene A. Riley, MMS, OTR, CHT; Susan Salzberg, MOT, OTR/L; Linda Scheirton, PhD; Lauren Sivula, OTS; Joan L. Sullivan, MA, OTR, CHT; Kris Vacek, OTD, OTR; Jean Wilwerding-Peck, OTR/L, CHT; and Aviva Wolff, OTR/L, CHT.

Preparing the artwork and filming for this book is time and labor intensive. We are grateful for the skills of Thomas H. Herbert (photographer) and J.R. Jasso (videographer) of the Creative Services department at Creighton University.

The editors at Elsevier have given steadfast support for this book. We are grateful for the guidance and assistance from Kathy Falk, Melissa Kuster, and Tom Pohlman.

We thank our families and friends for their continual support, encouragement, and patience. We also thank our students for enabling us to learn from them.

BMC
HL

CONTENTS

INTRODUCTION TO

Splinting

UNIT **ONE**

Splinting Foundations

CHAPTER 1

Foundations of Splinting

Brenda M. Coppard, PhD, OTR/L

Key Terms

Orthosis
Mobilization
Immobilization
Torque transmission
Dorsal
Volar
Evidence-based practice

Chapter Objectives

1. Define the terms *splint* and *orthosis*.
2. Identify the health professionals who may provide splinting services.
3. Appreciate the historical development of splinting as a therapeutic intervention.
4. Apply the Occupational Therapy Practice Framework (OTPF) to optimize evaluation and treatment for a client.
5. Describe how frame-of-reference approaches are applied to splinting.
6. Familiarize yourself with splint nomenclature of past and present.
7. List the purposes of immobilization (static) splints.
8. List the purposes of mobilization (dynamic) splints.
9. Describe the six splint designs.
10. Define *evidence-based practice*.
11. Describe the steps involved in evidence-based practice.
12. Cite the hierarchy of evidence for critical appraisals of research.

Determining splint design and fabricating hand splints are extremely important aspects in providing optimal care for persons with upper extremity injuries and functional deficits. Splint fabrication is a combination of science and art. Therapists must apply knowledge of occupation, pathology, physiology, kinesiology, anatomy, psychology, reimbursement systems, and biomechanics to best design splints for persons. In addition, therapists must consider and appreciate the aesthetic value of splints. Beginning splintmakers should be aware that each person is different, requiring a customized approach to splinting. The use of occupation-based and evidence-based approaches to splinting guides a therapist to consider a person's valued occupations. As a result, those occupations are used as both a means (e.g., as a medium for therapy) and an end to outcomes (e.g., therapeutic goals) [Gray 1998].

Therapists must also develop and use clinical reasoning skills to effectively evaluate and treat clients with upper extremity conditions, and when necessary splint them. This book emphasizes and fosters such skills for beginning splintmakers in general practice areas. After therapists are knowledgeable in the science of splint design and fabrication (including instructing clients on their use and on precautions regarding them, checking for proper fit, and making revisions as deemed appropriate), practical experience is essential for them to become comfortable and competent.

Definition of a Splint

Mosby's Medical, Nursing, and Allied Health Dictionary (2002) defines a *splint* as "an orthopedic device for immobilization, restraint, or support of any part of the body" (p. 1618). The text also defines *orthosis* as "a force system designed to control, correct, or compensate for a bone deformity, deforming forces, or forces absent from the body" (p. 1237).

Today, these health care field terms are often used synonymously. Technically, the term *splint* refers to a temporary device that is part of a treatment program, whereas the term *orthosis* refers to a permanent device to replace or substitute for loss of muscle function.

Note: This chapter includes content from previous contributions from Peggy Lynn, OTR, CHT.

Splints and orthoses not only immobilize but also mobilize, position, and protect a joint or specific body part. Splints range in design and fabrication from simple to complex, depending on the goals established for a particular condition.

Historical Synopsis of Splinting

Reports of primitive splints date back to ancient Egypt [Fess 2002]. Decades ago, blacksmiths and carpenters constructed the first splints. Materials used to make the splints were limited to cloth, wood, leather, and metal [War Department 1944]. Hand splinting became an important aspect of physical rehabilitation during World War II. Survival rates of injured troops dramatically increased because of medical, pharmacologic (e.g., the use of penicillin), and technological advances. During this period, occupational and physical therapists collaborated with orthotic technicians and physicians to provide splints to clients: "Sterling Bunnell, MD, was designated to organize and to oversee hand services at nine army hospitals in the United States" [Rossi 1987, p. 53]. In the mid 1940s, under the guidance of Dr. Bunnell many splints were made and sold commercially. During the 1950s, many children and adults needed splints to assist them in carrying out activities of daily living secondary to poliomyelitis [Rossi 1987]. During this time, orthotists made splints from high-temperature plastics. With the advent of low-temperature thermoplastics in the 1960s, hand splinting became a common practice in clinics.

Today, some therapists and clinics specialize in hand therapy. Hand therapy evolved from a group of therapists in the 1970s who were interested in researching and rehabilitating clients with hand injuries [Daus 1998]. In 1977, this group of therapy specialists established the American Society for Hand Therapy (ASHT). In 1991, the first certification examination in hand therapy was given. Those therapists who pass the certification examination are credentialed as certified hand therapists (CHTs).

Specialized organizations (e.g., American Society for Surgery of the Hand and ASHT) influence the practice, research, and education of upper extremity splinting [Fess et al. 2005]. For example, the ASHT Splint Classification System offered a uniform nomenclature in the area of splinting [Bailey et al. 1992].

Splintmakers

A variety of health care professionals design and fabricate splints. Occupational therapists (OTs) constitute a large population of health care providers whose services include splint design and fabrication. Certified occupational therapy assistants (COTAs) also provide splint services. Along with OTs and COTAs, physical therapists (PTs) specializing in hand rehabilitation often fabricate splints for their clients who have hand injuries. PTs are frequently involved in providing splints for the lower extremities. In addition, certified orthotists (COs) are trained and skilled in the design, construction, and fitting of braces and orthoses prescribed by physicians. Dentists frequently fabricate orthoses to address selective dental problems. Occasionally, nurses who have had special training fabricate splints.

Splint design must be based on scientific principles. A given diagnosis does not specify the splint the clinician will make. Splint fabrication often requires creative problem solving. Such factors as a client's occupational needs and interests influence a splint design, even among clients who have common diagnoses. Health care professionals who make splints must allow themselves to be creative and take calculated risks. Splintmaking requires practice for the clinician to be at ease with the design and fabrication process. Students or therapists beginning to design and fabricate splints should be aware of personal expectations and realize that their skills will likely evolve with practice. Therapists with experience in splinting tend to be more efficient with time and materials than novice students and therapists.

Occupational Therapy Theories, Models, and Frame-of-Reference Approaches for Splinting

The OTPF outlines the occupational therapy process of evaluation and intervention and highlights the emphasis on the use of occupation [AOTA 2002]. *Performance areas* of occupation as specified in the framework include the following: activities of daily living (ADL), instrumental activities of daily living (IADL), education, work, play, leisure, and social participation. Performance areas of occupation place demands on a person's *performance skills* (i.e., motor skills, process skills, and communication/interaction skills). Therapists must consider the influence of *performance patterns* on occupation. Such patterns include habits, routines, and roles. Contexts affect occupational participation. *Contexts* include cultural, physical, social, personal, spiritual, temporal, and virtual dimensions. The engagement in an occupation involves *activity demands* placed on the individual. Activity demands include objects used and their properties, space demands, social demands, sequencing and timing, and required actions, body functions, and body structures. *Client factors* relate to a person's body functions and body structures. Table 1-1 provides examples of how the framework assists one in thinking about splint provision to a client.

The practice of occupational therapy is guided by conceptual systems [Pedretti 1996]. One such conceptual system is the Occupational Performance Model, which consists of performance areas, components, and contexts. A therapist using the Occupational Performance Model may influence a client's performance area or component while considering the context in which the person must operate. The therapist is guided by several treatment approaches in providing

Table 1-1 Examples* of the Occupational Therapy Practice Framework and Splint Provision

CATEGORY	QUESTIONS
Performance in Areas of Occupation	
Activities of daily living (ADL)	What ADL will a person need to perform with a splint on? Will ADL need to be modified because of splint provision?
Instrumental activities of daily living (IADL)	What types of IADL will the person wearing a splint have to carry out (e.g., child care, shopping, and pet care)? Will IADL need to be modified because of splint provision?
Education	Can the person who just received a splint read the handout that explains the home program? What type of client education must be provided for optimum care?
Work	What paid or volunteer work does the client want or need to perform while wearing the splint? Will work activities need to be modified because of splint provision?
Play	Can a child who wears a splint interact with toys?
Leisure	Can the person who wears a splint engage in leisure activities? Do modifications in leisure equipment or activities need to be made for full participation?
Social participation	Will the splint provided cause an adolescent to withdraw from particular social situations because the splint draws unwanted attention?
Performance Skills	
Motor skills	Does the person have the coordination and strength to don and doff his new resting hand splint?
Process skills	Can the person who has developmental delays correctly complete the steps and sequence to don and doff a splint?
Communication/interaction skills	Will the person who communicates via sign language be hindered in communication while wearing a splint? Will the person feel like she can engage in sexual activity while wearing her splint?
Performance Patterns	
Habits	How will the therapist enable a habit for the person to take care of his splint?
Routines	How might ADL routines be interrupted because the splint interferes with established sequences?
Roles	What roles does the person fulfill and will any related behaviors be affected by wearing a splint?
Contexts	
Cultural	What if the person does not believe the splint will help his condition?
Physical	Does the client have accessibility to transportation to the clinic for follow-up visits?
Social	How might a caregiver be affected if the person receiving care is provided a splint?
Personal	What happens when a client needs a splint but has no means of paying for it?
Spiritual	How can the therapist tap into a client's motivation system to improve her outlook on the outcome of wearing a splint and receiving treatment?
Temporal	Should the client who has a six-month life prognosis be issued a splint?
Virtual	Will the person who wears a splint be able to access his e-mail?
Activity Demands	
Objects used and their properties	Will the teenager who is on the high school chess team be able to manipulate the chess pieces while wearing bilateral splints?
Space demands	Will wearing the splint impede a client's work tasks due to space restrictions?
Social demands	Will the teacher help the child don and doff a splint for participation in particular activities?
Sequencing and timing	Will the intensive care unit nursing staff be able to don and doff a client's splint according to the specified schedule?
Required actions	Can the client with arthritis thread the splint strap through the D-ring?
Required body functions	Does the client have the strength to lift her arm to dress while wearing an elbow splint?
Required body structures	How will the client with one arm amputated don and doff his splint?
Client Factors	
Body functions	Does the client have sensation to determine if a dynamic splint is exerting too much force on joints?

*Examples are inclusive, not exclusive.

assessment and treatment. The therapist may use the biomechanical, sensorimotor, and rehabilitative approaches. The biomechanical approach uses biomechanical principles of kinetics and forces acting on the body. Sensorimotor approaches are used to inhibit or facilitate normal motor responses in persons whose central nervous systems have been damaged. The rehabilitation approach focuses on abilities rather than disabilities and facilitates returning persons to maximal function using their capabilities [Pedretti 1996]. (See Self-Quiz 1-1.)

Each approach can incorporate splinting as a treatment intervention, depending on the rationale for splint provision. For example, if a person wears a tenodesis splint to recreate grasp and release to maximize function in activities of daily living, the therapist is using the rehabilitation approach [Hill and Presperin 1986]. If the therapist is using the biomechanical approach, a dynamic (mobilization) hand splint may be chosen to apply kinetic forces to the person's body. If the therapist chooses a sensorimotor approach, an antispasticity splint may be used to inhibit or reduce tone.

Pierce's notions [Pierce 2003] of contextual and subjective dimensions of occupation are powerful concepts for therapists who appropriately incorporate splinting into a client's care plan. Understanding how a splint affects a client's occupational engagement and participation are salient in terms of meeting the client's needs and goals, which may result in an increased probability of compliance. Contextual dimensions include spatial, temporal, and sociocultural contexts [Pierce 2003]. Subjective dimensions include restoration, pleasure, and productivity. Box 1-1 explicates both contextual and subjective dimensions of occupation. In Chapter 3, Pierce's framework is used to structure questions for a client interview.

Box 1-1 Contextual and Subjective Dimensions of Occupation

Contextual Dimensions
Temporal
Circadian rhythms
Social schedules
Time (clocks)
Patterns of occupations
Spatial
Physical body
Environmental conditions
Object use
Symbolic meanings of space
Sociocultural
Identity
Cultural diversity
Genders
Health care cultures
Relationships

Subjective Dimensions
Restoration
Eating
Sleeping
Self-care
Hobbies
Spirituality
Pleasure
Play
Leisure
Humor
Ritual
Productivity
Challenge to avoid boredom
Worth ethic
Work identity
Stress

SELF-QUIZ 1-1*

Match the approach used in each of the following scenarios.

a. Biomechanical approach
b. Sensorimotor approach
c. Rehabilitation approach

1. _________ This approach was used on a child who has cerebral palsy. The goal of the splint was to decrease the amount of tone present.
2. _________ This approach allowed a person who had a stroke to grasp the walker by using splints that were adapted to assist with grasp.
3. _________ This approach helped a person who had a tendon repair that resulted in flexor contractures of the metacarpophalangeal (MCP) joint to regain full range of motion.

*See Appendix A for the answer key.

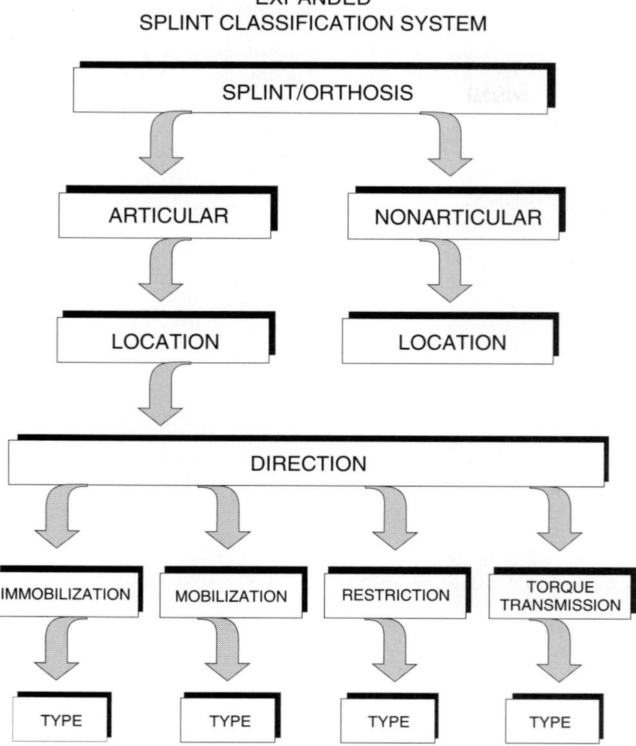

Figure 1-1 Expanded splint classification system division. [From Fess EE, Gettle KS, Philips CA, Janson JR (2005). *Hand and Upper Extremity Splinting: Principles and Methods, Third Edition.* St. Louis: Elsevier Mosby.]

Splint Categorization

According to the ASHT [1992], there are six splint classification divisions: (1) identification of articular or nonarticular, (2) location, (3) direction, (4) purpose, (5) type, and (6) total number of joints (Figure 1-1).

Articular/Nonarticular

The first element of the ASHT classification indicates whether or not a splint affects articular structures. Articular splints use three-point pressure systems "to affect a joint or joints by immobilizing, mobilizing, restricting, or transmitting torque" [Fess 2005, p. 124]. Most splints are articular, and the term *articular* is often not specified in the technical name of the splint.

Nonarticular splints use a two-point pressure force to stabilize or immobilize a body segment [Fess et al. 2005]. Thus, the term *nonarticular* should always be included in the name of the splint. Examples of nonarticular splints include those that affect the long bones of the body (e.g., humerus).

Location

Splints, whether articular or nonarticular, are classified further according to the location of primary anatomic parts included in the splint. For example, articular splints will include a joint name in the splint [e.g., elbow, thumb metacarpal (MP), index finger proximal interphalangeal (PIP)]. Nonarticular splints are associated with one of the long bones (e.g., ulna, humerus, radius).

Direction

Direction classifications are applicable to articular splints only. Because all nonarticular splints work in the same manner, the direction does not need to be specified. Direction is the primary kinematic function of splints. Such terms as *flexion*, *extension*, and *opposition* are used to classify splints according to direction. For example, a splint designed to flex the PIP joints of index, middle, ring, and small fingers would be named an *index–small-finger PIP flexion splint.*

Purpose

The fourth element in the ASHT classification system is purpose. There are four purposes of splints: (1) mobilization, (2) immobilization, (3) restriction, and (4) torque transmission. The purpose of the splint indicates how the splint works. Examples include the following:

- *Mobilization:* Wrist/finger-MP extension *mobilization* splint.
- *Immobilization:* Elbow *immobilization* splint.
- *Restriction:* Elbow extension *restriction* splint.
- *Torque transmission:* Finger PIP extension *torque transmission* splint, type 1 (2). (The number in parentheses indicates the total number of joints incorporated into the splint.)

Mobilization splints are designed to move or mobilize primary and secondary joints. Immobilization splints are designed to immobilize primary and secondary joints. Restrictive splints "limit a specific aspect of joint range of motion for the primary joints" [ASHT 1992, p. 9]. Torque transmission splints' purposes are to "(1) create motion of primary joints situated beyond the boundaries of the splint itself or (2) harness secondary 'driver' joint(s) to create motion of primary joints that may be situated longitudinally or transversely to the 'driver' joint(s)" [Fess et al. 2005, p. 126]. Torque transmission splints, illustrated in Figure 1-2, are also referred to as exercise splints.

Type

The classification of splint type specifies the secondary joints included in the splint. Secondary joints are often incorporated into the splint design to affect joints that are proximal, distal, or adjacent to the primary joint. There are 10 joints that comprise the upper extremity: shoulder, elbow, forearm, wrist, finger MP, finger PIP, finger distal interphalangeal (DIP), thumb carpometacarpal (CMC), thumb metacarpophalangeal (MP), and thumb interphalangeal (IP) levels. Only joint levels are counted, not the number of

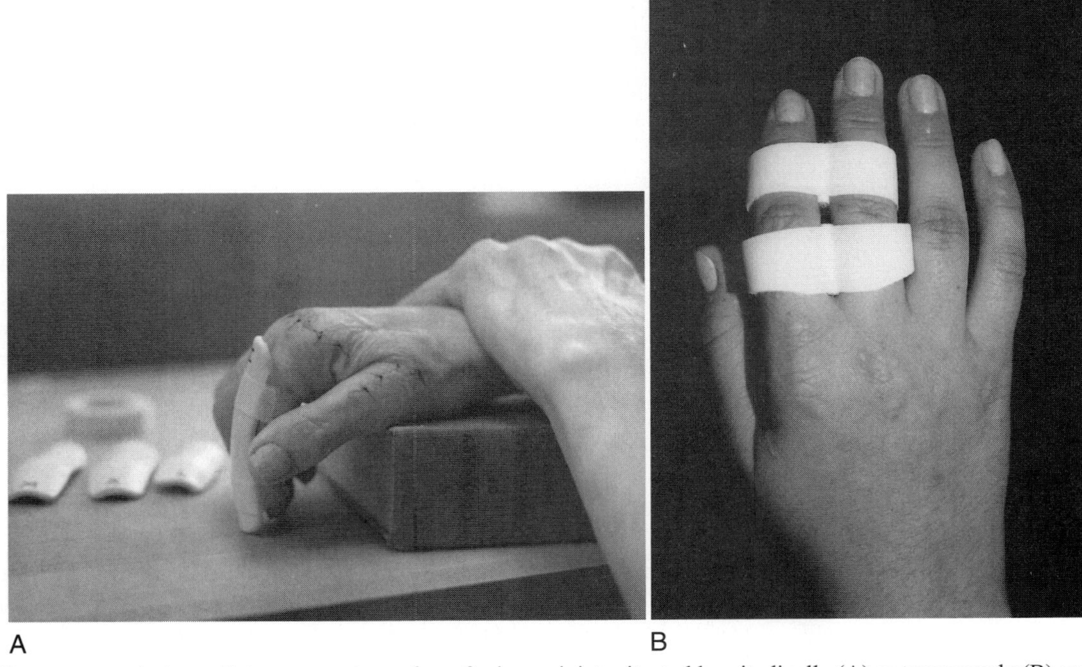

A B

Figure 1-2 Torque transmission splints may create motion of primary joints situated longitudinally (A) or transversely (B) according to secondary joints. [From Fess EE, Gettle KS, Philips CA, Janson JR (2005). *Hand and Upper Extremity Splinting: Principles and Methods, Third Edition*. St. Louis: Elsevier Mosby.]

individual joints. For example, if the wrist joint and multiple finger PIP joints are included as secondary joints in a splint the type is defined as *2* (PIP joints account for one level and the wrist joint accounts for another level, thus totaling two secondary joint levels). The technical name for a splint that flexes the MP joints of the index, middle, ring, and small fingers and incorporates the wrist and PIP joints is an *index–small-finger MP flexion mobilization splint, type 2*. If no secondary joints are included in the splint design, the joint level is type 0.

Total Number of Joints

The final ASHT classification level is the total number of individual joints incorporated into the splint design. The number of total joints incorporated in the splint follows the type indication. For example, if an elbow splint includes the wrist and MPs as secondary joints the splint would be called an *elbow flexion immobilization splint, type 2 (3)*. The number in parentheses indicates the total number of joints incorporated into the splint.

Splint Designs

In the past, splints were categorized as static or dynamic. This classification system has its problems and controversies. However, in some clinics ASHT splint terminology is not often used. Therefore, therapists must be familiar with the ASHT classification system as well as other commonly used nomenclature. Static splints have no movable parts [Cailliet 1994]. In addition, static splints place tissues in a stress-free position to enhance healing and to minimize friction [Schultz-Johnson 1996]. Dynamic splints have one or more movable parts [Malick 1982] and are synonymous with splints that employ elastics, springs, and wire, as well as with multipart splints.

The purpose of a splint as a therapeutic intervention assists the therapist in determining its design. Splinting design classifications include (1) static, (2) serial static, (3) dropout, (4) dynamic, and (5) static-progressive [Schultz-Johnson 1996].

A static splint (Figure 1-3) can maintain a position to hold anatomical structures at the end of available range of motion, thus exerting a mobilizing effect on a joint [Schultz-Johnson 1996]. For example, a therapist fabricates a splint to position the wrist in maximum tolerated extension to increase extension of a stiff wrist. Because the splint positions the shortened wrist flexors at maximum length and holds them there, the tissue remodels in a lengthened form [Schultz-Johnson 1996].

Serial static splinting (Figure 1-4) requires the remolding of a static splint. The serial static splint holds the joint or series of joints at the limit of tolerable range, thus promoting tissue remodeling. As the tissue remodels, the joint gains range and the clinician remolds the splint to once again place the joint at end range comfortably. Schultz-Johnson [1996]

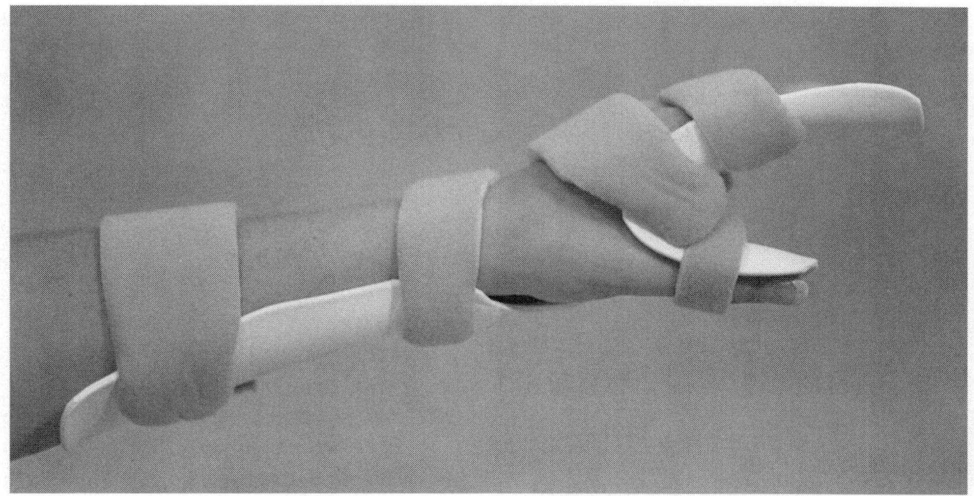

Figure 1-3 Static immobilization splint. This static splint immobilizes the thumb, fingers, and wrist.

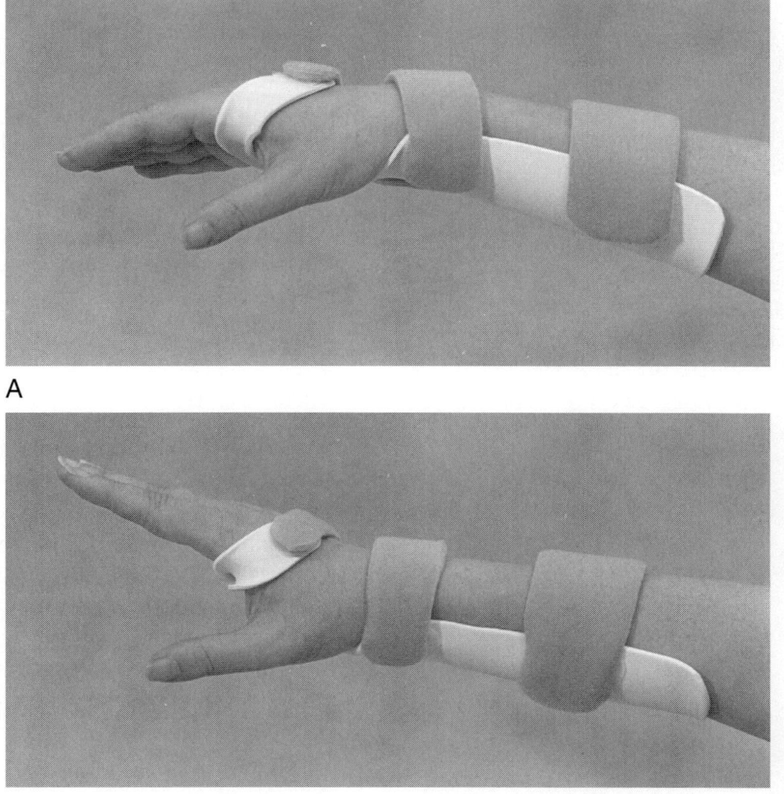

A

B

Figure 1-4 Serial static splints (A and B). The therapist intermittently remolds the splint as the client gains wrist extension motion.

pointed out that circumferential splints that are nonremovable require no cooperation from those who wear them, except to leave them on.

A dropout splint (Figure 1-5) allows motion in one direction while blocking motion in another [ASHT 1992]. This type of splint may help a person regain lost range of motion while preventing poor posture. For example, a splint may be designed to enhance wrist extension while blocking wrist flexion [Schultz-Johnson 1996].

Elastic tension dynamic (mobilization) splints (Figure 1-6) have self-adjusting or elastic components, which may include wire, rubber bands, or springs [Fess and Philips 1987]. A splint that applies an elastic tension force to straighten an index finger PIP flexion contracture exemplifies an elastic tension/traction dynamic (mobilization) splint.

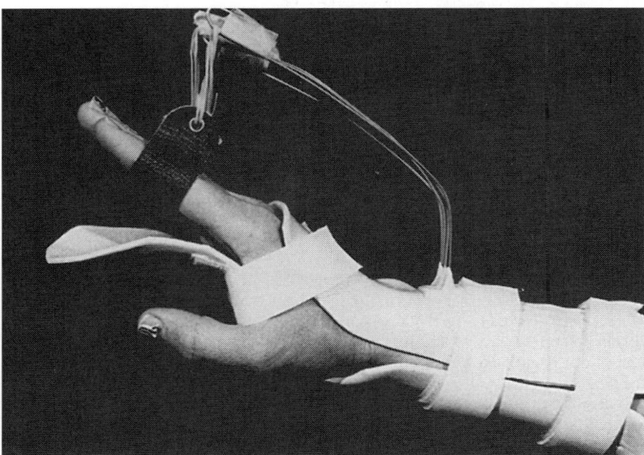

Figure 1-5 Dropout splint. A dorsal–forearm-based dynamic extension splint immobilizes the wrist and rests all fingers in a neutral position. A volar block permits only the predetermined MCP joint flexion. [From Evans RB, Burkhalter WE (1986). A study of the dynamic anatomy of extensor tendons and implications for treatment. Journal of Hand Surgery 11A:774.]

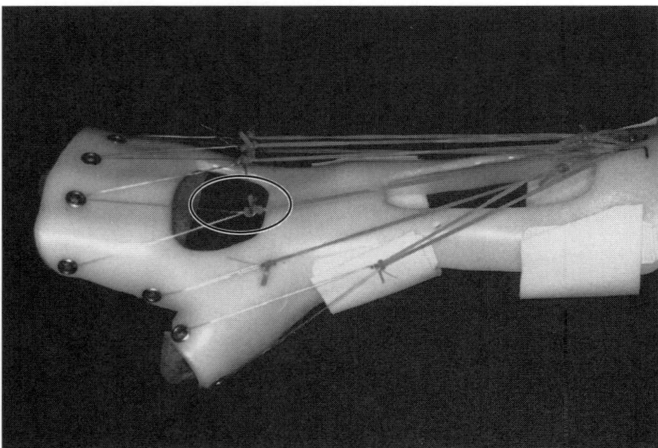

Figure 1-6 Elastic tension splint. This splint for radial nerve palsy has elastic rubber bands and inelastic filament traction. [Courtesy of Dominique Thomas, RPT, MCMK, Saint Martin Duriage, France, from Fess EE, Gettle KS, Philips CA, Janson JR (2005). *Hand and Upper Extremity Splinting: Principles and Methods, Third Edition*. St. Louis: Elsevier Mosby.]

Static progressive splints (Figure 1-7) are types of dynamic (mobilization) splints. They incorporate the use of inelastic components such as hook-and-loop tapes, outrigger line, progressive hinges, turnbuckles, and screws. The splint design incorporates the use of inelastic components to allow the client to adjust the line of tension so as to prevent overstressing of tissue [Schultz-Johnson 1995]. Chapter 11 more thoroughly addresses mobilization and torque transmission (dynamic) splints.

Many possibilities exist for splint design and fabrication. A therapist's creativity and skills are necessary for determining the best splint design. Therapists must stay updated on splinting techniques and materials, which change rapidly. Reading professional literature and manufacturers' technical information helps therapists maintain knowledge about materials and techniques. A personal collection of reference books is also beneficial, and continuing-education courses provide ongoing updates on the latest theories and techniques.

Evidence-Based Practice and Splinting

Calls for evidence-based practice have stemmed from medicine but have affected all of health care delivery, including splinting [Jansen 2002]. Sackett and colleagues [1996, pp. 71–72] defined evidence-based practice as "the conscientious, explicit, and judicious use of current best evidence in making decisions about the care of individual clients. The practice of evidence-based medicine means integrating individual clinical expertise with the best available external clinical evidence from systematic research."

The aim of applying evidence-based practice is to "ensure that the interventions used are the most effective and the safest options" [Taylor 1997, p. 470]. Essentially, therapists apply the research process during practice. This includes (1) formulating a clear question based on a client's problem, (2) searching the literature for pertinent research articles, (3) critically appraising the evidence for its validity and usefulness, and (4) implementing useful findings to the client case. Evidence-based practice is *not* about finding articles to support what a therapist does. Rather, it is reviewing a body of literature to guide the therapist in selecting the most appropriate assessment or treatment for an individual client.

Sackett et al. [1996] and Law [2002] outlined several myths of evidence-based practice and described the reality of each myth (Table 1-2). A misconception exists that evidence-based practice is impossible to practice or that it already exists. Although we know that keeping current on all health care literature is impossible, few practitioners consistently review research findings related to their specific practice. Instead, many practitioners rely on their training or

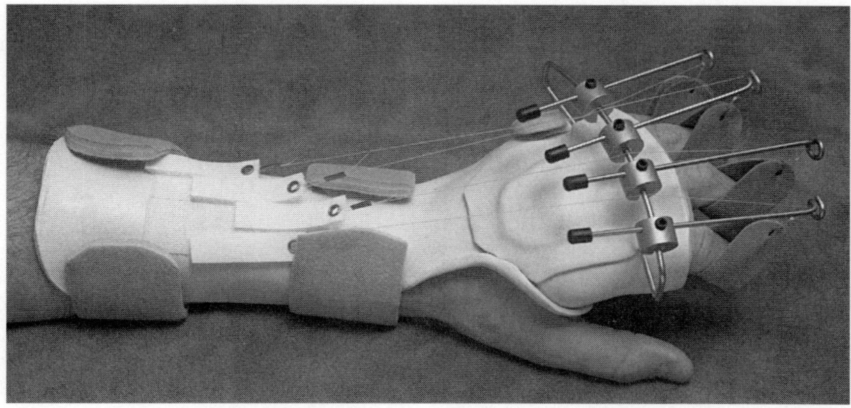

Figure 1-7 Static progressive splint. A splint to increase PIP extension uses hook-and-loop mechanisms for adjustable tension.

Table 1-2 Evidence-Based Practice Myths and Realities

MYTH	REALITY
Evidence-based practice exists	Practitioners spend too little time examining current research findings
Evidence-based practice is difficult to integrate into practice	Evidence-based practice can be implemented by busy practitioners
Evidence-based practice is a "cookie cutter" approach	Evidence-based practice requires extensive clinical experience
Evidence-based practice is focused on decreasing costs	Evidence-based practice emphasizes the best clinical evidence for individual clients

Table 1-3 Hierarchy of Evidence

STEP	DESCRIPTION
1A	Meta-analysis of randomized controlled trials
1B	One individual randomized controlled trial
2A	One well-designed nonrandomized controlled study
2B	Well-designed quasi-experimental study
3	Nonexperimental descriptive studies (comparative/case studies)
4	Respectable opinion

clinical experience to guide clinical decision making. Novel clinical situations present a need for evidence-based practice.

Some argue that evidence-based practice leads to a "cookie cutter" approach to clinical care. Evidence-based practice involves a critical appraisal of relevant research findings. It is not a top-down approach. Rather, it adopts a bottom-up approach that integrates external evidence with one's clinical experience and client choice. After reviewing the findings, practitioners must use clinical judgment to determine *if*, *why*, and *how* they will apply findings to an individual client case. Thus, evidence-based practice is not a *one-size-fits-all* approach because all client cases are different.

Evidence-based practice is not intended to be a mechanism whereby all clinical decisions must be backed by a random controlled trial. Rather, the intent is to address efficacy and safety using the best current evidence to guide intervention for a client in the safest way possible. It is important to realize that efficacy and safety do not always result in a cost decrease.

Important to evidence-based practice is the ability of practitioners to appraise the quality of the evidence available. A hierarchy of evidence is based on the certainty of causation and the need to control bias. Table 1-3 [Lloyd-Smith 1997] shows this hierarchy. The highest quality (gold standard) of evidence is the meta-analysis of randomized controlled studies. Next in the hierarchy is one study employing an individual random controlled trial. A well-designed nonrandomized study is next in the hierarchy, followed by quasi-experimental designs and nonexperimental descriptive studies. Last in the hierarchy is expert practitioner opinion. Box 1-2 presents a list of appraisal questions used to evaluate quantitative and qualitative research results.

Throughout this book, the authors made an explicit effort to present the research relevant to each chapter topic. Note that the evidence is limited to the timing of this publication. Students and practitioners should review literature to determine applicability of contemporary publications. The Cochrane Library, CINAHL (Cumulative Index of Nursing and Allied Health Literature), MEDLINE, EMBASE (comprehensive pharmacological and biomedical database), OT Index, HAPI (Health and Psychosocial Instruments), ASSIA (Applied Social Sciences Index of Abstracts), and HealthStar are useful databases to access during searches for research.

Box 1-2 Appraisal Questions Used to Evaluate Quantitative and Qualitative Research

Evaluating Quantitative Research
Was the assignment of clients to treatments randomized?
Were all subjects properly accounted for and attributed at the study's conclusion?
Were subjects, health workers, and research personnel blinded to treatment?
Were the groups similar to each other at the beginning of the trial?
Aside from experimental intervention, were the groups treated equally?
How large was the treatment effect?
How precise was the treatment effect?
Can the results be applied to my client care?
Were all clinically important outcomes considered?
Are the likely benefits worth the potential harms/costs?

Evaluating Qualitative Research
Are the results trustworthy?
Was the research question clearly articulated?
Was the setting in which the research took place described?
Were the sampling measures clearly described?
Were methods to ensure the credibility of research used?
Did the researchers address issues of confirmability and dependability?
Was the collection of data prolonged and varied?
Is there evidence of reflexivity?
Was the research process subjected to internal or external audits?
Were any steps taken to triangulate the outcomes?
Where were the primary findings?
Were the results of the research kept separate from the conclusions drawn?
If quantitative methods were appropriate as a supplement, were they used?
Will the results help me care for my clients?

Data from Gray JAM (1997). *Evidence-based Healthcare*. Edinburgh: Churchill Livingstone; Krefting L (1990). Rigour in qualitative research: The assessment of trustworthiness. American Journal of Occupational Therapy 45:214-222; Rosenberg W, Donald A (1995). Evidence-based medicine: An approach to clinical problem-solving. British Medical Journal 310:1122-1126.

CASE STUDY 1-1

*Read the following scenario and answer the questions based on information in this chapter.**

Renaldo is a new therapist working in an outpatient care setting. He has an order to make a wrist immobilization splint for a person with a diagnosis of carpal tunnel syndrome who needs a splint to provide rest and protection.

1. According to the ASHT splint terminology, which name would appropriately indicate the splint indicated in Figure 1-8.
   a. Forearm neutral mobilization splint, type 1 (2)
   b. Wrist neutral immobilization, type 1 (1)
   c. Wrist neutral immobilization, type 0 (1)
2. If Renaldo is focusing on the person's ability to perform activities of daily living with the splint, what is the guiding approach?
   a. Rehabilitation
   b. Biomechanical
   c. Sensorimotor
3. Listed below are several types of evidence. Rank the studies in descending order (1 = highest level, 2 next highest level, and so on).
   ___ a. Talking to a certified hand therapist about the protocol she believes is best for a particular client
   ___ b. A randomized control trial with one group of clients serving as the control group and another group of clients receiving a new type of treatment
   ___ c. A case study describing the treatment of an individual client

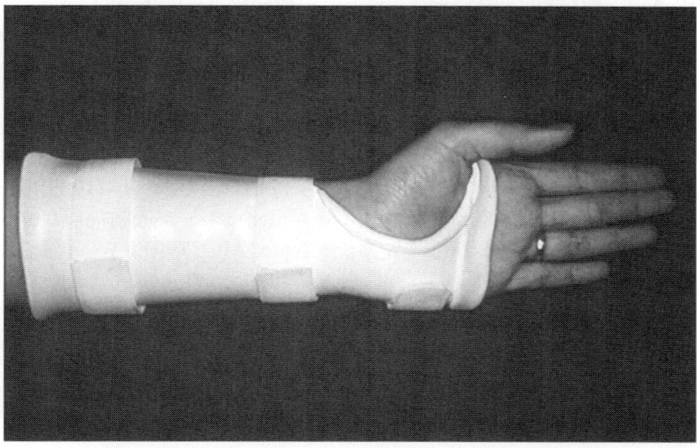

Figure 1-8

*See Appendix A for the answer key.

REVIEW QUESTIONS

1. What health care professionals provide splinting services to persons?
2. What are the three therapeutic approaches used in physical dysfunction? Give an example of how splinting could be used as a therapeutic intervention for each of the three approaches.
3. How might the Occupational Therapy Practice Framework assist a therapist in splint provision?
4. What are the six divisions of the ASHT splint classification system?
5. What purposes might a splint be used for as part of the therapeutic regimen?
6. What is evidence-based practice? How can it be applied to splint intervention?
7. In evidence-based practice, what is the hierarchy of evidence?

References

American Occupational Therapy Association (2002). Occupational therapy practice framework: Domain and process. American Journal of Occupational Therapy 56:609-639.

American Society of Hand Therapists (1992). Splint classification system. Garner, NC: The American Society of Hand Therapists.

Bailey J, Cannon N, Colditz J, Fess E, Gettle K, DeMott L, et al. (1992). *Splint Classification System*. Chicago: American Society of Hand Therapists.

Cailliet R (1994). *Hand Pain and Impairment, Fourth Edition*. Philadelphia: F. A. Davis.

Daus C (1998). Helping hands: A look at the progression of hand therapy over the past 20 years. Rehab Management 64-68.

Fess EE (2002). A history of splinting: To understand the present, view the past. Journal of Hand Therapy 15:97-132.

Fess EE, Gettle KS, Philips CA, Janson JR (2005). A history of splinting. In EE Fess, KS Gettle, CA Philips, JR Janson (eds.), *Hand and Upper Extremity Splinting: Principles and Methods*. St. Louis: Elsevier Mosby, pp. 3-43.

Fess EE, Philips CA (1987). *Hand Splinting Principles and Methods, Second Edition*. St. Louis: Mosby.

Gray JM (1998). Putting occupation into practice: Occupation as ends, occupation as means. American Journal of Occupational Therapy 52(5):354-364.

Hill J, Presperin J (1986). Deformity control. In S Intagliata (ed.), *Spinal Cord Injury: A Guide to Functional Outcomes in Occupational Therapy*. Rockville, MD: Aspen Publishers, pp. 49-81.

Jansen CWS (2002). Outcomes, treatment effectiveness, efficacy, and evidence-based practice. Journal of Hand Therapy 15:136-143.

Law M (2002). Introduction to evidence based practice. In M Law (ed.), *Evidence-based Rehabilitation*. Thorofare, NJ: Slack, pp. 3-12.

Lloyd-Smith W (1997). Evidence-based practice and occupational therapy. British Journal of Occupational Therapy 60:474-478.

Malick MH (1982). *Manual on Dynamic Hand Splinting with Thermoplastic Material, Second Edition*. Pittsburgh: Harmarville Rehabilitation Center.

Pedretti LW (1996). Occupational performance: A model for practice in physical dysfunction. In LW Pedretti (ed.), *Occupational Therapy: Practice Skills for Physical Dysfunction, Fourth Edition*. St. Louis: Mosby, pp. 3-12.

Pierce DE (2003). *Occupation by Design: Building Therapeutic Power*. Philadelphia: F. A. Davis.

Rossi J (1987). Concepts and current trends in hand splinting. Occupational Therapy in Health Care 4:53-68.

Sackett DL, Rosenberg WM, Gray JA, Haynes RB, Richardson WS (1996). Evidence-based medicine: What it is and what it isn't. British Medical Journal 312:71-72.

Schultz-Johnson K (1996). Splinting the wrist: Mobilization and protection. Journal of Hand Therapy 9(2):165-177.

Taylor MC (1997). What is evidenced-based practice? British Journal of Occupational Therapy 60:470-474.

War Department (1944). *Bandaging and Splinting*. Washington, D.C.: United States Government Printing Office.

CHAPTER 2

Occupation-Based Splinting

Debbie Amini, MEd, OTR/L, CHT
Deborah A. Rider, OTR/L, CHT

Key Terms

Occupation-based splinting
Client-centered treatment
Occupational profile
Context
Occupational deprivation
Occupational disruption
Treatment protocol

Chapter Objectives

1. Define occupation-based treatment as it relates to splint design and fabrication.
2. Describe the influence of a client's occupational needs on splint design and selection.
3. Review evidence to support preservation of occupational engagement through splinting.
4. Describe how to utilize an occupation-based approach to splinting.
5. Review specific hand pathologies that create the potential for occupational dysfunction.
6. Describe splint design options to promote occupational engagement.
7. Apply knowledge of application of occupation-based practice to a case study.

"Man, through the use of his hands as they are energized by mind and will, can influence the state of his own health" [Reilly 1962, p. 2].

As stated eloquently by Mary Reilly [1962], this phrase reminds us that the hand, as directed by the mind and spirit, is integral to function. Occupation-based splinting is an approach that promotes the ability of the individual with hand dysfunction to engage in desired life tasks and occupations [Amini 2005]. Occupation-based splinting is defined as "attention to the occupational desires and needs of the individual, paired with the knowledge of the effects (or potential effect) of pathological conditions of the hand, and managed through client-centered splint design and provision" [Amini 2005, p. 11].

Prior to starting the splinting process, the therapist must adopt a personal philosophy that supports occupation-based and client-centered practice. Multiple models of practice exist that adopt this paradigm, including the Canadian Model of Occupational Performance (COPM), The Contemporary Task-Oriented Approach [Kamm et al. 1990], and the Model of Human Occupation and Occupational Adaptation [Law 1998]. In addition, the occupational therapist should understand the tenets of the Occupational Therapy Practice Framework (OTPF) and its relationship to the International Classification of Functioning, Disability and Health (ICF).

The profession of occupational therapy adopted the use of splints, an ancient technique of immobilization and mobilization, in the mid part of the twentieth century [Fess 2002]. According to Fess, the most frequently recorded reasons for splinting include increasing function, preventing deformity, correcting deformity, protecting healing structures, restricting movement, and allowing tissue growth or remodeling [Fess et al. 2005]. Such reasons for splinting relate to changing the condition of the neuro-musculoskeletal system and body functions within the client factors category of the OTPF. However, body components comprise only a part of the overall occupational behavior of the client, and despite the importance of assisting the healing or mobility of the hand the therapist must immediately and concurrently tend to the needs of the client that transcend movement and strength of the body.

This chapter provides definitions of client-centered and occupation-based practice. The process of combining both approaches to splinting is presented, with suggested assessment tools and treatment approaches that are compatible with such practice approaches. Splinting options that promote occupational functioning are described.

Client-Centered versus Occupation-Based Approaches

Client-centered and occupation-based practice are compatible, but a distinction is made between the two [Pierce 2003]. Client-centered practice is defined as "an approach to service which embraces a philosophy of respect for, and partnership with, people receiving services" [Law et al. 1995, p. 253]. Law [1998] outlined concepts and actions of client-centered practice, which articulate the assumptions for shaping assessment and intervention with the client (Box 2-1).

Occupation-based practice is "the degree to which occupation is used with reflective insight into how it is experienced by the individual, how it is used in natural contexts for that individual, and how much the resulting changes in occupational patterns are valued by the client" [Goldstein-Lohman et al. 2003]. Methods of employing empathy, reflection, interview, observation, and rigorous qualitative inquiry assist in understanding the occupations of others [Pierce 2003]. Christiansen and Townsend [2004] described occupation-based occupational therapy as an approach to treatment that serves to facilitate engagement or participation in recognizable life endeavors. Pierce [2003] described occupation-based treatment as including two conditions: (1) the occupation as viewed from the client's perspective and (2) the occupation occurring within a relevant context. According to the OTPF, context relates "to a variety of interrelated conditions within and surrounding the client that influence performance" [AOTA 2002, p. 613]. Contexts include cultural, physical, social, personal, spiritual, temporal, and virtual aspects [AOTA 2002]. Thus, you should consider both factors when working with clients. Box 2-2 describes the contexts.

Box 2-1 Concepts and Actions of Client-Centered Practice

- Respect for clients and their families and choices they make
- Clients' and families' right to make decisions about daily occupations and therapy services
- A communication style that is focused on the person and includes provision of information, physical comfort, and emotional support
- Encourage client participation in all aspects of therapy service
- Individualized occupational therapy service delivery
- Enabling clients to solve occupational performance issues
- Attention to the person-environment-occupation relationship

Box 2-2 Description of Contexts

Cultural: The ethnicity, family values, attitudes, and beliefs of the individual
Physical: The physical environment in all respects
Social: Relationships the individual has with other individuals, groups, organizations, or systems
Personal: Features of the person specific to them (age, gender, socioeconomic status, and so on)
Spiritual: Belief in a higher being or purpose for existence
Temporal: Stages of life, time of day, time of year
Virtual: Realistic simulation of an environment and the ability to communicate is cyberspace

From American Occupational Therapy Association (2002). Occupational therapy practice framework: Domain and process. American Journal of Occupational Therapy 56:609-639.

Occupation-Based Splint Design and Fabrication

Occupation-based splinting is a treatment approach that supports the goals of the treatment plan to promote the ability of clients to engage in meaningful and relevant life endeavors. Unlike a more traditional model of splinting that may initially focus on body structures and processes, occupation-based splinting incorporates the client's occupational needs and desires, cognitive abilities, and motivation. When using occupation-based splinting, the therapist recognizes that the client is an *active* participant in the treatment and decision-making process [Amini 2005]. Splinting as occupation-based and client-centered treatment focuses on meeting client goals as opposed to therapist-designed or protocol-driven goals. Body structure healing is not the *main* priority. It is a priority *equal* to that of preservation of occupational engagement.

Occupation-based splinting can be viewed as part of a top-down versus bottom-up approach to occupational therapy intervention. According to Weinstock-Zlotnick and Hinojosa [2004], the therapist who engages in a top-down approach always begins treatment by examining a client's occupational performance and grounds treatment in a client-centered frame of reference. A therapist who uses a bottom-up approach first evaluates the pathology and then attempts to connect the body deficiencies to performance difficulties. To be truly holistic, one must never rely *solely* on one method or frame of reference for treatment. Treating a client's various *needs* is a first and foremost priority.

Occupation-Based Splinting and Contexts

According to the OTPF, occupational therapy is an approach that facilitates the individual's ability to engage in meaningful activities within specific performance areas of occupation and varied *contexts* of living [AOTA 2002]. The performance areas of occupation define the domain of occupational therapy and include activities of daily living (ADLs), instrumental activities of daily living (IADLs), leisure, play, work, education, and social participation [AOTA 2002]. Context is a strong component of occupational engagement that permeates all levels of treatment planning, intervention, and outcomes.

An often overlooked issue surrounding splinting is attention to the client's *cultural* needs. Unfortunately, to ignore culture is to potentially limit the involvement of clients in their splint programs. For example, there are cultures whereby the need to rely on a splint is viewed as an admission of vulnerability or as a weakness in character. Such feelings can exist due to large group beliefs or within smaller family dynamic units. Splinting within this context must involve a great deal of client education and possibly education of family members. Issuing small, unobtrusive splints that allow as much function as possible may diminish embarrassment and a sense of personal weakness [Salimbene 2000].

A knowledge of *physical* environments may contribute to an understanding of the need for splint provision. Physical environments may also hamper consistent use if clients are unable to engage in required or desired activities. For example, if a client needs to drive to work and is unable to drive while wearing a splint he might remove it despite the potential for reinjury. Figure 2-1A depicts a young woman wearing a splint because she sustained a flexor digitorum profundus injury. She found that typing at her workplace while wearing the splint was creating shoulder discomfort. She asked the therapist if she could remove her splint for work, and with physician approval the therapist created a modified protective splint (Figure 2-1B). The newly modified splint allowed improved function and protected the healing tendon.

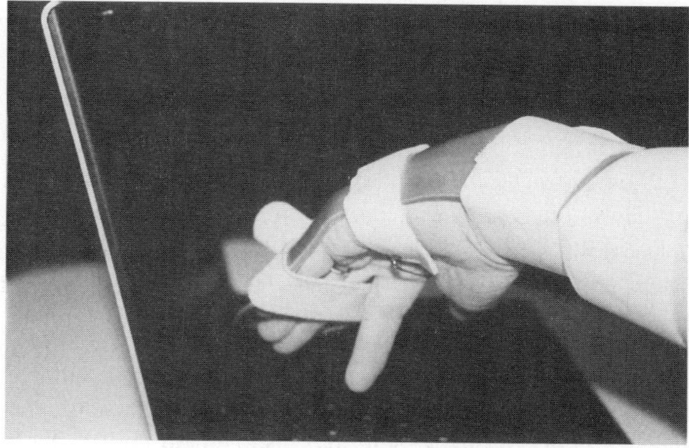

A

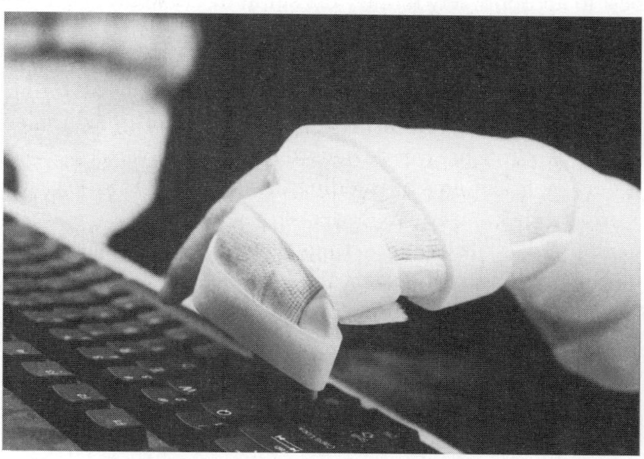

B

Figure 2-1 (A) Excessive pronation required to accurately press keys while using standard dorsal blocking splint. (B) Improved ability to work on computer using modified volar-based protective splint.

Social contexts pertain to the ability of clients to meet the demands of their specific group or family. Social contexts are taken into consideration with splint provision. For example, a new mother is recently diagnosed with de Quervain's tenosynovitis and is issued a thumb splint. The mother feels inadequate as a mother when she cannot cuddle and feed the infant without contacting the infant with a rigid splint. In such a case, a softer prefabricated splint or alternative wearing schedule is suggested to maximize compliance with the splint program (Figure 2-2).

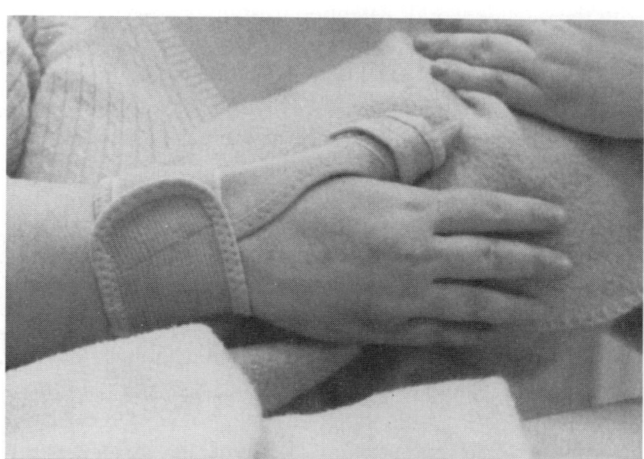

Figure 2-2 Prefabricated thumb immobilization splint. It improves comfort while holding the infant.

Personal context involves attention to such issues as age, gender, and educational and socioeconomic status. When clinicians who employ occupation-based splinting fabricate splints for older adults or children, they consider specific guidelines (see Chapters 15 and 16). The choices in material selection and color may be different based on age and gender. For example, a child may prefer a bright-colored splint whereas an adult executive may prefer a neutral-colored splint. Concerns may arise about the role educational level plays in splint design and provision. For clients who have difficulty understanding new and unfamiliar concepts, it is important to have a splint that is simple in design and can be donned and doffed easily. Precautions and instructions should be given in a clear manner.

Although it is typically considered a cognitive function, expression of *spirituality* can be potentially affected by changes to the physical body. For example, some clients are not able to pray or to attend religious services because parts of their bodies are restricted by splints. All clients should be asked if their splints are in any way inhibiting their ability to engage in any life experience. Almost all splints affect a person's ability to perform activities. The impact is a matter of degree, and consideration needs to be given to the trade-off between how it *enables clients* (if only in the future) and how it *disables* them. Therapists must be aware of the balance between enablement and disablement and do their best to appropriately modify the splint or the wearing schedule or to provide an adaptation to facilitate clients' occupational engagement.

Temporal concerns are addressed through attention to issues such as comfort of the splint during hot summer months or the use of devices during holidays or special events such as proms or weddings. An example is the case of a bride-to-be who was two weeks postoperative for a flexor tendon repair of the index finger. The young woman asked repeatedly if she could take off her splint for one hour during her wedding. A compromise reached between the therapist and the client ensured that her hand would be safe during the ceremony. A shiny new splint was made specifically for her wedding day to immobilize the injured finger and wrist (modified Duran protocol). The therapist discarded the rubber-band/finger-hook component (modified Kleinert protocol). This change made the splint smaller and less obvious. The client was a happy bride and her finger was well protected.

Virtual context addresses the ability to access and use electronic devices. The ability to access devices (e.g., computers, radios, PDAs, MP3 players, cell phones) plays an important role in many people's lives. Fine motor control is paramount when using these devices and should be preserved as much as possible to maximize electronic contact with the outside world. Attention to splint size and immobilizing only those joints required can facilitate the ability of clients to manipulate small buttons and dials required to use such devices. "While use of a keyboard tends to be a bilateral activity, many devices (such as radios, PDAs, and cell phones) do not require bilateral fine motor skill. As technology improves with cordless and voice-activated systems, the needs for fine motor skill in operation of some electronic devices may decrease. A therapist is the ideal person to introduce this technology to the client" [personal communication, K. Schultz-Johnson, October 5, 2005].

For a splint to be accepted as a legitimate holistic device, it must work for the client within the context(s). Splints might perpetuate dysfunction and may prolong the return to meaningful life engagement without attention to the specifics of how and where clients live their lives. To ignore the interconnection of function to where and how function plays out is to practice a reductionist form of treatment that emphasizes isolated skills and body structures, without regard to clients' engagement in selected activities.

Occupation-Based Splinting and Intervention Levels

Pedretti and Early [2001] described four intervention levels: adjunctive, enabling, purposeful activities, and occupations. Adjunctive methods prepare clients for purposeful activity and they do not imply activity or occupation. Examples include exercise, inhibition or facilitation techniques, and positioning devices. Enabling activities precede and simulate purposeful activity. For example, simulated activities (e.g., driving simulators) begin to prepare the client for participation in actually driving a vehicle. Purposeful activities are goal directed and have meaning and purpose to the client. In the case of driving, when a client actually gets into a vehicle and drives, the intervention level is considered purposeful activity. Occupation is the highest level of intervention. Clients participate in occupations in their natural context. The ability to drive to one's employment site is considered an occupation.

At first blush, splinting could appear to be less than occupation oriented because it is initiated prior to occupational engagement and discontinued when hand function resumes. From an occupation-based perspective, splinting is not a technique used *only* in preparation for occupation. For appropriate clients, splints are an integral part of ongoing intervention to support occupational engagement at all levels of intervention: adjunctive, enabling, purposeful activity, and occupation. For example, some clients may receive a splint to decrease pain while simultaneously being allowed engagement in work and leisure pursuits.

Splinting as a Therapeutic Approach

The OTPF intervention approaches are defined as "specific strategies selected to direct the process of intervention that are based on the client's desired outcome, evaluation data and evidence" [AOTA 2002, p. 632]. These treatment approaches include processes to (1) create or promote health, (2) establish or restore health, (3) maintain health, (4) modify through compensation and adaptation, and (5) prevent disability [AOTA 2002].

From an occupation-based perspective, when splints enable occupation it seems to elevate splint status to that of an integral *approach* to treatment versus an adjunctive technique. Custom fitted splints within the context of clients' occupational experience can promote health, remediate dysfunction, substitute for lost function, and prevent disability. When teamed with a full occupational analysis and knowledge of the appropriate use of splints for specific pathologies (supported by evidence of effectiveness), splinting options are selected to produce the outcomes that reach the goals collaboratively set by the client and the practitioner.

Splinting as a Facilitator of Therapeutic Outcomes

Within the context of occupation-based practice, splinting is a therapeutic approach interwoven through all levels of intervention. Splinting is a facilitator of purposeful and occupation-based activity. The OTPF describes specific therapeutic *outcomes* expected of intervention. Outcomes are occupational performance, client satisfaction, role competence, adaptation, health and wellness, prevention, and quality of life [AOTA 2002]. Positive outcomes in *occupational performance* are the effect of successful intervention. Such outcomes are demonstrated either by *improved* performance within the presence of continued deficits resulting from injury or disease or the *enhancement* of function when disease is not currently present.

Splinting addresses both types of occupational performance outcomes (improvement and enhancement). Splints that improve function in a person with pathology result in an "increased independence and function in an activity of daily living, instrumental activity of daily living, education, work, play, leisure, or social participation" [AOTA 2002, p. 628]. For example, a wrist immobilization splint is prescribed for a person who has carpal tunnel syndrome. The splint positions the wrist to rest the inflamed anatomical structures, thus decreasing pain and work performance improves. Splints that enhance function without specific pathology result in improved occupational performance from one's current status or prevention of potential problems. For example, some splints position the hands to prevent overuse syndromes resulting from hand-intensive repetitive or resistive tasks.

Satisfaction of the entire therapeutic process is increased when the client's needs are met. When clients are included as an integral part of the splinting process, they are more likely to comply and to use the splint. Inclusion of clients in treatment planning is important to creating splints that minimally inhibit function and take the client's lifestyle into consideration.

Role competence is the ability to satisfactorily complete desired roles (e.g., worker, parent, spouse, friend, and team member). Roles are maintained through splinting by minimizing the effects of pathology and facilitating upper extremity performance for role-specific activities. For example, a mother who wears a splint for carpal tunnel syndrome should be able to hold her child's hand without extreme pain. Holding the child's hand makes her feel like she is fulfilling her role as a mother.

Splints created to enhance *adaptation* to overcome occupational dysfunction address the dynamics of the challenges and the client's expected ability to overcome it. An example of splinting to improve adaptation might involve a client who experiences carpal ligament sprain but must continue working or risk losing employment. In this case, a wrist immobilization splint that allows for digital movements may enable continued hand functions while resting the involved ligament.

Health and wellness are collectively described as the absence of infirmity and a "state of physical, mental, and social well-being" [AOTA 2002, p. 628]. Splinting promotes health and wellness of clients by minimizing the effects of physical disruption through protection and substitution. Enabling a healthy lifestyle that allows clients to experience a sense of wellness facilitates motivation and engagement in all desired occupations [Christiansen 2000].

Prevention in the context of the OTPF involves the promotion of a healthy lifestyle at a policy creation, organizational, societal, or individual level [AOTA 2002]. When an external circumstance (e.g., environment, job requirement, and so on) exists with the potential for interference in occupational engagement, a splinting program may be a solution to prevent the ill effects of the situation. If it is not feasible to modify the job demands, clients may benefit from the use of splints in a preventative role. For example, a wrist immobilization splint and an elbow strap are fitted to prevent lateral epicondylitis of the elbow for a client who works in a job that involves repetitive and resistive lifting of the wrist with a clenched fist. In addition, the worker is educated on modifying motions and posture that contribute to the condition.

Of great concern is the concept of *quality of life* [Sabonis-Chafee and Hussey 1998]. Although listed as a separate therapeutic outcome within the OTPF, quality of life is a *subjective state of being* experienced by clients. Quality of life entails one's appraisal of abilities to engage in specific tasks that beneficially affect life and allow self-expressions that are socially valued [Christiansen 2000]. One's state of being is determined by the ability of the client to be satisfied, engage in occupations, adapt to novel situations, and maintain health and wellness. Ultimately, splinting focused on therapeutic outcomes will improve the quality of life through facilitating engagement in meaningful life occupations.

The Influence of Occupational Desires on Splint Design and Selection

The *occupational profile* phase of the evaluation process described in the OTPF involves learning about clients from a contextual and performance viewpoint [AOTA 2002]. For example, what are the interests and motivations of clients? Where do they work, live, and recreate? Tools (i.e., Canadian Occupational Performance Model; Disabilities of the Arm, Shoulder, and Hand; and the Patient-Rated Wrist Hand Evaluation) that offer clients the opportunity to discuss their injuries in the context of their daily lives lend insight into the needs that must be addressed. Table 2-1 lists such tools. When used in conjunction with traditional methods of hand and upper extremity assessment (e.g., goniometers, dynamometers, and volumeters), they help therapists learn about the specific clients they treat and assist in splint selection and design.

The assessment tools listed in Table 2-1 emphasize client occupations and functions as the focus of intervention. Information obtained from such assessments supports the

Table 2-1 Client-Centered Assessments

TOOL	GENERAL DESCRIPTION	CONTACT INFORMATION
Canadian Occupational Performance Measure (COPM) [Law et al. 1994]	The COPM is a client-centered approach to assessment of perceived functional abilities, interest, and satisfaction with occupations. This interview-based valid and reliable tool is scored and can be used to measure outcomes of treatment.	The COPM can be purchased through the Canadian Association of Occupational Therapists at *http://www.caot.ca.*
Disabilities of the Arm, Shoulder, and Hand (DASH) assessment [Hudak et al. 1996]	DASH is a condition-specific tool. The DASH consists of 30 predetermined questions addressing function within performance areas. Clients are asked to rate their recent ability to complete skills on a scale of 1 (no difficulty) to 5 (unable). The DASH assists with the development of the occupational profile through its valid and reliable measure of clients' functional abilities.	DASH/QuickDASH web site at *http://www.dash.iwh.on.ca.*
Patient-Rated Wrist/Hand Evaluation (PRWHE) [MacDermid and Tottenham 2004]	The PRWHE is a condition-specific tool through which the client rates pain and function in 15 preselected items.	MacDermid JC, Tottenham V (2004). Responsiveness of the disability of the arm, shoulder, and hand (DASH) and patient-rated wrist/hand evaluation (PRWHE) in evaluating change after hand therapy. Journal of Hand Therapy 17:18-23.

goal of occupation-based splinting, which is to improve the client's quality of life through the client's continued engagement in desired occupations.

A splint that focuses on client factors alone does not always treat the *functional* deficit. For example, a static splint to support the weak elbow of a client who has lost innervation of the biceps muscle protects the muscle yet allows only one angle of function of that joint. A dynamic flexion splint protects the muscle from end-range stretch yet allows the client the ability to change the arm angle through active extension and passive flexion. Assessment tools that measure physical client factors exclusively (e.g., goniometry, grip strength, volumeter, and so on) must remain as adjuncts to determine splint design because physical functioning is an adjunct to occupational engagement.

Canadian Occupational Performance Measure

The COPM is an interview-based assessment tool for use in a client-centered approach [Law et al. 1994]. The COPM assists the therapist in *identifying problems* in performance areas, such as those described by the OTPF. In addition, clients' perceptions of their *ability to perform* the identified problem area and their *satisfaction* with their abilities are determined when using the COPM [Law et al. 1994]. A therapist can use the COPM with clients from all age groups and with any type of disability. Parents or family members can serve as proxies if the client is unable to take part in the interview process (e.g., if the client has dementia). When the COPM is readministered, objective documentation of the functional effects of splinting through comparison of pre- and post-intervention scores is made.

When using the COPM, contextual issues will arise during the client interview about satisfaction with function. Clients may indicate why certain activities create personal dissatisfaction despite their ability to perform them. An example is the case of a woman who resides in an assisted living setting. During administration of the COPM, she identifies that she is able to don her splint by using her teeth to tighten and loosen the straps. She needs to remove the splint to use utensils during meals. However, she is embarrassed to do this in front of other residents while at the dining table. The use of the COPM uncovers issues that are pertinent to individual clients and must be considered by the therapist.

Disabilities of the Arm, Shoulder, and Hand

The Disabilities of the Arm, Shoulder, and Hand (DASH) is a condition-specific tool that measures a client's perception of how current upper extremity disability has impacted function [DASH 2005]. The DASH consists of 30 predetermined questions that explore function within performance areas. The client is asked to rate on a scale of 1 (no difficulty) to 5 (unable) his or her current ability to complete particular skills, such as opening a jar or turning a key. The DASH assists the therapist in gathering data for an occupational profile of functional abilities. The focus of the assessment is not on body structures or on the signs and symptoms of a particular diagnostic condition. Rather, the merit of the DASH is that the information obtained is about the client's functional abilities.

An interview, although not mandated by the DASH, should become part of the process to enhance the therapist's understanding of the identified problems. The therapist must also determine why a functional problem exists and how it may be affecting quality of life. The DASH is an objective means of measuring client outcomes when readministered following splint provision or other treatment interventions [Beaton et al. 2001].

When selecting the DASH as a measure of occupational performance, the therapist may consider several additional facts. For example, the performance areas measured are predetermined in the questionnaire and may limit the client's responses. In addition, the DASH does not specifically address contextual issues or client satisfaction or provide insight into the emotional state of the client. Additional information can be obtained through interview to gain insight needed for proper splint design and selection.

Patient-Rated Wrist Hand Evaluation

The Patient-Rated Wrist Hand Evaluation (PRWHE) is a condition-specific tool through which clients rate their pain and functional abilities in 15 preselected areas [MacDermid and Tottenham 2004]. PRWHE assists with the development of the occupational profile through obtaining information about clients' functional abilities. The functional areas identified in the PRWHE are generally much broader than those in the DASH. Similar to the DASH, the PRWHE's questions to elicit such information are not open-ended questions as in the COPM. Information about pain levels during activity and client satisfaction of the aesthetics of the upper limb are gathered during the PRWHE assessment.

The PRWHE does not specifically require an inquiry into the details of function, but such information would certainly assist the therapist and make the assessment process more occupation based. The PRWHE does not include questions related to context. Therefore, the therapist should include such questions in treatment planning discussions.

Following the data collection part of the evaluation process, the *analysis of occupational performance* can occur. If a therapist uses one of the aforementioned tools, analysis of the performance process has been initiated. Further questions will be asked based on the answers of previous questions. The therapist continues to gain specific insight into how splinting can be used to remediate the reported dysfunction.

During the analysis phase, the therapist may actually want to see the client perform several functions to gain additional insight into how activity affects, or is impacted by, the diagnosis or pathology. For example, a client states that he cannot write because of thumb carpometacarpal (CMC) joint pain. Therefore, the therapist asks the client to show how he is able to hold the pen while describing the type of discomfort experienced while writing. The therapist may begin splint design analysis by holding the client's thumb in a supported position to simulate the effect of a hand-based splint. The client will actively participate in the process by giving feedback to the therapist during splint design and fabrication.

After a client-centered occupation-based profile and analysis is completed, an occupation-based splinting intervention plan is developed. Measuring only physical factors to create a client profile will result in a therapist seeing only the upper extremity and not the *client*. The upper extremity does not dictate the quality of life. Rather, the mind, spirit, and body do so collectively! (See Self-Quiz 2-1.)

Evidence to Support Preservation of Occupational Engagement and Participation

Fundamental to occupational therapy treatment is the belief that individuals must retain their ability to engage in meaningful occupations or risk further detriment to their subjective experience of quality of life. If humans behaved as automatons–completing activities without drive, interest, or attention–correcting deficits would become reductionist and mechanical. A reductionistic approach could guarantee that an adaptive device or exercise could correct any problem and immediately lead to the continuation of the required task (much like replacing a spark plug to allow a car to start). Fortunately, humans are not automatons

SELF-QUIZ 2-1

Answer the following questions.

1. Consider a splinting plan with a client of a different culture than yourself. What factors of splint design and provision may need special attention to ensure acceptance, compliance, and understanding?

____

2. When designing splints to match the occupational needs of a young child, what performance areas and personal contextual factors will you be interested in addressing?

____

and occupational therapy exists to support the ability of the individual to engage in and maintain participation in desired occupations.

The literature supports the premise that any temporary or permanent disruption in the ability to engage in meaningful occupations can be detrimental [Christiansen and Townsend 2004]. For example, with a flexor tendon repair therapists must follow protocols to facilitate appropriate tissue healing. Such a protocol typically removes the hand from functional pursuits for a minimum of six to eight weeks. However, occupational dysfunction must be effectively minimized as soon as possible to maintain quality of life [McKee and Rivard 2004].

Evidence to Support Occupational Engagement

Supported by research, in addition to anecdotal experiences and reports of therapists, is the importance of multidimensional engagement in meaningful occupations. Originally described by Wilcock [1998], the term *occupational deprivation* is a state wherein clients are unable to engage in chosen meaningful life occupations due to factors *outside* their control. Disability, incarceration, and geographic isolation are but a few circumstances that create occupational deprivation. Depression, isolation, difficulty with social interaction, inactivity, and boredom leading to a diminished sense of self can result from occupational deprivation [Christiansen and Townsend 2004]. *Occupational disruption* is a temporary and less severe condition that is also caused by an unexpected change in the ability to engage in meaningful activities [Christiansen and Townsend 2004]. Additional studies conducted by behavioral scientists interested in how individual differences, personality, and lifestyle factors influence well-being have shown that engagement in occupations can influence happiness and life satisfaction [Christiansen et al. 1999].

Ecological models of adaptation suggest that people thrive when their personalities and needs are matched with environments or situations that enable them to remain engaged, interested, and challenged [Christiansen 1996]. Walters and Moore [2002] found that among the unemployed, involvement in *meaningful* leisure activities (not simply busy-work activities) decreased the sense of occupational deprivation.

Palmadottir [2003] completed a qualitative study that explored clients' perspectives on their occupational therapy experience. Positive outcomes of therapy were experienced by clients when treatment was client centered and held purpose and meaning for them. Thus, when a client who has an upper extremity functional deficit receives a splint the splint should meet the immediate needs of the injury while meeting the client's desire for occupational engagement.

According to Ludwig [1997], consistency and routine help older adult women maintain the ability to meet their obligations and maintain activity levels and overall health. In addition, routines control and balance ADLs, self-esteem, and intrinsic motivation for activities. Such consistency and routine can be maintained through splinting techniques that allow function while simultaneously decreasing the effects of pathology.

Research offers evidence that splints of all types and for all purposes are indeed effective in reaching the goals of improved function [Dunn et al. 2002, Li-Tsang et al. 2002, Schultz-Johnson 2002, Werner et al. 2005]. Four examples are presented to demonstrate such evidence. A study was conducted on the effects of splinting dental hygienists who had osteoarthritis. The researchers indicated that such splints can reduce the effect of pain on thumb function [Dunn et al. 2002]. Schultz-Johnson [2002] concluded that static progressive splints improve end-range motion and passive movements that cannot be obtained in any other way. Such splints make a difference in the lives of clients.

Li-Tsang et al. [2002] found splinting of finger flexion contractures caused by rheumatoid arthritis to be effective. Clients experienced statistically significant improvements in the areas of hand strength (pinch and grip) and active range of motion in both extension and flexion after a program of splinting [Li-Tsang et al. 2002]. Nocturnal wrist extension splinting was found to be effective in reducing the symptoms of carpal tunnel syndrome experienced by Midwestern auto assembly plant workers [Werner et al. 2005]. This evidence leads us to conclude that splinting with attention to occupational needs can and should be used to preserve quality of life.

Utilizing an Occupation-Based Approach to Splinting

With guiding philosophies in place, the therapist using an occupation-based approach to splinting will begin the following problem-solving process of splint design and fabrication.

Step 1: Referral

The clinical decision-making process begins with the referral. Some splint referrals come from physicians who specialize in hand conditions. A referral may contain details about the diagnosis or requested splint. However, some orders may be from physicians who do not specialize in the treatment of the hand. If this is the case, the physician may depend on the expertise of the therapist and may simply order a splint without detailing specifics. An order to splint a client with a condition may also rely on the knowledge and creativity of the therapist. At this step, the therapist must begin to consider the diagnosis, the contextual issues of the client, and the type of splint that must be fabricated.

Step 2: Client-Centered Occupation-Based Evaluation

Therapists use assessments such as the COPM, DASH, or PRWHE to learn which occupations the client desires to complete during splint wear, which occupations splinting can support, and which occupations the splint will eventually help the person accomplish. The therapist and the client use this information for goal prioritization and splint design in step 4.

Step 3: Understand/Assess the Condition and Consider Treatment Options

Review biology, cause, course, and traditional treatment of the person's condition, including protocols and healing timeframes. Assess the client's physical status. Research splint options and determine *possible* modifications to result in increased occupational engagement without sacrificing splint effectiveness. When a splint is ordered to prevent an injury, the therapist must analyze any activities that may be impacted by wearing the splint and determining how it may affect occupational performance.

Step 4: Analyze Assessment Findings for Splint Design

Analyze information about pathology and protocols to reconcile needs of tissue healing and function (occupational engagement). Consider whether the condition is acute or chronic. Acute injuries are those that have occurred recently and are expected to heal within a relatively brief time period. Acute conditions may require splinting to preserve and protect healing structures. Examples include tendon or nerve repair, fractures, carpal tunnel release, de Quervain's release, Dupuytren's release, or other immediate post-surgical conditions requiring mobilization or immobilization through splinting.

If the condition is acute, splint according to protocols and knowledge of client occupational status and desires. Determine if the client is able to engage in desired occupations within the splint. If the client can engage in occupations while wearing the splint, continue with a custom occupation-based treatment plan in addition to splinting.

Step 5: Determining Splint Design

If the client is unable to complete desired activities and functions within the splint, the therapist must determine modifications or alternative splint designs to facilitate function. Environmental modifications or adaptations may be needed to accommodate lack of function if no further changes can be made to the splint.

Figure 2-3A is an example of a hand-based trigger finger splint that allows unrestricted ability of the client to engage in a craft activity. Compare the splint shown in Figure 2-3B to the splint (shown in Figure 2-3C) previously issued, which limited mobility of the ulnar side of the hand and diminished comfort and activity satisfaction.

To ensure that an occupation-based approach to splinting has been undertaken, the occupation-based splinting (OBS) checklist can be used (Form 2-1). This checklist

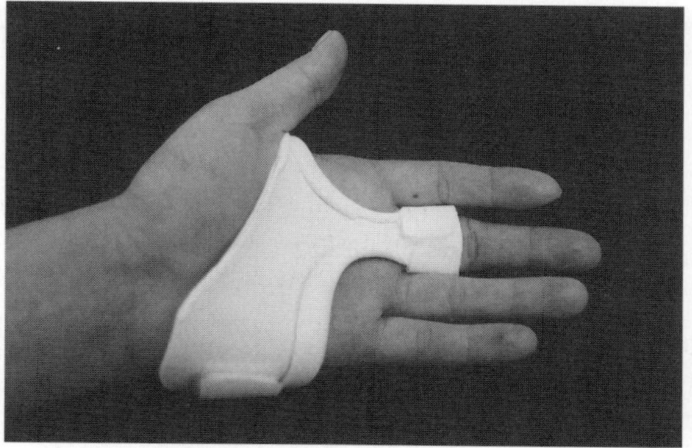

A

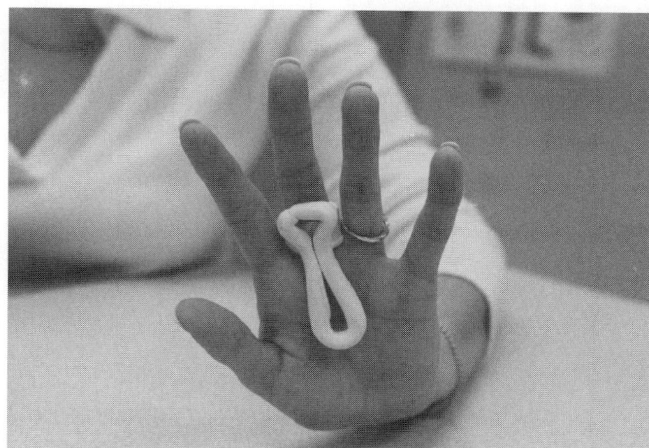

B

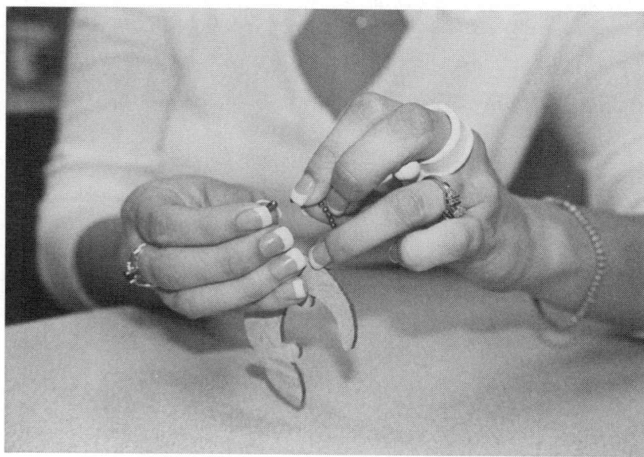

C

Figure 2-3 (A) Confining hand-based trigger finger splint. (B) Finger-based MP blocking trigger finger splint. (C) Functional ability while using finger-based trigger finger splint.

FORM 2-1 Occupation-based splinting (OBS) checklist

1. ______ Splint meets requirements of protocol for specific pathology; ensuring attention to bodily functions and structures.
2. ______ If indicated, splint design is approved with referring physician.
3. ______ Splint allows client to engage in all desired occupation-based tasks through support of activity demands.
4. ______ Splint supports client habits, roles, and routines.
5. ______ Splint design fits client's cultural needs.
6. ______ Splint design fits with temporal needs, including season, age of client, and duration of use.
7. ______ Splint design takes into consideration the client's physical environment.
8. ______ Splint design supports the client's social pursuits.
9. ______ Client's personal needs are addressed through splint design.
10. ______ Client is able to engage in the virtual world (e.g., cellular phone, PDA, computer use).
11. ______ Splint is comfortable.
12. ______ Client verbalizes understanding of splint use, care, precautions, and rationale for use.
13. ______ Client demonstrates the ability to don and doff splint.
14. ______ Adaptations to the physical environment are made to ensure function in desired occupations.
15. ______ Client indicates satisfaction with splint design and functionality within splint.

focuses the therapist's attention on client-centered occupation-based practice. Using the checklist helps ensure that the client does not experience occupational deprivation or disruption.

Splint Design Options to Promote Occupational Engagement and Participation

The characteristics of a splint will have an influence on a client's ability to function. The therapist faces the challenge of trying to help restore or protect the client's involved anatomic structure while preserving the client's performance. To achieve optimal occupational outcomes, specific designs and materials must be used to fabricate splints that are user friendly. The therapist must employ clinical reasoning that considers the impact on the injured tissue and the desires of the client. Such consideration will result in a splint that best protects the anatomic structure at the same time it preserves the contextual and functional needs of the client.

Summary

Engagement in relevant life activities to enhance and maintain quality of life is a concept to be considered with splint provision. The premise that splinting the hand and upper extremity can improve the overall function of the hand is supported in the literature. Hence, splinting that includes attention to the functional desires of the client is a valid occupation-based treatment approach that enhances life satisfaction and facilitates therapeutic outcomes.

CASE STUDY 2-1

Read the following scenario and use your clinical reasoning skills to answer the questions based on information in this chapter.

Henry is a 69-year-old man who is legally blind and is in the early stage of Alzheimer's disease. Henry underwent a palmar fasciectomy for Dupuytren's disease of the small and ring fingers three days ago. You have received an order to fabricate "forearm-based splint to position the wrist in neutral and the fingers in well-tolerated extension without tension on the incision(s)" for day and night use. Henry attends his first therapy appointment accompanied by his wife, who has become his primary caregiver.

1. During the initial interview, you attempt to conduct an interview using the COPM with Henry and his answers seem unrealistic and you suspect he is confabulating. What steps can you take to verify that the information you obtained is reflective of his current level of function?

   ____
   ____
   ____

2. How will you be certain that Henry is able to read and comprehend the printed splint care sheet?

   ____
   ____
   ____

3. How will you be certain that Henry is able to follow the home exercise program pamphlet?

   ____
   ____
   ____

CASE STUDY 2-2

Read the following scenario and use your clinical reasoning skills to answer the questions based on information in this chapter.

Malcolm, a 69-year-old man status post Guillain-Barré syndrome with residual hand and upper extremity dysfunction, was evaluated by an occupational therapist using goniometry, dynamometry, the nine-hole peg test, and the Canadian Occupational Performance Measure. The results of the ROM measurements indicate full passive motion, with 50% impairment of active flexion and full active extension. Grip strength testing indicated 25 pounds of force bilaterally with 3 pounds of lateral pinch strength. Nine-hole peg test indicated impaired fine motor coordination (FMC) due to a score of 45 seconds on left nondominant hand and 67 seconds on right hand.

Malcolm indicated three areas of functional concern from participating in the COPM, including the ability to sign his name on checks for independent bill paying, the ability to type on a computer to communicate with grandchildren via e-mail, and the ability to cut meat independently. Malcolm has scored his ability and satisfaction with these skills as follows (10 = high and 1 = low).

- Handwriting:
  - Performance: 3
  - Satisfaction: 1
- Typing
  - Performance: 4
  - Satisfaction: 2
- Meat cutting:
  - Performance: 3
  - Satisfaction: 1
- Average scores:
  - Performance: 11/3 = 3.6
  - Satisfaction: 4/3 = 1.3

1. According to the information presented previously, what areas should be addressed first to assist Malcolm with functional satisfaction? Why?

____

____

____

2. What approach to treatment will facilitate the most expedient return to function? Why?

____

____

____

3. What components of this assessment indicate a concern for the context of the client?

____

____

____

REVIEW QUESTIONS

1. According to this chapter, what is the definition of occupation-based splinting?
2. According to Fess [2002], what are the reasons therapists provide splints to clients who have upper extremity pathology?
3. Why is it important for the client to be an active participant in the splinting process?
4. Why is attention to the *context* of the client integral to occupation-based splinting?
5. Why should a therapist be knowledgeable about tissue healing and treatment protocols despite the fact that such factors do not imply occupation-based treatment?

References

American Occupational Therapy Association (2002). Occupational therapy practice framework: Domain and process. American Journal of Occupational Therapy 56:609-639.

Amini D (2005). The occupational basis for splinting. Advance for Occupational Therapy Practitioners 21:11.

Beaton DE, Katz JN, Fossel AH, Wright JG, Tarasuk V, Bombardier C (2001). Measuring the whole or parts? Validity, reliability and responsiveness of the disabilities of the arm, shoulder, and hand outcome measure in different regions of the upper extremity. Journal of Hand Therapy 14:128-146.

Christiansen C (1996). Three perspectives on balance in occupation. In R. Zemke & F. Clark (eds.), *Occupational Science: The Evolving Discipline* (pp. 431-451). Philadelphia: F. A. Davis.

Christiansen C (2000). Identity personal projects, and happiness: Self construction in everyday action. Journal of Occupational Science 7: 98-107.

Christiansen C, Backman C, Little B, Nguyen A (1999). Occupations and subjective well-being: A study of personal projects. American Journal of Occupational Therapy 53:91-100.

Christiansen C, Townsend E (2004). *Introduction to Occupation: The Art and Science of Living*. Upper Saddle River, NJ: Pearson Education.

DASH Outcome Measure, Institute for Work and Health. Retrieved February 13, 2005, from *www.dash.iwh.on.ca*.

Dunn J, Pearce O, Khoo CTK (2002). The adventures of a hygienist's hand: A case report and surgical review of the effects of osteoarthritis. Dental Health 41:6-9.

Fess E (2002). A history of splinting: To understand the present, view the past. Journal of Hand Therapy 15:97-132.

Fess EE, Gettle KS, Philips CA, Janson JR (2005). *Hand and Upper Extremity Splinting: Principles and Methods, Third Edition*. St. Louis: Elsevier Mosby.

Goldstein-Lohman H, Kratz A, Pierce D (2003). A study of occupation-based practice. In D Pierce (ed.), *Occupation by Design: Building Therapeutic Power*. Philadelphia: F. A. Davis, pp. 239-261.

Kamm K, Thelen E, Jensen JL (1990). A dynamical systems approach to motor development. Physical Therapy 70:763-775.

Law M (ed.), (1998). *Client-Centered Occupational Therapy*. Thorofare, NJ: Slack.

Law M, Baptiste S, Carswell A, McCall MA, Polatajko H, Pollock N (1994). *Canadian Occupational Performance Measure*. Ottawa, ON: CAOT.

Law M, Baptiste S, Mills J (1995). Client-centered practice: What does it mean and does it make a difference? Canadian Journal of Occupational Therapy 62:250-257.

Li-Tsang C, Hung L, Mak A (2002). The effect of corrective splinting on flexion contracture of rheumatoid fingers. Journal of Hand Therapy 15:185-191.

Ludwig F (1997). How routine facilitates wellbeing in older women. Occupational Therapy International 4:213-228.

MacDermid J, Tottenham V (2004). Responsiveness of the disability of the arm, shoulder and hand (DASH) and patient-rated wrist/hand evaluation (PRWHE) in evaluating change after hand therapy. Journal of Hand Therapy 17:18-23.

McKee P, Rivard A (2004). Orthoses as enablers of occupation: Client-centered splinting for better outcomes. Canadian Journal of Occupational Therapy 71:306-314.

Palmadottir G (2003). Client perspectives on occupational therapy in rehabilitation services. Scandinavian Journal of Occupational Therapy 10:157-166.

Pedretti LW, Early MB (2001). Occupational performance and models of practice for physical dysfunction. In LW Pedretti, MB Early (eds.), *Occupational Therapy Practice Skills for Physical Dysfunction*. St. Louis: Mosby, pp. 3-12.

Pierce D (2003). *Occupation by Design: Building Therapeutic Power*. Philadelphia: F. A. Davis.

Reilly M (1962). Occupational therapy can be one of the great ideas of 20th century medicine. American Journal of Occupational Therapy 16:2.

Sabonis-Chafee B, Hussey S (1998). *Introduction to Occupational Therapy, Second Edition*. St. Louis: Mosby.

Salimbene S (2000). *What Language Does Your Patient Hurt In?* St. Paul, MN: EMCParadigm.

Schultz-Johnson K (2002). Static progressive splinting. Journal of Hand Therapy 15:163-178.

Walters L, Moore K (2002). Reducing latent deprivation during unemployment: The role of meaningful leisure activity. Journal of Occupational and Organizational Psychology 75:15-18.

Weinstock-Zlotnick G, Hinojosa J (2004). Bottom-up or top-down evaluation: Is one better than the other? American Journal of Occupational Therapy 58:594-599.

Werner R, Franzblau A, Gell N (2005). Randomized controlled trial of nocturnal splinting for active workers with symptoms of carpal tunnel syndrome. Archives of Physical Medicine and Rehabilitation 86:1-7.

Wilcock A (1998). *An Occupational Perspective of Health*. Thorofare, NJ: Slack.

CHAPTER 3

Splinting Processes, Tools, and Techniques

Brenda M. Coppard, PhD, OTR/L
Shirley Blanchard, PhD, OTR/L

Key Terms

Thermoplastic material
Handling characteristics
Performance characteristics
Heat gun
Memory
Mechanoreceptors
Physical agent modalities
Superficial agents
Conduction
Convection

Chapter Objectives

1. Identify splint material properties.
2. Recognize tools commonly used in the splinting process.
3. Identify various methods to optimally prepare a client for splinting.
4. Explain the process of cutting and molding a splint.
5. List common splinting items that should be available to a therapist for splint provision.
6. List the advantages and disadvantages of using prefabricated splints.
7. Explain the reasons for selecting a soft splint over a prefabricated splint.
8. Explain three ways to adjust a static progressive force on prefabricated splints.
9. Relate an example of how a person's occupational performance might influence prefabricated splint selection.
10. Summarize the American Occupational Therapy Association's (AOTA's) position on occupational therapists' use of physical agent modalities (PAMs).
11. Define conduction and convection.
12. Describe the indications, contraindications, and safety precautions for the use of PAMs in preparation for splinting.

Splinting requires knowledge of a variety of processes, tools, and techniques. This chapter reviews commonly used processes, tools, and techniques related to splinting. Splints and their purposes needed to address a variety of clients who require custom-made or prefabricated splint intervention are discussed. This chapter also outlines how PAMs may be used to prepare a client for optimal positioning during the splinting process.

Thermoplastic Splinting Materials

Low-temperature thermoplastic (LTT) materials are the most commonly used to fabricate splints. The materials are considered "low temperature" because they soften in water heated between 135° and 180°F and the therapist can usually safely place them directly against a person's skin while the plastic is still moldable. These compare to high-temperature thermoplastics that become soft when warmed to greater than 250°F and cannot touch a person's skin while moldable without causing a thermal injury. When LTT is heated, it becomes pliable, and then hardens to its original rigidity after cooling. The first commonly available low-temperature thermoplastic material was Orthoplast. Currently, many types of thermoplastic materials are available from several companies. Types of materials used in clinics vary on the basis of patient population, diagnoses, therapists' preferences, and availability.

In addition to splint use, LTT material is commonly used to adapt devices for improving function. For example, thermoplastic material may be heated and wrapped around pens, handles, utensils, and other tools to build up the circumference and decrease the required range of motion needed to use such items.

Decisions regarding the best type of thermoplastic material to use for splint fabrication must be made. Decisions are based on such factors as cost, properties of the thermoplastic material, familiarity with splinting materials, and therapeutic goals. One type of thermoplastic material is not the best choice for every type or size of splint. If a therapist has not had experience with a particular type of thermoplastic material, it is beneficial to read the manufacturer's technical literature describing the material's content and properties. Therapists should practice using new materials *before* fabricating splints on clients.

Thermoplastic Material Content and Properties

Thermoplastic materials are elastic, plastic, a combination of plastic and rubberlike, and rubberlike [North Coast Medical 2006]. Thermoplastic materials that are elastic based have some amount of *memory*. (Memory is addressed in the properties discussion of this section.) Typically, elastic thermoplastic has a coating to prevent the material from adhering to itself. (Most thermoplastics have a nonstick coating, but there are a few that specify they do not.) Elastic materials have a longer working time than other types of materials and tend to shrink during the cooling phase.

Thermoplastics with a high plastic content tend to be drapable and have a low resistance to stretch. Plastic-based materials are often used because they result in a highly conforming splint. Such plastic requires great skill in handling the material (e.g., avoiding fingerprints and stretch) during heating, cutting, moving, positioning, draping, and molding. Thus, for novice splinters positioning the client in a gravity-assisted position is best to prevent overstretching of the material.

Thermoplastic materials described as rubbery or rubberlike tend to be more resistant to stretching and fingerprinting. These materials are less conforming than their drapier plastic counterparts. Therapists should not confuse resistance to stretch during the molding process with the rigidity of the splint upon completion. Materials that are quite drapey become extremely rigid when cooled and set, and the opposite is also true. In addition, the more contours a splint contains the more rigid it will be.

Some LTT materials are engineered to include an antimicrobial protection. Splints can create a moist surface on the skin where mold and mildew can form [Sammons et al. 2006]. When skin cells and perspiration remain in a relatively oxygen-free environment for hours at a time, it is conducive to microbe growth and results in odor. Daily isopropyl alcohol cleansing of the inside surface of the splint will effectively combat this problem. Splinting materials containing the antimicrobial protection offer a defense against microorganisms. The antimicrobial protection does not wash or peel off.

Each type of thermoplastic material has unique properties [Lee 1995] categorized by handling and performance characteristics. *Handling characteristics* refer to the thermoplastic material properties when heated and softened, and *performance characteristics* refer to the thermoplastic material properties after the material has cooled and hardened.

Handling Characteristics

Memory

Memory is a property that describes a material's ability to return to its preheated (original) shape, size, and thickness when reheated. The property ranges from 100% to little or no memory capabilities [North Coast Medical 1999]. Materials with 100% memory will return to their original size and thickness when reheated. Materials with little to no memory will not recover their original thickness and size when reheated.

Most materials with memory turn translucent (clear) during heating. Using the translucent quality as an indicator, the therapist can easily determine that the material is adequately heated and can prevent over- or underheating. The ability to see through the material also assists the therapist to properly position and contour the material on the client.

Memory allows therapists to reheat and reshape splints several times without the material stretching excessively. Materials with memory must be constantly molded throughout the cooling process to sustain maximal conformability to persons. Novice or inexperienced therapists who wish to correct errors in a poorly molded splint frequently use materials with memory. Material with memory will accommodate the need to redo or revise a splint multiple times while using the same piece of material over and over. LTT material with memory is often used to make splints for clients who have high tone or stiff joints, because the memory allows therapists to adjust or *serially splint* a joint(s) into a different position. Clinicians use a serial splinting approach when they intermittently remold to a person's limb to accommodate changes in range of motion.

Materials with memory may pose problems when one is attempting to make fine adjustments. For example, spot heating a small portion may inadvertently change the entire splint because of shrinkage. Therapists must carefully control duration of heat exposure. It may be best in these situations to either reimmerse the entire splint in water and repeat the molding process or prevent the problem and select a different type of LTT material.

Drapability

Drapability is the degree of ease with which a material conforms to the underlying shape without manual assistance.

The degree of drapability varies among different types of material. The duration of heating is important. The longer the material heats the softer it becomes and the more vulnerable it becomes to gravity and stretch. When a material with drapability is placed on a surface, gravity assists the material in draping and contouring to the underlying surface. Material exhibiting drapability must be handled with care after heating. A therapist should avoid holding the plastic in a manner in which gravity affects the plastic and results in a stretched, thin piece of plastic. Therefore, this type of plastic is best positioned on a clean countertop during cutting. Material with high drapability is difficult to use for large splints and is most successful on a cooperative person who can place the body part in a gravity-assisted position.

Thermoplastic materials with high drapability may be more difficult for beginning splintmakers because the materials must be handled gently and often novice splinters handle the material too aggressively. Successful molding requires therapists to refrain from pushing the material during shaping. Instead, the material should be lightly stroked into place. Light touch and constant movement of therapists' hands will result in splints that are cosmetically appealing. Materials with low drapability require firm pressure during the molding process. Therefore, persons with painful joints or soft-tissue damage will better tolerate materials with high drapability.

Elasticity

Elasticity is a material's resistance to stretch and its tendency to return to its original shape after stretch. Materials with memory have a slight tendency to rebound to their original shapes during molding. Materials with a high resistance to stretch can be worked more aggressively than materials that stretch easily. As a result, resistance to stretch is a helpful property when one is working with uncooperative persons, those with high tone, or when one splint includes multiple areas (i.e., forearm, wrist, ulnar border of hand, and thumb in one splint). Materials with little elasticity will stretch easily and become thin. Therefore, light touch must be used.

Bonding

Self-bonding or self-adherence is the degree to which material will stick to itself when properly heated. Some materials are coated; others are not. Materials that are coated always require surface preparation with a bonding agent or solvent. Self-bonding (uncoated) materials may not require surface preparation, but some thermoplastic materials have a coating that must be removed for bonding to occur. Coated materials tack at the edges because the coating covers only the surface and not the edges.

Often, the tacked edges can be pried apart after the material is completely cool. If a coated material is stretched, it becomes tackier and is more likely to bond. When heating self-bonding material, the therapist must take care that the material does not overlap on itself during the heating or draping process. If the material overlaps, it will stick to itself. Noncoated materials may adhere to paper towels, towels, bandages, and even the hair on a client's extremity! Thus, it may be necessary to apply an oil-based lotion to the client's extremity. To facilitate the therapist's handling of the material, wetting the hands and scissors with water or lotion can prevent sticking.

All thermoplastic material, whether coated or uncoated, forms stronger bonds if surfaces are prepared with a solvent or bonding agent (which removes the coating from the material). A bonding agent or solvent is a chemical that can be brushed onto both pieces of the softened plastic to be bonded. In some cases, therapists roughen the two surfaces that will have contact with each other. This procedure, called *scoring*, can be carefully done with the end of a scissors, an awl, or a utility knife. After surfaces have been scored, they are softened, brushed with a bonding agent, and adhered together. Self-adherence is an important characteristic for mobilization splinting when one must secure outriggers to splint bases (see Chapter 11) and when the plastic must attach to itself to provide support—for example, when wrapping around the thumb as in a thumb spica splint (see Chapter 8).

Self-finishing Edges

A self-finishing edge is a handling characteristic that allows any cut edge to seal and leave a smooth rounded surface if the material is cut when warm. This handling characteristic saves time for therapists because they do not have to manually roll or smooth the edges.

Other Considerations

Other handling characteristics to be considered are heating time, working time, and shrinkage. The time required to heat thermoplastic materials to a working temperature should be monitored closely because material left too long in hot water may become excessively soft and stretchy. Therapists should be cognizant of the temperature the material holds before applying it to a person's skin to prevent a burn or discomfort. After material that is ⅛ inch thick is sufficiently heated, it is usually pliable for approximately 3 to 5 minutes (S. Berger, personal communication, 1995). Some materials will allow up to 4 to 6 minutes of working time. Materials thinner than ⅛ inch and those that are perforated heat and cool more quickly.

Shrinkage is an important consideration when therapists are properly fitting any splint, but particularly with a circumferential design. Plastics shrink slightly as they cool. During the molding and cooling time, precautions should be taken to avoid a shrinkage-induced problem such as difficulty removing a thumb or finger from a circumferential component of a splint.

Performance Characteristics

Conformability

Conformability is a performance characteristic that refers to the ability of thermoplastic material to fit intimately into contoured areas. Material that is easily draped and has a high degree of conformability can pick up fingerprints and crease marks (as well as therapists' fingerprints). Splints that are intimately conformed to persons are more comfortable because they distribute pressure best and reduce the likelihood of the splint migrating on the extremity.

Flexibility

A thermoplastic material with a high degree of flexibility can take stresses repeatedly. Flexibility is an important characteristic for circumferential splints because these splints must be pulled open for application and removal.

Durability

Durability is the length of time splint material will last. Rubber-based materials are more likely to become brittle with age.

Rigidity

Materials that have a high degree of rigidity are strong and resistant to repeated stress. Rigidity is especially important when therapists make medium to large splints (such as splints for elbows or forearms). Large splints require rigid material to support the weight at larger joints. In smaller splints, rigidity is important if the plastic must stabilize a joint. Rigidity can be enhanced by contouring a splint intimately to the underlying body shape [Wilton 1997]. Most LTT materials cannot tolerate the repeated forces involved in weight bearing on a splint, as in foot orthoses. Most foot orthoses will have fatigue cracks within a few weeks [McKee and Morgan 1998].

Perforations

Theoretically, perforations in material allow for air exchange to the underlying skin. Various perforation patterns are available (e.g., mini-, maxi-, and micro-perforated) [PSR 2006]. Perforated materials are also designed to reduce the weight of splints. Several precautions must be taken if one is working with perforated materials [Wilton 1997]. Perforated material should not be stretched because stretching will enlarge the holes in the plastic and thereby decrease its strength and pressure distribution. When cutting a pattern out of perforated material, therapists should attempt to cut between the perforations to prevent uneven or sharp edges. If this cannot be avoided, the edges of the splint should be smoothed.

Finish, Colors, and Thickness

Finish refers to the texture of the end product. Some thermoplastics have a smooth finish, whereas others have a grainy texture. Generally, coated materials are easier to keep clean because the coating resists soiling [McKee and Morgan 1998].

The color of the thermoplastic material may affect a person's acceptance and satisfaction with the splint and compliance with the wearing schedule. Darker-colored splints tend to show less soiling and appear cleaner than white splints. Brightly colored splints tend to be popular with children and youth. Colored materials may be used to help a person with unilateral neglect call attention to one side of the body [McKee and Morgan 1998]. In addition, colored splints are easily seen and therefore useful in preventing loss in institutional settings. For example, it is easier to see a blue splint in white bed linen than to see a white splint in white bed linen.

A common thickness for thermoplastic material is ⅛ inch. However, if the weight of the entire splint is a concern a thinner plastic may be used—reducing the bulkiness of the splint and possibly increasing the person's comfort and improving compliance with the wearing schedule. Some thermoplastic materials are available in thicknesses of 1⁄16, 3⁄32, and 3⁄16 inch. Thinner thermoplastic materials are commonly used for small splints and for arthritis and pediatric splints, whereas the 3⁄16-inch thickness is commonly used for lower extremity splints and fracture braces [Melvin 1989, Sammons et al. 2006]. Therapists should keep in mind that plastics thinner than ⅛ inch will soften and harden more quickly than thicker materials. Therefore, therapists who are novices in splinting may find it easier to splint with ⅛-inch-thick materials than with thinner materials [McKee and Morgan 1998]. Table 3-1 lists property guidelines for thermoplastic materials. (See also Laboratory Exercise 3-1.)

Process: Making the Splint

Splint Patterns

Making a good pattern for a splint is necessary for success. Giving time and attention to the making of a well-fitting pattern will save the splintmaker's time and materials involved in making adjustments or an entirely new splint. A pattern should be made for each person who needs a splint. Generic patterns rarely fit persons correctly without adjustments. Having several sizes of generic patterns cut out of aluminum foil for trial fittings may speed up the pattern process. A standard pattern can be reduced on a copy machine for pediatric sizes.

To make a custom pattern, the therapist traces the outline of the person's hand (or corresponding body part) on a paper towel (or foil), making certain that the hand is flat and in a neutral position. If the person's hand is unable to flatten on the paper, the contralateral hand may be used to draw the pattern and fit the pattern. If the contralateral hand cannot be used, the therapist may hold the paper in a manner so as to contour to the hand position. The therapist marks on the paper any hand landmarks needed for the pattern before the hand is removed. The therapist then draws the splint pattern over the outline of the hand, cuts out the pattern with scissors, and completes final sizing.

Fitting the Pattern to the Client

As shown in Figure 3-1, moistening the paper and applying it to the person's hand helps the therapist determine which adjustments are required. Patterns made from aluminum foil work well to contour the pattern to the extremity. If the

Table 3-1 Thermoplastic Property Guidelines*

THERMOPLASTIC NAME	DEGREE OF HEATING TEMPERATURE (°F)	THERMOPLASTIC NAME	DEGREE OF HEATING TEMPERATURE (°F)
Memory		NCM Clinic	160
Aquaplast-T	160–170	NCM Preferred	160
Watercolors	160–170	NCM Spectrum	140–145
Aquaplast Resilient T	160–170	Prism	140–160
Aquaplast ProDrape-T	160–170	Watercolors	160–170
Encore	140–160		
NCM Spectrum	140–145	**Resistance to Drape**	
Omega Max	140–160	Aquaplast Resilient T	160–170
Omega Plus	140–160	Caraform	140–145
Orfit Soft	135	Synergy	160–170
Orfit Stiff	135	Omega Plus	140–160
Prism	140–160		
		Resistance to Stretch	
Rigidity		Aquaplast Original Resilient	160–170
Ezeform	160–170	Aquaplast Resilient T	160–170
NCM Clinic	160	Ezeform	160–170
NCM Clinic D	160	Synergy	160–170
NCM Preferred	160	San-splint	160–175
Omega Max	140–160	Omega Max	140–160
Omega Plus	140–160	Omega Plus	140–160
Polyform	150–160		
		Self-adherence	
Conformability, Drapability		Aquaplast Original	160–170
Aquaplast ProDrape-T	160–170	Contour Colors	140–145
Contour Form	140–145	Contour Form	140–145
Ezeform	160–170	Encore	140–160
Polyform	150–160	Ezeform	160–170
Polyform Light	150–160	NCM Spectrum	140–145
Polyflex II	150–160	Omega Max	140–160
Polyflex Light	150–160	Orfit Soft	135
Orfit Soft	135	Orfit Stiff	135
Orthoplast II	150–160	Prism	140–160
Encore	140–160	Spectrum	160
NCM Clinic D	160	Synergy	160–170
Omega Max	140–160		
Orfit	135	**Antimicrobial Defense**	
Watercolors	160–170	• Polyform with antimicrobial built in	
		• Aquaplast ProDrape-T with antimicrobial built in	
Moderate Drapability		• Polyflex II with antimicrobial built in	
Aquaplast-T	160–170	• Aquaplast-T with antimicrobial built in	
Ezeform	160–170	• TaylorSplint with antimicrobial built in	
Ezeform Light	150–160		

*Not all-inclusive.
Courtesy Serena Berger, Smith & Nephew Rolyan, Inc., Germantown, Wisconsin, and North Coast Medical, Inc., San Jose, California.

pattern is too large in areas, the therapist can make adjustments by marking the pattern with a pen and cutting or folding the paper. Sometimes it is necessary to make a new pattern or to retrace a pattern that is too small or that requires major adjustments. The therapist ensures that the pattern fits the person before tracing it onto and cutting it out of the thermoplastic material. It is well worth the time to make an accurate pattern because any ill-fitting pattern directly affects the finished product.

Throughout this book, detailed instructions are provided for making different splint patterns. One should keep in mind that therapists with experience and competency may find it unnecessary to identify all landmarks as indicated by the detailed instructions. Form 3-1 lists suggestions

Laboratory Exercise 3-1 Low-temperature Thermoplastics

Cut small squares of different thermoplastic materials. Soften them in water, and experiment with the plastics so that you can answer the following questions for each type of thermoplastic.

Name of thermoplastic material: ______________________________

1. Does it contour and drape to the hand?	Yes	❍	No	❍
2. Does it appear to be strong when cool?	Yes	❍	No	❍
3. Can its edges be rolled easily?	Yes	❍	No	❍
4. Does it discolor when heated?	Yes	❍	No	❍
5. Does it take fingerprints easily?	Yes	❍	No	❍
6. Does it bond to itself?	Yes	❍	No	❍
7. Can it revert to original shape after being reheated several times?	Yes	❍	No	❍

helpful to a beginning splintmaker when drawing and fitting patterns.

Tracing, Heating, and Cutting

After making and fitting the pattern to the client, the therapist places it on the sheet of thermoplastic material in such a way as to conserve material and then traces the pattern on the thermoplastic material with a pencil. (Conserving materials will ultimately save expenses for the clinic or hospital.) Pencil lines do not show up on all plastics. Using an awl to "scratch" the pattern outline on the plastics works well. Another option is to use grease pencils or china pencils. Caution should be taken when a therapist uses an ink pen, as the ink may smear onto the plastic. However, the ink may be removed with chlorine.

Once the pattern is outlined on a sheet of material, a rectangle slightly larger than the pattern is cut with a utility knife (Figure 3-2). After the cut is made, the material is folded over the edge of a countertop. If unbroken, the material can be turned over to the other side and folded over the countertop's edge. Any unbroken line can then be cut with a utility knife or scissors.

Heating the Thermoplastic Material

Thermoplastic material is softened in an electric fry pan, commercially available splint pan, or hydrocollator filled with water heated to approximately 135° to 180°F (Figure 3-3). (Some materials can be heated in a microwave oven or in a fry pan without water.) To ensure temperature consistency, the temperature dial should be marked to indicate the correct setting of 160°F by using a hook-and-loop (Velcro) dot or piece of tape. When softening materials vertically in a hydrocollator, the therapist must realize the potential for problems associated with material stretching due to gravity's effects. If a fry pan is used, the water height in the pan should be a minimum of three-fourths full (approximately 2 inches deep).

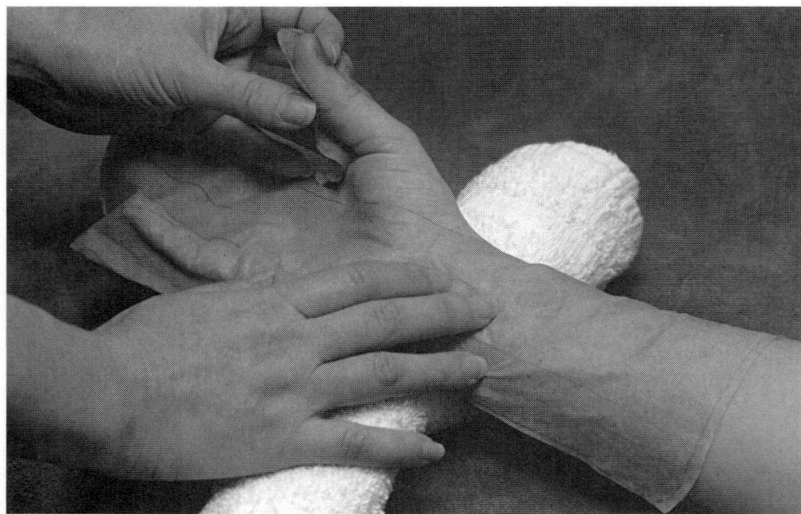

Figure 3-1 To make pattern adjustments, moisten the paper and apply it to the extremity during fitting.

FORM 3-1* Hints for Drawing and Fitting a Splint Pattern

- ○ Explain the pattern-making process to the person.
- ○ Ask or assist the person to remove any jewelry from the area to be splinted.
- ○ Wash the area to be splinted if it is dirty.
- ○ If splinting over bandages or foam, cover the extremity with stockinette or a moist paper towel to prevent the plastic from sticking to the bandages.
- ○ Position the affected extremity on a paper towel in a flat, natural resting position. The wrist should be in a neutral position with a slight ulnar deviation. The fingers should be extended and slightly abducted.
- ○ To trace the outline of the person's extremity, keep the pencil at a 90-degree angle to the paper.
- ○ Mark the landmarks needed to draw the pattern *before* the person removes the extremity from the paper.
- ○ For a more accurate pattern, the paper towel can be wet and placed on the area for evaluation of the pattern, or aluminum foil can be used.
- ○ Folding the paper towel to mark adjustments in the pattern can help with evaluation of the pattern.
- ○ When evaluating the pattern fit of a forearm-based splint on the person, look for the following:
  - Half the circumference of body parts for the width of troughs
  - Two-thirds the length of the forearm
  - The length and width of metacarpal or palmar bars
  - The correct use of hand creases for landmarks
  - The amount of support to the wrist, fingers, and thenar and hypothenar eminencies
- ○ When tracing the pattern onto the thermoplastic material, do not use an ink pen because the ink may smear when the material is placed in the hot water to soften. Rather, use a pencil, grease pencil, or awl to mark the pattern outline on the material.

*See Appendix B for a perforated copy of this form.

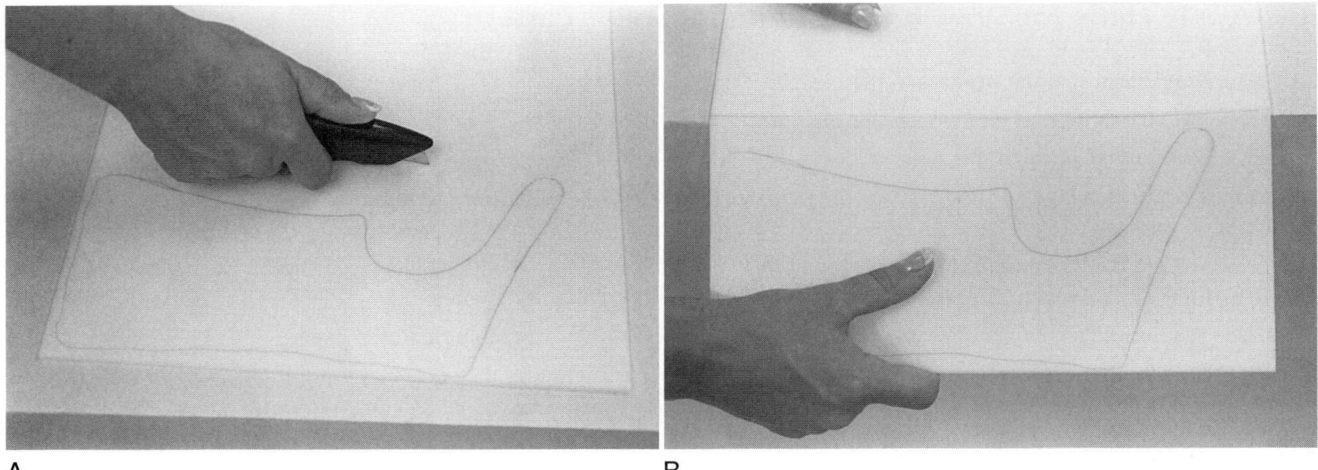

Figure 3-2 (A) A utility knife is used to cut the sheet of material with the pattern outline on it in such a way that the thermoplastic material fits in the hydrocollator or fry pan. (B) The score from the utility knife is pressed against a countertop.

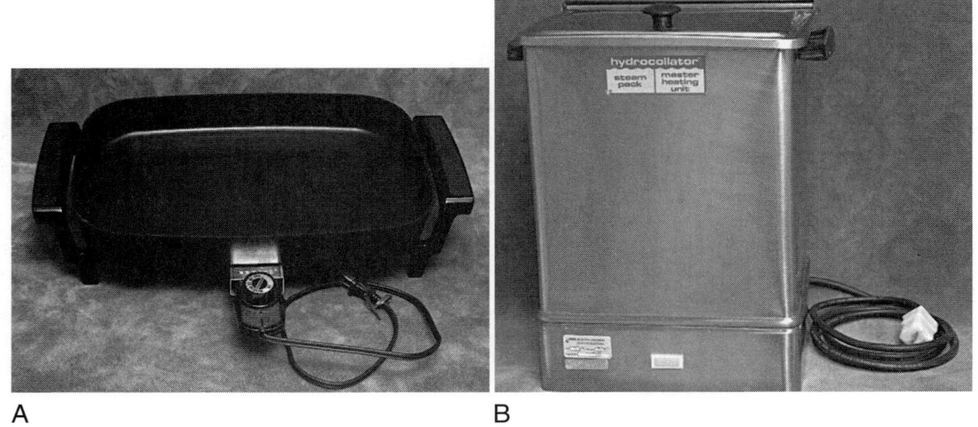

Figure 3-3 Soften thermoplastic material in (A) an electric fry pan or (B) a hydrocollator.

Adequate water height allows a therapist to submerge portions of the splint later when making adjustments. If the thermoplastic material is larger than the fry pan, a portion of the material should be heated. When the material is soft, a paper towel is placed on the heated portion and the rest of the material is folded on the paper towel. A nonstick mesh may be placed in the bottom of a fry pan to prevent the plastic from sticking to any materials or particles. However, it can create a mesh imprint on the plastic. When the thermoplastic piece is large (and especially when it is a high-stretch material), it is a great advantage to lift the thermoplastic material out of the splint pan on the mesh. This keeps the plastic flat and minimizes stretch.

Cutting the Thermoplastic Material

After removing the thermoplastic material from the water with a spatula or on the mesh, the therapist cuts the material with either round- or flat-edged scissors (Figure 3-4). The therapist uses sharp scissors and cuts with long blade strokes (as opposed to using only the tips of the scissors). Scissors should be sharpened at least once each year, and possibly more often, depending on use. Dedicating scissors for specific materials will prolong the edge of the blade. For example, one pair of scissors should be used to cut plastic, another for paper, another for adhesive-backed products, and so on. Sharp scissors in a variety of sizes are helpful for difficult contoured cutting and trimming. Splinting solvent or adhesive removers will remove adhesive that builds up on scissor blades.

Reheating the Thermoplastic Material

After the pattern is cut from the material, it is reheated. During reheating, the therapist positions the person to the desired joint position(s). If the therapist anticipates positioning challenges and needs to spend time solving problems, positioning should be done before the material is reheated to prevent the material from overheating [personal communication, K. Schultz-Johnson, 1999]. During this time frame, the

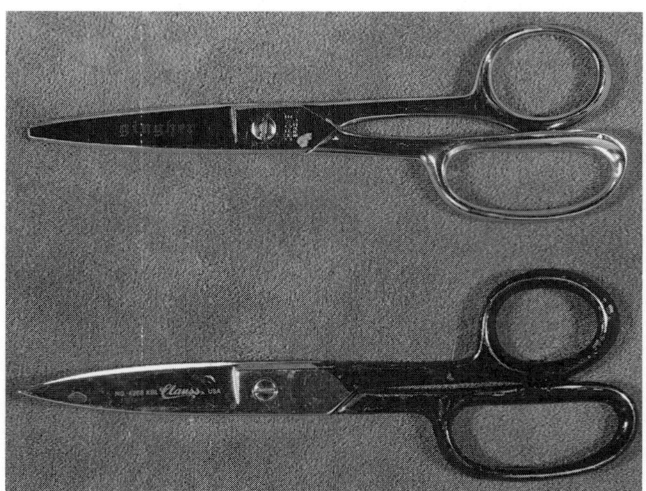

Figure 3-4 Sharp round- or flat-edged scissors work well for cutting thermoplastic.

therapist explains that the material will be warm and that if it is too intolerable the client should notify the therapist. The therapist completes any pre-padding of boney prominences and covers dressings and padding (the LTT will stick to these if not covered with stockinette) prior to the molding process.

Positioning the Client for Splinting

There are several client positioning options. The client is placed in a position that is comfortable, especially for the shoulder and elbow. A therapist may use a gravity-assisted position for hand splinting by having the person rest the dorsal wrist area on a towel roll while the forearm is in supination to maintain proper wrist positioning. Alternatively, a therapist may ask the person to rest the elbow on a table and splint the hand while it is in a vertical position.

For persons with stiffness, a warm water soak or whirlpool, ultrasound, paraffin dip, or hot pack can be used before splinting. Splinting is easiest when persons take their pain medication 30 to 60 minutes before the session. For persons with hypertonicity, it may be effective to use a hot pack on the joint to be splinted. Then the joint should be positioned and splinted in a submaximal range. When splinting is done after warming or after a treatment session, the joints are usually more mobile. However, the splint may not be tolerated after the preconditioning effect wears off. Thus, the therapist must find a balance to complete a gentle warm-up and avoid aggressive preconditioning treatments [personal communication, K. Schultz-Johnson, 1999]. Goniometers are used, when possible, to measure joint angles for optimal therapeutic positioning.

Molding the Splint to the Client

Once positioning is accomplished, the therapist retrieves the softened thermoplastic material. Any hot water is wiped off on a paper towel, a fabric towel, or a pillow that has a dark-colored pillowcase on it. (The dark-colored pillowcase helps identify any small scraps or snips of material from previous splinting activities that may adhere to the thermoplastic material.) The therapist checks the temperature of the softened plastic and finally applies the thermoplastic material to the person's extremity. The thermoplastic material may be extremely warm, and thus the therapist should use caution to prevent skin burn or discomfort. For persons with fragile skin who are at risk of burns, the extremity may be covered with stockinette before the splinting material is applied. Some thermoplastic materials will stick to hair on the person's skin, but this situation can be avoided by using stockinette or lotion on the skin before application of the splinting material.

Therapists may choose to hasten the cooling process to maintain joint position and splint shape. Several options are available. First, a therapist can use an environmentally friendly cold spray. Cold spray is an agent that serves as a surface coolant. Cold spray should not be used near persons who have severe allergies or who have respiratory problems. Because the spray is flammable, it should be properly stored. A second option is to dip the person's extremity with the splint into a tub of cold water. This must be done cautiously with persons who have hypertonicity because the cold temperature could cause a rapid increase in the amount of tone, thus altering joint position. Similar to using a tub of cold water, the therapist may carefully walk the person wearing the splint to a sink and run cold water over the splint. Third, a therapist can use frozen Theraband and wrap it around the splint to hasten cooling. An Ace bandage immersed in ice water and then wrapped around the splint may also speed cooling [Wilton 1997]. However, Ace bandages often leave their imprints on the splinting material.

Making Adjustments

Adjustments can be made to a splint by using a variety of techniques and equipment. While the thermoplastic material is still warm, therapists can make adjustments to splints—such as marking a trim line with their fingernails or a pencil or stretching small areas of the splint. The amount of allowable stretch depends on the property of the material and the cooling time that has elapsed. If the plastic is too cool to cut with scissors, the therapist can quickly dip the area in hot water. A professional-grade metal turkey baster or ladle assists in directly applying hot water to modify a small or difficult-to-immerse area of the splint.

A heat gun (Figure 3-5) may also be used to make adjustments. A heat gun has a switch for *off*, *cool*, and *hot*. After using a heat gun, before turning it to the *off* position the therapist sets the switch to the *cool* setting. This allows the motor to cool down and protects the motor from overheating. When a heat gun is on the *hot* setting, caution must be used to avoid burning materials surrounding it and reaching over the flow of the hot air.

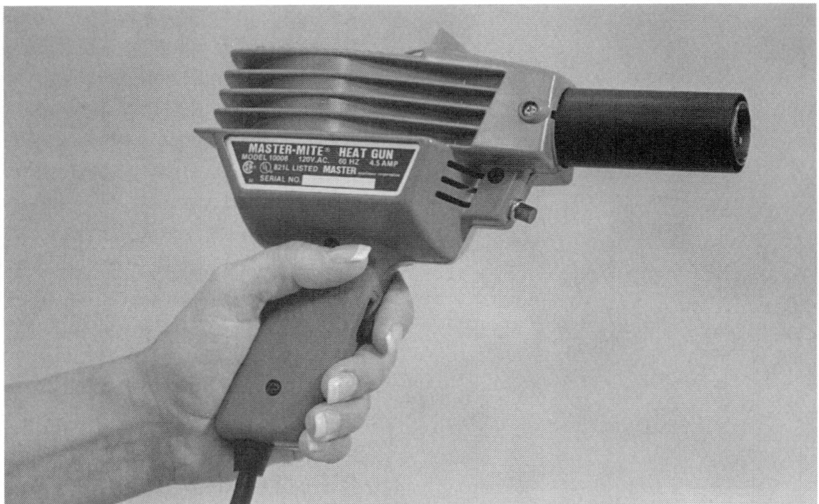

Figure 3-5 A heat gun is used for spot heating.

Heat guns must be used with care. Because heat guns warm unevenly, therapists should not use them for major heating and trimming. Use of heat guns to soften a large area on a splint may result in a buckle or a hot/cold line. A hot/cold line develops when a portion of plastic is heated and its adjacent line or area is cool. A buckle can form where the hot area stretched and the cooled material did not. Heat guns are helpful for warming small focused areas for finishing touches. When using a heat gun, it is best to continually move the heat gun's air projection on the area of the splint to be softened. In addition, the area to be softened should be heated on both sides of the plastic. Attachments for the heat gun's nozzle are available to focus the direction of hot air flow. Small heat guns are available and may assist in spot heating thinner plastics and areas of the splint that have attachments that cannot be exposed to heat (i.e., splint line) [personal communication, K. Schultz-Johnson, 1999 and 2006].

Strapping

After achieving a correct fit, the therapist uses strapping materials to secure the splint onto the person's extremity. Many strapping materials are available commercially. Velcro hook and loop, with or without an adhesive backing, is commonly used for portions of the strapping mechanism. Velcro is available in a variety of colors and widths. Therapists trim Velcro to a desired width or shape. For cutting self-adhesive Velcro, sharp scissors other than those used to cut thermoplastic material should be used. The adhesive backing from strapping materials often accumulates on the scissor blades and makes the scissors a poor cutting tool. The adhesive can be removed with solvent. When a self-adhesive Velcro hook is used, the corners should be rounded. Rounded corners decrease the chance of corners peeling off the splint. Precut self-adhesive Velcro hook dots can be purchased and save therapists' time not only in cutting and rounding corners but in keeping adhesive off scissors. A clinic may have an aid or volunteer cut self-adhesive Velcro hook pieces that have rounded corners to save therapists' time. Briefly heating the adhesive backing and the site of attachment on the splint with a heat gun increases the bond of the hook or loop to the thermoplastic material.

Alternative pressure-sensitive straps, which attach to the Velcro hook, are available. Strapping materials are often padded to add comfort, but these tend to be less durable than Velcro loop. Some padded strapping materials, when cut, have a self-sealing or more finished look than others. Soft straps without self-sealing edges tend to tear apart with use over time. The therapist may cut extra straps and give them to the client to take home if necessary. Commercially sold splint strapping packs provide all the straps needed for a forearm-based splint in one convenient package.

Spiral or continuous strapping can be employed to evenly distribute pressure along the splint. A spiral or continuous strap is a piece of soft strapping that is spiraled around the forearm portion of a splint. Rather than several pieces of Velcro hook being cut to attach to selected sites on the splint, both sides of the forearm trough can be the sites for placement of a long strip of Velcro hook. The spiral or continuous strap attaches to the Velcro hook. Spiral or continuous straps can be used in conjunction with compression gloves for persons who have edematous hands. The spiral strapping and glove prevent the trapping of distal edema.

To prevent the person wearing the splint from losing straps, the therapist may attach one end of the strap to the splint with a rivet or strong adhesive glue. Another helpful technique is to heat the end of a metal butter knife with a heat gun and push it through the splinting material to make a slit. The area is cooled and the knife is removed. The therapist threads the strap through the slit, folds the strap end over itself, and sews the strap together (Figure 3-6A).

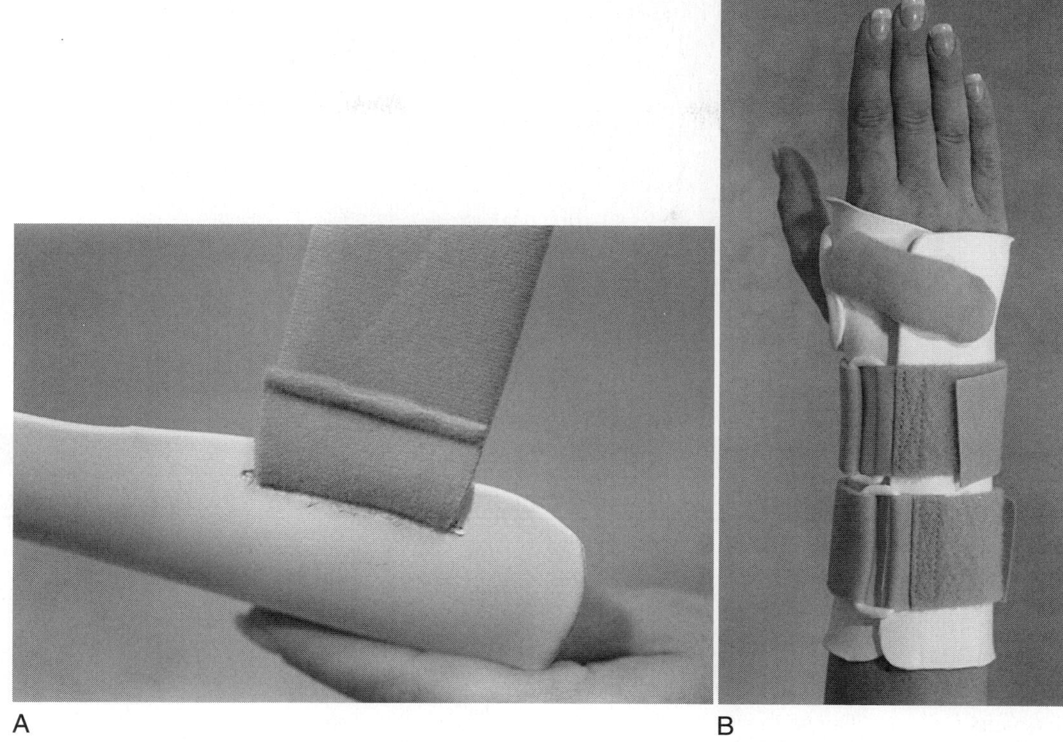

Figure 3-6 (A) Strap is threaded through a slit in forearm trough. The strap is overlapped upon itself and securely sewn. (B) D-ring strapping mechanism.

D-ring straps are available commercially. This type of strapping material affords the greatest control over strap tension and splint migration (Figure 3-6B).

Strap placement is critical to a proper fit. Many therapists fail to place the straps strategically for joint control and render the splint useless. [personal communication, K. Schultz-Johnson, 1999] particularly stresses wrist strap placement *at* the wrist, rather than *proximal* to the wrist.

Padding and Avoiding Pressure Areas

Therapists attempt to remediate portions of splints that may potentially cause pressure areas or irritations. The therapist can use a heat gun to push out areas of the thermoplastic material that may irritate bony prominences. Any bony prominences should be padded before splint formation. Padding should not be added as an afterthought. Padding over these areas or lining of an entire splint may also be considered to prevent irritation. Sufficient space must be made available for the thickness of the padding. Otherwise, the pressure may actually increase over the area.

Use of a self-adhesive gel disk (other paddings will work as well) is helpful in cushioning bony prominences, such as the ulnar head. To use gel disks, the therapist adheres the disk to the person's skin and then forms the splint over the gel disk. Upon cooling of the splint, the gel disk is removed from the person and adhered to the corresponding area inside the splint. To bubble out or dome areas over bony prominences, a therapist can place elastomer putty over the prominence before applying the warm thermoplastic material.

If an entire splint is to be lined with padding, the therapist can use the splint pattern to cut out the padding needed. The therapist can trace the pattern ¼ to ½ inch larger on the padding if the intention is to overlap the self-adhesive padding onto the splint's edges, as shown in Figure 3-7.

Gel lining is often used within the interior of the splint to assist in managing scars. Two types of gel lining are available: silicone gel and polymer gel. Silicone gel sheets, which are flexible and washable, can be cut with scissors into any shape. The silicone gel sheets are often positioned in conjunction with pressure garments or splints or positioned with Coban. Persons using silicone gel sheets must be monitored for the development of rashes, skin irritations, and maceration. Polymer gel sheets are filled with mineral oil, which is released into the skin to soften "normal," hypertrophic, or keloid scars. Polymer gel sheets adhere to the skin and can be used with pressure garments or splints.

Various padding systems are commercially available in a variety of densities, durabilities, cell structures, and surface textures [North Coast Medical 1999]. A self-adhesive backing is available with some types of padding, which saves the therapist time and materials because glue does not have to

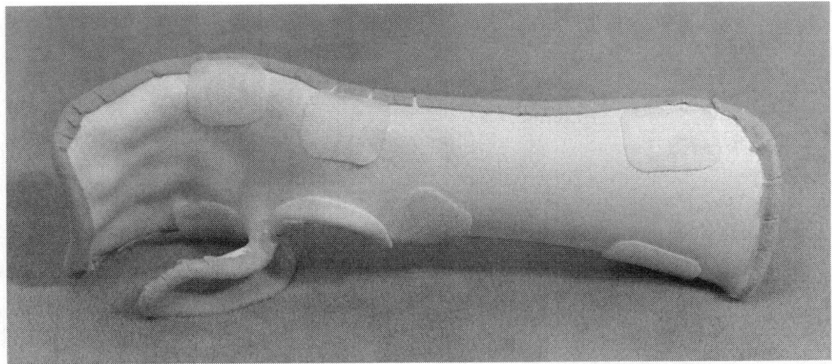

Figure 3-7 Moleskin overlaps the splint's edges.

Table 3-2 Padding Categorization Guidelines

PADDING NAME	DENSITY	DURABILITY	SURFACE TEXTURE	SELF-ADHESIVE
Orthopedic adhesive	Dense	Long	Semi-soft	Yes
Moleskin	Thin	Long	Soft	Yes
Soft splint padding	Thin	Medium	Soft	Yes
Orthopedic felt	Dense	Long	Semi-soft	No
Terry cushion	Thin	Long	Textured	Yes
Luxafoam	Semi-dense	Medium	Soft	Yes
Elasto-gel splint pads	Dense	Medium	Semi-soft	Yes
Contour foam	Semi-dense	Medium	Textured	Yes
Slo-Foam padding	Semi-dense	Medium	Textured	No
Silopad pressure	Dense	Long	Semi-soft	Yes
Splint cushion	Semi-dense	Medium	Semi-soft	Yes
Splint pad	Semi-dense	Long	Textured	Yes
Sorbothane	Dense	Medium	Semi-soft	No
Firm foam padding	Dense	Long	Semi-soft	Yes
Reston foam padding	Thin	Short	Semi-soft	Yes
BioPad	Thin	Short	Soft	Yes
Microtape	Thin	Medium	Soft	Yes
Plastizote padding	Semi-dense	Medium	Semi-soft	No

From North Coast Medical *Hand Therapy Catalog* (1999), San Jose, California.

be used to adhere the padding to a splint. Some cushioning and padding materials have an adhesive backing for easy application. Other types of padding are applied to any flat sheet of thermoplastic material and put in a heavyweight sealable plastic bag before immersion in hot water. The padding and thermoplastic material are adhered prior to molding the splint on the client. Putting the plastic with the padding adhered to it in a plastic bag prevents the padding from getting wet and can save the therapist time. Table 3-2 outlines available padding products.

Padding has either closed or open cells. Closed-cell padding resists absorption of odors and perspiration, and can easily be wiped clean. Open-cell padding allows for absorption. Because of low durability and soiling, padding used in a splint may require periodic replacement. Some types of padding are virtually impossible to remove from a splint. Thus, when padding needs replacement so does the splint.

Edge Finishing

Edges of a splint should be smooth and rolled or flared to prevent pressure areas on the person's extremity. The therapist may use a heat gun or heated water in a fry pan or hydrocollator to heat, soften, and smooth edges. Fingertips moistened with water or lotion help avoid finger imprints on the plastic. Most of the newer thermoplastic materials have self-finishing edges. When the warm plastic is cut, it does not require detailed finishing other than that necessary to flare the edges slightly.

Reinforcement

Strength of a splint increases when the plastic is curved. Thus, a plastic that has curves will be stronger than a flat piece of thermoplastic material. When the thermoplastic

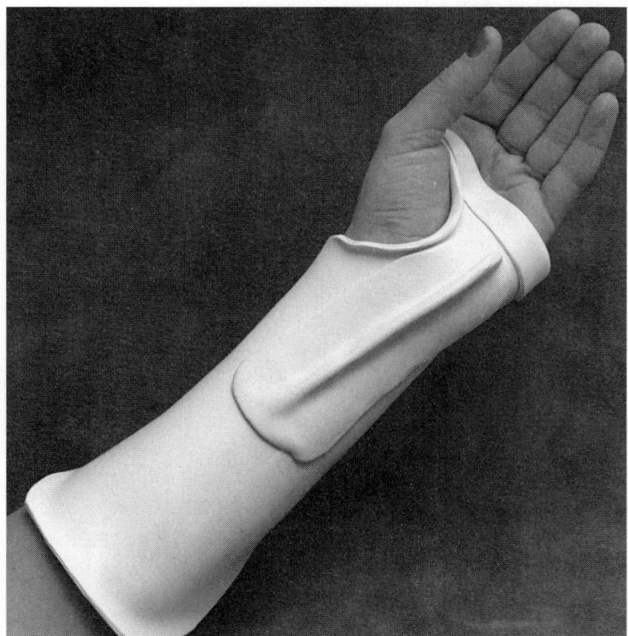

Figure 3-8 Splint reinforcement. This ridge on the reinforcement piece adds strength.

material has been stretched too thin or is too flexible to provide adequate support to an area such as the wrist, it must be reinforced. If an area of a splint requires reinforcement, an additional piece of material bonded to the outside of the splint will increase the strength. A ridge molded in the reinforcement piece provides additional strength (Figure 3-8).

Prefabricated Splints

In addition to making a custom-made splint, therapists have options to use prefabricated splints. The manufacturing of commercially available prefabricated splints is market driven. Therefore, changes in style or materials may appear from year to year. Styles and materials are also affected by the manufacturing processes. Manufacturers are slow to change materials and design even when the market requests it. When a prefabricated splint's material, cut, or style does not sell well, it may be discontinued or replaced with a different design. Vendors often attempt to manufacture prefabricated splints for broad populations.

Manufacturing for a specific population is often costly and not financially rewarding unless that "specific population" has a large market. Improvements in the quality of prefabricated splints are affected by market economics, which stimulate companies to manufacture better products in terms of comfort, durability, and therapeutics. Current catalogs serve as the ultimate reference to what is available. Vendors selling prefabricated splints are listed at the end of this chapter.

In addition to market economics, the proliferation of various styles of prefabricated splints can be attributed to two factors. First, the proliferation of prefabricated splints is influenced by third-party payers' willingness to reimburse for splints. For example, the variety of soft hand and wrist splints for the elderly is an outgrowth of Medicare reimbursement policies during the 1980s and early 1990s. In contrast, because pediatric splints are typically not well reimbursed (except for orthopedic injuries) the market is small. Pediatric splints marketed for orthopedic needs tend to be smaller versions of adult-size splints.

Another reason for the proliferation of prefabricated splints involves the conceptual advances in design and the recognition that a need for these types of splints exists. For example, the refinement of wrist and thumb prefabricated splints has been influenced by the advancement of ergonomic knowledge and the public's awareness of the incidence and effects of cumulative trauma disorders.

Prefabricated splints are available from numerous vendors in a variety of styles, materials, and sizes. Prefabricated splints are available for the head, neck, joints of the upper and lower extremities, and trunk. Typically, prefabricated splints are ordered by size—and in some cases for right or left extremities. Some splints have a universal size, meaning that one splint fits the right or left hand. Before deciding to provide a prefabricated splint for a client, the therapist must be aware of the advantages and disadvantages of prefabricated splints.

Advantages and Disadvantages of Prefabricated Splints

The advantages and disadvantages of using prefabricated splints are listed in Box 3-1.

Box 3-1 Advantages and Disadvantages of Using Soft and Prefabricated Splints

Advantages

- May save time and effort (if the splint fits the person well)
- Immediate feedback from client in terms of satisfaction and therapeutic fit
- Variety of material choices
- Some clients prefer sports-brace appearance

Disadvantages

- Unique fit is often compromised
- Little control over therapeutic positioning of joints
- Expensive to stock a variety of sizes and designs
- Prefabricated and soft splints usually made for a few target populations (cannot address all conditions requiring unique or creative splint designs)

Advantages

An obvious advantage of using a prefabricated splint is saving of the therapist's time and effort. The time required to design a pattern, trace and cut the pattern from plastic, and mold the splint to the person is saved when a prefabricated splint is used. However, one should keep in mind the time and expense involved in ordering and paying for the prefabricated splints. The costs and wage-hours involved in processing an order through a large facility are considerable. Maintaining inventory takes time and space.

If a prefabricated splint is in a clinic's inventory, the ability to immediately assess the splint in terms of therapeutics and customer satisfaction is an advantage. After splint application, the client is readily able to see and feel the splint. When fabricating a custom splint, the therapist may find that it does not meet the client's expectations or needs. When this occurs, a considerable amount of time and effort is expended in modifying the current splint or in designing and fabricating an entirely new splint. With prefabricated splints, an educated trial-and-error process can be used to find the best splint to meet the client's goals and therapeutic needs.

A third advantage is the variety of materials used to make prefabricated splints. Many prefabricated splint materials offer sophisticated technology that cannot be duplicated in the clinic. For example, a prefabricated splint made from high-temperature thermoplastic material is often more durable than a counterpart made of low-temperature thermoplastic material. Softer materials (combinations of fabric and foam) may be more acceptable to persons, especially those with rheumatoid arthritis.

Soft splints can be more comfortable than the LTT ones usually used for custom splinting. In a study comparing soft versus hard resting hand splints in 39 persons with rheumatoid arthritis, Callinan and Mathiowetz [1996] found that compliance with the splint wearing was significantly better with the soft splint (82%) than with the hard splint (67%). However, therapists must realize that a person who needs rigid immobilization for comfort will not prefer a soft splint because soft splints allow some mobility to occur. Some clients may think that the sports-brace appearance of a prefabricated splint is more aesthetically pleasing than the medical appearance of a custom-fabricated splint. For these clients, wearing compliance may increase.

Disadvantages

Several disadvantages must be noted with regard to prefabricated splints. A major disadvantage of using a prefabricated splint is that a custom, unique fit is often compromised. Soft prefabricated splints vary in how much they can be adjusted. If a high degree of conformity or a specialized design is needed, a prefabricated splint will usually not meet the person's needs. LTT prefabricated splints can be spot heated and adjusted somewhat (Figure 3-9), but they will never conform like a custom-made splint of the same material. Some prefabricated splints require adjustments.

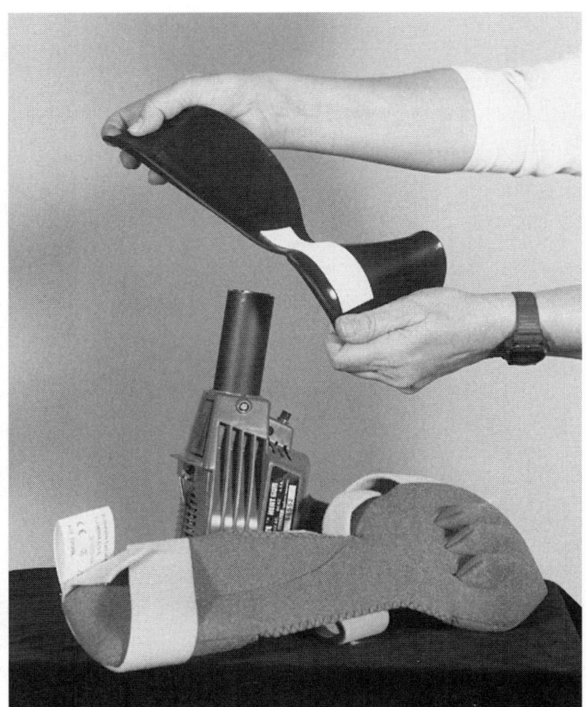

Figure 3-9 Adjustments can be made to commercial LTT splints with the use of a heat gun. [Courtesy Medical Media Service, Veterans Administration Medical Center, Durham, North Carolina.]

For example, thumb splints may require adjustment of the palmar bar to prevent chafing in the thumb web space. Other preformed splints must be adjusted by trimming the forearm troughs for proper strap application.

The second disadvantage of prefabricated splints is related to the therapist's lack of control over customization. When using prefabricated splints, therapists often have little or no control over joint angle positioning. Often a therapeutic protocol or specific client need prescribes a specific joint angle for positioning. In such instances, the therapist must select a prefabricated splint that is designed with the appropriate joint angle(s) or choose one that can be adjusted to the correct angle. If unavailable, a custom splint is warranted. For example, therapists must use prefabricated splints cautiously with persons who have fluctuating edema. The splint and its strapping system must be able to accommodate the extremity's changing size. In addition, when conditions require therapists to create unique splint designs the desired prefabricated splints may not always be commercially available.

A third disadvantage of using a prefabricated splint is that the splint may not be stocked in the clinic and may have to be ordered. Many clinics cannot afford to stock a wide variety of prefabricated splints because of cost and storage restrictions. When a splint must be applied immediately and the prefabricated splint is not in the clinic's stock, a time delay for ordering it is unacceptable. A custom-made splint should be fabricated instead of waiting for the prefabricated splint to arrive.

Once the advantages and disadvantages have been weighed, a decision must be made regarding whether to use a prefabricated or a custom-made splint. The therapist engages in a clinical reasoning process to select the most appropriate splint.

Selecting a Splint

Therapists rarely use custom or prefabricated splints for 100% of their clientele. The therapist uses clinical reasoning based on a frame of reference to select the most appropriate splint. There is little outcome research addressing custom and prefabricated splint usage. To determine whether to use a prefabricated or a custom-made splint, the therapist must know the specific splinting needs of the person and determine how best to accomplish them. Would a soft material or an LTT best meet the person's needs? How would the function and fit of a prefabricated splint compare with that of a custom-made splint? To properly evaluate whether a prefabricated splint or a custom-made splint would best meet a person's needs, the factors and questions discussed in the following sections must be considered and answered.

Diagnosis

Is a prefabricated splint available for the diagnosis? Which splint design meets the therapeutic goals? Is there a match between the therapeutic goals and the design of a prefabricated or soft splint? For example, if a therapist must provide a splint to immobilize a wrist joint in neutral a commercial splint must have the ability to position and immobilize the wrist in a neutral position.

Age of the Person

Is the client at an age where he or she may have an opinion about the splint's cosmesis? What special considerations are there for a geriatric or pediatric person? (See Chapters 15 and 16.) For example, an adolescent may be unwilling to wear a custom-made elastic tension radial nerve splint at school because of its appearance. However, the adolescent might agree to wear a prefabricated wrist splint because of its less conspicuous sports-brace appearance.

Medical Complications

Does the person have compromised skin integrity, vascular supply, or sensation? Is the person experiencing pain, edema, or contractures? Medical conditions must be considered because they may influence splint design. For example, the therapist may choose a splint with wide elastic straps to accommodate the change in the extremity's circumference for a person who has fluctuating edema.

Goals

What are the client's goals? What are the therapeutic goals? The therapist determines the client's priorities and goals from an interview. The therapist can facilitate clients' compliance by understanding each person's capabilities and expectations.

Splint Design

Which joints must be immobilized or mobilized? Will the splint achieve the desired therapeutic goals? Avoid over-splinting. Do not immobilize unnecessary joints. Any splint that limits active range of motion may result in joint stiffness and muscle weakness. For example, if only the hand is involved use a prefabricated hand-based splint to avoid limiting wrist motion.

Occupational Performance

Does the splint affect the client's occupational performance? Does the splint maintain, improve, or eliminate occupational performance? Does wearing the splint interfere with participation in valued activities? Occupational performance should be considered, regardless of the age of the client. Stern et al. [1996] studied 42 persons with rheumatoid arthritis and reported that the "major use of wrist orthoses occurs during instrumental activities of daily living where greater stresses are placed on the wrist" (p. 30). Therapists should observe or ask the client about his or her occupational participation while wearing the splint. Functional problems that occur while the splint is being worn require problem solving. Resolution of functional problems may lead to a modification of performance technique, an adjustment in the wearing schedule, or a change in the splint's design.

Person's or Caregiver's Ability to Comply with Splinting Instructions

Is the person or caregiver capable of following written and verbal instruction? Is the person motivated to comply with the wearing schedule? Are there any factors that may influence compliance? Forgetfulness, fear, cultural beliefs, values, therapeutic priorities, and confusion about the splint's purpose and schedule may influence compliance. A therapist should consider a person's motivation, cognitive functioning, and physical ability when determining a splint design and schedule.

Compliance tends to increase with proper education [Agnew and Maas 1995]. For example, persons receiving education often have a better outcome if instructions are presented in verbal and written formats [Schneiders et al. 1998]. Therapists often explain to clients that long-term gains are usually worth short-term inconvenience. When compliance is a problem, the splint program may have to be modified.

Independence with Splint Regimen

If there is no caregiver, can the person independently apply and remove the splint? Can the person monitor for precautions, such as the development of numbness, reddened areas, pressure sores, rash, and so on? For example, Fred (an 80-year-old man) is in need of bilateral resting hand splints to reduce pain from a rheumatoid arthritis exacerbation. His 79-year-old wife is forgetful. Fred's therapist designs a wearing schedule so that Fred can elicit assistance from his wife. The therapist recommends putting the splints on the bed so that Fred can remind his wife to assist him in donning the splints before bedtime.

Comfort

Does the person report that the splint is comfortable? Does the person have any condition, such as rhumatoid arthritis, that may warrant special attention to comfort? Are there insensate areas that may be potentially harmed by the splint? A therapist should monitor the comfort of a commercial splint on each client. If the splint is not comfortable, a person is not likely to wear it. In studying three prefabricated wrist supports for persons with rheumatoid arthritis, Stern et al. [1997] concluded that "satisfaction … appears to be based not only on therapeutic effect, but also the comfort and ease of its use" (p. 27).

Environment

In what type of environment will the person be wearing the splint? How might the environment affect splint wear and care?

Industrial Settings. Industrial settings may warrant splints made of more durable materials such as leather, Kydex, or metal. For example, splints may need extra cushioning to buffer vibration from machinery or tools that often aggravate cumulative trauma disorders.

Long-Term Care Settings. Therapists providing commercial splints to residents in long-term care settings must consider the influence of multiple caretakers and the fragile skin of many elders. The following suggestions may assist in dealing with multiple caretakers and elders' fragile skin. Splints should be labeled with the person's name. To avoid strap loss, consider attaching them to the splint or choose a splint with attached straps. Select splints made from materials that are durable and easy to keep clean. Colored commercial splints provide a contrast and may be more easily identified and distinguished from white or neutral-colored backgrounds.

School Settings. Several factors relating to pediatric splints must be considered by the therapist. Pediatric prefabricated splints should be made of materials that are easy to clean. Splints for children should be durable. Consider attaching straps to the splint or choose a splint with attached straps. Because multiple caretakers (parents and school personnel) are typically involved in the application and wear schedule, instructions for wear and care should be clear and easy to follow. When the child is old enough, personal preferences as well as parental preferences should be considered during splint selection. If the splint is for long-term use, the therapist must remember that the child will grow. If possible, the therapist should select a splint that can be adjusted to avoid the expense of purchasing a new splint. In addition, splints with components that may scratch or be swallowed by the child should be avoided.

Education Format

What education do the client and caregiver need to adhere to the splint-wearing schedule? What is the learning style of the person and caregiver? How can the therapist adjust educational format to match the person's and caregiver's learning styles? Educating clients and caregivers in methods consistent with their preferred learning style may increase compliance. Learning styles include kinesthetic, visual, and auditory [Fleming and Mills 1993].

Written instructions should include the splint's purpose, wearing schedule, care, and precautions. Because correct use of a splint affects treatment outcome, the client should demonstrate an understanding of instructions in the presence of the therapist. A therapist may complete a follow-up phone call at a suitable interval to detect any problems encountered by the client or caregiver in regard to the prefabricated splint [Racelis et al. 1998]. (See also Chapter 6.)

Fitting and Making Adjustments

If a decision is made to use a prefabricated splint and a selection is made, the therapist must evaluate it for size, fit, and function. Just as with custom splints, a particular prefabricated splint design does not work for every client. As professionals who provide splints to clients, therapists have an obligation and duty to fit the splint to the client rather than fitting the client to the splint! The implications of this duty suggest that clinics should stock a variety of commercial splint designs. Although a large clinic's overhead is expensive, limiting choices may result in poor client compliance [Stern et al. 1997]. When a variety of splint designs are available, a trial-and-error approach can be used with commercial splints because most clients are able to report their preference for a splint after a few minutes of wear. When fitting a client with a commercial splint, the therapist should ask the following questions [Stern et al. 1997]:

- Does the splint feel secure on your extremity?
- Does the splint or its straps rub or irritate you anywhere?
- When wearing the splint, does your skin feel too hot?
- What activities will you be doing while wearing your splint?
- When you move your extremity while wearing the splint, do you experience any pain?
- Does the splint feel comfortable after wearing it for 20 to 30 minutes?

In addition to fit and size, therapists must evaluate the prefabricated splint's effect on function. Stern et al. [1996] investigated three commercial wrist splints for their effect on finger dexterity and hand function. Dexterity was reduced similarly across the three splints. In addition, dexterity was significantly affected when the splints were used during tasks that required maximum dexterity. In such cases, therapists and clients should decide whether dexterity reduction outweighs the known benefits of splinting.

Jansen et al.'s [1997] research indicated that grip strength decreased when clients wore wrist splints. However, for women with rheumatoid arthritis grip strength increased during splint wear [Nordenskiöld 1990]. A reduction in grip strength occurs because wrist splints prevent the amount of wrist extension required to generate maximal grip strength in the "normal" population. Those with rheumatoid arthritis have poor wrist stability. Thus, the splints allow them to generate improved grip strength because of improved stability. Prefabricated splints often require adjustments to appropriately fit the person and condition.

Technical Tips for Custom Adjustments to Prefabricated Splints

The following points describe common adjustments made to commercial splints.

- Therapists should ensure that splints do not irritate soft tissue, reduce circulation, or cause paresthesias [Stern et al. 1997]. Adjustments may include flaring ends, bubbling out pressure areas, or addition of padding.
- Although soft splints are intended to be used as is, minor modifications to customize the fit to a person can be accomplished. Some soft splints can be trimmed with scissors to customize fit. If a soft splint has stitching to hold layers together, it will need to be resewn. (Note that it is beneficial to have a sewing machine in the clinic.)
- Modification methods for preformed splints include heating, cutting, or reshaping portions of the LTT splint. Minor modifications can be made with the use of a heat gun, fry pan, or hydrocollator to soften LTT preformed splints for trimming or slight stretching.
- Some elastic traction/tension prefabricated splints may be adjusted by bending and repositioning portions of wire, metal, or foam splint components. Occasionally, technical literature accompanying the splint describes how to make adjustments in the amount of traction. Often traction can be adjusted with the use of an Allen wrench on the rotating wheels on a hinge joint, as shown in Figure 3-10. When there are no instructions describing how to make adjustments on prefabricated splints, the therapist must use creative problem-solving skills to accomplish the desired changes.
- When a static prefabricated splint is used and serial adjustments are required to accommodate increases in passive range of motion (PROM), the splint must be reheated and remolded to the client. It is advantageous to select a prefabricated splint made of material that has memory properties to allow for the serial adjustments.
- The amount of force provided by some static-progressive splints is made through mechanical adjustment of the force-generating device. Force may be adjusted by manipulating the splint's turnbuckle, bolt, or hinge.
- The force exerted by elastic traction components of a prefabricated splint is also made through adjustments of the force-generating device. Therapists can adjust the forces by changing elastic component length by gradually moving the placement of the neoprene or rubber band–like straps on a splint throughout the day, as shown in Figure 3-11.
- Adding components to prefabricated splints can be helpful. For example, putty-elastomer inserts that serve as finger separators can be used in a resting hand splint. Finger separators add contour in the hand area to maintain the arches. A therapist may choose to add other components, such as wicking lining or padding.
- Prefabricated splints can be modified by replacing parts of them with more adjustable materials. For example, if a wrist splint has a metal stay replacing it with an LTT stay results in a custom fit with the correct therapeutic position.

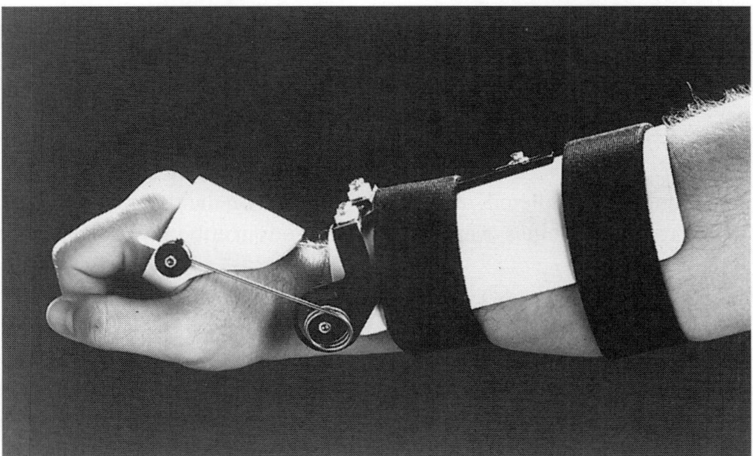

Figure 3-10 Tension is adjusted with an Allen wrench on the rotating wheels on the hinge joint of this splint.

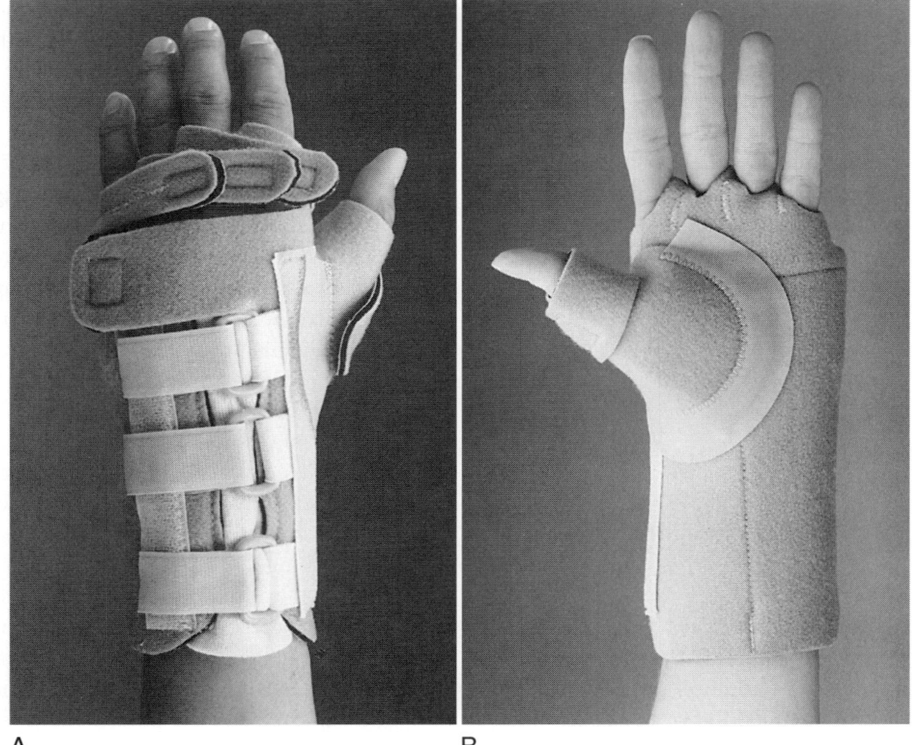

Figure 3-11 (A) The Rolyan In-Line splint with thumb support can be adjusted by loosening or tightening the neoprene straps. (B) Volar view of the Rolyan In-Line splint with thumb support. [Courtesy Rehabilitation Division of Smith & Nephew, Germantown, Wisconsin.]

- It is often necessary to customize strapping mechanisms for prefabricated splints. The number and placement of straps are adjusted to best secure the splint on the person. Straps must be secured properly, but not so tightly as to restrict circulation. Straps coursing through web spaces must not irritate soft tissue. The research by Stern et al. [1997] on commercial wrist splints indicates that clients with stiff joints experienced difficulty threading straps through D-rings. Clients reported having to use their teeth to manipulate straps. Straps that are too long also appear to be troublesome because they catch on clothing [Stern et al. 1997].
- Stern et al. [1994] showed that although commercial splints are often critiqued for being too short, some persons prefer shorter forearm troughs. Shorter splints seem to be preferred by clients when wrist support, not immobilization, is needed.

After the necessary adjustments are completed and a proper fit is accomplished, a therapist determines wearing schedule.

Wearing Schedule

Although there are no easy answers about wearing protocols, experienced therapists have several guidelines for decision making as they tailor wearing schedules to each client [Schultz-Johnson 1992].

- For splints designed to increase PROM, light tension exerted by a splint over a long period of time is preferable to high tension for short periods of time.
- For joints with hard end feels and PROM limitations, more hours of splint wear are warranted than for joints with soft end feels.
- Persons tolerate static splints (including serial and static-progressive splints) better than dynamic splints during sleep.
- When treatment goals are being considered, wearing schedules should allow for facilitation of active motion and functional use of joints when appropriate.

As with any splint provision, the splint-wearing schedule should be given in verbal and written formats to the person and caregiver(s). The wearing schedule depends on the person's condition and dysfunction and the severity (chronic or acute) of the problem. The wearing schedule also depends on the therapeutic goal of the splint, the demands of the environment, and the ability of the person and caregiver(s).

Care of Prefabricated Splints

Always check the manufacturer's instructions for cleaning the splint. Give the client the manufacturer's instructions on splint care. If a client is visually impaired, make an enlarged copy of the instructions. For soft splints, the manufacturer usually recommends hand washing and air drying because the agitation and heat of some washers and dryers can ruin soft splints. Because air drying of soft splints takes time, occasionally two of the same splint are provided so that the person can alternate wear during cleaning and drying. The inside of LTT splints should be wiped out with rubbing alcohol. The outside of LTT splints can be cleaned with toothpaste or nonabrasive cleaning agents and rinsed with tepid water. Clients and caregivers should be reminded that LTT splints soften in extreme heat, as in a car interior or on a windowsill or radiator.

Precautions

In addition to selecting, fitting, and scheduling the wear of a prefabricated splint, the therapist must educate the client or caregiver about any precautions and how to monitor for them. There are several precautions to be aware of with the use of commercial splints. These are discussed in the section following.

Dermatological Issues Related to Splinting

Latex Sensitivity. Some prefabricated splints contain latex. More latex-sensitive people, including clients and medical professionals, are being identified [Jack 1994, Personius 1995]. Therapists should request a list of both latex and latex-free products from the suppliers of commercial splints used.

Allergic Contact Dermatitis. Recently, dermatologic issues related to neoprene splinting have come to therapists' attention. Allergic contact dermatitis (ACD) and miliaria rubra (prickly heat) are associated in some persons with the wearing of neoprene (also known as polychloroprene) splints [Stern et al. 1998]. ACD symptoms include itching, skin eruptions, swelling, and skin hemorrhages. Miliaria rubra presents with small, red, elevated, inflamed papules and a tingling and burning sensation. Before using commercial or custom neoprene splints, therapists should question clients about dermatologic reactions and allergies. If a person reacts to a neoprene splint, wear should be discontinued and the therapist should notify the manufacturer. An interface such as polypropylene stockinette may also serve to resolve the problem.

Clients need to be instructed not only in proper splint care but in hygiene of the body part being splinted. Intermittent removal of the splint to wash the body part, the application of cornstarch, or the provision of wicking liners may help minimize dermatologic problems. Time of year and ambient temperatures need to be considered by the therapist. For example, neoprene may provide desired warmth to stiff joints and increase comfort while improving active and passive range of motion. However, during extreme summer temperatures the neoprene splint may cause more perspiration and increase the risk of skin maceration if inappropriately monitored.

Ordering Commercial Splints

A variety of vendors sell prefabricated splints. Companies may sell similar splint designs, but the splint names can be quite different. To keep abreast of the newest commercial splints, therapists should browse through vendor catalogs, communicate with vendor sales representatives, and seek out vendor exhibits during meetings and conferences for the ideal "hands-on" experience.

It is most beneficial to the therapist and the client when a clinic has a variety of commercial splint designs and sizes for right and left extremities. Keeping a large stock in a clinic can be expensive. To cover the overhead expense of stocking and storing prefabricated splints, a percentage markup of the prefabricated splint is often charged in addition to the therapist's time and materials used for adjustments.

Splint Workroom or Cart

Having a well-organized and stocked splinting area will benefit the therapist who must make decisions about the splint design and construct the splint in a timely manner. Clients who need splint intervention will also benefit from a well-stocked splint and splinting supply inventory. Readily available splinting materials and tools will expedite the splinting process.

Clinics should consider the services commonly rendered and stock their materials accordingly. In addition to a stocked splinting room, therapists may find it useful to have a splint cart organized for splinting in a client's room or in another portion of the health care setting. The cart can assist the therapist in readily transporting splinting supplies to the client, rather than a client coming to the therapist. For therapists who travel from clinic to clinic, splinting supply suitcases on rollers are ideal. Splinting carts or cases should contain such items as the following:

- Paper towels
- Pencils/awl
- Masking tape
- Thermoplastic material
- Fry pan
- Scissors
- Strapping materials, including Ace bandages
- Padding materials
- Heat gun
- Spatula, metal turkey baster
- Thermometer
- Pliers
- Revolving hole punch
- Glue
- Goniometer
- Solvent or bonding agent
- Other specialized supplies as needed (e.g., finger loops, outrigger wire, outrigger line, springs, turnbuckles, rubber bands, and so on)

Documentation and Reassessment

Splint provision must be well documented. Documentation assists in third-party reimbursement, communication to other health care providers, and demonstration of efficacy of the intervention. Splint documentation should include several elements, such as the type, purpose, and anatomic location of the splint. Therapists should document that they have communicated in oral and written formats with the person receiving the splint. Topics addressed with each person include the wearing schedule, splint care, precautions, and any home program activities.

In follow-up visits, documentation should include any changes in the splint's design and wearing schedule. In addition, the therapist should note whether problems with compliance are apparent. The therapist should determine whether the range of motion is increasing with splint wearing time and draw conclusions about splint efficacy or compliance with the program. Function in and out of the splint should be documented. For example, the therapist determines whether the person can independently perform some type of function as a result of wearing the splint. The therapist must listen to the client's reports of functional problems and solve problems to remediate or compensate for the functional deficit. If function or range of motion is not increased, the therapist will need to consider splint revision or redesign or counsel the client on the importance of splint wear.

The therapist should perform splint reassessments regularly until the person is weaned from the splint or discharged from services. Facilities use different methods of documentation, and the therapist should be familiar with the routine method of the facility. (Refer to the documentation portion of Chapter 6 for more information.)

Physical Agent Modalities

PAMs are defined as those modalities that produce a biophysiologic response through the use of light, water, temperature, sound, electricity, or mechanical devices [AOTA 2003, p. 1]. The AOTA's PAM position paper indicates that "physical agent modalities may be used by occupational therapy practitioners as an adjunct to or in preparation for intervention that ultimately enhances engagement in occupation; physical agents may only be applied by occupational therapists who have documented evidence of possessing the theoretical background for safe and competent integration into the therapy treatment plan" [AOTA 2003, p. 1]. Therapists must comply with their respective state's scope of practice requirements regarding the use of PAMs as preparation for splinting.

Experienced therapists often use PAMs as an adjunctive method to effect a change in musculoskeletal tissue. Select PAMs may be used before, during, or after splint provision for management of pain, to increase soft-tissue extensibility, reduce edema, increase tendon excursion, promote wound healing, and decrease scar tissue. Occasionally, PAMs are used to prepare the upper extremity for optimal positioning for splinting. Prior to using any PAM, the therapist must develop and use clinical reasoning skills to effectively select and evaluate the appropriate modality; identify safety precautions, indications, and contraindications; and facilitate individualized treatment outcomes.

The type of PAM selected and the parameter setting(s) affects the neuromuscular system and tissue response. Changes in tissue response depend on how sensory information is processed to produce a motor response. Thermotherapy (heat) and cryotherapy (cold) have a significant effect on the peripheral nervous system and on neuromuscular control, and may enhance sensory and motor function when applied as an adjunctive method.

Therapists who use PAMs to effect a change in soft tissue, joint structure, tendons and ligaments, sensation, and pain level must consider the agent's effects on superficial structures within the skin (i.e., epidermis, dermis, and hypodermis). Because splints are usually applied to an extremity (e.g., hand or foot), therapists must consider which sensory structures are stimulated and which motor responses are expected when applying a PAM prior to splinting. PAMs can be generally categorized in numerous ways. An overview of superficial agents commonly used to position the client for splinting follows.

Superficial Agents

Superficial agents penetrate the skin to a depth of 1 to 2 cm [Cameron 2003]. These heating agents or thermotherapy agents include moist hot packs, fluidotherapy, paraffin wax therapy, and cryotherapy. Table 3-3 lists superficial agents and their physiologic responses, indications, contraindications, and precautions.

Heat Agents

Heat is transferred to the skin and subcutaneous tissue by *conduction* or by *convection*. Conduction transfers heat from one object to another. Heat is conducted from the higher-temperature object to the lower-temperature material (such as moist heat packs or paraffin). Table 3-4 lists the temperature ranges for heat application.

Hot Packs

Superficial heat may be used for the relief of pain with noninflammatory conditions, general relaxation, and to stretch contractures and improve range of motion prior to splinting. For example, a client fractures her wrist and upon removal of the cast demonstrates limited wrist extension. The therapist intends to gain wrist extension by applying a moist hot pack to her wrist to increase the extensibility of the soft tissue. After application of the heat, the therapist is able to range the wrist into 10 degrees of wrist extension (an improvement from neutral). The client is splinted in slight

Table 3-3 Superficial Agents

TYPE OF PAM	PHYSIOLOGIC RESPONSE	INDICATIONS	CONTRAINDICATIONS	PRECAUTIONS
Hot packs (conduction)	• Increased collagen extensibility • Increased activity of thermoreceptors • Increased blood flow increases nutrients to the area and facilitates removal of prostaglandin, bradykinin, and histamine • Changes muscle spindle firing rate • Increased sensory nerve conduction velocity	• Clients with subacute and chronic conditions that experience stiffness and/or pain that interferes with positioning needed for splinting	• Do not use with clients who have absent sensation or decreased circulation.	• Use tongs to remove the hot pads. • Clients should not lie on top of heat packs. • Do not use in presence of severe edema. • Be careful with clients who have decreased sensation.
Fluidiotherapy (convection)	• Increased collagen extensibility • Increased activity of thermoreceptors • Increased blood flow increases nutrients to the area and facilitates removal of prostaglandin, bradykinin, and histamine • Changes muscle spindle firing rate • Increased sensory nerve conduction velocity	• Clients with subacute and chronic conditions that experience stiffness and/or pain that interferes with positioning needed for splinting • Have clients complete AROM while in the fluidiotherapy machine	• Do not use with clients who have open wounds or draining wounds.	• Be cautious with clients who have decreased sensation and circulation. • Caution needed when used with persons who have asthma or respiratory problems.
Paraffin (conduction)	• Increased collagen extensibility • Increased activity of thermoreceptors • Increased blood flow increases nutrients to the area and facilitates removal of prostaglandin, bradykinin, and histamine • Changes muscle spindle firing rate • Increased sensory nerve conduction velocity	• Clients with subacute and chronic conditions that experience stiffness and/or pain that interferes with positioning needed for splinting	• Do not use with clients who have open wounds, infections or absent sensation.	• Check the thermostat on machine. • Keep a CO_2 fire extinguisher available. • Be careful with clients who have decreased sensation or circulation.
Cold cryotherapy: • Ice packs • Ice towels • Vapo-coolant sprays	• Vasoconstriction • Decreased velocity of nerve conduction • Decreased metabolism • Increased pain threshold • Reduced spasticity due to decreased muscle spindle activity	• Decreased pain, edema, and spasticity	• Cardiac dysfunction • Chronic or deep open wounds, arterial insufficiency • Hypersensitivity to cold • Impaired sensation • Regenerating peripheral nerves • Elders who have decreased tolerance to cold	

Table 3-4 Temperature Ranges for Heat Application

TEMPERATURE RANGE	°F	°C
Normal temperature	98.6	37
Mild heating	98.6–104	37–40
Vigorous heating	104–110	40–43
Tissue damage	>110	>43

Data from Bracciano A. *Physical Agent Modalities: Theory and Application for the Occupational Therapist.* Thorofare, NJ: Slack 2002.

wrist extension. A serial static splinting approach is used to gain a functional level of wrist extension.

Heat may be used to decrease muscle spasms by increasing nerve conduction velocity. According to Cameron [2003, p.159]: "Nerve conduction velocity has been reported to increase by approximately 2 meters/second for every 1°C (1.8°F) increase in temperature. Elevation of muscle tissue to 42°C (108°F) has been shown to decrease firing rate of the alpha motor neurons resulting in decreased muscle spasm." Thus, in some cases heat is applied to reduce muscle spasms with a client who needs a splint.

Fluidotherapy

Convection transfers heat between a surface and a moving medium or agent. Examples of convection include fluidotherapy and whirlpool (hydrotherapy). Fludiotherapy is a form of dry heat consisting of ground cellulose particles made from corn husks. Circulated air heated to 100° to 118°F suspends the particles, creating agitation that functions much like a whirlpool turbine. Fluidotherapy is frequently used for pain control and desensitization and sensory stimulation. It is also used to increase soft tissue extensibility and joint range of motion and to reduce adhesions. Fluidotherapy is often used prior to applying static and dynamic hand splints for increasing soft-tissue extensibility. Fluidotherapy can increase edema due to the heat and dependent positioning of the upper extremity. Caution must be taken when using fluidotherapy on those who have asthma or when using fluidotherapy around those near the machine who have respiratory conditions, as particles can trigger a respiratory attack.

Paraffin Wax Therapy

Heated paraffin wax is another source of superficial warmth that transfers heat by conduction. The melting point of paraffin wax is 54.5°C (131°F). Administration includes dipping the clean hand in the wax for 10 consecutive immersions. The hand is then wrapped in a plastic bag and covered with a towel. Clients with open wounds, infections, or absent sensation should not receive paraffin therapy. Clients with chronic conditions such as rheumatoid arthritis may benefit from paraffin therapy to reduce stiffness prior to splinting.

Cryotherapy

Cryotherapy is defined as the therapeutic use of cold modalities. Cold is considered a superficial modality that penetrates to a depth of 1 to 2 cm and produces a decrease in tissue temperature. Cold is transferred to the skin and subcutaneous tissue by conduction. Examples of cold modalities include cold packs, ice packs, ice towels, ice massage, and vapor sprays. Cold packs are usually stored at –5°C (23°F) and treatment time is 10 to 15 minutes. The effectiveness of the cold modality used depends on intensity, duration, and frequency of application.

There are four sensations of cold associated with reduced pain and inflammation: cold, burning, aching, and numbness. Hayes [2000] suggested that cold modalities used to reduce swelling and slow metabolism must be mild. To block pain, cold must be very cold. Duration of cold application depends on the targeted tissue. Deeper tissues must be cooled for longer periods of time. The colder the medium the shorter the duration. Cryotherapy may be used in the treatment of acute injury or to control bleeding associated with recent wounds. Other therapeutic benefits of cold include increased vasoconstriction, decreased metabolic response (reduces oxygen and thus decreases inflammation), decreased nerve conduction velocity, increased pain threshold, decreased muscle spindle activity, and reduced spasticity.

Cryotherapy is contraindicated for clients with cardiac dysfunction, chronic or deep open wounds, arterial insufficiency, hypersensitivity to cold, impaired sensation, and regenerating peripheral nerves. Elders with decreased tolerance to cold may be unable to tolerate even brief applications of therapeutic cold modalities [Belanger 2002, Bracciano 2002, Cameron 2003, Hayes 2000, Kahn 2000, Shankar and Randall 2002, Sussman and Bates-Jensen 1998].

Cold modalities may be used to decrease edema, pain, and spasticity during range of motion prior to splint application. Cryotherapy does not increase soft-tissue extensibility and may reduce circulation, oxygen, and nutrition to healing tissues. Refer to Table 3-3 for a comparison of the therapeutic effects of cryotherapy and thermotherapy.

Vendors

Advanced Therapy Products
P.O. Box 34320
Glen Allen, VA 23058
1-800-548-4550

AliMed
297 High St.
Dedham, MA 02026
1-800-225-2610

Benik Corporation
11871 Silverdale Way NW
Silverdale, WA 98383
1-800-442-8910

Biodex Medical Systems
101 Technology Dr.
Bethlehem, PA 18015
1-800-971-2468

Bio Technologies
2160 N. Central Rd.
Suite 204
Fort Lee, NJ 07024
1-800-971-2468

Chattanooga Group
4717 Adams Rd., P.O. Box 489
Hixton, TN 37343
1-800-592-7329

Core Products International, Inc.
808 Prospect Ave.
Osceola, WI 54020
1-800-365-3047

DeRoyal/LMB
200 DeBusk Lane
Posell, TN 37849
1-800-251-9864

Dynasplint
770 Ritchie Hwy.
Suite W 21
Severna Park, MD 21146-3937
1-800-638-6771

Empi
599 Cardigan Rd.
St. Paul, MN 55126-4099
1-800-328-2536, ext. 1773

Joint Active Systems
2600 S. Raney St.
Effingham, IL 62401
1-800-879-0117

Joint Jack Company
108 Britt Rd.
East Hartford, CT 06118
1-800-568-7338

Medassist-OP, Inc.
P.O. Box 758
Palm Harbor, FL 34682
1-800-521-6664

Medical Designs, Inc.
2820 N. Sylvania Ave.
Fort Worth, TX 76111
1-817-834-3300

North Coast Medical, Inc.
187 Stauffer Blvd.
San Jose, CA 95125
1-800-821-9319

OrthoLogic/Sutter Corporation
1275 W. Washington St.
Tempe, AZ 85281
1-800-225-1814

Restorative Care of America, Inc. (RCAI)
11236 47th St. North
Clearwater, FL 33762
1-800-627-1595

Sammons Preston
P.O. Box 5071
Bollingbrook, IL 60440
1-800-323-5547

Silver Ring Splint Company
P.O. Box 2586
Charlottesville, VA 22902
1-804-971-4052

Smith & Nephew, Inc.
One Quality Dr.
P.O. Box 1005
Germantown, WI 53022
1-800-545-7758

Tetra Medical Supply Corporation
6364 West Gross Point Rd.
Niles, IL 60713-3916
1-800-621-4041

Therakinetics
55 Carnegie Plaza
Cherry Hill, NJ 08003-1020
1-800-800-4276

3-Point Products
1610 Pincay Court
Annapolis, MD 21401-5644
1-410-349-2649

U.E. Tech
P.O. Box 2145
Edwards, CO 81632
1-800-736-1894

REVIEW QUESTIONS

1. What are six handling characteristics of thermoplastics?
2. What are six performance characteristics of thermoplastics?

3. At what temperature range are low-temperature thermoplastics softened?
4. What steps are involved in making a splint pattern?
5. What equipment can be used to soften thermoplastic materials?
6. How can a therapist prevent a tacky thermoplastic from sticking to the hair on a person's arms?
7. What are the purposes of using a heat gun?
8. Why should a therapist use a bonding agent?
9. Why should the edges of a splint be rolled or flared?
10. What is the AOTA position on the use of PAMs by occupational therapy practitioners?
11. What is the depth of penetration to skin and subcutaneous obtained with superficial agents?
12. How can PAMs be used in preparation for splinting?

References

Agnew PJ, Maas F (1995). Compliance in wearing wrist working splints in rheumatoid arthritis. Occupational Therapy Journal of Research 15(3):165-180.

American Occupational Therapy Association (2003). Position paper: Physical agent modalities. American Journal of Occupational Therapy 57:650.

Belanger AY (2002). *Evidenced-based Guide to Therapeutic Physical Agents*. Philadelphia: Lippincott Williams & Wilkins.

Bracciano A (2002). *Physical Agent Modalities: Theory and Application for the Occupational Therapist*. Thorofare, NJ: Slack.

Callinan N, Mathiowetz V (1996). Soft versus hard resting hand splints in rheumatoid arthritis: Pain relief, preference and compliance. American Journal of Occupational Therapy 50(5): 347-353.

Cameron M (2003). *Physical Agents in Rehabilitation: From Research to Practice*. St. Louis: Elsevier Saunders.

Fleming ND, Mills C (1993). Helping students understand how they learn. The Teaching Professor [volume]:3-4.

Hayes KW (2000). *Manual for Physical Agents, Fifth Edition*. Upper Saddle River, NJ: Prentice-Hall.

Jack M (1994). Latex allergies: A new infection control issue. Canadian Journal of Infection Control 9(3):67-70.

Jansen CWS, Olson SL, Hasson SM (1997). The effect of use of a wrist orthosis during functional activities on surface electromyography of the wrist extensors in normal subjects. Journal of Hand Therapy 10(4):283-289.

Kahn J (2000). *Principles and Practices of Electrotherapy, Fourth Edition*. Philadelphia: Churchill Livingstone.

Lee DB (1995). Objective and subjective observations of low-temperature thermoplastic materials. Journal of Hand Therapy 8(2): 138-143.

McKee P, Morgan L (1998). Orthotic materials. In P McKee, L Morgan (eds.), *Orthotics in Rehabilitation*. Philadelphia: F. A. Davis.

Melvin JL (1989). *Rheumatic Disease in the Adult and Child: Occupational Therapy and Rehabilitation*. Philadelphia: F. A. Davis.

Nordenskiöld U (1990). Elastic wrist orthoses: Reduction of pain and increase in grip force for women with rheumatoid arthritis. Arthritis Care and Research 3(3):158-162.

North Coast Medical (1999). Hand Therapy Catalog, San Jose, CA.

North Coast Medical (2006). Hand Therapy Catalog, San Jose, CA.

Personius CD (1995). Patients, health care workers, and latex allergy. Medical Laboratory Observer 27(3):30-32.

Preston Sammons Rolyan (PSR) (2006). *Hand Rehab Products for Hand Rehabilitation*. Bolingbrook, IL: Patterson Medical Products.

Racelis MC, Lombardo K, Verdin J (1998). Impact of telephone reinforcement of risk reduction education on patient compliance. Journal of Vascular Nursing 16(1):16-20.

Schneiders AG, Zusman M, Singer KP (1998). Exercise therapy compliance in acute low back pain patients. Manual Therapy 3(3):147-152.

Schultz-Johnson K (1992). Splinting: A problem-solving approach. In BG Stanley, SM Tribuzi (eds.), *Concepts in Hand Rehabilitation*. Philadelphia: F. A. Davis.

Shankar K, Randall KD (2002). *Therapeutic Physical Modalities*. Philadelphia: Hanley & Belfus.

Stern EB, Callinan N, Hank M, Lewis EJ, Schousboe JT, Ytterberg SR (1998). Neoprene splinting: Dermatological issues. American Journal of Occupational Therapy 52(7):573-578.

Stern EB, Sines B, Teague TR (1994). Commercial wrist extensor orthoses: Hand function, comfort and interference across five styles. Journal of Hand Therapy 7:237-244.

Stern EB, Ytterberg S, Krug HE, Mahowald ML (1996). Arthritis Care and Research 9(3):197-205.

Stern EB, Ytterberg S, Larson L, Portoghese C, Kratz W, Mahowald M (1997). Commercial wrist extensor orthoses: A descriptive study of use and preference in patients with rheumatoid arthritis. Arthritis Care and Research 10(1):27-35.

Sussman C, Bates-Jensen BM (1998). *Wound Care: A Collaborative Practice Manual for Physical Therapists and Nurses*. Philadelphia: Lippincott Williams & Wilkins.

Wilton JC (1997). *Hand Splinting Principles of Design and Fabrication*. Philadelphia: Saunders.

CHAPTER 4

Anatomic and Biomechanical Principles Related to Splinting

Brenda M. Coppard, PhD, OTR/L

Key Terms

Volar
Dorsal
Radial
Ulnar
Zones of the hand
Aponeurosis
Prehension
Grasp
Degrees of freedom
Torque
Three-point pressure
Mechanical advantage
Pressure
Stress
Plasticity
Viscoelasticity

Chapter Objectives

1. Define the anatomical terminology used in splint prescriptions.
2. Relate anatomy of the upper extremity to splint design.
3. Identify arches of the hand.
4. Identify creases of the hand.
5. Articulate the importance of the hand's arches and creases to splinting.
6. Recall actions and nerve innervations of upper extremity musculature.
7. Differentiate prehensile and grasp patterns of the hand.
8. Apply basic biomechanical principles to splint design.
9. Describe the correct width and length for a forearm splint.
10. Describe uses of padding in a splint.
11. Explain the reason splint edges should be rolled or flared.
12. Relate contour to splint fabrication.
13. Describe the change in skin and soft tissue mechanics with scar tissue, material application, edema, contractures, wounds, and infection.

Basic Anatomical Review for Splinting

Splinting requires sound knowledge of anatomic terminology and structures, biomechanics, and the way in which pathologic conditions impair function. Knowledge of anatomic structures is necessary in the choice and fabrication of a splint. This knowledge also influences the therapeutic regimen and home program. The following is a brief overview of anatomic terminology, proximal-to-distal structures, and landmarks of the upper extremity pertinent to the splinting process. It is neither comprehensive nor all-inclusive. For more depth and breadth in anatomic review, access an anatomy text, anatomic atlas, or compact disk [Colditz and McGrouther 1998] showing anatomic structures.

Terminology

Knowing anatomic location terms is extremely important when a therapist receives a splint prescription or is reading professional literature. In rehabilitation settings, the word *arm* usually refers to the area from the shoulder to the elbow (humerus). The term *antecubital fossa* refers to the depression at the bend of the elbow. *Forearm* is used to describe the area from the elbow to the wrist, which includes the radius and ulna. *Carpal* or *carpus* refers to the wrist or the carpal bones. Different terminology can be used to refer to the thumb and fingers. Narrative names include thumb, index, middle or long, ring, and little fingers. A numbering system is used to refer to the digits (Figure 4-1). The thumb is digit 1, the index finger is digit II, the middle (or long) finger is digit III, the ring finger is digit IV, and the little finger is digit V.

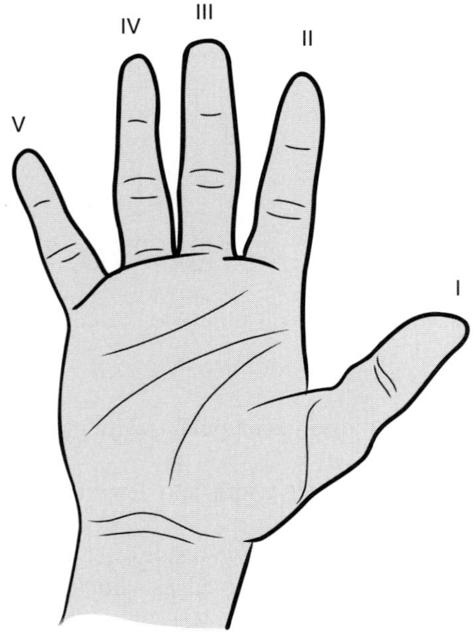

Figure 4-1 Numbering system used for the digits of the hand.

The terms *palmar* and *volar* are used interchangeably and refer to the front or anterior aspect of the hand and forearm in relationship to the anatomic position. The term *dorsal* refers to the back or posterior aspect of the hand and forearm in relationship to the anatomic position. *Radial* indicates the thumb side, and *ulnar* refers to the side of the fifth digit (little finger). Therefore, if a therapist receives an order for a dorsal wrist splint the physician has ordered a splint that is to be applied on the back of the hand and wrist. Another example of location terminology in a splint prescription is a radial gutter thumb spica splint. The therapist applies this type of splint to the thumb side of the hand and forearm.

Literature addressing hand injuries and rehabilitation protocols often refers to zones of the hand. Figure 4-2 diagrams the zones of the hand [Kleinert et al. 1981]. Table 4-1 presents the zones' borders. Therapists should be familiar with these zones for understanding literature, conversing with other health providers, and documenting pertinent information.

Shoulder Joint

The shoulder complex comprises seven joints, including the glenohumeral, suprahumeral, acromioclavicular, scapulocostal, sternoclavicular, costosternal, and costovertebral joints [Cailliet 1981]. The suprahumeral and scapulocostal joints are pseudojoints, but they contribute to the shoulder's function. Mobility of the shoulder is a compilation of all seven joints. Because the shoulder is extremely mobile, stability is sacrificed. This is evident when one considers that

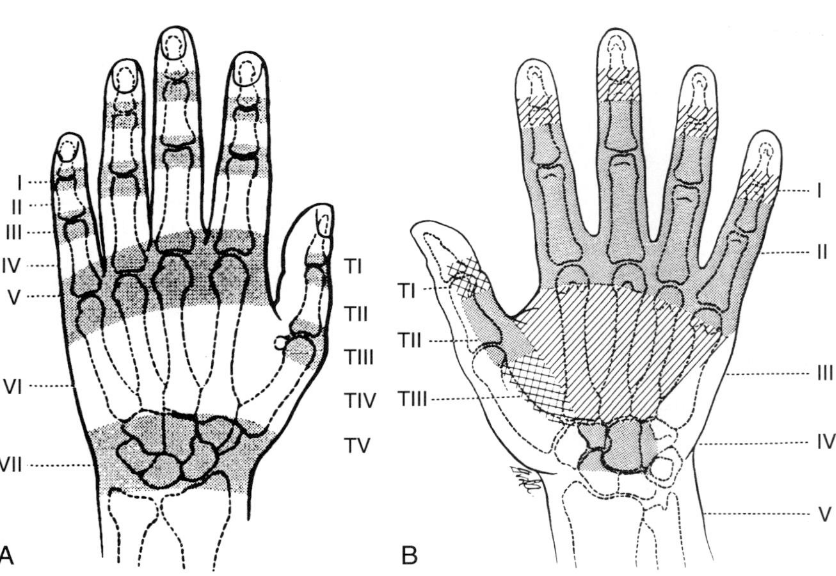

Figure 4-2 Zones of the hand for (A) extensor and (B) flexor tendons. [From Kleinert HE, Schepel S, Gill T (1981). Flexor tendon injuries. Surgical Clinics of North America 61:267.]

Table 4-1 Tendon Injury Zones of the Hand

	FLEXOR TENDON ZONE BORDERS	EXTENSOR TENDON ZONE BORDERS
Zone I	Extends flexor digitorum profundus distal to flexor digitorum superficialis on middle phalanx	Over the distal interphalangeal joints
Zone II (no man's land)	Extends from proximal end of the digital fibrous sheath to the distal end of the A_1 pulley	Over the middle phalanx
Zone III	Extends from proximal end of the finger pulley system to the distal end of the transverse carpal ligament	Over the apex of the proximal interphalangeal joint
Zone IV	Entails the carpal tunnel, extending from the distal to the proximal borders of the transverse carpal ligament	Over the proximal phalanx
Zone V	Extends from the proximal border of the transverse carpal ligament to the musculotendinous junctions of the flexor tendons	Over the apex of the metacarpophalangeal joint
Zone VI		Over the dorsum of the hand
Zone VII		Under the extensor tendon retinaculum
Zone VIII		The distal forearm
Thumb zone TI	Distal to the interphalangeal joint	Over the interphalangeal joint
Thumb zone TII	Annular ligament to interphalangeal joint	Over the proximal phalanx
Thumb zone TIII	The thenar eminence	Over the metacarpophalangeal joint
Thumb zone TIV		Over the first metacarpal
Thumb zone V		Under the extensor tendon retinaculum
Thumb zone VI		The distal forearm

the head of the humerus articulates with approximately a third of the glenoid fossa. The shoulder complex allows motion in three planes, including flexion, extension, abduction, adduction, and internal and external rotation.

The scapula is intimately involved with movement at the shoulder. *Scapulohumeral rhythm* is a term used to describe the coordinated series of synchronous motions, such as shoulder abduction and elevation.

A complex of ligaments and tendons provides stability to the shoulder. Shoulder ligaments are named according to the bones they connect. The ligaments of the shoulder complex include the coracohumeral ligament and the superior, middle, and inferior glenohumeral ligaments [Kapandji 1970]. The rotator cuff muscles contribute to the dynamic stability of the shoulder by compressing the humeral head into the glenoid fossa [Wu 1996]. The rotator cuff muscles include the supraspinatus, infraspinatus, teres minor, and subscapularis. Table 4-2 lists the muscles involved with scapular and shoulder movements.

Elbow Joint

The elbow joint complex consists of the humeroradial, humeroulnar, and proximal radioulnar joints. The humeroradial joint is an articulation between the humerus and the radius. The humeroradial joint has two degrees of freedom that allow for elbow flexion and extension and forearm supination and pronation. The humerus articulates with the ulna at the humeroulnar joint. Flexion and extension movements take place at the humeroulnar joint. Elbow flexion and extension are limited by the articular surfaces of the trochlea of the ulna and the capitulum of the humerus.

The medial and lateral collateral ligaments strengthen the elbow capsule. The radial collateral, lateral ulnar, accessory lateral collateral, and annular ligaments constitute the ligamentous structure of the elbow.

Muscles acting on the elbow can be categorized as functional groups: flexors, extensors, flexor-pronators, and extensor-supinators. Table 4-3 lists the muscles in these groups and their innervation.

Wrist Joint

The wrist joint is frequently incorporated into a splint's design. A therapist must be knowledgeable of the wrist joint structure to appropriately choose and fabricate a splint that meets therapeutic objectives. The osseous structure of the wrist and hand consists of the ulna, radius, and eight carpal bones. Several joints are associated with the wrist complex, including the radiocarpal, midcarpal, and distal radioulnar joints.

The carpal bones are arranged in two rows (Figure 4-3). The proximal row of carpal bones includes the scaphoid (navicular), lunate, and triquetrum. The pisiform bone is considered a sesamoid bone [Wu 1996]. The distal row of carpal bones comprises the trapezium, trapezoid, capitate, and hamate. The distal row of carpal bones articulates with the metacarpals.

Table 4-2 Muscles Contributing to Scapular and Shoulder Motions

MOVEMENT	MUSCLES	INNERVATION
Scapular elevation	Upper trapezius	Accessory, CN 1
	Levator scapulae	3rd and 4th cervical; dorsal scapular
Scapular depression	Lower trapezius	Accessory CN 1
Scapular lateral rotation	Serratus anterior	Long thoracic
Scapular medial rotation	Rhomboids	Dorsal scapular
Scapular abduction	Serratus anterior	Long thoracic
Scapular adduction	Middle and lower trapezius	Accessory CN 1
	Rhomboids	Dorsal scapular
Shoulder flexion	Anterior deltoid	Axillary
	Coracobrachialis	Musculocutaneous
Shoulder extension	Teres major	Lower subscapular
	Latissimus dorsi	Thoracodorsal
Shoulder abduction	Middle deltoid	Axillary
	Supraspinatus	Suprascapular
Shoulder adduction	Pectoralis major	Medial and lateral
	Latissimus dorsi	Pectoral
	Teres major	Thoracodorsal
	Coracobrachialis	Lower subscapular
		Musculocutaneous
Shoulder external rotation	Infraspinatus	Suprascapular
	Teres minor	Axillary
Shoulder internal rotation	Subscapularis	Upper and lower subscapular

Table 4-3 Elbow and Forearm Musculature Actions and Nerve Supply

MUSCLE GROUP	INNERVATION
Flexors	
Biceps	Musculocutaneous
Brachialis	Musculocutaneous, radial
Brachioradialis	Radial
Extensors	
Triceps	Radial
Anconeus	Radial
Supinatorsm	
Supinator	Posterior
Interosseous branch of supinator	Radial
Pronators	
Pronator teres	Median
Pronator quadratus	Anterior
Interosseous branch of pronator quadratus	Median

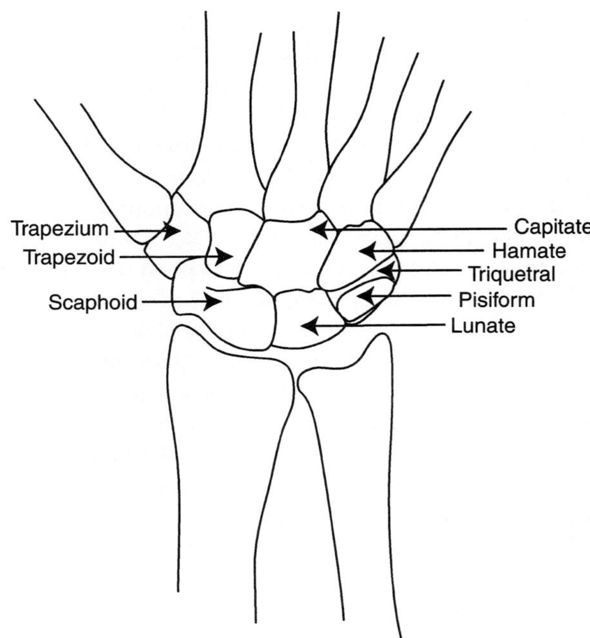

Figure 4-3 Carpal bones. Proximal row: scaphoid, lunate, pisiform, and triquetrum. Distal row: trapezium, trapezoid, capitate, and hamate. [From Pedretti LW (ed.), (1996). *Occupational Therapy: Practice Skills for Physical Dysfunction, Fourth Edition*. St. Louis: Mosby, p. 320.]

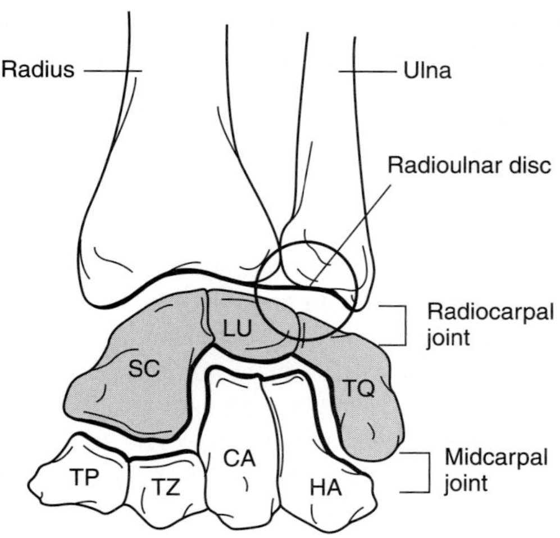

Figure 4-4 Radiocarpal and midcarpal joints. [From Norkin C, Levangie P (1983). *Joint Structure and Function: A Comprehensive Analysis*. Philadelphia: F. A. Davis, p. 217.]

The radius articulates with the lunate and scaphoid in the proximal row of carpal bones. This articulation is the radiocarpal joint, which is mobile. The radiocarpal joint (Figure 4-4) is formed by the articulation of the distal head of the radius and the scaphoid and lunate bones. The ulnar styloid is attached to the triquetrum by a complex of ligaments and fibrocartilage. The ligaments bridge the ulna and radius and separate the distal radioulnar joint and the ulna from the radiocarpal joint. Motions of the radiocarpal joint include flexion, extension, and radial and ulnar deviation. The majority of wrist extension occurs at the midcarpal joint, with less movement occurring at the radiocarpal joint [Kapandji 1970].

The midcarpal joint (Figure 4-4) is the articulation between the distal and proximal carpal rows. The joint exists, although there are no interosseous ligaments between the proximal and distal rows of carpals [Buck 1995]. The joint capsules remain separate. However, the radiocarpal joint capsule attaches to the edge of the articular disk, which is distal to the ulna [Pratt 1991]. The wrist motions of flexion, extension, and radial and ulnar deviation also take place at this joint. The majority of wrist flexion occurs at the radiocarpal joint. The midcarpal joint contributes less movement for wrist flexion [Kapandji 1970].

The distal radioulnar joint is an articulation between the head of the ulna and the distal radius. Forearm supination and pronation occur at the distal radioulnar joint.

Wrist stability is provided by the close-packed positions of the carpal bones and the interosseous ligaments [Wu 1996]. The intrinsic intercarpal ligaments connect carpal bone to carpal bone. The extrinsic ligaments of the carpal bones connect with the radius, ulna, and metacarpals. The ligaments on the volar aspect of the wrist are thick and strong, providing stability. The dorsal ligaments are thin and less developed [Wu 1996]. In addition, the intercarpal ligaments of the distal row form a stable fixed transverse arch [Chase 1990]. Ligaments of the wrist cover the volar, dorsal, radial, and ulnar areas. The ligaments in the wrist serve to stabilize joints, guide motion, limit motion, and transmit forces to the hand and forearm. These ligaments also assist in prevention of dislocations. The wrist contributes to the hand's mobility and stability. Having two *degrees of freedom* (movements occur in two planes), the wrist is capable of flexing, extending, and deviating radially and ulnarly.

Finger and Thumb Joints

Cutaneous and Connective Coverings of the Hand

The skin is the protective covering of the body. There are unique characteristics of volar and dorsal skin, which are functionally relevant. The skin on the palmar surface of the hand is thick, immobile, and hairless. It contains sensory receptors and sweat glands. The palmar skin attaches to the underlying palmar aponeurosis, which facilitates grasp [Bowers and Tribuzi 1992]. Palmar skin is different from the skin on the dorsal surface of the hand. The dorsal skin is thin, supple, and quite mobile. Thus, it is often the site for edema accumulation. The skin on the dorsum of the hand accommodates to the extremes of the fingers' flexion and extension movements. The hair follicles on the dorsum of the hand assist in protecting as well as activating touch receptors when the hair is moved slightly [Bowers and Tribuzi 1992].

Palmar Fascia

The superficial layer of palmar fascia in the hand is thin. Its composition is highly fibrous and is tightly bound to the deep fascia. The deep fascia thickens at the wrist and forms the palmar carpal ligament and the flexor retinaculum. The fascia thins over the thenar and hypothenar eminences but thickens over the midpalmar area and on the volar surfaces of the fingers. The fascia forms the palmar aponeurosis and the fibrous digital sheaths [Buck 1995].

The superficial palmar aponeurosis consists of longitudinal fibers that are continuous with the flexor retinaculum and palmaris longus tendon. The flexor tendons course under the flexor retinaculum. With absence of the flexor retinaculum, as in carpal tunnel release, bowstringing (Figure 4-5) of the tendons may occur at the wrist level. The distal borders of the superficial palmar aponeurosis fuse with the fibrous digital sheaths. The deep layer of the aponeurosis consists of transverse fibers, which are continuous with the thenar and hypothenar fascias. Distally, the deep layer forms the superficial transverse metacarpal ligament [Buck 1995]. The extensor retinaculum is a fibrous band that bridges over the extensor tendons. The deep and superficial layers of the aponeurosis form this retinaculum.

Functionally, the fascial structure of the hand protects, cushions, restrains, conforms, and maintains the hand's arches

[Bowers and Tribuzi 1992]. Therapists may splint persons with Dupuytren's disease, in which the palmar fascia thickens and shortens.

Joint Structure

Splints often immobilize or mobilize joints of the fingers and thumb. Therefore, a therapist must have knowledge of these joints. The hand skeleton comprises five polyarticulated rays (Figure 4-6). The radial ray or first ray (thumb) is the shortest and includes three bones: a metacarpal and two phalanges. Joints of the thumb include the carpometacarpal (CMC) joint, the metacarpophalangeal (MCP) joint, and the interphalangeal (IP) joint (Figure 4-6). Functionally, the thumb is the most mobile of the digits. The thumb significantly enhances functional ability by its ability to oppose the pads of the fingers, which is needed for prehension and grasp. The thumb has three degrees of freedom, allowing for flexion, extension, abduction, adduction, and opposition. The second through fifth rays comprise four bones: a metacarpal and three phalanges. Joints of the fingers include the MCP joint, proximal interphalangeal (PIP) joint, and the distal interphalangeal (DIP) joint. The digits are unequal in length. However, their respective lengths contribute to the hand's functional capabilities.

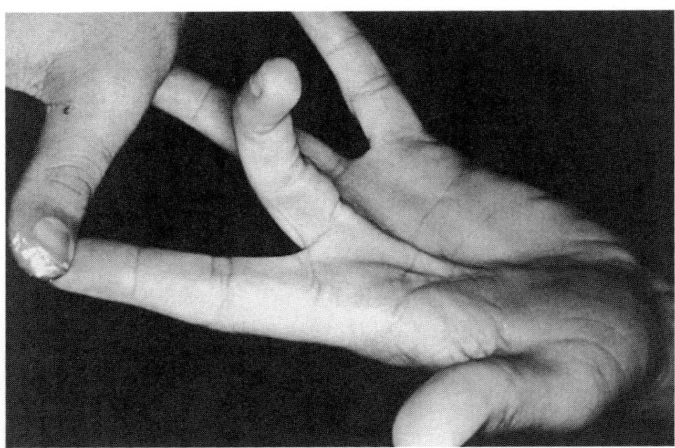

Figure 4-5 Bowstringing of the flexor tendons. [From Stewart-Pettengill KM, van Strien G (2002). Postoperative management of flexor tendon injuries. In EJ Mackin, AD Callahan, TM Skirven, LH Schneider, AL Osterman (eds.), *Rehabilitation of the Hand: Surgery and Therapy, Fifth Edition*. St. Louis: Mosby, p. 434.]

The thumb's metacarpotrapezial or CMC joint is saddle shaped and has two degrees of freedom, allowing for flexion, extension, abduction, and adduction movements. The CMC joints of the fingers have one degree of freedom to allow for small amounts of flexion and extension.

The fingers' and thumb's MCP joints have two degrees of freedom: flexion, extension, abduction, and adduction. The convex metacarpal heads articulate with shallow concave bases of the proximal phalanges. Fibrocartilaginous volar plates extend the articular surfaces on the base of the phalanges. As the finger's MCP joint is flexed, the volar plate slides proximally under the metacarpal. This mechanism allows for significant range of motion. The volar plate movement is controlled by accessory collateral ligaments and the metacarpal pulley for the long flexor tendons to blend with these structures.

During extension, the MCP joint is able to move medially and laterally. During MCP extension, collateral ligaments

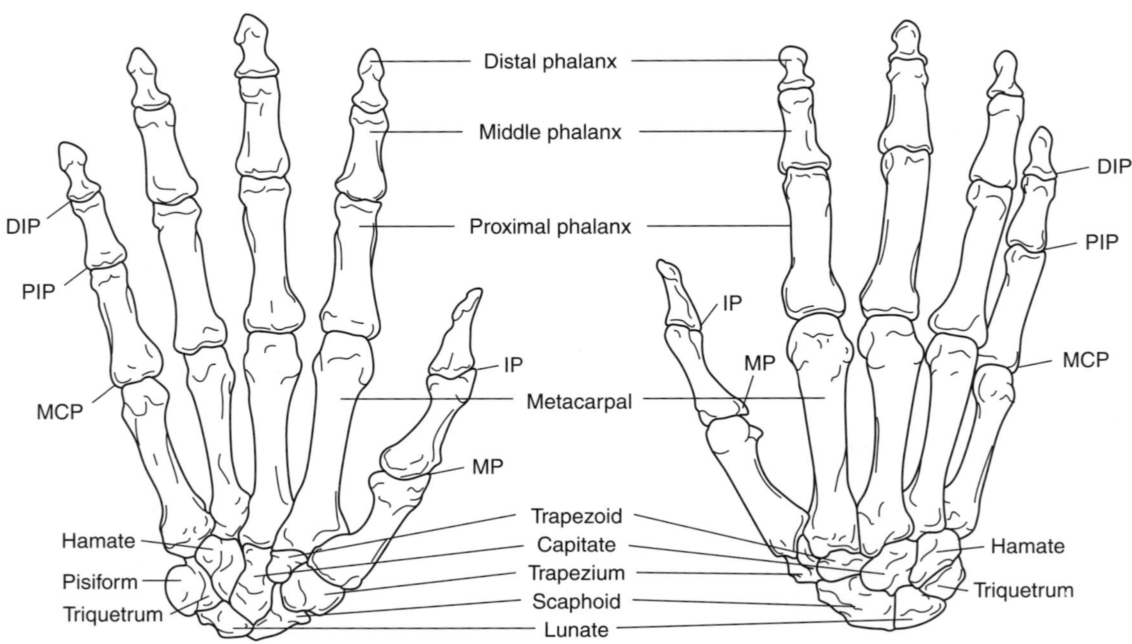

Figure 4-6 Joints of the fingers and thumb.

are slack. When digits II through V are extended at the MCP joints, finger abduction movement is free. Conversely, when the MCP joints of digits II through V are flexed abduction is extremely limited. The medial and lateral collateral ligaments of the metacarpal heads become taut and limit the distance by which the heads can be separated for abduction to occur. Mechanically, this provides stability during grasp.

Digits II through V have two interphalangeal joints: a PIP joint and a DIP joint. The thumb has only one IP joint. The IP joints have one degree of freedom, contributing to flexion and extension motions. IP joints have a volar plate mechanism similar to the MCP joints, with the addition of check reign ligaments. The check reign ligaments limit hyperextension.

Table 4-4 provides a review of muscle actions and nerve supply of the wrist and hand [Clarkson and Gilewich 1989]. Muscles originating in the forearm are referred to as extrinsic muscles. Intrinsic muscles originate within the hand. Each group contributes to upper extremity function.

Extrinsic Muscles of the Hand

Extrinsic muscles acting on the wrist and hand can be further categorized as extensor and flexor groups. Extrinsic muscles of the wrist and hand are listed in Box 4-1. Extrinsic flexor muscles are most prominent on the medial side of the upper forearm. The function of extrinsic flexor muscles includes flexion of joints between the muscles' respective origin and insertion. Extrinsic muscles of the hand and forearm accomplish flexion and extension of the wrist and the phalanges (fingers). For example, the flexor digitorum superficialis flexes the PIP joints of digits II through V, whereas the flexor digitorum profundus primarily flexes the DIP joints of digits II through V.

Because these tendons pass on the palmar side of the MCP joints, they tend to produce flexion of these joints. During grasp, flexion of the MCPs is necessary to obtain the proper shape of the hand. However, flexion of the wrist is

Table 4-4 Wrist and Hand Musculature Actions and Nerve Supply

MUSCLE	ACTIONS	NERVE
Flexor carpi radialis	Wrist flexion Wrist radial deviation	Median
Palmaris longus	Wrist flexion Tenses palmar fascia	Median
Flexor carpi ulnaris	Wrist flexion Wrist ulnar deviation	Ulnar
Extensor carpi radialis longus	Wrist radial deviation Wrist extension	 Radial
Extensor carpi radialis brevis	Wrist extension Wrist radial deviation	Radial
Extensor carpi ulnaris	Wrist ulnar deviation Wrist extension	Radial
Flexor digitorum superficialis	Finger PIP flexion	Median
Flexor digitorum profundus	Finger DIP flexion	Median Ulnar
Extensor digitorum communis	Finger MCP extension	Radial
Extensor indicis proprius	Index finger MCP extension	Radial
Extensor digiti minimi	Little finger MCP extension	Radial
Interosseous	Finger MCP abduction	Ulnar
Dorsal Palmar	Finger MCP adduction	Ulnar
Lumbricales	Finger MCP flexion and IP extension	Ulnar Median
Abductor digiti minimi	Little finger MCP abduction	Ulnar
Opponens digiti minimi	Little finger opposition	Ulnar
Flexor digiti minimi	Little finger MCP flexion	Ulnar
Flexor pollicus longus	Thumb IP flexion	Median
Flexor pollicus brevis	Thumb MCP flexion	Median Ulnar
Extensor pollicis longus	Thumb IP extension	Radial
Extensor pollicis brevis	Thumb MCP extension	Radial
Abductor pollicis longus	Thumb radial abduction	Radial
Abductor pollicis brevis	Thumb palmar abduction	Median
Adductor pollicis	Thumb adduction	Ulnar
Opponens pollicis	Thumb opposition	Median

Box 4-1 Extrinsic Muscles of the Wrist and Hand

Extensor digitorum
Extensor pollicis longus
Flexor digitorum profundus
Flexor pollicis longus
Extensor digiti minimi
Extensor carpi radialis longus
Extensor carpi ulnaris
Palmaris longus
Flexor digitorum superficialis
Extensor pollicis brevis
Extensor indicis proprius
Abductor pollicis longus
Extensor carpi radialis brevis
Flexor carpi radialis
Flexor carpi ulnaris

undesirable because it decreases the grip force. The synergic contraction of the wrist extensors during finger flexion prevents wrist flexion during grasp.

The force of the extensor contraction is proportionate to the strength of the grip. The stronger the grip the stronger the contraction of the wrist extensors [Smith et al. 1996]. Digit extension and flexion are a combined effort from extrinsic and intrinsic muscles.

At the level of the wrist, the extensor tendons organize into six compartments [Fess et al. 2005]. The first compartment consists of tendons from the abductor pollicis longus (APL) and extensor pollicis brevis (EPB). When the radial side of the wrist is palpated, it is possible to feel the taut tendons of the APL and EPB.

The second compartment contains tendons of the extensor carpi radialis longus (ECRL) and brevis (ECRB). A therapist can palpate the tendons on the dorsoradial aspect of the wrist by applying resistance to an extended wrist.

The third compartment houses the tendon of the extensor pollicis longus (EPL). This tendon passes around Lister's tubercle of the radius and inserts on the dorsal base of the distal phalanx of the thumb.

The fourth compartment includes the four communis extensor (EDC) tendons and the extensor indicis proprius (EIP) tendon, which are the MCP joint extensors of the fingers.

The fifth compartment includes the extensor digiti minimi (EDM), which extends the little finger's MCP joint. The EDM acts alone to extend the little finger.

The sixth compartment consists of the extensor carpi ulnaris (ECU), which inserts at the dorsal base of the fifth metacarpal. A taut tendon can be palpated over the ulnar side of the wrist just distal to the ulnar head.

Unlike the other fingers, the index and little fingers have dual extensor systems comprising the EIP and the EDM in conjunction with the extensor digitorum communis. The EIP and EDM tendons lie on the ulnar side of the extensor

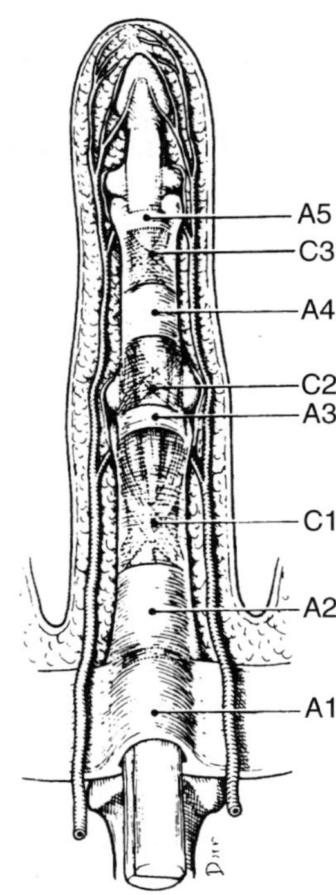

Figure 4-7 Annular (A) and cruciate (C) pulley system of the hand. The digital flexor sheath is formed by five annular (A) pulleys and three cruciate (C) bands. The second and fourth annular pulleys are the most important for function. [From Tubiana R, Thomine JM, Mackin E (1996). *Examination of the Hand and Wrist*. St. Louis: Mosby, p. 81.]

digitorum communis tendons. Each finger has a flexor digitorum superficialis (FDS) and flexor digitorum profundus (FDP) tendon. Five annular (or *A*) pulleys and four cruciate (or *C*) pulleys prevent the flexor tendons from bowstringing (Figure 4-7).

In relationship to splinting, when pathology affects extrinsic musculature the splint design often incorporates the wrist and hand. This wrist-hand splint design is necessary because the extrinsic muscles cross the wrist and hand joints.

Intrinsic Muscles of the Hand and Wrist

The intrinsic muscles of the thumb and fingers are listed in Box 4-2. The intrinsic muscles are the muscles of the thenar and hypothenar eminences, the lumbricals, and the interossei. Intrinsic muscles can be grouped according to those of the thenar eminence, the hypothenar eminence, and the central muscles between the thenar and hypothenar eminences. The function of these intrinsic hand muscles produces flexion of the proximal phalanx and extension of the middle and distal phalanges, which contribute to the precise finger movements required for coordination.

The thenar eminence comprises the opponens pollicis, flexor pollicis brevis, adductor pollicis, and abductor pollicis brevis. The thenar eminence contributes to thumb opposition,

Box 4-2 Intrinsic Muscles of the Hand

Central Compartment Muscles:
Lumbricals
Palmar interossei
Dorsal interossei

Thenar Compartment Muscles:
Opponens pollicis
Abductor pollicis brevis
Adductor pollicis
Flexor pollicis brevis

Hypothenar Compartment Muscles:
Opponens digiti minimi
Abductor digiti minimi
Flexor digiti minimi brevis
Palmaris brevis

which functionally allows for grasp and prehensile patterns. The thumb seldom acts alone except when pressing objects and playing instruments [Smith et al. 1996]. However, without a thumb the hand is virtually nonfunctional.

The hypothenar eminence includes the abductor digiti minimi, the flexor digiti minimi, the palmaris brevis, and the opponens digiti minimi. Similar to the thenar muscles, the hypothenar muscles also assist in rotating the fifth digit during grasp [Aulicino 1995].

The muscles of the central compartment include lumbricals and palmar and dorsal interossei. The interossei muscles are complex, with variations in their origins and insertions [Aulicino 1995]. There are four dorsal interossei and three palmar interossei muscles. The four lumbricals are weaker than the interossei. The lumbricals originate on the radial aspect of the flexor digitorum profundus tendons and insert on the extensor expansion of the finger. They are the only muscles in the human body with a moving origin and insertion. The primary function of the lumbricals is to flex the MCP joints [Wu 1996].

Normally, the interossei extend the PIP and DIP joints when the MCP joint is in extension. The dorsal interossei produce finger abduction, and the palmar interossei produce finger adduction. Functionally, the first dorsal interossei is a strong abductor of the index finger, which assists in properly positioning the hand for pinching. Research shows the interossei are active during grasp and power grip in addition to pinch [Long et al. 1970]. With function of the interossei and lumbricals, a person is able to place the hand in an *intrinsic plus position*. An intrinsic plus position is established when the MCP joints are flexed and the PIP joints are fully extended (Figure 4-8). Some injuries may result in an *intrinsic minus* hand (Figure 4-9) caused by paralysis or contractures. With an intrinsic minus hand, the person loses the cupping shape of the hand [Aulicino 1995]. In addition, the intrinsic musculature may waste or atrophy. In relationship to splinting, if intrinsic muscles are solely affected the splint design will often involve only immobilizing or mobilizing the finger joints as opposed to incorporating the wrist. To facilitate function and prevent deformity, joint positioning in splints frequently warrants an intrinsic plus posture rather than an intrinsic minus position.

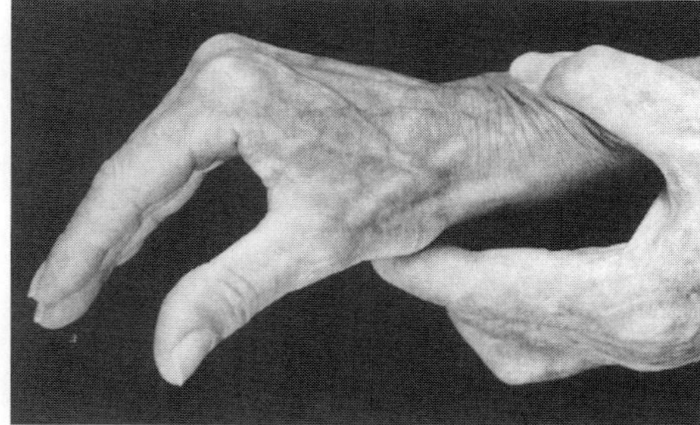

Figure 4-8 Intrinsic plus position of the hand. MCP flexion with PIP extension. [From Tubiana R, Thomine JM, Mackin E (1996). *Examination of the Peripheral Nerve Function in the Upper Extremity*. St. Louis: Mosby, p. 308.]

Arches of the Hand

To have a strong functional grasp, the hand uses the following three arches: (1) the longitudinal arch, (2) the distal transverse arch, and (3) the proximal transverse arch (Figure 4-10). Because of their functional significance, these arches require care during the splinting process for their preservation. The therapist should never splint a hand in a flat position because doing so compromises function and creates deformity. Especially in cases of muscle atrophy (as with a tendon or nerve injury), the splint should maintain integrity and mobility of the arches.

The proximal transverse arch is fixed and consists of the distal row of carpal bones. It is a rigid arch acting as a stable pivot point for the wrist and long-finger flexor muscles [Chase 1990]. The transverse carpal ligament and the bones of the proximal transverse arch form the carpal tunnel. The finger flexor tendons pass beneath the transverse carpal ligament. The transverse carpal ligament provides mechanical advantage to the finger flexor tendons by serving as a pulley [Andrews and Bouvette 1996].

The distal transverse arch, which deepens with flexion of the fingers, is mobile and passes through the metacarpal heads [Malick 1972]. A splint must allow for the functional movement of the distal arch to maintain or increase normal hand function [Chase 1990].

The longitudinal arch allows the DIP, PIP, and MCP joints to flex [Fess et al. 2005]. This arch follows the longitudinal axes of each finger. Because of the mobility of their base, the first, fourth, and fifth metacarpals move in relationship to the shape and size of an object placed in the palm. Grasp is the result of holding an object against the rigid portion of the hand provided by the second and third digits.

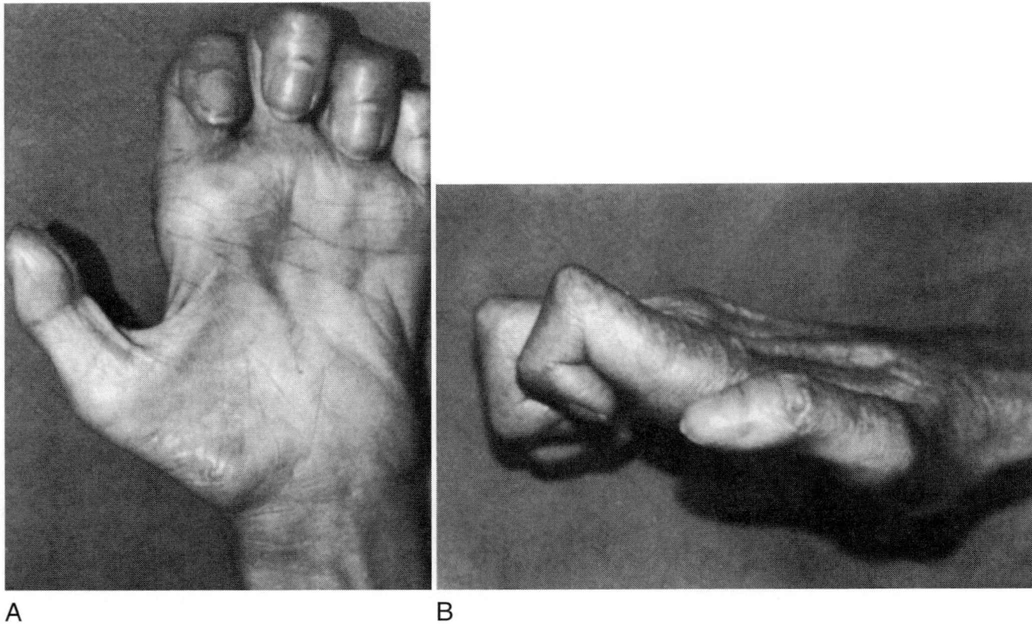

Figure 4-9 (A) Intrinsic minus position of the hand. (B) Notice loss of normal arches of the hand and wasting of all intrinsic musculature resulting from a long-standing low median and ulnar nerve palsy. [From Aulicino PL (2002). Clinical examination of the hand. In EJ Mackin, AD Callahan, TM Skirven, LH Schneider, AL Osterman (eds.), *Rehabilitation of the Hand: Surgery and Therapy, Fifth Edition*. St. Louis: Mosby, p. 130.]

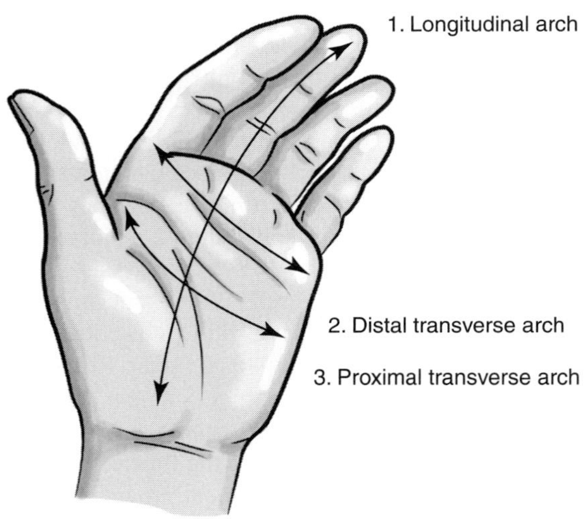

Figure 4-10 Arches of the hand: longitudinal arch (1), distal transverse arch (2), and proximal transverse arch (3).

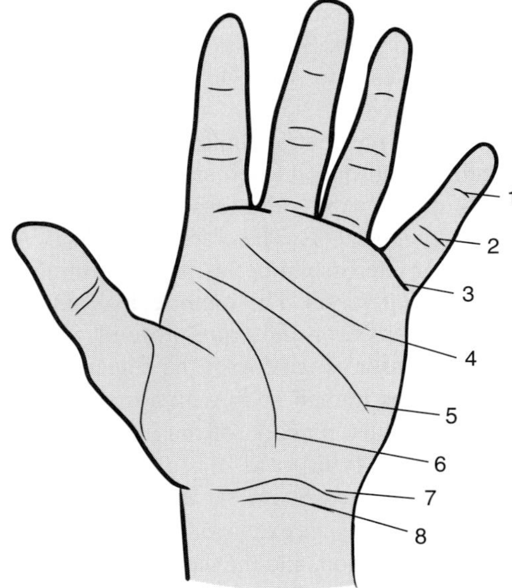

Figure 4-11 Creases of the hand: distal digital (DIP) crease (1), middle digital (PIP) crease (2), proximal digital (MCP) crease (3), distal palmar crease (4), proximal palmar crease (5), thenar crease (6), distal wrist crease (7), and proximal wrist crease (8).

The flattening and cupping motions of the palm allow the hand to pick up and handle objects of various sizes.

Anatomic Landmarks of the Hand

Creases of the Hand

The creases of the hand are critical landmarks for splint pattern making and molding. Therefore, knowledge of the creases and their functional implications is important. Three flexion creases are located on the palmar surface of digits II through V, and additional creases are located on the palmar surface of the hand and wrist (Figure 4-11).

The three primary palmar creases are the distal, proximal, and thenar creases. As shown in Figure 4-11, the distal palmar crease extends transversely from the fifth MCP joint to a point midway between the third and second MCP joints [Cailliet 1994]. This crease is the landmark for the distal edge of the palmar portion of a splint intended to immobilize the wrist while allowing motion of the MCPs. By positioning the splint proximal to this crease, the therapist makes full MCP joint flexion possible. Below the distal palmar crease is the proximal palmar crease, which is used as a guide during splint fabrication. A splint must be proximal to the proximal palmar crease at the index finger or the MCP joint will not be free to move into flexion.

The thenar crease begins at the proximal palmar crease and curves around the base of the thenar eminence (see Figure 4-11) [Cailliet 1994]. To allow thumb motion, this crease should define the limit of the splint's edge. If the splint extends beyond the thenar crease toward the thumb, thumb opposition and palmar abduction of the CMC joint are inhibited.

The two palmar (or volar) wrist creases are the distal and proximal wrist creases. The distal wrist crease extends from the pisiform bone to the tubercle of the trapezium (see Figure 4-11) and forms a line that separates the proximal and distal rows of the carpal bones. The proximal wrist crease corresponds to the radiocarpal joint and delineates the proximal border of the carpal bones, which articulates with the distal radius [Cailliet 1994]. The distal and proximal wrist creases assist in locating the axis of the wrist motion [Clarkson and Gilewich 1989].

The three digital palmar flexion creases are on the palmar aspect of digits II through V (see Figure 4-11). The distal digital crease (or DIP crease) marks the DIP joint axis, and the middle digital crease (or PIP crease) marks the PIP joint axis. The proximal digital crease (or MCP crease) is distal to the MCP joint axis at the base of the proximal phalanx. The creation of the proximal and distal palmar creases results from the thick palmar skin folding due to the force allowing full MCP flexion [Malick 1972]. The flexion axis of the IP joint of the thumb corresponds to the IP crease of the thumb. Similarly, the MCP crease describes the axis of thumb MCP joint flexion.

The creases are close to but not always directly over bony joints [Chase 1990]. When splinting to immobilize a particular joint, the therapist must be sure to include the corresponding joint flexion crease within the splint so as to provide adequate support for immobilization. Conversely, when attempting to mobilize a specific joint the therapist must not incorporate the corresponding flexion crease in the splint to allow for full range of motion [Fess et al. 2005]. When one is working with persons who have moderate to severe edema, the creases may dissipate. Creases may also dissipate with disuse associated with paralysis or disuse resulting from pain, stiffness, or psychological problems.

Grasp and Prehensile Patterns

The normal hand can perform many prehensile patterns in which the thumb is a crucial factor. Therapists must be knowledgeable about prehensile and grasp patterns, especially when splinting to assist the performance of these patterns.

Even though hand movements are extremely complex, they can be categorized into several basic prehensile and grasp patterns, including fingertip prehension, palmar prehension, lateral prehension, cylindrical grasp, spherical grasp, hook grasp [Smith et al. 1996], and intrinsic plus grasp [Belkin and English 1996]. Figure 4-12 depicts these types of prehensile and grip patterns. Therapists should keep in mind that finer prehensile movements require less strength than grasp movements. Pedretti [1990, p. 405] remarked, "The grasp and prehension patterns that may be provided by hand splinting are determined by the muscles that are functioning, potential and present deformities, and how the hand is to be used."

Fingertip prehension is the contact of the pad of the index or middle finger with the pad of the thumb [Smith et al. 1996]. This movement, which clients use to pick up small objects such as beads and pins, is the weakest of the pinch patterns and requires fine motor coordination. A splint to facilitate the fingertip prehension for a person with arthritis may include a static splint to block (stabilize) the thumb IP joint in slight flexion (Figure 4-13) [Belkin and English 1996].

Palmar prehension, also known as the *tripod* or *three jaw chuck* pinch [Clarkson and Gilewich 1989, Belkin and

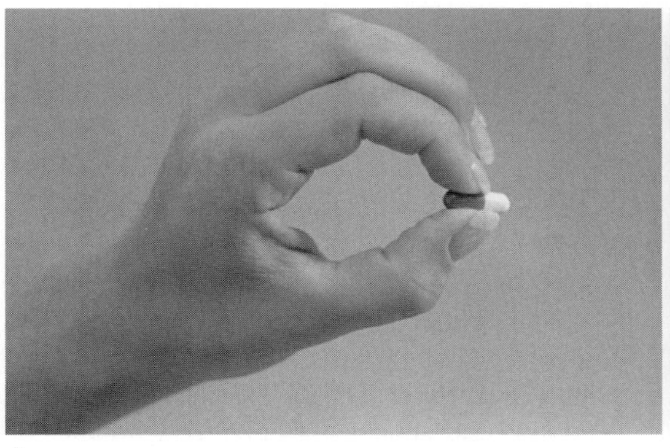

A

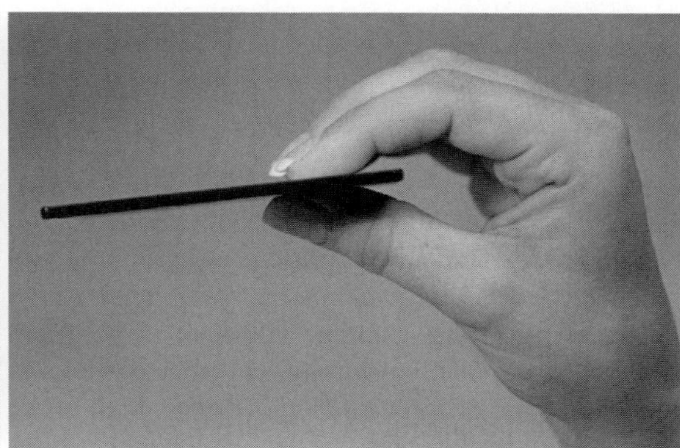

B

Figure 4-12 Prehensile and grip patterns of the hand. (A) Fingertip prehension, (B) palmar prehension,

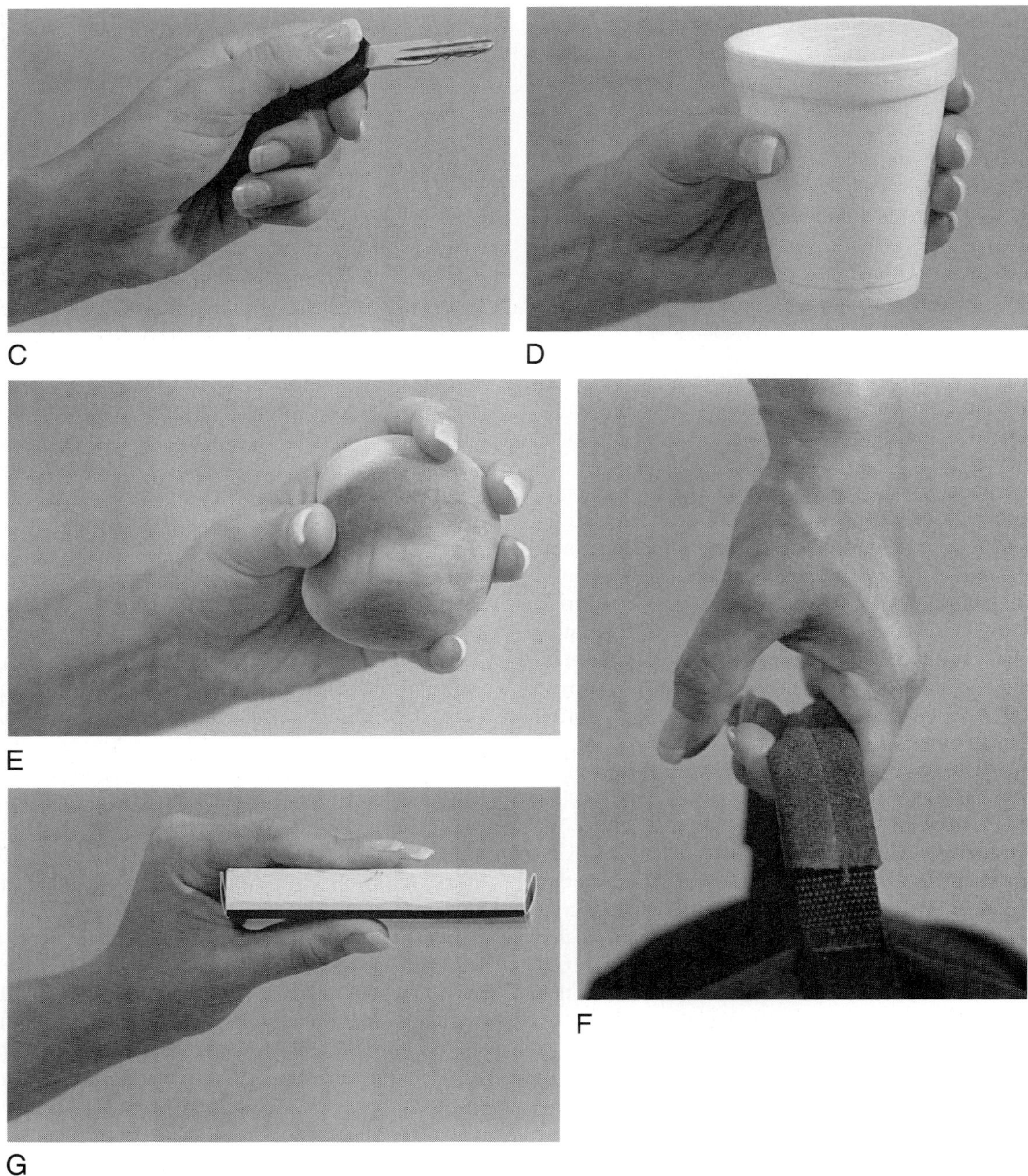

Figure 4-12, cont'd (C) lateral prehension, (D) cylindrical grasp, (E) spherical grasp, (F) hook grasp, and (G) intrinsic plus grasp.

English 1996], is the contact of the thumb pad with the pads of the middle and index fingers. People use palmar prehension for holding pencils and picking up small spherical objects. Splints to facilitate palmar prehension include thumb spica splints that position the thumb in palmar abduction, which may be hand or forearm based (Figure 4-14).

Lateral prehension, the strongest of the pinch patterns, is the contact between the thumb pad and the lateral aspect of the index finger [Smith et al. 1996]. Clients typically use this pattern for holding keys. Splints that position the hand for lateral prehension include thumb spica splints that place the thumb in slight radial abduction (Figure 4-15).

Cylindrical grasp is used for holding cylindrical-shaped objects such as soda cans, pan handles, and cylindrical tools [Smith et al. 1996]. The object rests against the palm of the hand, and the adducted fingers flex around the object to maintain a grasp. Splinting to encourage such motions as thumb opposition or finger and thumb joint flexion may

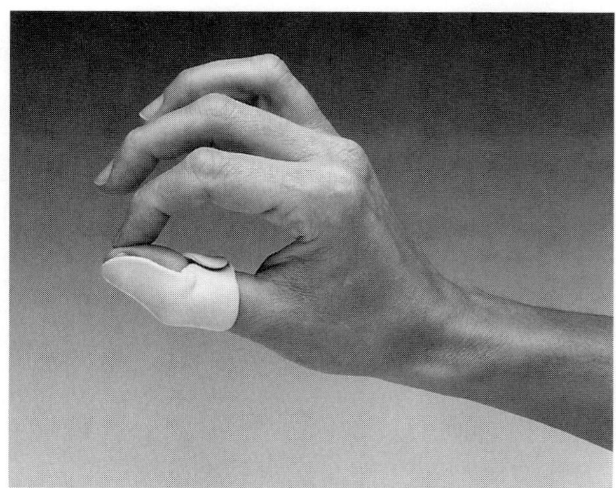

Figure 4-13 Static splint to block the thumb IP joint in slight flexion to facilitate tip pinch. [From Pedretti LW (ed.), (1996). *Occupational Therapy: Practice Skills for Physical Dysfunction, Fourth Edition*. St. Louis: Mosby, p. 327.]

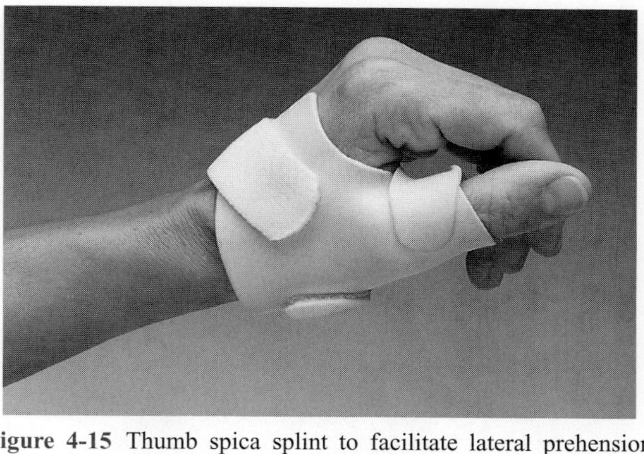

Figure 4-15 Thumb spica splint to facilitate lateral prehension by positioning the thumb in lateral opposition to the index finger. [From Pedretti LW (ed.), (1996). *Occupational Therapy: Practice Skills for Physical Dysfunction, Fourth Edition*. St. Louis: Mosby, p. 327.]

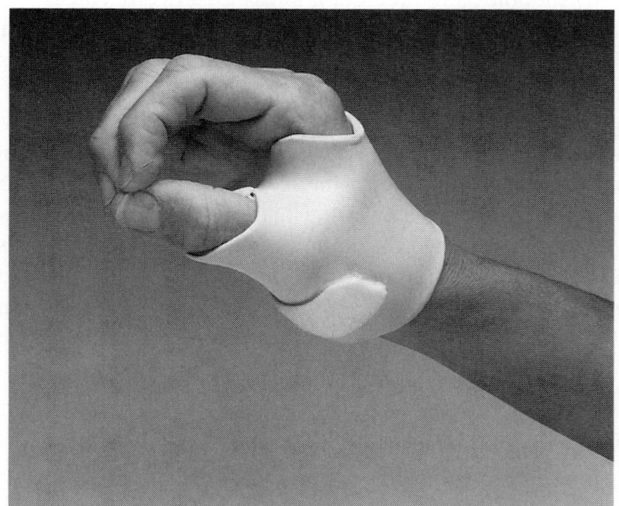

Figure 4-14 Thumb spica splint to facilitate palmar prehension by positioning the thumb in opposition to the index and long fingers. [From Pedretti LW (ed.), (1996). *Occupational Therapy: Practice Skills for Physical Dysfunction, Fourth Edition*. St. Louis: Mosby, p. 327.]

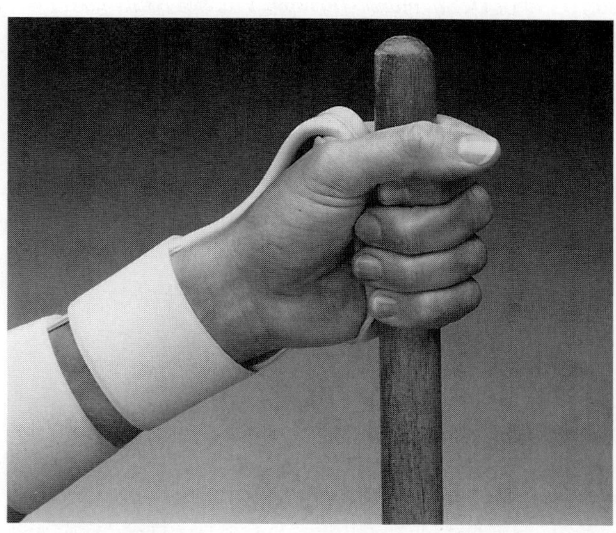

Figure 4-16 This dorsal wrist splint stabilizes the wrist to increase grip force and minimizes coverage of the palm. [From Pedretti LW (ed.), (1996). *Occupational Therapy: Practice Skills for Physical Dysfunction, Fourth Edition*. St. Louis: Mosby, p. 328.]

contribute to a person's ability to regain cylindrical grasp (Figure 4-16).

The spherical grasp is used to hold round objects such as tennis balls and baseballs [Smith et al. 1996]. The object rests against the palm of the hand, and the abducted five digits flex around the object. Splinting to enhance spherical grasp may include splints addressing such motions as finger and thumb abduction (Figure 4-17).

The hook grasp, which is accomplished with the fingers only, involves the carrying of such items as briefcases and suitcases by the handles [Smith et al. 1996]. The PIPs and DIPs flex around the object, and the thumb often remains passive in this type of grasp. With ulnar and median nerve damage, this position may be avoided rather than encouraged. However, for PIP and DIP joints lacking flexion a therapist may fabricate dynamic flexion splints to gain range of motion in these joints.

The intrinsic plus grip is characterized by MCP flexion and PIP and DIP extension. The thumb is positioned in palmar abduction for opposition with the third and fourth fingers [Belkin and English 1996]. This grasp is helpful in holding flat objects such as books, trays, or sandwiches.

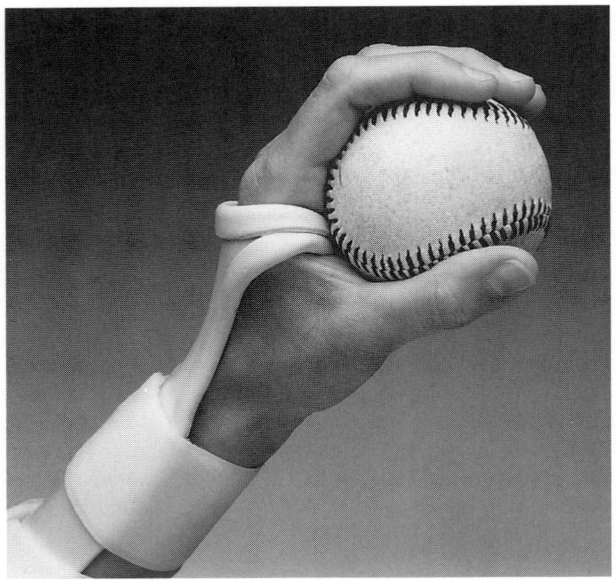

Figure 4-17 This dorsal wrist splint stabilizes the wrist and allows MCP mobility required for a spherical grasp. [From Pedretti LW (ed.), (1996). *Occupational Therapy: Practice Skills for Physical Dysfunction, Fourth Edition*. St. Louis: Mosby, p. 328.]

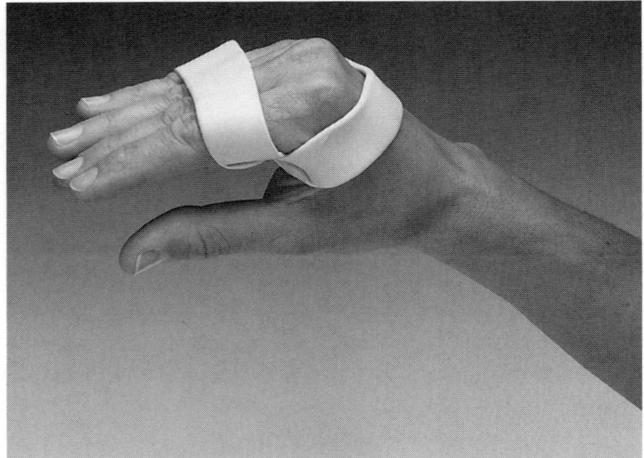

Figure 4-18 Figure-of-eight splint to facilitate an intrinsic plus grasp. [From Pedretti LW (ed.), (1996). *Occupational Therapy: Practice Skills for Physical Dysfunction, Fourth Edition*. St. Louis: Mosby, p. 328.]

The intrinsic plus grip is not present with ulnar and median nerve injuries. A therapist may facilitate the grasp by using a figure-of-eight splint, shown in Figure 4-18.

Biomechanical Principles of Splinting

Splinting involves application of external forces on the hand, and thus understanding basic biomechanical principles is important for the therapist when constructing and fitting a splint. Correct biomechanics of a splint design results in an optimal fit and reduces risks of skin irritation and pressure areas, which ultimately may lead to client comfort, compliance, and function. In addition, knowledgeable manipulation of biomechanics increases splint efficiency and improves splint durability while decreasing cost and frustration [Fess 1995].

Three-point Pressure

Most splints use a *three-point pressure* system to affect a joint motion. A three-point pressure system consists of three individual linear forces in which the middle force is directed in an opposite direction from the other two forces, as depicted in Figure 4-19. Three-point pressure systems in splints are used for different purposes [Fess 1995, Andrews and Bouvette 1996]. For example, a splint affecting extension or flexion of a joint exerts forces in one plane or unidirectionally, as shown in Figure 4-20. Three-point systems can be applied to multiple directions. In other words, a splint may immobilize one joint while mobilizing an adjacent joint. An example of a multidirectional three-point pressure system is a circumferential wrist splint, shown in Figure 4-21.

Mechanical Advantage

Splints incorporate lever systems, which incorporate forces, resistance, axes of motion, and moment arms. Splints serving as levers use a proximal input force (F_i), two moment arms, and an axis or fulcrum to move a distal output force [Fess 1995]. Similar to a teeter-totter, the force side of a splint lever equals the resistance side of the lever. The sum of the proximal (F_i) and the distal (F_o) forces equals the magnitude (F_m) of the middle opposing force. The system's balance is defined as:

$$F_i \times d_i = F_o \times d_o.$$

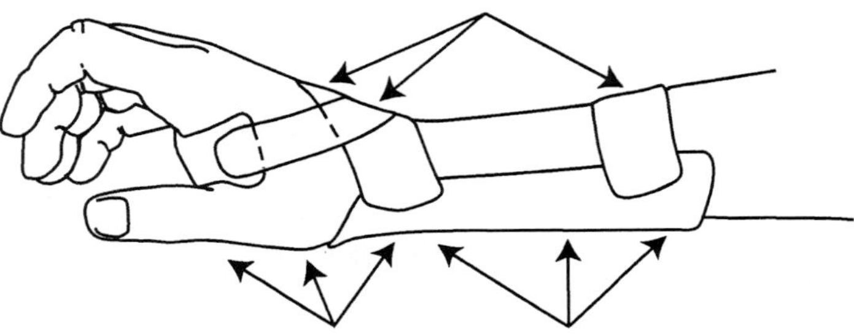

Figure 4-19 Three-point pressure system is created by a splint's surface and properly placed straps to secure the splint and ensure proper force for immobilization. [From Pedretti LW (ed.), (1996). *Occupational Therapy: Practice Skills for Physical Dysfunction, Fourth Edition*. St. Louis: Mosby, p. 336.]

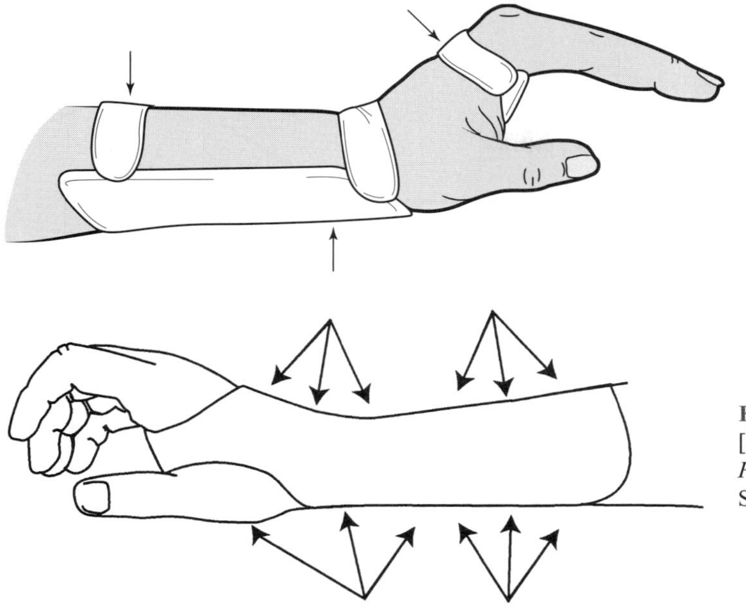

Figure 4-20 Unidirectional three-point pressure system. [From Fess EE, Philips CA (1987). *Hand Splinting: Principles and Methods, Second Edition*. St. Louis: Mosby, p. 4.]

Figure 4-21 Multidirectional three-point pressure systems. [From Pedretti LW (ed.), (1996). *Occupational Therapy: Practice Skills for Physical Dysfunction, Fourth Edition*. St. Louis: Mosby, p. 336.]

In this equation, F_i is the input force and d_i is the input distance (or the proximal force moment arm). F_o is the resistance (or output) force, and d_o is the output distance (or the resistance moment arm). Mechanical advantage is defined as:

$$\frac{d_i}{d_o}$$

Mechanical advantage principles can be applied and adjusted when one is designing a splint. For example, when designing a volar-based wrist cock-up splint increasing the length of the forearm trough will decrease force on the proximal anterior forearm (Figure 4-22). This results in a more comfortable splint for the client. Application of this concept involves consideration of the anatomic segment length in designing the splint. The length of a splint's forearm trough should be approximately two-thirds the length of the forearm. Persons wearing volar-based splints should be able to flex their elbows without interference with full motion [Barr and Swan 1988]. The width of a thumb or forearm trough should be half the circumference of the thumb or forearm. The muscle bulk of an extremity gradually increases more proximal to the body, and the splint trough should widen proportionately in the proximal area. When making a splint pattern, the therapist attempts to maintain one-half the circumference of the thumb or forearm for a correct fit.

Torque

Torque is a biomechanical principle defined as the rotational effect of a mechanism. Other terms used synonymously include *moment arm* or *moment of force*. Torque is the product of the applied force (F) multiplied by the perpendicular distance from the axis of rotation to the line of application of force (d). The equation for torque is:

$$\text{Torque} = F \times d$$

It is important to consider torque for dynamic or mobilization splinting (see Chapter 11).

Pressure and Stress

There are four ways in which skin and soft tissue can be damaged by force or pressure: (1) degree, (2) duration, (3) repetition, and (4) direction.

Degree and Duration of Stress

Generally, low stress can be tolerated for longer periods of time, whereas high stress over long periods of time will cause damage [Bell-Krotoski et al. 1995]. It must be noted that *low stress* and *high stress* are generic and imprecise terms. A therapist should remember that generally the tissue that least tolerates pressure is the skin. Skin becomes ischemic as load increases. Low stress can be damaging if it is continuous and can eventually cause capillary damage and lead to ischemia. The effects of continuous low force from constricting circumferential bandages and splints and their straps can be damaging at times. However, if a system can be devised to distribute pressure over a larger area of skin a higher load can be exerted on a ligament, adhesion, tendon, or muscle. Such a splint system may include a longer trough or a circumferential component.

Repetitive Stress

If a stress is repetitively applied in moderate amounts, it can lead to inflammation and skin breakdown [Bell-Krotoski

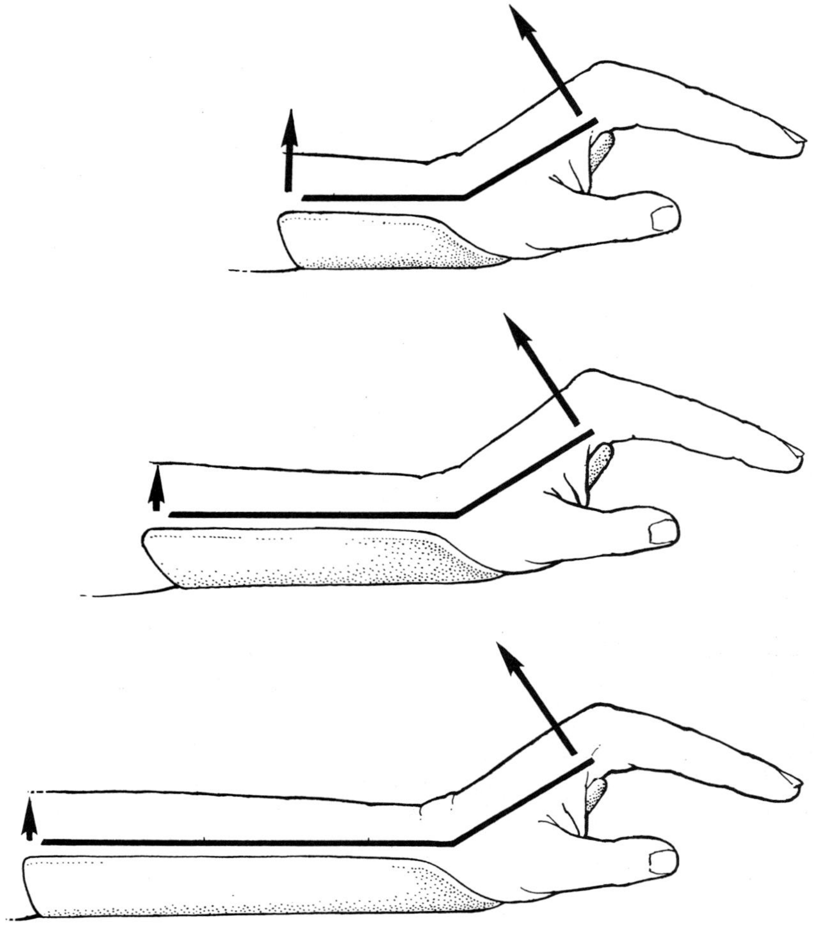

Figure 4-22 A longer forearm trough decreases the resultant pressure caused by the proximally transferred weight of the hand to the anterior forearm. [From Fess EE, Gettle KS, Philips CA, Janson JR (2005). Mechanical principles. In EE Fess, CA Philips (eds.), *Hand Splinting: Principles and Methods, Third Edition*. St. Louis: Mosby, p. 167.]

et al. 1995]. An example of a repetitive stress may be seen in a person wearing a dynamic flexion splint that has rubber band traction. If the person continually flexes the finger against the tension, the tissue may become inflamed after some time. If inflammation or redness occurs, the therapist adjusts the tension by relaxing the traction. A therapist must realize that persons with traumatic hand injuries or pathology may not be able to tolerate the repetitive amounts of stress a normal person could tolerate. Poor tolerance is usually a result of damaged vascular and lymph structures.

High stress may quickly result in tissue damage [Bell-Krotoski et al. 1995]. High stress can be applied to the skin from any object, such as a splint or bandage. The smaller or sharper the object the greater the amount of stress produced. High stress should be avoided at all times. For example, if a dynamic splint is applying too much stress to a joint, circulation may be restricted (potentially leading to tissue damage).

Direction of Stress

During splinting, consider the direction of stress or force on the skin and soft tissue. There are three directions of force to consider: (1) tension, (2) compression, and (3) shear [Fess 1995]. Tension occurs when forces on an object are applied opposite each other (Figure 4-23A). Compression stress results from forces pressing inwardly on an object (Figure 4-23B). Shear force occurs "when parallel forces are applied in an equal and opposite direction across opposite faces of a structure" [Fess 1995, p. 126] (Figure 4-23C). Research suggests that shear stress is the most damaging to skin [Bell-Krotoski et al. 1995].

Therapists must be astute in recognizing and knowing how to use the stress of splints in such a way as to not create soft-tissue damage. Generally, therapists avoid excessive stress or pressure from splints by employing wide troughs placed far from the fulcrum of movement while using an appropriate amount of tension on structures [Andrews and Bouvette 1996]. To determine the appropriate amount of tension on structures, the splint's tension should be sufficient to take the joint to a comfortable joint end range. This means that the tension in the splint should bring the joint just to the maximum comfortable position (flexion, extension, deviation, or rotation) that is tolerable. This should be a position the client can tolerate for long periods of time. The client may need to work up to long wearing time, but the goal is usually at least four hours per day.

Ideally, the four hours will be continuous, but it can be broken up as necessary. Clients can be asked to try to wear

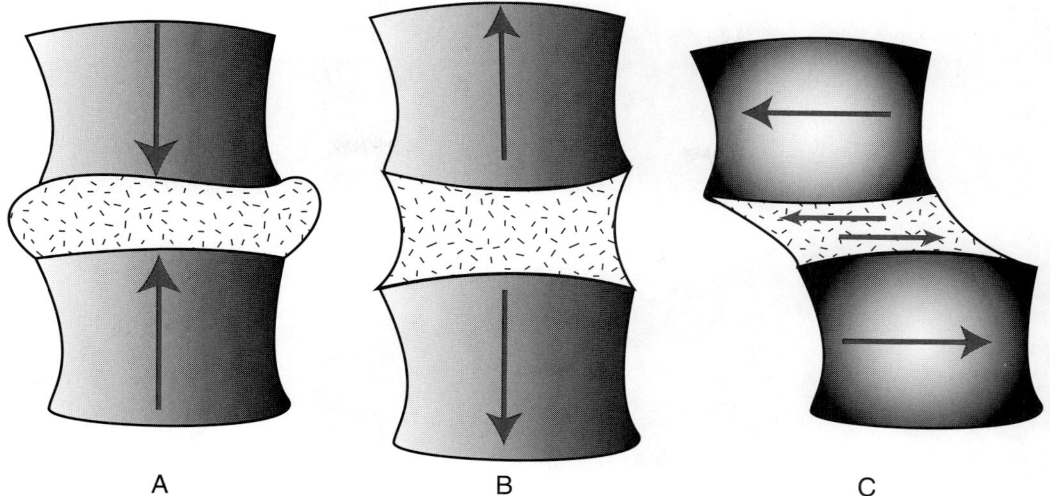

Figure 4-23 (A) Tension occurs when forces pull in opposite directions (tensile forces). (B) Compression is a force pushing tissues together. (C) Shear forces are parallel to the surfaces they affect. [From Greene DP, Roberts SL (2005). *Kinesiology Movement in the Context of Activity, Second Edition*. St. Louis: Mosby, p. 21.]

their splints to improve passive range of motion (PROM) during sleep. However, this depends on their cognitive, sensory, and substance abuse status. The rationale for this wearing schedule is based on studies that show that low-load prolonged stress at the end range is very effective in increasing PROM. Technically, for dense scars or for tissue that has adaptively shortened over a long period of time higher tension forces can be used as long as the pressure is well distributed along the skin. The skin is the structure that is the "weak link." The skin cannot tolerate the tension in the splint and becomes ischemic and therefore painful. If the pressure is well distributed, higher forces can be used and the tissue will lengthen more quickly as a result.

Several examples may explicate the effects of force on soft tissues [Fess 1995]. For example, after repair of a tendon rupture a therapist may employ early mobilization with a small amount of tension to facilitate the alignment of collagen fibers for improving tensile strength of the healing tendon. The tendon may be re-ruptured if the tension and repetition applied are not well controlled. A splint may be applied to assist in controlling fluctuating edema in the upper extremity. However, if the splint applies too much compression force on the underlying soft tissue over too much time the splint may restrict vascularity, possibly leading to soft-tissue necrosis. Shear stress between a healing tendon and its sheath must be carefully monitored to minimize and control adhesion shape.

The concepts of stress are considered when splinting. Splints and straps apply external forces on tissues that in turn affect forces or stresses exerted internally [Fess 1995]. The formula for pressure is:

$$\text{Pressure} = \frac{\text{Total force}}{\text{Area of force application}}$$

Ideally, splints should be contoured and cover a large surface area to decrease pressure and the risk of pressure sores [Cannon et al. 1985]. Straps should be as wide as possible to distribute pressure appropriately and to prevent restriction of circulation or trapping of edema.

Thermoplastic splints can cause pressure points over areas with minimal soft tissue or over bony prominences. To avoid this risk, the therapist should use a splint design that is wider and longer [Fess et al. 2005]. A larger design is more comfortable because it decreases the force concentrated on the hand and arm by increasing the surface area of the splint's force application.

Continuous well-distributed pressure is the goal of a splint, but pressure over any bony prominence should be nonexistent [Cailliet 1994]. Therapists should be cautious of pressure over bony prominences, such as the radial and ulnar styloids and the dorsal-aspect MCPs and the PIPs (Figure 4-24). Therapists can use heat guns to alleviate pressure exerted by the splint. This is done by heating the plastic in problem areas and pushing the plastic away from the bony prominence. Another technique for avoiding pressure on bony prominences is to splint over padding, gel pads, or elastomer positioned over bony prominences. A frequent mistake in splinting occurs when a pad is placed over the localized pressure area after the splint is formed [Bell-Krotoski et al. 1995]. Therapists should keep in mind that padding takes up space, reducing the circumference measurement of the splint and increasing the pressure over an area. Planning must be done before application of the thermoplastic material. The splint's design must accommodate the thickness of the padding.

Moist substances, such as perspiration and wound drainage, can cause skin maceration, irritation, and breakdown. Bandages help absorb the moisture but require frequent

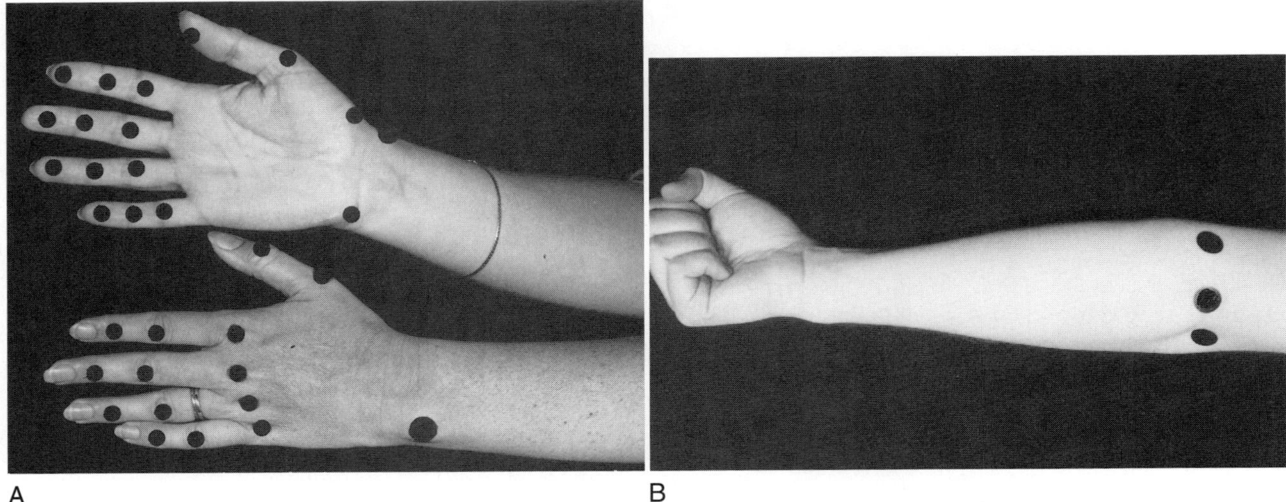

Figure 4-24 (A and B) Bony sites susceptible to pressure, which may cause soft-tissue damage. [From Fess EE, Gettle KS, Philips CA, Janson JR (2005). Principles of fit. In EE Fess, CA Philips (eds.), *Hand Splinting: Principles and Methods, Third Edition*. St. Louis: Mosby, p. 261.]

changing for infection control [Agency for Health Care Policy and Research 1992]. Some types of stockinette are more effective in wicking moisture away from skin. Polypropylene and thick terry liners are much more effective than cotton or common synthetic stockinette. Therapists can fabricate splints over extremities covered with stockinette or bandages, but the splint should be altered if the bulk of dressings or bandages changes.

Rolled or round edges on the proximal and distal ends of splints cause less pressure than straight edges [Cailliet 1994]. Imperfect edges are potential causes of pressure areas and therefore should be smoothed.

Contour

When flat, thermoplastic materials are more flexible and can be bent. Curving and contouring thermoplastic material to an underlying surface will change the mechanical characteristics of the material [Wilton 1997]. Contoured thermoplastic material is stronger and is better able to handle externally applied forces (Figure 4-25). Thermoplastic materials have varying degrees of drapability and conformity properties, which may affect the degree of contour the therapist is able to obtain in a splint.

Mechanics of Skin and Soft Tissue

Therapists often use splints to effect a change in the skin and soft tissue, which may address a client's performance deficit. It is important to have a basic understanding of the mechanics of normal soft tissue and skin. In addition, one should know when and how the mechanics change in the presence of scar tissue, materials (bandages, splints, cuffs), edema, contractures, wounds, and infection.

Normal skin and soft tissue have properties of *plasticity* and *viscoelasticity*, which allow them to resist breakdown

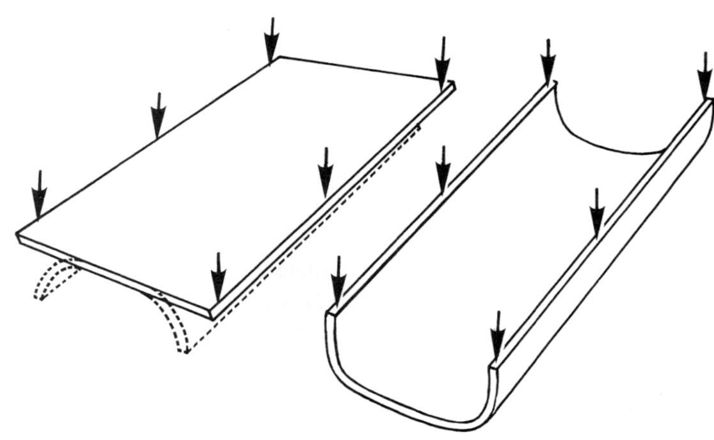

Figure 4-25 Contour mechanically increases the material's strength. [From Fess EE, Gettle KS, Philips CA, Janson JR (2005). Mechanical principles. In EE Fess, CA Philips (eds.), *Hand Splinting: Principles and Methods, Third Edition*. St. Louis: Mosby, p. 178.]

under stress in normal situations [Bell-Krotoski et al. 1995]. *Plasticity* refers to the extent the skin can mold and reshape to different surfaces. *Viscoelasticity* refers the skin's degree of viscosity and elasticity, which enables the skin to resist stress. The skin and soft tissue are able to tolerate some force or stress, but beyond a certain point the skin will break down [Yamada 1970].

When edema is present, the hand's normal soft tissue undergoes mechanical changes because of the volume of viscous fluid present [Villeco et al. 2002, Bell-Krotoski et al. 1995]. Prolonged or excessive edema can lead to permanent deformity. Therefore, edema must be managed in conjunction with splint application. Splints often assist in controlling edema. Because of the increase in volume of fluid, swollen skin, joints, and tendons have an increase in friction in relation to the resistance to movement. "Swollen tissue, then, in addition to its increased viscosity, is limited in its ability to be elongated, compressed, or compliant. This is why a hand will never have a normal range of motion as long as there is edema in the tissue in and under the skin" [Bell-Krotoski et al. 1995, p. 159].

Properties of thermoplastic material should be selected carefully. For example, soft splints with some flexibility and pliability may be more common in the future—once the properties of such materials are better understood [Bell-Krotoski et al. 1995]. According to Schultz-Johnson [personal communication, March 3, 1999], soft splints may be limited in use for additional reasons. In Europe, high levels of immobilization are not deemed as valuable as they are in the United States. The limited use of soft splints may be related to philosophy of care, prior training, physician bias, and therapists' habits.

Elastic bandages have the potential to apply high amounts of stress and may lead to constriction in the vascular and lymphatic circulation. A therapist must consider the amount of pressure applied to skin and tissue, especially when a second wrap of an elastic bandage covers an initial wrap. The pressure applied by the second wrap is doubled. This occurs even when bandages are applied in a figure-of-eight fashion. Another consideration is the effect bandages have on motion. Movement while bandages are being worn can further concentrate pressure, particularly over bony prominences. If appropriate, bandages should be removed while exercises are being performed.

Finger cuffs or loops used with dynamic splinting increase pressure on the underlying skin and tissue. Bell-Krotoski et al. [1995] caution that using very flexible finger cuffs could increase the shear stress on fingers. Leather finger loops may be an appropriate choice because they simulate normal skin by being flexible while providing some firmness to decrease the shear stress. Finger loops should be as wide as possible to avoid edge shear and to distribute pressure (Figure 4-26). Chapter 11 addresses finger loops in more depth.

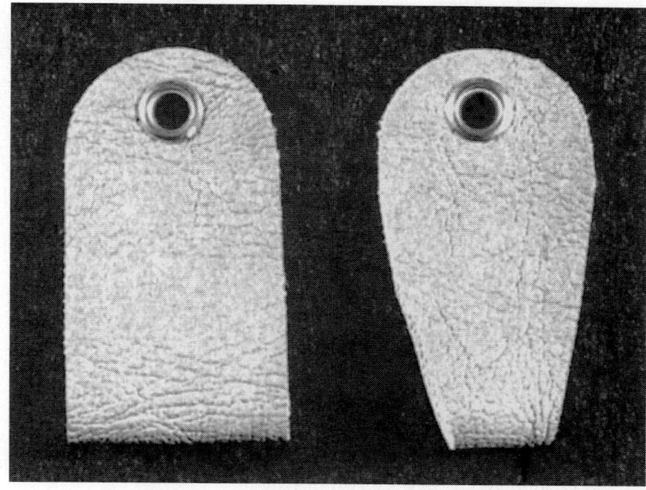

Figure 4-26 Finger loops apply pressure to the underlying surface. They should be as wide as possible without limiting adjacent joint mobility. [From Fess EE, Gettle KS, Philips CA, Janson JR (2005). Principles of fit. In EE Fess, CA Philips (eds.), *Hand Splinting: Principles and Methods, Third Edition*. St. Louis: Mosby, p. 274.]

In joints with flexion contractures, skin on the dorsum of the joints grows with elongation tension on the skin [Bell-Krotoski et al. 1995]. Skin on the volar surface of the joints is reabsorbed by a reduction in the elongation tension. There is a natural balance of tension in the skin and muscles. Skin will adjust to the tension required of it. Not only will skin lose length (contracture) but grow new cells to lengthen. The use of stretch *gradually* produces these changes. If skin is stretched to the point of microtrauma, a scar forms. When skin stretches, it releases proteins that result in scar formation. The scar tissue decreases the elasticity of the skin. To counteract excessive scarring, therapists use scar massage, mobilization techniques, and gentle stretch. Optimal regrowth involves the use of continuous (or almost continuous) tension [Bell-Krotoski et al. 1995].

New healing tissue can be negatively affected by mechanical stress. Tension of a wound site may "reduce the rate of repair, compromise tensile strength, and increase the final width of the scar" [Evans and McAuliffe 2002]. Rather than simply removing a splint and returning the extremity to function, Bell-Krotoski et al. [1995] suggested that immobilization splints should be gradually weaned as the affected skin and tissue become more mobile.

When working with a person who has infected tissues, caution must be taken to avoid mechanical stress from motion (as from a dynamic splint). Blood and interstitial fluids are forced into motion, and this pushes infection into deeper tissue and results in a more widespread infection and delay in healing. In the presence of infection, it is best to immobilize a joint with a splint for a few days and then remove the splint to maintain normal or partial range of motion.

SELF-QUIZ 4-1*

Answer the following.

Part I

Match the following with the correct splints.

a. Based on the palmar surface of the hand and forearm
b. Based on the dorsal surface of the hand and forearm
c. Based on the thumb side of the hand and forearm
d. Based on the little finger side of the hand and forearm

1. Ulnar gutter wrist cock-up splint
2. Volar- or palmar-based dynamic flexion splint
3. Dorsal MCP protection splint
4. Palmar-based wrist cock-up splint
5. Radial gutter dynamic extension splint

Part II

From the following diagram, label the creases of the hand.

1.
2.
3.
4.
5.

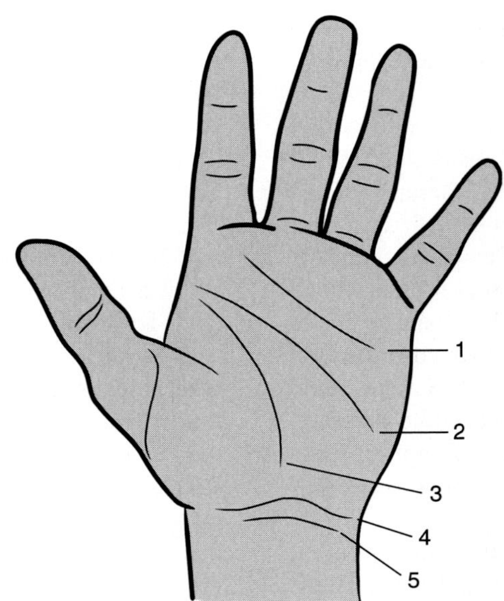

*See Appendix A for the answer key.

Part III

From the following diagram, label the arches of the hand.

1.
2.
3.

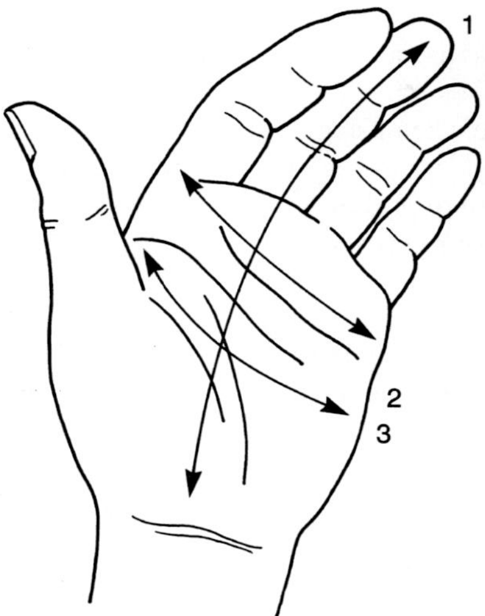

SELF-QUIZ 4-2*

Determine whether the following statements are true or false.

1. T F The forearm trough should be two-thirds the circumference of the forearm.
2. T F Short, narrow splints apply less pressure to the skin's surface than long, wide splints and are therefore better.
3. T F A splint should be approximately two-thirds the length of the forearm.
4. T F Avoidance of pressure over a bony prominence is preferable to unequal pressure.
5. T F A person uses a spherical grasp when holding a soda can.
6. T F A splint's design must accommodate padding thickness.
7. T F In joints with flexion contractures, the skin on the dorsum of the joint shortens and exerts tension.
8. T F In the splinting of persons with infection, caution is taken to avoid mechanical stress from motion such as dynamic splinting.
9. T F Contour of a splint increases its strength.
10. T F Shear force results from forces pressing inwardly on an object.

*See Appendix A for the answer key.

Summary

A therapist's knowledge of anatomic and biomechanical principles is important during the entire splinting process. One must be familiar with terminology to interpret medical reports, therapy prescriptions, and professional literature. In addition, the therapist uses medical terminology in documenting evaluation and treatment. The application of biomechanical principles to splint design and construction results in better fitting splints and thus contributes to compliance with therapeutic regimens. Ultimately, adherence to such principles impacts therapeutic outcomes.

REVIEW QUESTIONS

1. To what do the terms *palmar*, *dorsal*, and *radial* (or *ulnar*) refer in regard to splint fabrication?
2. What are the three arches of the hand?
3. Why is support for the hand's arches important when therapists splint a hand?
4. What is the significance of the distal palmar crease when therapists fabricate a hand splint?
5. If a splint's edge does not extend beyond the thenar crease toward the thumb, what thumb motions can occur?

6. What is an example of each of the following prehensile or grasp patterns: fingertip prehension, palmar prehension, lateral prehension, cylindrical grasp, spherical grasp, hook grasp, and intrinsic plus grasp?
7. How can a therapist determine the correct length of a forearm splint?
8. What is the correct width for a splint that has a forearm or thumb trough?
9. What precautions should a therapist take when using padding on a splint?
10. What are two methods a therapist can use to prevent the edges of a splint from causing a pressure sore?
11. Why is it important to consider contour when fabricating a splint?
12. How do skin and soft-tissue mechanics change in the presence of scar tissue, material application, edema, contractures, wounds, and infection?

References

Agency for Health Care Policy and Research (1992). *Pressure ulcers in adults: Prediction and prevention* (No. 92-0047). Rockville, MD: U.S. Department of Health and Human Services.

Andrews KL, Bouvette KA (1996). Anatomy for management and fitting of prosthetics and orthotics. Physical Medicine and Rehabilitation: State of the Art Reviews 10(3):489-507.

Aulicino PL (1995). Clinical examination of the hand. In JM Hunter, EJ Mackin, AD Callahan (eds.), *Rehabilitation of the Hand: Surgery and Therapy, Fourth Edition*. St. Louis: Mosby.

Barr NR, Swan D (1988). *The Hand*. Boston: Butterworth.

Belkin J, English CB (1996). Hand splinting: Principles, practice, and decision making. In LW Pedretti (ed.), *Occupational Therapy: Practice Skills for Physical Dysfunction, Fourth Edition*. St. Louis: Mosby.

Bell-Krotoski JA, Breger-Lee DE, Beach RB (1995). Biomechanics and evaluation of the hand. In JM Hunter, EJ Mackin, AD Callahan (eds.), *Rehabilitation of the Hand: Surgery and Therapy, Fourth Edition*. St. Louis: Mosby.

Bowers WH, Tribuzi SM (1992). Functional anatomy. In BG Stanely, SM Tribuzi (eds.), *Concepts in Hand Rehabilitation*. Philadelphia: F. A. Davis.

Buck WR (1995). *Human Gross Anatomy Lecture Guide*. Erie, PA: Lake Erie College of Osteopathic Medicine.

Cailliet R (1994). *Hand Pain and Impairment, Fourth Edition*. Philadelphia: F. A. Davis.

Cailliet R (1981). *Shoulder Pain, Second Edition*. Philadelphia: F. A. Davis.

Cannon NM, Foltz RW, Koepfer JM, Lauck MF, Simpson DM, Bromley RS (1985). *Manual of Hand Splinting*. New York: Churchill Livingstone.

Chase RA (1990). Anatomy and kinesiology of the hand. In JM Hunter, LH Schneider, EJ Mackin, AD Callahan (eds.), *Rehabilitation of the Hand: Surgery and Therapy, Third Edition*. St. Louis: Mosby.

Clarkson HM, Gilewich GB (1989). *Musculoskeletal Assessment: Joint Range of Motion and Manual Muscle Strength*. Baltimore: Williams & Wilkins.

Colditz JC, McGrouther DA (1998). *Interactive Hand: Therapy Edition CD-ROM*. London: Primal Pictures.

Evans, RB, McAuliffe, JA (2002). Wound classification and management. In EJ Mackin, AD Callahan, TM Skirven, LH Schneider, L Osterman (eds.), *Rehabilitation of the Hand and Upper Extremity, Fifth Edition*. St. Louis: Mosby.

Fess EE (1995). Splints: Mechanics versus convention. Journal of Hand Therapy 9(1):124-130.

Fess EE, Gettle KS, Philips CA, Janson JR (2005). *Hand and Upper Extremity Splinting: Principles and Methods, Third Edition*. St. Louis: Elsevier Mosby.

Kapandji IA (1970). *The Physiology of the Joints*. London: E&S Livingstone.

Kleinert HE, Schepel S, Gill T (1981). Flexor tendon injuries. Surgical Clinics of North America 61(2):267-286.

Long C, Conrad PW, Hall EA (1970). Intrinsic-extrinsic muscle control of the hand in power grip and precision handling: An electromyographic study. Journal of Bone Joint Surgery 52:853.

Malick MH (1972). *Manual on Static Hand Splinting*. Pittsburgh: Hamarville Rehabilitation Center.

Pedretti LW (1990). Hand splinting. In LW Pedretti, B Zoltan (eds.), *Occupational Therapy: Practice Skills for Physical Dysfunction, Third Edition*. St. Louis: Mosby, pp. 18-39.

Smith LK, Weiss EL, Lehmkuhl LD (1996). *Brunnstrom's Clinical Kinesiology, Fifth Edition*. Philadelphia: F. A. Davis.

Villeco JP, Mackin EJ, Hunter JM (2002). Edema: Therapist's management. In EJ Mackin, AD Callahan, TM Skirven, LH Schneider, AL Osterman (eds.), *Rehabilitation of the Hand and Upper Extremities, Fifth Edition*. St. Louis: Mosby, pp. 183-193.

Wilton JC (1997). *Hand Splinting Principles of Design and Fabrication*. Philadelphia: W. B. Saunders.

Wu PBJ (1996). Functional anatomy of the upper extremity. Physical Medicine and Rehabilitation: State of the Art Reviews, 10(3):587-600.

Yamada H (1970). *Strength of Biological Materials*. Baltimore: Williams & Wilkins.

CHAPTER 5

Clinical Examination for Splinting

Brenda M. Coppard, PhD, OTR/L

Key Terms

Protocols
Validity
Reliability
Responsiveness
Verbal analog scale
Visual analog scale
Canadian Occupational Performance Measure
Assessment of motor and process skills

Chapter Objectives

1. List components of a clinical examination for splinting.
2. Describe components of a history, an observation, and palpation.
3. Describe the resting hand posture.
4. Relate how skin, vein, bone, joint, muscle, tendon, and nerve assessments are relevant to splinting.
5. Identify specific assessments that can be used in a clinical examination before splinting.
6. Explain the three phases of wound healing.
7. Recognize the identifying signs of abnormal illness behavior.
8. Explain how a therapist can assess a person's knowledge of splint precautions and wear and care instructions.

Clinical Examination

A thoughtfully selected battery of clinical assessments is crucial to therapists' and physicians' treatment plans. A thorough, organized, and clearly documented examination is the basis for the development of a treatment plan and splint design. In today's health care system, a therapist completes examinations that are time and cost efficient. This chapter addresses components of the assessment in relationship to the splinting process.

Time-efficient informal assessments may indicate the level of hand function initially and the results may prompt the therapist to select more sophisticated testing procedures, as indicated by the person's condition [Fess 1995]. Generally, initial and discharge evaluations are most comprehensive in scope, whereas regular reassessments are usually more focused.

Reassessments are typically conducted at consistent intervals of time. For example, if Joe is evaluated at his Monday appointment the therapist may reevaluate Joe every Monday or every other Monday thereafter. On some occasions, a case manager may request the therapist to reevaluate a client. However, the time span between assessments is based on the person's condition and progress. For example, a person with a peripheral nerve injury may be reevaluated once every three weeks because of the slow nature of nerve healing. Another person being rehabilitated after a burn injury may be reevaluated every week because his condition changes more quickly, thereby affecting his functional ability.

The assessment process for the upper extremity should incorporate data from an interview, observation, palpation, and a selection of tests that are objective, valid, and reliable. Form 5-1 is a check-off sheet therapists can use when evaluating a person with upper extremity dysfunction.

History

Beginning with a medical history, the therapist gathers data from various sources. Depending on the setting, the therapist may have access to the person's medical chart, surgical or radiologic reports, and the physician's referral or prescription. The person's age, gender, and diagnosis are typically easy to obtain from these sources. Client age is important

FORM 5-1* Hand evaluation check-off sheet

Person's History: Interviews, Chart Review, and Reports:

- Age
- Vocation
- Date of injury and surgery
- Method of injury
- Hand dominance
- Treatment rendered to date (surgery, therapy, and so on)
- Medication
- Previous injury
- General health
- Avocational interests
- Family composition
- Subjective complaints
- Support systems
- Activities of daily living responsibilities before and after injury
- Impact of injury on family, economic status, and social well-being
- Reimbursement
- Motivation

Observation:

- Walking, posture
- Facial movements
- Speech patterns
- Affect
- Hand posture
- Cognition

Palpation:

- Muscle tone
- Muscle symmetry
- Scar density/excursion
- Tendon nodules
- Masses (ganglia, fistulas)

Assessments For:

- Pain
- Skin and allergies
- Wound healing/wound status
- Bone
- Joint and ligament
- Muscle and tendon
- Nerve/sensation
- Vascular status
- Skin turgor and trophic status
- Range of motion
- Strength
- Coordination and dexterity
- Function
- Reimbursement source
- Vocation

Follow-up Considerations:

- Splint fit
- Compliance

*See Appendix B for a perforated copy of this form.

because some congenital anomalies and diagnoses are unique to certain age groups. Age may also affect prognosis or length of recovery. Some problems are unique to gender.

From available sources, the therapist seeks out the person's past medical history and the dates of occurrences, as well as current medical status and treatment. This includes invasive and noninvasive treatments. Conditions such as diabetes, epilepsy, kidney or liver dysfunction, arthritis, and gout should be reported because they can directly or indirectly influence rehabilitation (including splinting). The therapist determines whether the current upper extremity problem is the result of neurologic or orthopedic dysfunction or from an orthopedic problem or trauma affecting soft tissue (i.e., tendon laceration, burn). The nature of dysfunction helps the therapist determine the splinting approach.

With postoperative persons, therapists must know the anatomic structures involved and the surgical procedures performed. Therapists should be aware that physicians may prefer to follow conventional rehabilitative programs for certain diagnostic populations. Other physicians may prefer to follow different rehabilitative programs they have developed for specific postoperative diagnostic populations. Whether standardized or nonstandardized, these programs are known as *protocols*. Protocols delineate which types of splint, exercise, and therapeutic interventions are appropriate in rehabilitation programs. Protocols also indicate the timing of interventions.

Interview

The therapist collects the person's history at the time of the initial evaluation. The goal of the interview is for the therapist to determine the impact of the condition on the person's functioning, family, economic status, and social/emotional well-being. It is beneficial to complete introductions and explain what occupational therapy is and what the purpose of evaluation and treatment are at the beginning of the interview. In addition, the therapist should create a teaching/learning environment directed at the client's learning style. For example, a therapist may tell a person that he or she should feel comfortable about asking any questions concerning therapy, evaluation, or treatment.

Co-histories are obtained from family, parents, friends, and caretakers of children and persons who are unable to communicate or who have cognitive impairments and are unreliable or questionable self-reporters. The therapist should obtain the following information by asking the person a variety of questions.

- Age
- Date of injury
- Hand dominance
- Avocation interests
- Subjective complaints
- Support systems
- Vocation
- Method of injury
- Functional abilities
- Family composition
- Social history
- Treatment to date

Therapists ask about general health as well as about any prior orthopedic, neurologic, psychologic, or cardiopulmonary conditions [Ellem 1995]. Habits and conditions such as smoking [Mosely and Finseth 1977, Siana et al. 1989], stress [Ebrecht et al. 2004], obesity [Wilson and Clark 2004], and depression [Tarrier et al. 2005] may influence rehabilitation [Ramadan 1997]. The therapist asks the client about any previous upper extremity conditions and their dates of onset in order to assess the current condition. The therapist inquires about any prior treatments and their results. The therapist can determine clients' insight into their condition by asking them to describe what they understand about their condition.

Observation

Observations are noted immediately when the person walks into a clinic or during the first meeting between the therapist and client. For example, the therapist should observe how the person carries the upper extremity, looking for reduced reciprocal arm swing, guarding postures, and involuntary movements such as tremors or tics [Smith and Bruner 1998]. For example, facial tics may be a sign of a neurologic or psychological problem. Further information is gleaned from observing facial movements, speech patterns, and affect. For example, if there is a facial droop the therapist may suspect that the client has Bell's palsy or has had a stroke. In addition, the therapist should always observe whether the person is able to answer questions and follow instructions.

A general inspection of the person's upper quarter (including the neck, shoulder, elbow, forearm, wrist, and hand) is completed, and joint attitude is noted. The therapist notes the posture of the affected extremity and looks for any postural asymmetry and guarded or protective positioning. A normal hand at rest assumes a posture of 10 to 20 degrees of wrist extension, 10 degrees of ulnar deviation, slight flexion and abduction of the thumb, and approximately 15 to 20 degrees of flexion of the metacarpophalangeal (MCP) joints. The fingers in a resting posture exhibit a greater composite flexion to the radial side of the hand (scaphoid bone), as shown in Figure 5-1 [Aulicino and DuPuy 1990]. The thumbnail usually lies perpendicular to the index finger. These hand postures are a useful basis for splint fabrication because a person's hand often deviates from the normal resting posture when injury or disease is present.

A variety of presentations can be observed by the therapist and will contribute to the overall clinical picture of the person. The following are noteworthy observational points [Ellem 1995].

- Position of hand in relationship to the body: protective or guarding posture
- Diminished or absent reciprocal arm swing

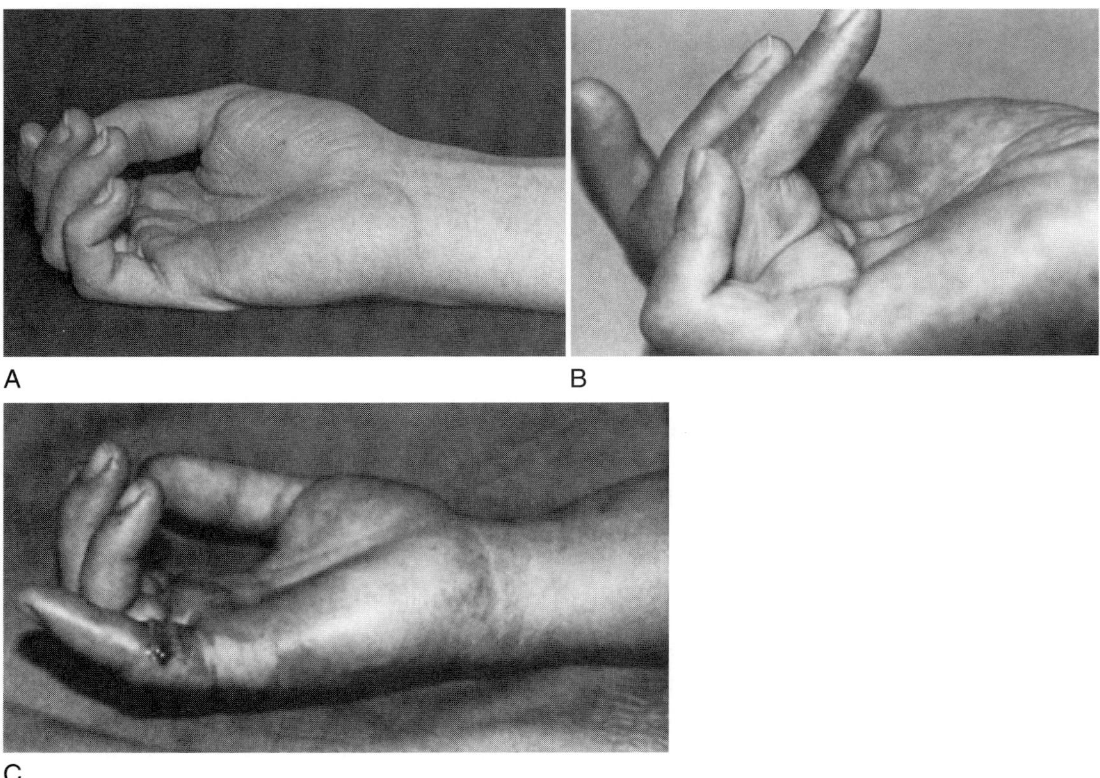

Figure 5-1 (A) Normal resting posture of the hand. Note that the fingers are progressively more flexed from the radial aspect to the ulnar aspect of the hand. (B) This normal hand posture is lost because of contractures of the digits as a result of Dupuytren's disease. (C) Loss of the normal hand posture is due to a laceration of the flexor tendons of the fifth digit. [From Hunter JM, Mackin EJ, Callahan AD (eds.), (1996). *Rehabilitation of the Hand: Surgery and Therapy, Fourth Edition*. St. Louis: Mosby, p. 55.]

- Normal hand arches
- Muscular atrophy
- Contractures
- Nails: ridged or smooth
- Finger pads: thin or smooth (loss of rugal folds, fingerprint lines)
- Lesions: scars, abrasions, burns, wounds
- Abnormal web spaces
- Heberden's or Bouchard's nodes
- Neurologic deficit postures: claw hand, wrist drop, monkey hand
- Color: pale, red, blue
- Grafts or sutures
- External devices: percutaneous pins, external fixator, splints, slings, braces
- Deformities: boutonniere, mallet finger, intrinsic minus hand, swan neck
- Pilomotor signs: appearance of "goose pimples" or hair standing on end
- Joint deviation or abnormal rotation

Palpation

After a general inspection of the client, palpation of the affected areas is completed when appropriate. A therapist palpates any area in which the person describes symptoms, including any area that is swollen or abnormal [Smith and Bruner 1998]. Muscle bulk is palpated on each extremity to compare proximal and distal muscles, as well as to compare right and left. Muscle tone is best assessed through passive range of motion (PROM). When assessing tone, the therapist should coach the client to relax the muscles so that the most accurate results can be obtained. The client's skin should be examined by the therapist. In the presence of ulcers, gangrene, inflammation, or neural or vascular impairment, skin temperature may change and can be felt during palpation [Ramadan 1997]. In the presence of infection, draining wounds, or sutured sites, therapists wear sterile gloves and follow universal precautions.

Assessments

Assessment selection is a critical step in formulating appropriate treatment interventions. There are more than 100 assessments in the musculoskeletal literature [Suk et al. 2005]. Several factors must be considered in selecting an assessment, including content, methodology, and clinical utility [Suk et al. 2005]. In order to critically choose assessment tools used for practice, one must understand the psychometric development of such tools.

Table 5-1 Definitions of Types of Validity

TYPE OF VALIDITY	DEFINITION
Construct validity	The degree to which a theoretical construct is measured by the tool
Content validity	The degree to which the items in a tool reflect the content domain being measured
Face validity	Determination if a tool appears to be measuring what it is intended to measure
Criterion validity	The degree to which a tool correlates with a "gold standard" or criterion test (it can be assessed as concurrent or predictive validity)
Concurrent validity	The degree to which the scores from a tool correlate with a criterion test when both tools are administered relatively at the same time
Predictive validity	The degree to which a measure will be a valid predictor of a future performance

Table 5-2 Definitions of Types of Reliability

TYPE OF RELIABILITY	DEFINITION
Inter-rater reliability	The degree to which two raters can obtain the same ratings for a given variable
Test/retest reliability	The degree to which a test is stable based on repeated administrations of the test to the same individuals over a specified time interval
Internal consistency	The degree to which each item of a test measures the same trait
Intra-rater reliability	The degree to which one rater can reproduce the same score in administering the tool on multiple occasions to the same individual

Content of an assessment is what the tool is attempting to measure. Content can be separated into three categories: type, scale, and interpretation. The type of content can be focused on data gathered by the clinician or data reported by the client. The scale of the content refers to the measurements or questions that constitute the tool and how they are measured. Content interpretation addresses how scores or measures pertain to "excellent" or "poor" outcomes [Suk et al. 2005].

Methodology of the tool relates to validity, reliability, and responsiveness. Validity is the extent to which the assessment measures what it intends to measure. Table 5-1 lists and defines the various types of validity. Reliability is the consistency of the assessment. Table 5-2 lists and defines the types of reliability. Responsiveness refers to the assessment's sensitivity to measure differences in status [Suk et al. 2005].

Clinical utility refers to the degree the tool is easy to administer by the therapist and the degree of ease the client experiences in completing the assessment. Utility is a subjective component addressing the degree to which the tool is acceptable to the client and the degree to which the tool is feasible to the therapist. Factors that impact clinical utility include training on administration, cost and administration, documentation, and interpretation time [Suk et al. 2005].

Assessment tools can be categorized in several ways. There are standardized and nonstandardized assessment tools. Some assessments are norm based, whereas others are criterion based. Bear-Lehman and Abreu [1989] suggest that evaluation is a quantitative and qualitative process. Thus, therapists who select assessments that produce precise, objective, and quantitative measurement decrease subjective judgments and increase their ability to obtain reproducible findings. However, therapists are cautioned to reject the tendency to neglect important information about their clients that may not be quantifiable [Bear-Lehman and Abreu 1989]. Qualitative information—such as attitude, pain response, coping mechanisms, and locus of control (center of responsibility for one's behavior)—influence the evaluation process. "The selection of the hand assessment tools to be used, the art of human interaction between the therapist and the client, the art of evaluating the client's hand as a part, but also as an integrated whole, are part of the subjective processes involved in hand assessment" [Bear-Lehman and Abreu 1989, p. 1025]. Even *objective* evaluation tools require the comprehension and motivation of the client.

Unfortunately, there is no universally accepted upper extremity assessment tool. Depending on the setting, a battery of assessments may be developed by the facility or department. In other settings, therapists use their clinical reasoning to determine what battery of assessments will be used with each person. Therapists should keep in mind that a theoretical perspective as well as a diagnostic population can influence the evaluation selection [Bear-Lehman and Abreu 1989]. For example, one facility's assessment reflects a biomechanical perspective whereas another facility's assessment reflects a neurodevelopmental perspective.

The sections that follow explore common assessments performed as part of an upper extremity battery of evaluations. There is a gamut of assessments for particular conditions not presented in this text.

Pain

The therapist has several options for evaluating pain, including interview questions, rating scales, body diagrams, and questionnaires. Box 5-1 lists questions a therapist can ask the person in relationship to pain [Fedorczyk and

Michlovitz 1995]. Therapists often use a combination of pain measures to obtain an accurate representation of the client's pain [Kahl and Cleland 2005].

The Verbal Analog Scale (VeAS) can be used to determine the person's perception of pain intensity. The person is asked to rate pain on a scale from 0 to 10 (0 refers to no pain and 10 refers to the worst pain ever experienced). Reliability scores for retesting under the VeAS are moderate to high, ranging from 0.67 to 0.96 [Good et al. 2001, Finch et al. 2002]. When correlated with the Visual Analog Scale (ViAS), the VeAS had a reliability score of 0.79 to 0.95 [Good et al. 2001, Finch et al. 2002]. Finch et al. [2002] reported that a three-point change in score is necessary to establish a true pain intensity change. Thus, the VeAS may be limited in detecting small changes, and clients with cognitive deficits may have trouble following instructions to complete the VeAS [Flaherty 1996, Finch et al. 2002].

A ViAS can also be used to rate pain intensity. A person is asked to look at a 10-cm horizontal line. The left side of the line represents "no pain" and the right side represents "pain as bad as it could be." The person indicates pain level by marking a slash on the line, which represents the pain experienced. The distance from *no pain* to the slash is measured and recorded in centimeters (Figure 5-2). The ViAS "may have a high failure rate because patients may have difficulty interpreting the instructions" [Weiss and Falkenstein 2005, p. 63]. Errors can occur due to changes in length of the line resulting from photocopying [Kahl and Cleland 2005]. Both VeAS and ViAS are unidimensional assessments of pain (i.e., intensity) [Kahl and Cleland 2005]. Although test-retest is not applicable to self-reported measures, studies have demonstrated a high range of test-retest reliability (ICC = 0.71 to 0.99) [Enebo 1998, Good et al. 2001, Finch et al. 2002]. When compared to the VaAS, concurrent validity measures ranged from 0.71 to 0.78 [Enebo 1998].

A body diagram consists of outlines of a body with front and back views, as shown in Figure 5-3. The person is asked to shade or color in the location of pain that corresponds to the body part experiencing pain. Colored pencils corresponding to a legend can be used to represent different intensities or types of pain, such as numbness, pins and needles, burning, aching, throbbing, and superficial.

Therapists may choose to use a more formal assessment, such as the McGill Pain Questionnaire (MPQ) [Fedorczyk and Michlovitz 1995] or the Schultz Pain Assessment [Weiss and Falkenstein 2005]. Although formal assessments usually take more time to administer than screening tools, they comprehensively assess many aspects of pain [Ross and LaStayo 1997].

Melzack [1975] developed the MPQ, which is widely used in clinical practice and for research purposes. The MPQ consists of a pain rating index, total number of word descriptors, and a present pain index. In its original version, the MPQ required 10 to 15 minutes to administer. The MPQ is a valid and reliable assessment tool. High internal consistency within the MPQ was demonstrated, with correlations

Box 5-1 Assessment Questions Relating to Pain*

Location and Nature of Pain

Where do you feel uncomfortable (pain)?
Does your discomfort (pain) feel deep or superficial?
Is your problem (pain) constant or intermittent? If constant, does it vary in intensity?
How long does your discomfort (pain) last?
What is the frequency of your discomfort (pain)?
How long have you had this problem (pain)?
Are you experiencing discomfort (pain) right now?

Pain Manifestations

How would you describe your discomfort (pain): throbbing, aching/sharp, dull, electrical, and so on?
Does the discomfort (pain) move or spread to other areas?
Does movement aggravate the discomfort (pain)?
Do certain positions aggravate the discomfort (pain)? If yes, can you show me the movement or postures that cause the discomfort (pain)?
Do you have stiffness with your discomfort (pain)?
Do you have discomfort (pain) at rest?
Do you have discomfort (pain) during the morning or night?
Does the discomfort (pain) wake you from sleep?
Do you have discomfort (pain) during particular activities?
Do you experience discomfort (pain) after performing particular activities?
What makes your discomfort (pain) worse?
What helps relieve your discomfort (pain)?
What have you tried to reduce your discomfort (pain)?
What worked to reduce your discomfort (pain)?

*Therapists working with persons experiencing chronic pain may find that focusing on pain and repeating the word *pain* over and over is not beneficial. Therapists may select questions according to their judgment and substitute alternative words for *pain* when necessary.

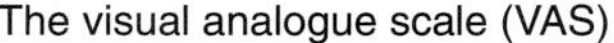

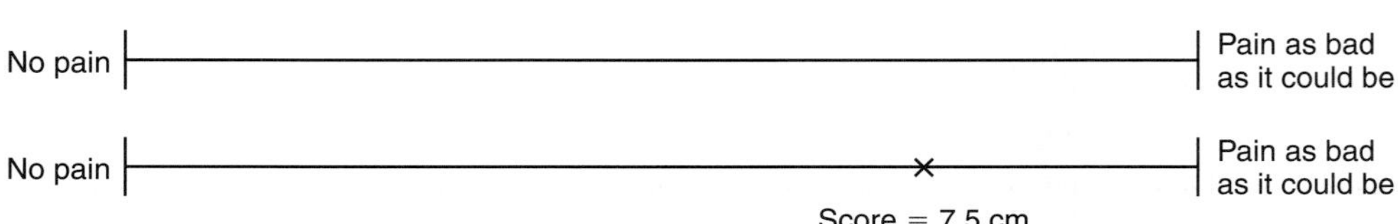

Figure 5-2 The Visual Analog Scale (ViAS) and an example of a completed ViAS with a score of 7.5.

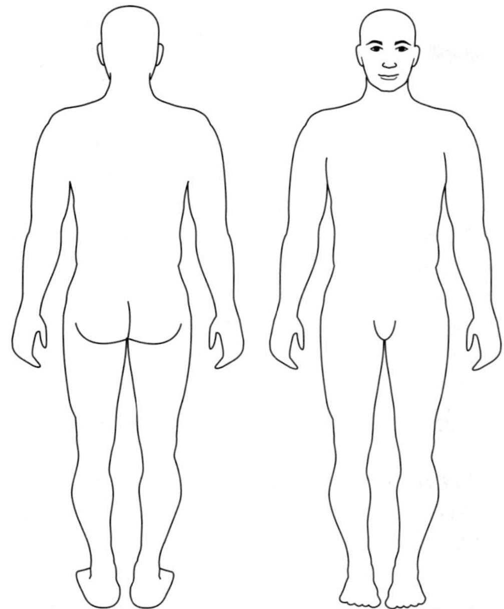

Figure 5-3 Example of a body diagram.

Table 5-3 Children's Report of Pain

AGE	REPORT
2 years	Presence and location of pain
3-4 years	Presence, location, and intensity of pain • 3 years: use a three-level pain intensity scale • 4 years: use a four- to five-item scale
5 years	Begin to use pain rating scales
8 years	Rate quality of pain

Data from O'Rourke D (2004). The measurement of pain in infants, children, and adolescents: From policy to practice. Physical Therapy 84:560-570.

of 0.89 to 0.90 [Melzack 1975]. Test-retest reliability scores for the MPQ are reported as 70.3% [Melzack 1975].

For assessment of pediatric pain, self-reporting measures are considered the *gold standard* [O'Rourke 2004]. A therapist must determine the child's concepts of quantification, classification, and matching prior to administering simple pain intensity scales [Chapman et al. 1998]. Nonverbal scales using facial expressions and the ViAS are commonly used. Children can report pain according to various aspects of child development. Table 5-3 outlines ages and recommendations associated with the various types of reporting in children.

Skin

A thorough examination of the surface condition and contour of the extremity may define possible pathologic conditions, which may influence splint design. During the examination the therapist observes and documents the skin's color, temperature, and texture. The therapist also observes the skin for muscle atrophy, scarring, edema, hair patterns, sweat patterns, and abnormal masses. Persons having fragile skin (especially persons who are older, who have been taking steroids for a long time, or who have diabetes) require careful monitoring. For these persons, the therapist carefully considers the splinting material so as to prevent harm to the already fragile skin (see Chapter 15).

With regard to skin, many clients are aware of skin allergies they have. Some are allergic to bandages, adhesive, and latex (all of which can be used in the splinting process). To avoid skin reactions, the therapist should ask each client to disclose any types of allergy before choosing splinting materials. When persons are unsure of skin allergies, the therapist should be aware that thermoplastic material, padding, and strapping supplies may create an allergic reaction. Therapists educate persons to monitor for any rashes or other skin reactions that develop from wearing a splint. The client experiencing a reaction should generally discontinue wearing the splint and report immediately to the therapist.

Veins and Lymphatics

Normally the veins on the dorsum of the hand are easy to see and palpate. They are cordlike structures. Any tenderness, pain, redness, or firmness along the course of veins should be noted [Ramadan 1997]. Venous thrombosis, subcutaneous fibrosis, and lymphatic obstruction will cause edema [Neviaser 1978].

Wounds

The therapist measures wounds or incisions (usually in centimeters) and assesses discharge from wounds for color, amount, and odor. If there is concern about the discharge being a sign of infection, a wound culture is obtained by the medical staff to identify the source of infection, and appropriate medication is prescribed. Wounds can be classified by color: black, yellow, or red [Cuzzell 1988]. A black wound consists of dark, thick eschar, which impedes epithelialization. A yellow wound may range in color from ivory to green-yellow (e.g., colonization with *pseudomonas*). Typically, yellow wounds are covered with purulent discharge. A red wound indicates the presence of granulation tissue and is normal.

Many wounds consist of a variety of colors [Cuzzell 1988]. Treatment focuses on treating the most serious color initially. For example, in the presence of eschar (commonly seen after thermal and crush injuries) a wound takes on a white or yellow-white color. Part of the treatment regimen for eschar is mechanical, chemical, or surgical debridement, which usually must be done before splinting. Debridement may result in a yellow wound. The yellow wound is managed by cleansing and dressing techniques to assist in the removal of debris. Once the desired red wound bed is achieved, it is protected by dressings [Walsh and Muntzer 1992].

Because open wounds threaten exposure to the person's body fluids, the therapist follows universal precautions.

The following precautions were derived from the Centers for Disease Control (CDC) [Singer et al. 1995].

- Gloves are worn for all procedures that may involve contact with body fluids.
- Gloves are changed after contact with each person.
- Masks are worn for procedures that may produce aerosols or splashing.
- Protective eyewear or face shields are worn for procedures generating droplets or splashing.
- Gowns or aprons are worn for procedures that may produce splashing or contamination of clothing.
- Hands are washed immediately after removal of gloves, after contact with each person.
- Torn gloves are replaced immediately.
- Gloves are replaced after punctures, and the instrument of puncture wounds is discarded.
- Areas of skin are cleansed with soap and water immediately if contaminated with blood or body fluids.
- Mouthpieces, resuscitation bags, and other ventilatory devices must be available for resuscitation to reduce the need for mouth-to-mouth resuscitation techniques.
- Extra care is taken when using sharps (especially needles and scalpels).
- All used disposable sharps are placed in puncture-resistant containers.

Many upper extremity injuries result in wounds, whether from trauma or surgery. Therefore, therapists must know the stages of wound healing. The healing of wounds is a cellar process [Evans and McAuliffe 2002]. Experts have identified three overlapping stages [Staley et al. 1988, Smith 1990], which consist of the (1) inflammatory or epithelialization, (2) proliferative or fibroblastic, and (3) maturation and remodeling phases [Smith 1990, 1995; Evans and McAuliffe 2002].

The first stage is the inflammatory (epithelialization) phase (Staley et al. 1988, Smith 1990, 1995], which begins immediately after trauma and lasts three to six days in a clean wound. Vasoconstriction occurs during the first 5 to 10 minutes of this stage, leading to platelet adhesion of the damaged vessel wall and resulting in clot formation. This activity stimulates fibroblast proliferation. During the inflammatory phase for a repaired tendon, cells proliferate on the outer edge of the tendon bundles during the first four days [Smith 1992]. By day seven, these cells migrate into the substance of the tendon. In addition, there is vascular proliferation within the tendon, which provides the basis for intrinsic tendon healing [DeKlerk and Jouck 1982]. Extrinsic repair of the tendon occurs when the adjacent tissues provide collagen-producing fibroblasts and blood vessels [Lindsay 1987]. Fibrovascular tissue that infiltrates from tissues surrounding the tendon can become future adhesions. Adhesions will prevent tendon excursion if allowed to mature with immobilization [Smith 1992].

The second stage is the proliferative (fibroblastic) phase, which begins two to three days after the injury and lasts about two to six weeks [Staley et al. 1988, Smith 1990, 1995]. During this stage, epithelial cells migrate to the wound bed. Fibroblasts begin to multiply 24 to 36 hours after the injury. The fibroblasts initiate the process of collagen synthesis [Evans and McAuliffe 2002]. The fibers link closely and increase tensile strength. A balanced interplay between collagen synthesis and its remodeling and reorganization prevents hypertrophic scarring. During tendon healing, the proliferative phase begins by day seven and is marked by collagen synthesis [Smith 1992]. In a tendon repair where there is no gap between the tendon ends, collagen appears to bridge the repair [Smith 1992]. Collagen fibers and fibroblasts are initially oriented perpendicularly to the axis of the tendon. However, by day 10 the new collagen fibers begin to align parallel to the longitudinal collagen bundles of the tendon ends [Lindsay 1987].

The final stage is the maturation (remodeling) phase, which can last up to one or two years after the injury [Staley et al. 1988; Smith, 1990, 1995]. During this stage the tensile strength continues to increase. Initially, the scar may appear red, raised, and thick, but with maturation a normal scar softens and becomes more pliable. The maturation phase for healing tendons is lengthier than time needed for skin or muscle because the blood supply to the tendons is much less [Smith 1992]. Tendon strength increases in a predictable fashion [Smith 1992]. Smith [1992] points out that in 1941 Mason and Allen first described how tensile strength of a repaired tendon progresses. From 3 to 12 weeks after tendon repair, mobilized tendons appear to be twice as strong as immobilized tendons. At 12 weeks, immobilized tendons have approximately 20% of normal tendon strength. In comparison, mobilized tendons at 12 weeks have 50% of normal tendon strength.

Bone

When assessing a person who has a skeletal injury, the therapist reviews the surgery and radiology reports. The therapist places importance on knowing the stability level of the fracture reduction, the method the physician used to maintain good alignment, the amount of time since the fracture's repair, and fixation devices still present in the upper extremity. A physician may request that the therapist fabricate a splint after the fracture heals. On occasion, the therapist may fabricate a custom splint or use a commercial fracture brace to stabilize the fracture before healing is complete. For example, for a person with a humeral fracture a commercially available humeral cuff may be prescribed.

The rationale for using a commercially fabricated fracture brace rather than fabricating a custom splint is based on time, client comfort, ease of application, and cost. Custom fabrication of fracture braces can be challenging because the client is typically in pain and the custom splint involves the use of large pieces of thermoplastic material, which can be difficult to control. The commercial fracture brace saves the therapist's time and therefore minimizes expense. A commercial brace also minimizes donning and doffing for fitting, which can also be uncomfortable for the client.

Indications for fabricating a custom fracture brace may include bracing extremely small or large extremities.

Joint and Ligament

Joint stability is important to assess and is evaluated by carefully applying a manual stress to any specific ligament. Each digital articulation achieves its stability through the collateral ligaments and a dense palmar plate [Cailliet 1994]. The therapist should carefully assess the continuity, length, and glide of these ligaments. Joint play or accessory motion of a joint is assessed by grading the elicited symptoms upon passive movement. The grading system is as follows: 0 = ankylosis, 1 = extremely hypomobile, 2 = slightly hypomobile, 3 = normal, 4 = slightly hypermobile, 5 = extremely hypermobile, and 6 = unstable [Wadsworth 1983]. Unstable joints, subluxations, dislocations, and limited PROM directly affect splint application. Lateral stress on finger joints should be avoided. In addition, the person may wear a splint to prevent unequal stress on the collateral ligaments [Cannon et al. 1985].

Muscle and Tendon

Tensile strength is the amount of long-axis force a muscle or tendon can withstand [Fess et al. 2005]. When a tendon is damaged or undergoes surgical repair, tensile strength directly affects the amount of force a splint should provide. Tensile strength also mandates which exercises or activities the person can safely perform.

Therapists should keep in mind that proximal musculature can affect distal musculature tension in persons experiencing spasticity. For example, wrist position can influence the amount of tension placed on finger musculature. When the therapist is attempting to increase wrist extension in the presence of spasticity, the wrist, hand, and fingers must be incorporated into the splint's design. If the splint design addresses only wrist extension, the result may be increased finger flexion. Conversely, if the splint design addresses only the fingers, the wrist may move into greater flexion (see Chapter 14).

Nerve

Sensory evaluations are important to determine areas of diminished or absent sensibility. Conventional tests for protective sensibility include the sharp/dull and hot/cold assessments. Discriminatory sensibilities include assessment for stereognosis, proprioception, kinesthesia, tactile location, and light touch. Aulicino and DuPuy [1990] recommend two-point discrimination testing (Figure 5-4) as a quick screening for sensibility. In addition, the American Society for Surgery of the Hand recommends static and moving

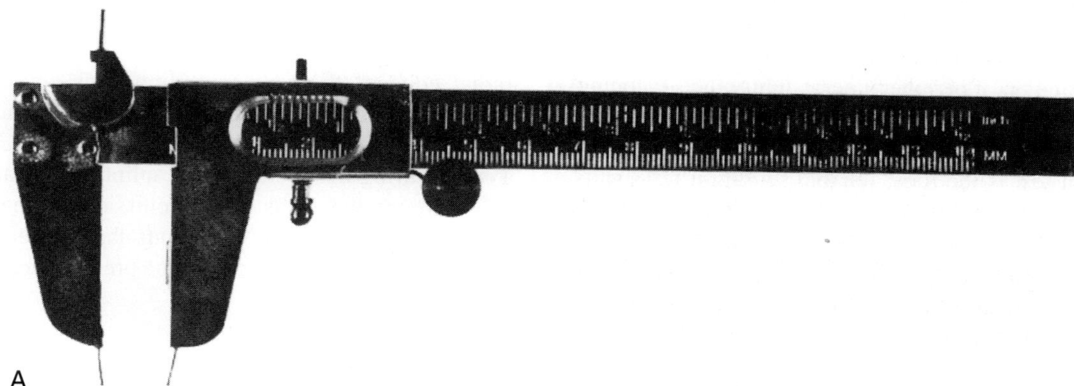

A

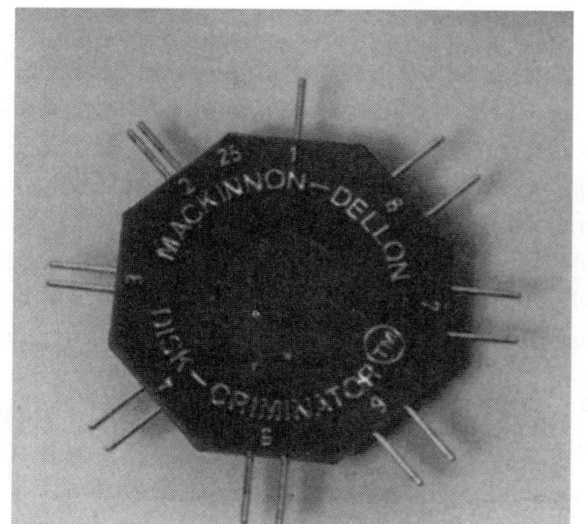

B

Figure 5-4 The recommended instruments for testing two-point discrimination include the Boley Gauge (A) and the Disk-Criminator (B). [From Hunter JM, Mackin EJ, Callahan AD (eds.), (1996). *Rehabilitation of the Hand: Surgery and Therapy, Fourth Edition*. St. Louis: Mosby, p. 146.]

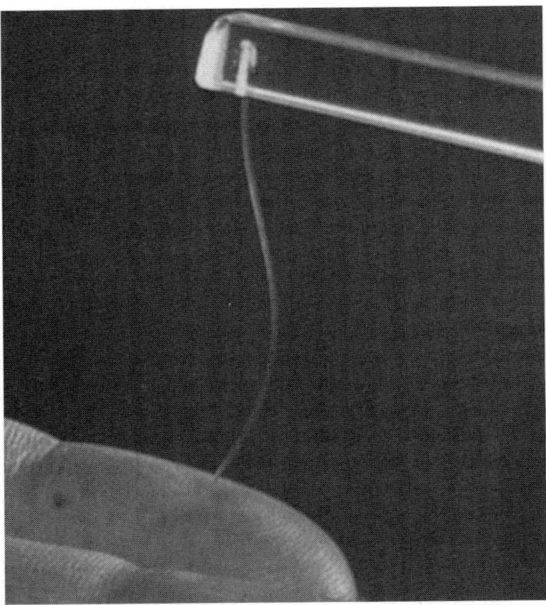

Figure 5-5 The monofilament collapses when a force dependent on filament diameter and length is reached, controlling the magnitude of the applied touch pressure. [From Hunter JM, Mackin EJ, Callahan AD (eds.), (1996). *Rehabilitation of the Hand: Surgery and Therapy, Fourth Edition*. St. Louis: Mosby, p. 76.]

two-point discrimination tests. The Semmes-Weinstein Monofilament test (Figure 5-5) provides useful detailed mapping of the level of functional sensibility, particularly during rehabilitation of peripheral nerve injury. This mapping is useful to physicians, therapists, clients, case managers, and employers [Tomancik 1987]. The Semmes-Weinstein Monofilament test is the most reliable sensation test available and is often used as the comparison for concurrent validity studies [Dannenbaum et al. 2002].

Therapists searching for objective sensory assessment data should be aware that "tests that were considered objective in the past can be demonstrated to be subjective in application dependent on the technique of the examiner" [Bell-Krotoski 1995, p. 109; Bell-Krotoski and Buford 1997]. For example, when administering the Semmes-Weinstein Monofilament test if the stimulus is applied too quickly "the force can result in an overshoot beyond the desired stimulus" [Bell-Krotoski and Buford 1997, p. 304] and affect the test results. In addition, even when the Semmes-Weinstein Monofilament test is administered with excellent technique the cooperation and comprehension of the client are required.

When peripheral nerve injuries have occurred or are suspected, a Tinel's test can be conducted. Tinel's test can be performed in two ways. The first method involves gently tapping over the suspected entrapment site to help determine whether entrapment is present. The second method consists of tapping the nerve distal to proximal. The location where the paresthesias are felt is considered the level to which a nerve has regenerated after Wallerian degeneration has occurred. A person is said to have a positive Tinel's sign if he or she experiences tingling or shooting sensations in one of two areas: at the site of tapping or in a direction distally from the tapped area [Ramadan 1997]. If the person experiences paresthesia or hyperparesthesia in a direction proximal to the tapped area, the Tinel's test is negative.

A Phalen's sign is present if a person feels similar symptoms when resting elbows on the table while flexing the wrists for 1 minute [American Society for Surgery of the Hand 1983]. Phalen's sign may indicate a median nerve problem. One should be aware that Tinel's and Phalen's signs can be positive in normal subjects [Smith and Bruner 1998].

Cervical nerve problems must be ruled out before a diagnosis of peripheral nerve injury can be made. For example, a person may have signs similar to carpal tunnel syndrome in conjunction with complaints of neck pain. In the absence of a cervical nerve screen, the person may have a misdiagnosis of carpal tunnel syndrome but actually have cervical nerve involvement. In the absence of electrical studies, many surgeons still make the diagnosis of nerve compression.

During the fitting process, hand splints may cause pressure and friction on vulnerable areas with impaired sensibility. If a person has decreased sensibility, the therapist uses a splint design with long, well-molded components. The reason for using such a splint is to distribute the forces of the splint over as much surface area as possible, thereby decreasing the potential for pressure areas.

When splinting occurs across the wrist, the superficial branch of the radial nerve is at risk of compression. If the radial edge of the forearm splint stops beyond the mid-lateral forearm near the dorsum of the thumb, the superficial branch of the radial nerve can be compressed [Cannon et al. 1985]. During the evaluation of splint fit, therapists should be aware of the signs of compression of the superficial branch of the radial nerve. Splints that cause compression require adjustments to decrease the pressure near the dorsum of the thumb.

Vascular Status

To understand the vascular status of a diseased or injured hand, the therapist monitors the skin's color and temperature and checks for edema. The therapist clearly defines areas of questionable tissue viability and adapts splints to prevent obstruction of arterial and venous circulation. To assess radial and ulnar artery patency, the therapist uses Allen's test [American Society for Surgery of the Hand 1983].

A therapist can take circumferential measurements proximal and distal to the location of a splint's application. Then, after applying the splint to the extremity the therapist measures the same areas and compares them with the previous measurements. An increase in measurements taken while the splint is on indicates that the splint is exerting too much force on the underlying tissues. This situation poses a risk for circulation. When fluctuating edema is present, the therapist should make the splint design larger. A well-fitting circumferential splint, sometimes in conjunction with a pressure garment, can control or eliminate fluctuating edema. In addition, fluctuating edema may signal poor compliance with elevation. A sling and education about its use may assist in edema control.

The therapist can also use the Fingernail Blanch Test to assess circulation [Aulicino and DuPuy 1990]. Long-lasting blanched areas of the fingertips indicate restricted circulation.

When a therapist applies a splint to the upper extremity, the skin should maintain its natural color. Red or purple areas indicate obstructed venous circulation. Dusky or white areas indicate obstructed arterial circulation. Splints causing circulation problems must be modified or discontinued.

Range of Motion and Strength

The therapist records active and passive motions when no contraindications are present (Figure 5-6), and takes measurements on both extremities for a baseline data comparison. The therapist also records total active motion (TAM) and total passive motion (TPM) [American Society for Surgery of the Hand 1983]. Grasp and pinch strengths are completed and documented only when no contraindications are present (Figures 5-7 and 5-8). Manual muscle testing (MMT) assesses muscle strength but should be done only when there are no contraindications. For example, if a person with rheumatoid arthritis in an exacerbated state is being evaluated, MMT should be avoided to prevent further exacerbation of pain and swelling.

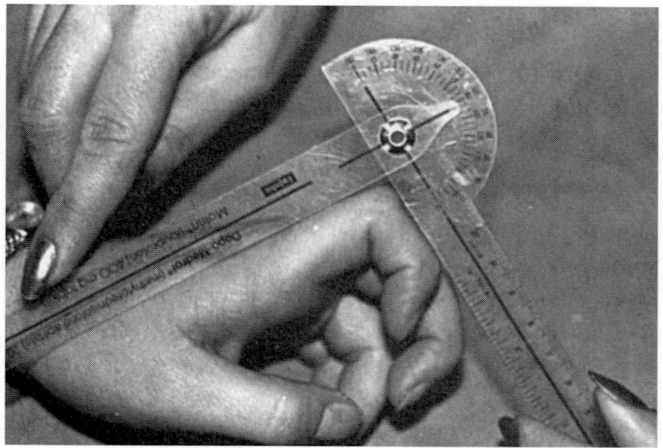

Figure 5-6 Goniometric measurements of active and passive motion are taken regularly when no contraindications are present. [From Hunter JM, Mackin EJ, Callahan AD (eds.), (1996). *Rehabilitation of the Hand: Surgery and Therapy, Fourth Edition*. St. Louis: Mosby, p. 34.]

Coordination and Dexterity

Hand coordination and dexterity are needed for many functional performance tasks, and it is important to evaluate them. Many standardized tests for coordination and dexterity exist, including the Nine Hole Peg Test (Figure 5-9), the Minnesota Rate of Manipulation Test, the Crawford Small Parts Dexterity Test, the Purdue Peg Board Test, the Rosenbusch Test of Dexterity, and the Valpar Tests. Most dexterity tests are based on time measurements, and normative data are available for all of these tests. In particular, the Valpar work samples use methods time measurement (MTM). MTM is a method of analyzing work tasks to determine how long a trained worker will require to complete a certain task at a rate that can be sustained for an eight-hour workday.

The Sequential Occupational Dexterity Assessment (SODA) was developed in the Netherlands [Van Lankveld et al. 1996]. The SODA is a test to measure hand dexterity and the client's perception of difficulty and pain while performing four unilateral and eight bilateral activities of daily living (ADL) tasks [Massey-Westropp et al. 2004]. In a study conducted by Massey-Westropp et al. [2004] on 62 clients with rheumatoid arthritis, they concluded that "The SODA is also valid and reliable for assessing disability in a clinical situation that cannot be generalized to the home" (p. 1996). More research should be conducted to test such findings.

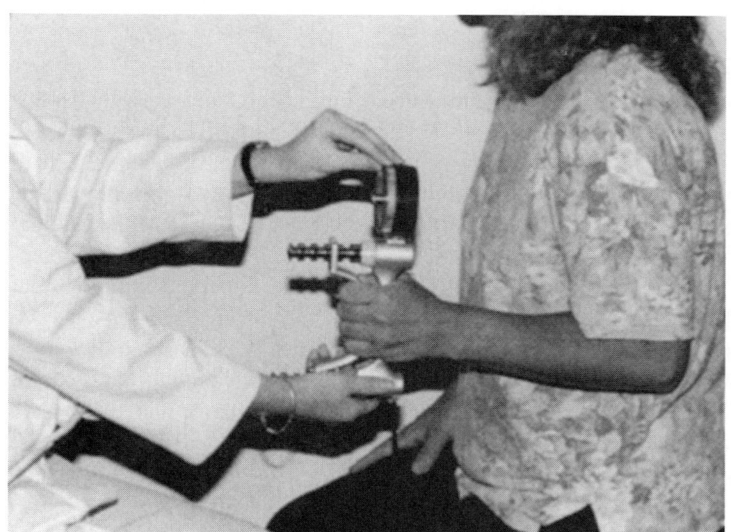

Figure 5-7 Therapists use the Jamar dynamometer to obtain reliable and accurate grip strength measurements. [From Tubiana R, Thomine JM, Mackin E (1996). *Examination of the Hand and Wrist*. St. Louis: Mosby, p. 344.]

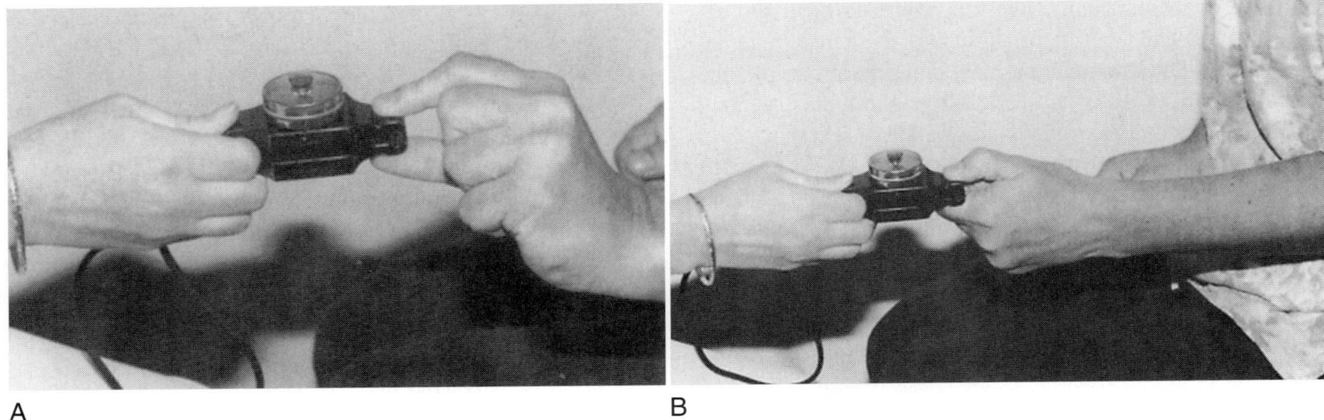

Figure 5-8 The pinch meter measures pulp pinch (A) and lateral pinch (B). [From Tubiana R, Thomine JM, Mackin E (1996). *Examination of the Hand and Wrist*. St. Louis: Mosby, p. 344.]

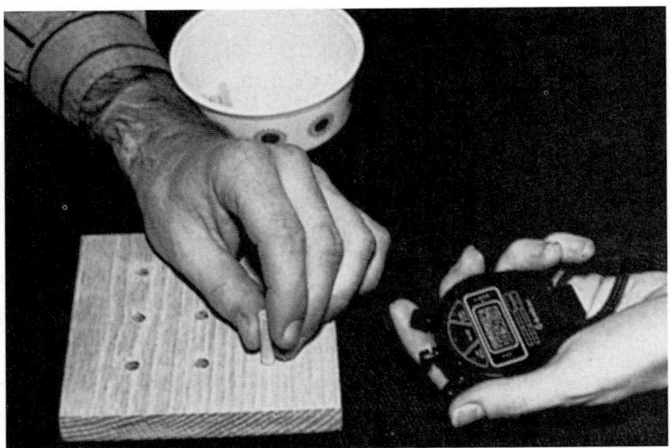

Figure 5-9 The Nine Hole Peg Test is a quick test for coordination. [From Hunter JM, Mackin EJ, Callahan AD (eds.), (1996). *Rehabilitation of the Hand: Surgery and Therapy, Fourth Edition*. St. Louis: Mosby, p. 1158.]

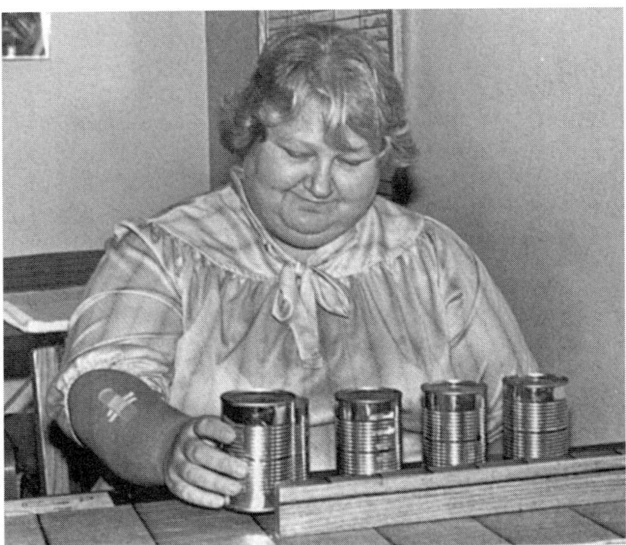

Figure 5-10 The Jebsen-Taylor Hand Test assesses the ability to perform prehension tasks. [From Hunter JM, Mackin EJ, Callahan AD (eds.), (1996). *Rehabilitation of the Hand: Surgery and Therapy, Fourth Edition*. St. Louis: Mosby, p. 98.]

Function

Function can be assessed by observation, interview, task performance, and standardized testing. Close observation during the interview and splint fabrication gives the therapist information regarding the person's views of the injury and disability. The therapist also observes the person for protected or guarded positioning, abnormal hand movements, muscle substitutions, and pain involvement during functional tasks. During evaluation, the person's willingness for the therapist to touch and move the affected extremity is noted.

During the initial interview, the therapist questions the person about the status of ADL, instrumental activities of daily living (IADL), and avocational and vocational activities. The therapist notes problem areas. Having clients perform tasks as part of an evaluation may result in more information, particularly when self-reporting is questioned by the therapist.

The therapist may use standardized hand function assessments. The Jebsen-Taylor Hand Function Test (Figure 5-10) is helpful because it gives objective measurements of standardized tasks with norms the therapist uses for comparison [Jebsen et al. 1969]. The Dellon modification of the Moberg Pick-up Test evaluates hand function when the person grasps common objects (Figure 5-11) [Moberg 1958]. Similar objects in the test require the person to have sensory discrimination and prehensile abilities [Callahan 1990].

Other functional outcome assessments that may be used include the Canadian Occupational Performance Measure (COPM); the Assessment of Motor and Process Skills (AMPS); the Disability of Arm, Shoulder and Hand (DASH), and the Short Form-36 (SF-36).

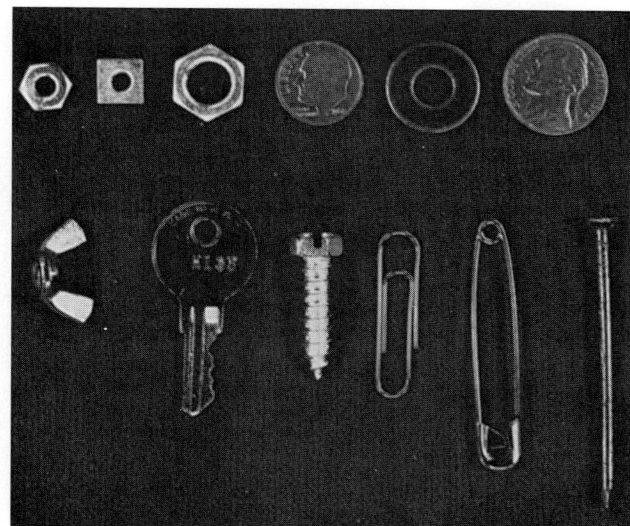

Figure 5-11 Items used in the Dellon modification of the Moberg Pick-up Test. [From Hunter JM, Mackin EJ, Callahan AD (eds.), (1990). *Rehabilitation of the Hand: Surgery and Therapy, Third Edition*. St. Louis: Mosby, p. 608.]

The COPM is a client-centered outcome measure used to assess self-care, productivity, and leisure [Law et al. 1990]. Clients rate their performance and satisfaction with performance on a 1 to 10 point scale. The result is a weighted individualized client goal plan (Law et al. 1998). It is a top-down assessment, which is done before administration of tests to evaluate performance components. Test-retest reliability was reported as ICC = 0.63 for performance and ICC = 0.84 for satisfaction (as cited in Case-Smith, 2003) (Sanford et al. 1994). "Validity was estimated by correlating COPM change scores with changes in overall function as rated by caregivers ($r = 0.55$, $r = 0.56$), therapist ($r = 0.30$, $r = 0.33$), and clients ($r = 0.26$, $r = 0.53$)" (Case-Smith, 2003, p. 501).

The DASH is a standardized questionnaire rating disability and symptoms related to upper extremity conditions. The DASH includes 30 pre-determined questions that explore function within performance areas. The client rates on a scale of 1 (no difficulty) to 5 (unable) his or her current ability to complete particular skills, such as opening a jar or turning a key. Beaton, Katz, Fossel, Wright, Tarasuk and Bombardier (2001) studied reliability and validity of the DASH. Excellent test-retest reliability was reported (ICC = 0.96) in a study of 86 clients. Concurrent validity was established with correlations with other pain and function measures ($r > 0.69$).

The Short Form-36 (SF-36) measures eight aspects of health that contribute to quality of life [Ware et al. 2000]. The SF-36 "yields an eight scale profile of functional health and well being scores, as well as psychometrically based physical and mental health summary measures and a preference based health utility index" [Ware 2004, p. 693]. Reliability scores range from $r = 0.43$ to $r = 0.96$ [Brazier et al. 1992]. Evidence of content, concurrent, criterion, construct, and predictive evidence of validity have been established [Ware 2004]. The tool has been translated for use in more than 60 countries and languages.

Both the COPM and AMPS may take more time to administer than screening tools. However, the assessments are focused on functional performance. In addition, therapists using these tests should be trained in their administration, scoring, and interpretation.

Work

Evaluations of paid and unpaid work entail assessment of the work to be done and how the work is performed [Mueller et al. 1997]. It is estimated that 36% of all functional capacity evaluations (FCEs) are conducted because of upper extremity and hand injuries [Mueller et al. 1997]. Some facilities use a specific type of FCE system, such as the Blankenship System or the Key Method. Standardized testing includes the Work Evaluations Systems Technologies II (WEST II), the EPIC Lift Capacity (ELC), the Bennett Hand Tool Dexterity Test, the Purdue Pegboard, the Minnesota Rate of Manipulation Test (MRMT), and the Valpar Component Work Samples (VCWS). Commercially available computerized tests can be administered in work evaluations. Isometric, isoinertional, and isokinetic tests can be performed on equipment tools manufactured by Cybex, Biodex, and Baltimore Therapeutic Equipment (BTE). FCEs frequently assess abnormal illness behavior and often include observation, psychometric testing, and physical or functional testing. New and experienced therapists should have specialized training in administering and interpreting FCEs because of the standardized nature of the examination and the legal implications of these assessments [Mueller et al. 1997].

Other Considerations

The person's motivation, ability to understand and carry out instructions, and compliance may affect the type of splint the therapist chooses. The therapist considers a person's vocational and avocational interests when designing a splint. Some persons wear more than one splint throughout the day to allow for completion of various activities. In addition, some persons wear one splint design during the day and a different design at night.

Related to motivation may be the presence or absence of a third-party reimbursement source. Whenever possible, the therapist discusses reimbursement issues with the client before completing the initial visit. If a third party is paying for the client's services, the therapist first determines whether that source intends to pay for any or all of the splint fabrication services. At times, some clients will be very motivated to comply with the rehabilitation program if they have to pay for the services. In other cases, where third-party reimbursement is quite good and the client is temporarily on a medical leave from work, the client may be less motivated and perhaps show signs of abnormal illness behavior. Terms such as *malingering*, *secondary gain*, *hypochondriases*, *hysterical neurosis*, *conversion*, *somatization disorder*, *functional overlay*, and *nonorganic pain* have been used to describe abnormal illness behaviors [Mueller et al. 1997]. Gatchel et al. [1986] reported the following *red flags*, which can assist the therapist in identifying such abnormal behaviors [Blankenship 1989].

- Client agitates other clients with disruptive behaviors
- Client has no future work plan or changes to previous work plan
- Client is applying for or receiving Social Security or long-term disability
- Client opposes psychological services and refuses to answer questions or fill out forms
- Client has obvious psychosis
- Client has significant cognitive or neuropsychological deficits
- Client expresses excessive anger at persons involved in case
- Client is a substance abuser
- Client's family is resistant to his or her recovery or return to work
- Client has young children at home or has a short-term work history for primarily financial reasons
- Client perpetually complains about the facility, staff, and program rather than being willing to deal with related physical and psychological issues
- Client is chronically late to therapy and is noncompliant, with excuses that do not check out
- Client focuses on pain complaints in counseling sessions rather than dealing with psychological issues

Splinting Precautions

During the splint assessment, the therapist must be aware of splinting precautions. An ill-fitting splint can harm a person. Several precautions are outlined in Form 5-2, which a therapist can use as a check-off sheet. The therapist must not only educate a client about appropriate precautions but evaluate the client's understanding of them. The client's understanding can be assessed by having him or her repeat important precautions to follow or by role-playing (e.g., if this happens, what will you do?). In follow-up visits, the client can be questioned again to determine whether precautions are understood. Form 5-3 lists splint fabrication hints to follow. Adherence to the hints will assist in avoiding situations that result in clients experiencing problems with their splints.

Pressure Areas

After fabricating a splint, the therapist does not allow the person to leave until the splint has been evaluated for problem areas. A general guideline is to have the person wear the splint at least 20 to 30 minutes after fabrication. Red areas should not be present 20 minutes after removal of the splint. Splints often require some adjustment. After receiving assurance that no pressure areas are present, the therapist instructs the person to remove the splint and to call if any problems arise. Persons with fragile skin are at high risk of developing pressure areas. The therapist provides the person with thorough written and verbal instructions on the wear and care of the splint. The instructions should include a phone number for emergencies. During follow-up visits, the therapist inquires about the splint's fit to determine whether adjustments are necessary in the design or wearing schedule.

Edema

The therapist completes an evaluation for excessive tightness of the splint or straps. Often edema is caused by inappropriate strapping, especially at the wrist or over the MCP joints. Strapping systems should be evaluated and modified if they are contributing to increased edema. If the splint is too narrow, it may also inadvertently contribute to increased edema. Persons can usually wear splints over pressure garments if necessary. However, therapists should monitor circulation closely.

The therapist assesses edema by taking circumferential or volumetric measurements (Figure 5-12). When taking volumetric measurements, the therapist administers the test according to the testing protocol and then compares the involved extremity measurement with that of the uninvolved extremity. If edema fluctuates throughout the day, it is best to fabricate the splint when edema is present so as to ensure that the splint will accommodate the edema fluctuation. When edema is minimal but fluctuates during the day, the splint design must be wider to accommodate the edema [Cannon et al. 1985].

Splint Regimen

Upon provision of a splint, the therapist determines a wearing schedule for the client. *Most* diagnoses allow persons to remove the splints for some type of exercise and hygiene. The therapist provides a written splint schedule and reviews the schedule with the person, nurse, and caregiver responsible for putting on and taking off the splint. If the person is confused, the therapist is responsible for instructing the appropriate caregiver regarding proper splint wear and care. The therapist must evaluate the client or caregiver's understanding of the wearing schedule.

Clients wearing mobilizing (dynamic) splints should follow several general precautions. A therapist must be cautious when instructing a client to wear a mobilizing (dynamic) splint during sleep. Because of moving parts on mobilization splints, the person could accidentally scratch, poke, or cut himself or herself. Therefore, therapists must design splints with no sharp edges and must consider the possibility of using elastic traction (see Chapter 11).

FORM 5-2* Splint precaution check-off sheet

- ○ Account for bony prominences such as the following:
  - Metacarpophalangeal (MCP), proximal interphalangeal (PIP), and distal interphalangeal (DIP) joints
  - Pisiform bone
  - Radial and ulnar styloids
  - Lateral and medial epicondyles of the elbow
- ○ Identify fragile skin and select the splinting material carefully. Monitor the temperature of the thermoplastic closely before applying the material to the fragile skin.
- ○ Identify skin areas having impaired sensation. The splint design should not impinge on these sites.
- ○ If fluctuating edema is a problem, consider pressure garment wear in conjunction with a splint.
- ○ Do not compress the superficial branch of the radial nerve. If the radial edge of a forearm splint impinges beyond the middle of the forearm near the dorsal side of the thumb, the branch of the radial nerve may be compressed.

*See Appendix B for a perforated copy of this form.

FORM 5-3* Hints for splint provision

- ○ Give the person oral and written instructions regarding the following:
  - Wearing schedule
  - Care of splint
  - Purpose of splint
  - Responsibility in therapy program
  - Phone number of contact person if problems arise
  - Actions to take if skin reactions such as the following occur: rashes, numbness, reddened areas, pain increase because of splint application
- ○ Evaluate the splint after the person wears it at least 20 to 30 minutes and make necessary adjustments.
- ○ Position all joints incorporated into the splint at the correct therapeutic angle(s).
- ○ Design the splint to account for bony prominences such as the following:
  - MCP, PIP, and DIP joints
  - Pisiform
  - Radial and ulnar styloids
  - Lateral and medial epicondyles of the elbow
- ○ If fluctuating edema is a problem, make certain the splint design can accommodate the problem by using a wider design. Consider pressure garment to wear under splint.
- ○ Make certain the splint design does not mobilize or immobilize unnecessary joint(s).
- ○ Make certain the splint does not impede or restrict motions of joints adjacent to the splint.
- ○ Make certain the splint supports the arches of the hand.
- ○ Take into consideration the creases of the hand for allowing immobilization or mobilization, depending on the purpose of the splint.
- ○ Make certain the splint does not restrict circulation.
- ○ Make certain application and removal of the splint are easy.
- ○ Secure the splint to the person's extremity using a well-designed strapping mechanism.
- ○ Make certain the appropriate edges of the splint are flared or rolled.

*See Appendix B for a perforated copy of this form.

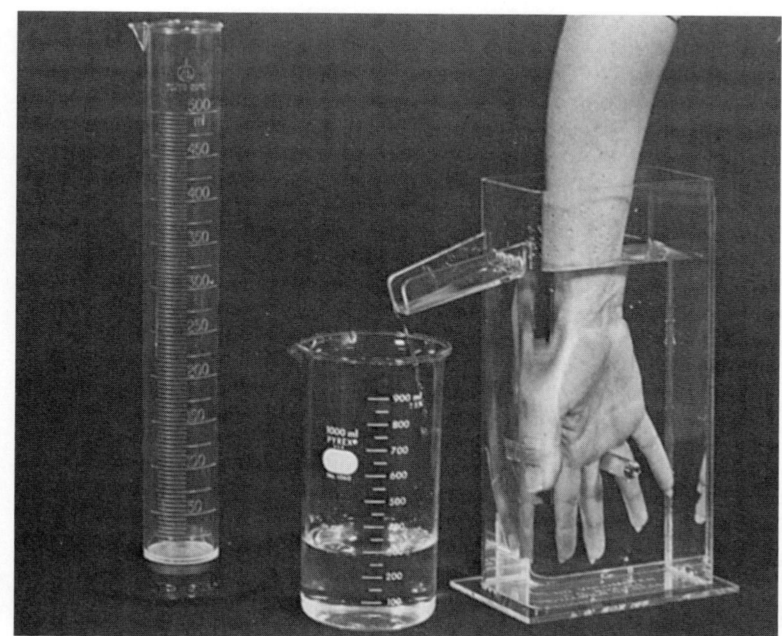

Figure 5-12 The volumeter measures composite hand mass via water displacement. [From Hunter JM, Mackin EJ, Callahan AD (eds.), (1990). *Rehabilitation of the Hand: Surgery and Therapy, Third Edition*. St. Louis: Mosby, p. 63.]

Typically, persons should wear mobilizing (dynamic) splints for a few minutes out of each hour and gradually work up to longer time periods. As with all splints, a therapist never fabricates a mobilizing (dynamic) splint without checking its effect on the person. The therapist also considers the diagnosis and appropriately schedules splint wearing. Often, but not always, a splint regimen will allow for times of rest, exercise, hygiene, and skin relief. The therapist considers the client's daily activity schedule when designing the splint regimen. However, treatment goals must sometimes supersede the desire for the client to perform activities. In addition, the therapist uses clinical judgment to determine and adjust the splint-wearing schedule and reevaluates the splint consistently to alter the treatment plan as necessary.

Compliance

On the basis of the initial interview and statements from conversations, the therapist must determine whether compliance with the wearing schedule and rehabilitation program is a problem. (Chapter 6 contains strategies to help persons with compliance and acceptance.) If the hand demonstrates that the splint is not achieving its goal, the therapist must check that the splint is well designed and fits properly and then determine whether the splint is being worn. If the therapist is certain about the design and fit, compliance is probably poor. Clients returning for follow-up visits must bring their splints. The therapist can generally determine whether a client is wearing the splint by looking for signs of normal wear and tear. Signs include dirty areas or scratches in the plastic, soiled straps, and nappy straps (caused by pulling the strap off the Velcro hook).

Splint Care

Therapists are responsible for educating persons about splint care. An evaluation of a person's understanding of splint care must be completed before the client leaves the clinic. Assessment is accomplished by asking the client to repeat instructions or demonstrate splint care. To keep the splint clean, washing the hand with warm water and a mild soap and cleansing the splint with rubbing alcohol are effective. The person or caregiver should thoroughly dry the hand and splint before reapplication. Chlorine occasionally removes ink marks on the splint. Rubbing alcohol, chlorine bleach, and hydrogen peroxide are good disinfectants to use on the splint for infection control.

Persons should be aware that heat may melt their splints and should be careful not to leave their splints in hot cars, on sunny windowsills, or on radiators. Therapists should discourage persons from making self-adjustments, including the heating of splints in microwave ovens (which may cause splints to soften, fold in on themselves, and adhere). If the person successfully softens the plastic, a burn could result from the application of hot plastic to the skin. However, clients should be encouraged to make suggestions to improve a splint. Therapists, especially novice therapists, tend to ignore the client's ideas. Not only does this send a negative message to the client but clients often have wonderful ideas that are too beneficial to discount.

Summary

Evaluation before splint provision is an integral part of the splinting process. The evaluation process includes report

SELF-QUIZ 5-1*

For the following questions, circle either true (T) or false (F).

1. T F All physicians follow the same protocol for postoperative conditions.
2. T F Motivation may affect the person's compliance for wearing a splint, and thus determining the person's motivational level is an important task for the therapist.
3. T F The resting hand posture is 10 to 20 degrees of wrist extension, 10 degrees of ulnar deviation, 15 to 20 degrees of MCP flexion, and partial flexion and abduction of the thumb.
4. T F Proximal musculature never affects distal musculature.
5. T F Therapists should encourage persons to carry their affected extremities in guarded or protective positions to ensure that no further harm is done to the injury.
6. T F A general guideline for evaluating splint fit is to have the person wear the splint for 20 minutes and then remove the splint. If no reddened areas are present after 20 minutes of splint removal, no adjustments are necessary.
7. T F All splints require 24 hours of wearing to be most effective.
8. T F Every person should receive a splint-wearing schedule in written and verbal forms.
9. T F For infection control purposes, persons and therapists should use extremely hot water to clean splints.
10. T F Strength of a healing tendon is stronger when the tendon is immobilized rather than mobilized.
11. T F A red wound is a healthy wound.
12. T F A score of 10 on a Verbal Analog Scale would indicate that pain does not need to be addressed in the treatment plan.
13. T F Strapping, padding, and thermoplastic materials may cause a skin allergic reaction in some persons.
14. T F Assessments of function include the Nine Hole Peg Test and the Semmes-Weinstein Monofilament Test.

*See Appendix A for the answer key.

reading, observation, interview, palpation, and formal and informal assessments. Evaluation before, during, and after splint provision results in the therapist's ability to understand how the splint affects function and how function affects the splint. A thorough evaluation process ultimately results in client satisfaction.

REVIEW QUESTIONS

1. What are components of a thorough hand examination before splint fabrication?
2. What is the posture of a resting hand?
3. What information should a therapist obtain about the person's history?
4. What sources can therapists use to obtain information about persons and their conditions?
5. What should a therapist be noting when palpating a client?
6. What observations should be made when a client first enters a clinic?
7. What types of formal upper extremity assessments for function are available?
8. What procedure can a therapist use when assessing whether a newly fabricated splint fits well on a person?
9. What precautions should a therapist keep in mind when designing and fabricating a splint?
10. How can a therapist evaluate a client's understanding of a splint-wearing schedule?
11. What safeguard can a therapist employ to avoid skin reactions from splinting materials?

References

American Society for Surgery of the Hand (1983). *The Hand.* New York: Churchill Livingstone.

Aulicino PL, DuPuy TE (1990). Clinical examination of the hand. In JM Hunter, LH Schneider, EJ Mackin, AD Callahan (eds.), *Rehabilitation of the Hand: Surgery and Therapy, Third Edition.* St. Louis: Mosby.

Bear-Lehman J, Abreu BC (1989). Evaluating the hand: Issues in reliability and validity. Physical Therapy 69(12):1025-1031.

Beaton DE, Katz JN, Fossel AH, Wright JG, Tarasuk V, Bombardier C (2001). Measuring the whole or the parts? Validity, reliability, and responsiveness of the Disabilities of the Arm, Shoulder and Hand outcome measure in different regions of the upper extremity. Journal of Hand Therapy 14(2):128-146.

Bell-Krotoski JA (1995). Sensibility testing: Current concepts. In JM Hunter, EJ Mackin, AD Callahan (eds.), *Rehabilitation of the Hand, Fourth Edition.* St. Louis: Mosby.

Bell-Krotoski JA, Buford WL (1997). The force/time relationship of clinically used sensory testing instruments. Journal of Hand Therapy 10(4):297-309.

Blankenship KL (1989). *The Blankenship System: Functional Capacity Evaluation, The Procedure Manual.* Macon, GA: Blankenship Corporation, Panaprint.

Brazier JE, Harper R, Jones N, O'Cathain A, Thomas KJ, Usherwood T (1992). Validating the SF-36 Health Survey Questionnaire: new outcome measure for primary care. British Medical Journal 305:160-164.

Cailliet R (1994). *Hand Pain and Impairment, Fourth Edition*. Philadelphia: F. A. Davis.

Callahan AD (1990). Sensibility testing: Clinical methods. In JM Hunter, LH Schneider, EJ Macklin, AD Callahan (eds.), *Rehabilitation of the Hand: Surgery and Therapy, Third Edition*. St. Louis: Mosby.

Cannon NM, Foltz RW, Koepfer JM, Lauck MF, Simpson DM, Bromley RS (1985). *Manual of Hand Splinting*. New York: Churchill Livingstone.

Case-Smith, 1993

Chapman GD, Goodenough B, von Baeyer C, Thomas W (1998). Measurement of pain by self-report. In GA Finley, PJ McGrath (eds.), *Measurement of Pain in Infants and Children*. Seattle: IASP Press, pp. 123-160.

Cuzzell JZ (1988). The new RYB color code: Next time you assess an open wound, remember to protect red, cleanse yellow and debride black. American Journal of Nursing 88(10):1342-1346.

Dannenbaum RM, Michaelsen SM, Desrosiers J, Levin MF (2002). Development and validation of two new sensory tests of the hand for patients with stroke. Clinical Rehabilitation 16:630-639.

DeKlerk AJ, Jouck LM (1982). Primary tendon healing: An experimental study. South African Medical Journal 62(9):276.

Ebrecht M, Hextall J, Kirtley LG, Taylor A, Dyson M, Weinman J (2004). Perceived stress and cortisol levels predict speed of wound healing in healthy male adults. Psychoneuroendocrinology 29:798-809.

Ellem D (1995). Assessment of the wrist, hand and finger complex. Journal of Manual and Manipulative Therapy 3(1):9-14.

Enebo BA (1998). Outcome measures for low back pain: Pain inventories and functional disability questionnaires. Journal of Chiropractic Technique 10:68-74.

Evans RB, McAuliffe JA (2002). Wound classification and management. In EJ Mackin, AD Callahan, TM Skirven, LH Schneider, AL Osterman (eds.), *Rehabilitation of the Hand and Upper Extremity, Fifth Edition*. St. Louis: Mosby, pp. 311-330.

Fedorczyk JM, Michlovitz SL (1995). Pain control: Putting modalities in perspective. In JM Hunter, EJ Mackin, AD Callahan (eds.), *Rehabilitation of the Hand, Fourth Edition*. St. Louis: Mosby.

Fess EE (1995). Documentation: Essential elements of an upper extremity assessment battery. In JM Hunter, EJ Mackin, AD Callahan (eds.), *Rehabilitation of the Hand, Fourth Edition*. St. Louis: Mosby.

Fess EE, Gettle KS, Philips CA, Janson JR (2005). *Hand and Upper Extremity Splinting: Principles and Methods, Third Edition*. St. Louis: Elsevier Mosby.

Finch E, Brooks D, Stratford PW, Mayo N (2002). *Physical Rehabilitation Outcome Measures: A Guide to Enhanced Clinical Decision Making, Second Edition*. Baltimore: Lippincott, Williams & Wilkins.

Fisher AG (1995). *Assessment of Motor and Process Skills Manual*. Fort Collins, CO: Three Star Press.

Flaherty SA (1996). Pain measurement tools for clinical practice and research. AANA Journal 64:133-140.

Gatchel R, Mayer T, Capra P, Barnett J (1986). Million behavioral health inventory: Predicting physical function in patients with low back pain. Archives of Physical Medicine and Rehabilitation 67:879-882.

Good M, Stiller C, Zauszniewski JA, Anderson GC, Stanton-Hicks M, Grass JA (2001). Sensation and distress of pain scales: Reliability, validity, and sensitivity. Journal of Nursing Measurement 9:219-238.

Jebsen RH, Taylor N, Trieschmann RB, Trotter MJ, Howard LA (1969). An objective and standardized test of hand function. Archives of Physical Medicine and Rehabilitation 50(6):311-319.

Kahl C, Cleland JA (2005). Visual analogue scale, numeric pain rating scale and the McGill Pain Questionnaire: An overview of psychometric properties. Physical Therapy Reviews 10:123-128.

Law M, Baptiste S, Carswell A, McColl M, Polatajko H, Pollock N (1998). *Canadian Occupational Performance Measures, Third Edition*, Ottowa, Ontario: CAOT.

Law M, Baptiste S, McColl M, Opzoomer A, Polatajko H, Pollock N (1990). The Canadian Occupational Performance Measure: An outcome measure for occupational therapy. Canadian Journal of Occupational Therapy 57(2):82-87.

Lindsay WK (1987). Cellular biology of flexor tendon healing. In JM Hunter, LH Schneider, EJ Mackin (eds.), *Tendon Surgery in the Hand*. St. Louis: Mosby.

Massy-Westropp N, Krishnan J, Ahern M (2004). Comparing the AUSCAN osteoarthritis hand index, Michigan hand outcomes questionnaire, and sequential occupational dexterity assessment for patients with rheumatoid arthritis. The Journal of Rheumatology 31:1996-2001.

Melzack R (1975). The McGill pain questionnaire: Major properties and scoring methods. Pain 1:277-299.

Moberg E (1958). Objective methods for determining the functional value of sensibility in the hand. Journal of Bone and Joint Surgery 40:454-476.

Mosely LH, Finseth F (1977). Cigarette smoking: Impairment of digital blood flow and wound healing in the hand. Hand 9:97-101.

Mueller BA, Adams ED, Isaac CA (1997). Work activities. In J Van Deusen, D Brunt (eds.), *Assessment in Occupational Therapy and Physical Therapy*. Philadelphia: W. B. Saunders.

Neviaser RJ (1978). Closed tendon sheath irrigation for pyogenic flexor tenosynovitis. Journal of Hand Surgery 3:462-466.

O'Rourke D (2004). The measurement of pain in infants, children, and adolescents: From policy to practice. Physical Therapy 84:560-570.

Ramadan AM (1997). Hand analysis. In J Van Deusen, D Brunt (eds.), *Assessment in Occupational Therapy and Physical Therapy*. Philadelphia: W. B. Saunders.

Ross RG, LaStayo PC (1997). Clinical assessment of pain. In J Van Deusen, D Brunt (eds.), *Assessment in Occupational Therapy and Physical Therapy*. Philadelphia: W. B. Saunders.

Sanford J, Law M, Swanson L, Guyant G (1994). Assessing clinically important change on an outcome of rehabilitation in older adults. Paper presented at the Conference of the American Society of Aging. San Francisco.

Siana JE, Rex S, Gottrup F (1989). The effect of cigarette smoking on wound healing. Scandinavian Journal of Plastic Reconstructive Surgery & Hand Surgery 23:207-209.

Singer DI, Moore JH, Byron PM (1995). Management of skin grafts and flaps. In JM Hunter, EJ Mackin, AD Callahan (eds.), *Rehabilitation of the Hand: Surgery and Therapy, Fourth Edition*. St. Louis: Mosby.

Smith GN, Bruner AT (1998). The neurologic examination of the upper extremity. Physical Medicine and Rehabilitation: State of the Art Reviews 12(2):225-241.

Smith KL (1990). Wound care for the hand patient. In JM Hunter, LH Schneider, EJ Macklin, AD Callahan (eds.), *Rehabilitation of the Hand: Surgery and Therapy, Third Edition*. St. Louis: Mosby.

Smith KL (1995). Wound care for the hand patient. In JM Hunter, EJ Mackin, AD Callahan (eds.), *Rehabilitation of the Hand: Surgery and Therapy, Fourth Edition*. St. Louis: Mosby.

Smith KL (1992). Wound healing. In BG Stanley, SM Tribuzi (eds.), *Concepts in Hand Rehabilitation*. Philadelphia: F. A. Davis.

Staley MJ, Richard RL, Falkel JE (1988). Burns. In SB O'Sullivan, TJ Schmidtz (eds.), *Physical Rehabilitation: Assessment and Treatment, Third Edition*. Philadelphia: F. A. Davis.

Suk M, Hanson B, Norvell D, Helfelt D (2005). *Musculoskeletal Outcome Measures and Instruments*. Switzerland: AO Publishing.

Tarrier N, Gregg L, Edwards J, Dunn K (2005). The influence of pre-existing psychiatric illness on recovery in burn injury patients: The impact of psychosis and depression. Burns 31:45-49.

Tomancik L (1987). *Directions for Using Semmes-Weinstein Monofilaments*. San Jose, CA: North Coast Medical.

Van Lankveld W, van't Pad Bosch P, Bakker J, Terwindt S, Franssen M, van Riel P (1996). Sequential occupational dexterity assessment (SODA): A new test to measure hand disability. Journal of Hand Therapy 9(1):27-32.

Wadsworth CT (1983). Wrist and hand examination and interpretation. The Journal of Orthopaedic and Sports Physical Therapy 5(3): 108-120.

Walsh M, Muntzer E (1992). Wound management. In BG Stanley, SM Tribuzzi (eds.), *Concepts in Hand Rehabilitation*. Philadelphia: F. A. Davis.

Ware JE (2004). SF-36 Health Survey update. In ME Maruish (editor), *The Use of Psychological Testing for Treatment Planning and Outcomes Assessment, Third Edition*, volume 3, pp. 693-718. Mahwah, NJ: Lawrence Erlbaum Associates.

Ware JE, Snow KK, Kosinski M, Gandek B (2000). *SF-36 Health Survey: Manual and Interpretation Guide*. Lincoln, RI: QualityMetric, Inc.

Weiss S, Falkenstein N (2005). *Hand Rehabilitation: A Quick Reference Guide and Review, Second Edition*. St. Louis: Mosby.

Wilson JA, Clark JJ (2004). Obesity: Impediment to postsurgical wound healing. Adv Skin Wound Care 17:426-435.

CHAPTER 6

Clinical Reasoning for Splint Fabrication

Helene Lohman, MA, OTD, OTR/L
Linda S. Scheirton, PhD

Key Terms

Clinical reasoning
Compliance
Treatment process
Health Insurance Portability and Accountability Act (HIPPA)
Documentation
Splint error
Client safety

Chapter Objectives

1. Describe clinical reasoning approaches and how they apply to splinting.
2. Identify essential components of a splint referral.
3. Discuss reasons for the importance of communication with the physician about a splint referral.
4. Discuss diagnostic implications for splint provision.
5. List helpful hints regarding the hand evaluation.
6. Explain factors the therapist considers when selecting a splinting approach and design.
7. Describe what therapists problem solve during splint fabrication.
8. Describe areas that require monitoring after splint fabrication is completed.
9. Describe the reflection process of the therapist before, during, and after splint fabrication.
10. Discuss important considerations concerning a splint-wearing schedule.
11. Identify conditions that determine splint discontinuation.
12. Identify patient safety issues to consider when splinting errors occur
13. Discuss factors about splint cost and reimbursement.
14. Discuss how Health Insurance Portability and Accountability Act (HIPAA) regulations influence splint provision in a clinic.
15. Discuss documentation with splint fabrication.

Note: This chapter includes content from previous contributions from Sally E. Poole, MA, OTR, CHT and Joan L. Sullivan, MA, OTR, CHT.

In clinical practice there is no simple design or type of splint that applies to all diagnoses. Splint design and wearing protocols vary because each injury is unique. Clinical reasoning regarding which splint to fabricate involves considering the physician's referral, the physician's surgical and rehabilitation protocol, the therapist's conceptual model, the therapist's assessment of the person's needs based on objective and subjective data gathered during the evaluation process, and knowledge about the reimbursement source.

Instructors sometimes teach students only one way to do something when in reality there may be multiple ways to achieve a goal. For example, this book emphasizes the typical methods that generalist clinicians use to fabricate common splints. Learning a foundation for splint fabrication is important. In clinical practice, however, the therapist should use a problem-solving approach and apply clinical reasoning to address each person who needs a splint. Clinical reasoning may include integration of knowledge of biomechanics, anatomy, kinesiology, psychology, conceptual models, pathology, splinting protocols and techniques, clinical experience, and awareness of the person's motivation, compliance, and lifestyle (occupational) needs.

This chapter first overviews clinical reasoning models and then addresses approaches to clinical reasoning from the moment the therapist obtains a splint referral until the person's discharge. This chapter also presents prime questions to facilitate the clinical reasoning process the therapist undertakes during treatment planning throughout the person's course of therapy.

Clinical Reasoning Models

Clinical reasoning helps therapists deal with the complexities of clinical practice. It involves professional thinking during evaluation and treatment interventions [Neistadt 1998]. Professional thinking is the ability to distinctly and critically analyze the reasons for whatever actions therapists make and to reflect on the decisions afterward [Parham 1987]. Skilled therapists reflect throughout the entire splinting process (reflection in action), not solely after the splint is completed (reflection on action) [Schon 1987]. Clinical reasoning also entails understanding the meaning a disability, such as a hand injury, has for each person from the person's perspective [Mattingly 1991]. Various approaches to clinical reasoning have been depicted in the literature, including interactive, narrative, pragmatic, conditional, and procedural reasoning. Although each of these approaches is distinctive, experienced therapists often shift from one type of thinking to another to critically analyze complex clinical problems [Fleming 1991] such as splinting.

Interactive reasoning involves getting to know the person as a human being so as to understand the impact the hand condition has had on the person's life [Fleming 1991]. Understanding this can help identify the proper splint to fabricate. For example, for a person who is very sensitive about his or her appearance after a hand injury the therapist may select a skin-tone splinting material that blends with the skin and attracts less attention than a white splinting material.

With narrative reasoning, the therapist reflects on the person's occupational story (or life history), taking into consideration activities, habits, and roles [Neistadt 1998]. For assessment and treatment, the therapist first takes a top-down approach [Trombly 1993] by considering the roles the person had prior to the hand condition and the meaning of occupations in the person's life. The therapist also considers the person's future and the impact the therapist and the person can have on it [Fleming 1991]. For example, through discussion or a formal assessment interview a therapist learns that continuation of work activities is important to a person with carpal tunnel syndrome. Therefore, the therapist fabricates a wrist immobilization splint positioned in neutral and has the person practice typing while wearing the splint.

With pragmatic reasoning, the therapist considers practical factors such as reimbursement, public policy regulations, documentation, availability of equipment, and the expected discharge environment. This type of reasoning includes the pragmatic considerations of the therapist's values, knowledge, and skills [Schell and Cervero 1993, Neistadt 1998]. For example, a therapist may need to review the literature and research evidence if he or she does not know about a particular diagnosis that requires a splint. If a therapist does not have the expertise to splint a client with a complicated injury, he or she might consider referring the person to a therapist who does have the expertise.

In addition, a therapist may need to make an ethical decision such as whether to fabricate a splint for a terminally ill 98-year-old person. This ethical decision would involve the therapist's values about age and terminal conditions. In today's ever-changing health care environment, there is a trend toward cost containment. Budgetary shortages may require therapists to ration their clinical services. Prospective payment systems for reimbursing the costs of rehabilitation, such as in skilled nursing facilities (SNFs), are a reality. Therapists fabricate splints quickly and efficiently to save costs. The information provided throughout this book may assist with pragmatic reasoning.

With conditional reasoning, the therapist reflects on the person's "whole condition" by considering the person's life before the injury, the disease or trauma, current status, and possible future life status [Mattingly and Fleming 1994]. Reflection is multidimensional and includes the condition that requires splinting, the meaning of having the condition or dysfunction, and the social and physical environments in which the person lives [Fleming 1994]. The therapist then envisions how the person's condition might change as a result of splint provision and therapy. Finally, the therapist realizes that success or failure of the treatment will ultimately depend on the person's cooperation [Fleming 1991, Neistadt 1998]. Evaluation and treatment with this clinical reasoning model begin with a top-down approach, considering the meaning of having an injury in the context of a person's life.

Procedural reasoning involves finding the best splinting approach to improve functional performance, taking into consideration the person's diagnostically related performance areas, components, and contexts [Fleming 1991, 1994; Neistadt 1998]. Much of the material in this chapter, which summarizes the treatment process from referral to discontinuation of a splint, can be used with procedural reasoning. To demonstrate clinical reasoning, Table 6-1 summarizes each approach and includes questions for the therapist to either ask the person or reflect on during splint provision and fabrication. As stated at the beginning of this discussion, each approach is explained separately. However, experienced therapists combine these approaches, moving easily from one to another [Mattingly and Fleming 1994].

Clinical Reasoning Throughout the Treatment Process

The following information assists with pragmatic and procedural reasoning.

Essentials of Splint Referral

The first step in the problem-solving process is consideration of the splint referral. The ideal situation is to receive the

Table 6-1 Clinical Reasoning Approaches

SUMMARY OF APPROACH	KEY QUESTIONS FOR SPLINT PROVISION
Interactive reasoning: Getting to know the person through understanding the impact the hand condition has had on the person's life. The focus of this approach is the person's perspective.	Questions directed to person: • How are you coping with having a hand condition? • How has your hand condition impacted all areas of your lifes? • How will you go about following a splint schedule based on your lifestyle? • What type of support do you need to help you with your splint and hand injury?
Narrative reasoning: Consider the person's occupational story (or life history), taking into consideration activities, habits, and roles. The focus of this approach is the person's perspective.	Questions directed to person: • How have you dealt with difficult situations in your life? • What was your typical daily routine before and after the injury? • How do you deal with changes in your schedule? • What roles (such as parent, friend, professional, hobbyist, volunteer) do you have in your life? • What activities have interested you throughout your life? • What activities are difficult for you to perform? • What activities would you like to continue after treatment is over?
Pragmatic reasoning: Consider practical factors such as reimbursement, documentation, equipment availability, and the expected discharge environment. Also consider the therapist's values, knowledge, and skills.	Questions directed to therapist for self-reflection: • Do I have adequate skills to fabricate this splint? • Where can I get more information to best fabricate the splint? • Are there any ethical issues I will need to address with the provision of this splint? • How long will I be working with this person? • What is the reimbursement source for splint coverage? • If it is a managed care source, have I received proper preauthorization and precertification? • Have I clearly communicated the need for this splint with all appropriate medical personnel, such as case managers? • Have I documented succinctly with adequate detail? • Is my documentation functionally based? • Am I basing the splinting protocol on evidence-based practice? • Have I considered the legal aspects of documentation? • What are the proper supplies to fabricate this splint? • Are there ways I can be more timely and cost-effective in fabricating this splint? • What is the person's discharge environment and how will that impact splint provision?
Conditional reasoning: Reflect on the person's whole condition, taking into consideration the person's life before the condition happened, current status, and possible future status. Consider the condition and meaning of having it, social and physical environments, and cooperation of the person.	Questions directed to the person: • What is your medical history? • What is your social history? Questions directed to the therapist for self-reflection: • What is the person's current medical and functional status? • How will splinting impact the person's functional status? • Will the splint provided assist the client in carrying out valued occupations for activities of daily living (ADL), work, and leisure? • What is the person's expected discharge environment and how can this splint help with the person's discharge plans? • Does the person have adequate resources to attend therapy or follow through with a home program? • Describe the person's level of cooperation. • If the person is not cooperative with wearing the splint, how will that be addressed?
Procedural reasoning: Problem solving the best splinting approach, taking into consideration the person's diagnostically related performance areas, components, and contexts.	Questions directed to therapist: • What in the person's medical history warrants a splint? • What conceptual model will I use to approach splint fabrication? • What problems have I identified from the evaluation that will need to be addressed with splinting? • What problems could occur if the hand is or is not splinted?

Continued

Table 6-1 Clinical Reasoning Approaches—cont'd

SUMMARY OF APPROACH	KEY QUESTIONS FOR SPLINT PROVISION
	• What is the person's rehabilitation potential as a result of getting a splint? • Am I basing the splinting protocol on evidence-based practice? • Am I basing the splinting protocol on functional outcomes? • What is the purpose of this splint (prevention, immobilization, protection, correction of deformity, control/modify scar formation, substitution, exercise)? • Will a fabricated or prefabricated splint best meet the needs of the person? • What will be my splinting approach (immobilization, mobilization, restriction, torque transmission)? • How many joints will be splinted? • What precautions will I follow? • What precautions should the person follow? • Have I developed an appropriate home program? • How is the person's function progressing as a result of the splinting regimen? • Do I need to make adjustments with the splinting protocol? • What would I do differently to fabricate this splint next time?

Examples are inclusive, not exclusive.

splint referral from the physician's office early to allow ample time for preparation. In reality, however, the first time the therapist sees the referral is often when the person arrives for the appointment. In these situations the therapist makes quick clinical decisions. Aside from client demographics, Fess et al. [2005] suggest that therapists also need or should determine the following information.

- Diagnosis
- Date of the condition's onset
- Medical or surgical management
- Purpose of the splint
- Type of splint (immobilization, mobilization, restriction, torque transmission)
- Anatomical parts the therapist should immobilize or mobilize
- Precautions and other instructions
- Timing for splint wear
- Wearing schedule

Therapist/Physician Communication About Splint Referral

A problem that many therapists encounter is an incomplete splint referral that lacks a clear diagnosis. Even an experienced therapist becomes frustrated upon receiving a referral that states "Splint." Splint what? For what purpose? For how long? An open line of communication between the physician and the therapist is essential for good splint selection and fabrication. Most physicians welcome calls from the treating therapist when those calls are specific. If the physician's splint referral does not contain the pertinent information, the therapist is responsible for requesting this information. The therapist prepares a list of questions before calling, and if the physician is not available the therapist conveys the list to the physician's secretary or nurse and agrees on a specific time to call again. Sometimes the secretary or nurse can read the chart notes or fax an operative report to the therapist. The therapist must never rely solely on the client's perception of the diagnosis and splint requirements.

In some cases, the physician expects the therapist to have the clinical reasoning skills to select the appropriate splint for the specific clinical diagnosis. Sometimes a therapist receives a physician's order for an inappropriate splint, a nontherapeutic wearing schedule, or a less than optimal material. It is the therapist's responsibility to always scrutinize each physician referral. If the referral is inappropriate, the therapist should apply clinical reasoning skills to determine the appropriate splinting approach. The therapist makes successful independent decisions with a knowledge base about the fundamentals of splinting and with the ability to locate additional information. Then the therapist calls the physician's office and diplomatically explains the problem with the referral and suggests a better splinting approach and rationale. See Boxes 6-1 and 6-2 for examples of complete and incomplete splinting referrals. Reflect on what you would do if you received the incomplete splint referral.

Diagnostic Implications for Splint Provision

The therapist identifies the person's diagnosis after reviewing the splint order. Often, the therapist can begin the clinical reasoning process by using a categorical splinting approach according to the diagnosis. The first category involves chronic conditions, such as hemiplegia. In such a situation, a splint may prevent skin maceration or contracture. The second category involves a traumatic or acute condition that may encompass surgical or nonsurgical

Box 6-1 Example of an Incomplete Splint Referral

From the Office of Dr. S.
Name: Mrs. P. MR. Number: 415672 Age: 51 Diagnosis: De Quervain's tenosynovitis
Date: August 12th
Fabricate a left hand splint
Dr. S.

Box 6-2 Example of a Complete Splint Referral

From the Office of Dr. S.
Date: August 12th
Name: Mrs. P. MR. Number: 415672 Age: 51 Diagnosis: De Quervain's tenosynovitis
Fabricate a volar-based thumb immobilization splint L U/E with the wrist in 15 degrees dorsiflexion, the thumb CMC joint in 40 degrees palmar abduction and the MCP joint in 10 degrees flexion.
Dr. S.

CMC, Carpometacarpal. *LUE,* Left upper extremity. *MCP,* Metacarpophalangeal.

intervention. For example, the person may have tendinitis and require a nonsurgical splint intervention for the affected extremity.

Regardless of whether the condition is acute or chronic, it is very important that the therapist have an adequate knowledge of diagnostic protocols. By knowing protocols, therapists are aware of any precautions for splinting. For example, for a person with carpal tunnel syndrome the therapist knows to splint the wrist in a neutral position. If the therapist splinted the wrist in a functional position of 30 degrees of extension it could actually harm the person by putting too much pressure on the median nerve. Therapists should keep abreast of current treatment trends through literature, continuing education, and communication with physicians. In all cases, the splint provision approach is individually tailored to each client, beginning with categorization by diagnosis and then adapting the approach according to the client's performance, cognition, and physical environment.

Factors Influencing the Splint Approach

The sections that follow offer specific hints that elaborate on areas of the splinting evaluation the therapist can use with clinical reasoning. (See Chapter 5 for essential components to include in a thorough hand evaluation.)

Age

The person's age is important for many reasons. Barring other problems, most children, adolescents, and adults can wear splints according to the respective protocol. An infant or toddler, however, can usually get out of any splint at any time or place. Extraordinary and creative methods are often necessary to keep splints on these youngsters [Armstrong 2005]. Older persons, especially those with diminished functional capacities, may require careful monitoring by the caregiver to ensure a proper fit and compliance with the wearing schedule.

Occupation

From the interview with the person, family, and caregiver (and from the medical record review), the therapist obtains information about the impact a splint may have on occupational function, economic status, and social well-being. The therapist should carefully consider the meaning the condition has for the person, how the person has dealt with medical conditions in the past, how the person's condition may change as a result of the splint provision, and the person's social environment. Thus, when choosing the splint design and material the therapist considers the person's lifestyle needs. The following are some specific questions to reflect on when determining lifestyle needs.

- What valued occupations, such as work or sports, will the person engage in while wearing the splint?
- Do special considerations exist because of rules and regulations for work or sports?
- In what type of environment will the person wear the splint? For example, will the splint be used in extreme temperatures? Will the splint get wet?
- Will the splint impede a hand function necessary to the person's job or home activities?
- What is the person's normal schedule and how will wearing a splint impact that schedule?

If a physician refers a person for a wrist immobilization splint because of wrist strain, the therapist might contemplate the following question: Is the person a construction worker who does heavy manual work or a computer operator who does light, repetitious work? A construction worker may require a splint of stronger material with extremely secure strapping. The computer operator may benefit from lighter, thinner splint material with wide soft straps. In some situations the person may best benefit from a prefabricated splint.

The therapist determines the person's activity status, including when the person is wearing a splint that does not allow for function or movement (such as a positioning splint). If the person must return to work immediately, albeit in a limited capacity, the splint must always be secure. Proper instructions regarding appropriate care of the limb and the splint are necessary. This care may involve elevation of the affected extremity, wound management, and periodic range-of-motion exercises while the person is working.

When the person plans to continue in a sports program (professional, school, or community based), the therapist checks the rules and regulations governing that particular sport. Rules and regulations usually prevent athletes from wearing hard splint material during participation in the sport, unless the splint design includes exterior and interior padding. Therapists need to communicate with the coach or referee to determine appropriateness of a splint [Wright and Rettig 2005].

Expected Environment

The therapist must consider the person's discharge environment. Some persons return to their own homes and have families and friends who can lend assistance if necessary. For those persons returning to inpatient units or nursing homes, therapists consider instructing the staff in the care and use of the splints. If persons return to psychiatric units or prison wards, therapists consider whether supervision is necessary so that persons cannot use their splints as potential weapons to harm themselves or others.

Activities of Daily Living Responsibilities

The therapist considers the following question: Is the person able to successfully complete all activities of daily living (ADL) and instrumental activities of daily living (IADL) if a splint needs to be worn? For example, the therapist may consider how a person can successfully prepare a meal wearing a splint that immobilizes one extremity. In that case, the therapist may address one-handed meal-preparation techniques.

Person Motivation and Compliance

There has been a limited amount of research investigating compliance issues with splint provision. Only recently have experts considered compliance as it relates to persons with hand injuries [Groth and Wilder 1994, Kirwan et al. 2002]. Many considerations affect compliance with a treatment regimen, including such external factors as socioeconomic status and family support (and such internal factors as the person's perception of the severity of the condition). Knowledge, beliefs, and attitudes about the condition also influence compliance [Bower 1985, Groth and Wulf 1995].

Another factor addressed in research is the psychosocial construct of locus of control, which proposes a relationship between a person's perception of control over treatment outcomes and the likelihood the person will comply with treatment. This perception of control can be internally or externally based [Bower 1985]. For example, an internally motivated person would follow a splint schedule on his or her own motivation. An externally motivated person may need encouragement from the therapist or caregiver to follow a splint-wearing schedule. Often not discussed with compliance are organizational variables and clinic environment issues such as transportation problems, interference with daily schedule, wait time, differing therapists, and clinic location [Kirwan et al. 2002].

The therapist can positively influence the person's compliance and motivation to wear a splint. Establishing goals together may help invest the person in the treatment. Perhaps doing an occupation-focused assessment such as the Canadian Occupational Performance Measure (COPM) can help invest the client in wearing the splint [Law et al. 1998]. If the goals determined by the COPM are improvement of hand function, the therapist discusses how the splint will meet this goal. Furthermore, it is important for the therapist to examine her own treatment goals in relation to the client's goals because there might be disparity between them [Kirwan et al. 2002]. Sometimes the client will have input about the splint design, which should be considered seriously by the therapist. Therapists should convey to clients that success with rehabilitation and splints involves shared responsibility. To attain the splint goal, the therapist must always clarify the person's responsibilities in the treatment plans.

In addition, the therapist should perceive the person as a whole individual with a lifestyle beyond the clinic, not just as a person with an injury. Paramount to compliance is education about the medical necessity of wearing splints, in which the therapist should consider the person's perspectives on the ways the splints would affect his or her lifestyle. Education should be repetitive throughout the time the person wears the splint [Southam and Dunbar 1987, Groth and Wulf 1995]. When the therapist and the physician communicate clearly about the type of splint necessary, the person receives consistent information regarding the rationale for wearing the splint. Showing the way the splint works and explaining the goal of the splint enhance client compliance.

Rather than labeling the person as noncompliant or uncooperative, trained personnel must make a serious attempt to help the person better cope with the injury. The therapist should be an empathetic listener as the person learns to adjust to the diagnosis and to the splint. Compliance also involves both therapist and client [Kirwan et al. 2002]. Box 6-3 presents some of the many factors that may influence compliance with splint wear. Box 6-4 provides some suggested questions that may assist the therapist in eliciting pertinent information from clients about splint compliance, fit, and follow-up.

Others can also have an impact on client compliance. Sometimes a peer wearing a splint can be a role model to help a person who is noncompliant. A supportive spouse or caregiver encourages compliance, and physician support influences compliance. Sometimes a person may need more structured psychosocial support from mental health personnel.

Selection of an appropriate design may alleviate a person's difficulty in adjusting to an injury and wearing a splint. Therapists should ask themselves many questions as they consider the best design. (See the questions listed in the section on procedural reasoning in Table 6-1.)

In addition to splint design, material selection (e.g., soft instead of hard) may influence satisfaction with a splint [Callinan and Mathiowetz 1996]. People with rheumatoid arthritis who wear a soft prefabricated splint consider comfort and ease of use when involved in activities important factors for splint satisfaction [Stern et al. 1997]. (See the discussion of advantages and disadvantages of prefabricated soft splints in Chapter 5.)

Box 6-3 Examples of Factors That May Influence Compliance with Splint Wear

Organizational/Clinic Environment
Time involved with splint wear
Interference with life tasks
Inconsistent therapists
Transportation issues
Long wait time for treatment
Inconvenient clinic location
Noisy clinic with little privacy

Client
Belief in the efficacy of wearing a splint
Belief in one's ability to follow through with the splint-wearing schedule
Poor social support

Treatment
Splint is uncomfortable
Splint is cumbersome
Splint is poorly made

Therapeutic Relationship and Communication
Inconsistent communication between therapists and physicians concerning the splint
Poor understanding, difficulty reading, or being forgetful about instructions on splint wear and care

Adapted from Kirwan T, Tooth L, Harkin C (2002). Compliance with hand therapy programs: Therapists' and patients' perceptions. Journal of Hand Therapy 15(1):31-40.

Making the splint aesthetically pleasing helps with a person's compliance. A person is less likely to wear a splint that is messy or sloppy. This is especially true of children and adolescents, for whom personal appearance is often an important issue.

Splint and strapping materials are now available in a variety of colors. Persons, both children and adults, who are coping successfully with the injury may want to have fun with the splint and select one or more colors. However, a person who is having a difficult time adjusting to the injury may not want to wear a splint in public at all, let alone a splint with a color that draws more attention.

Finally, fabrication of a correct-fitting splint on the first attempt eases a person's anxiety. The therapist is responsible for listening to the person's complaints and adjusting the splint. A therapist's attitude about splint adjustments makes a difference. If the therapist seems relaxed, the person may consider adjustment time a normal part of the splintmaking process. Encouraging effective communication with the person facilitates understanding and satisfaction about splint provision.

Cognitive Status

When a person is unable to attend the therapy program and follow the splinting regimen because of his or her cognitive status, the therapist must educate the family, caregiver, or staff members. Education includes medical reasons for the splint provision, wearing schedule, home program, splint precautions, and splint cleaning. This leads to better cooperation. Sometimes the therapist chooses designs and techniques to maximize the person's independence. For example, instructions are written directly on the splint. Such symbols as suns and moons to represent the time of day can be used in written instructions [personal communication, K. Schultz-Johnson, March 1999]. Simple communication strategies such as showing the client a sheet with a smiley face, neutral face, or frowning face can be used to determine how the client feels about splint comfort.

Box 6-4 Questions for Follow-up Telephone Calls or E-mail Communication Regarding Clients with Splints

The following open- and closed-ended questions may assist you in eliciting pertinent information from clients about splint compliance, fit, and follow-up. Closed-ended questions usually elicit a brief response, often a yes or no.

- Have you been wearing your splint according to the schedule I gave you? If no, why aren't you wearing your splint?
- Have you noticed any reddened or painful areas after removing your splint? If so, where?
- Is the splint easy to put on and take off?
- Are there any tasks you want to do but cannot do when wearing your splint?
- Do you have any concerns about your splint-wearing schedule or care?
- Are there any broken or faulty components on your splint?
- Do you have any questions for me?
- Do you know how to reach me?
- Have you noticed any increased swelling or pain since you've been wearing the splint?

Open-ended questions elicit a qualitative response that may give the therapist more information.

- Will you tell me about a typical day and when you put your splint on and take it off?
- What concerns, if any, might you have about your splint-wear and care schedule?
- What precautions have you been taking in regard to monitoring your splint wear?
- How is the splint affecting your activities at home and at work?
- Are there any areas to improve with our clinic management, which would help with your follow-through with splint wear?
- Can you tell me how you would contact me if you need to do so?
- Do you have any questions for me?

Splinting Approach and Design Considerations

The five approaches to splint design are dorsal, palmar, radial, ulnar, and circumferential. The therapist must determine the type of splint to fabricate, such as a mobilization splint or immobilization splint. Understanding the purpose of the splint clarifies these decisions. For example, when working with a person who has a radial nerve injury the therapist may choose to fabricate a dorsal torque transmission splint (wrist flexion: index-small finger MP extension/index-small finger MP flexion, wrist extension torque transmission splint, ASHT, 1992) to substitute for the loss of motor function in the wrist and MCP extensors. On the basis of clinical reasoning, the therapist may choose in addition to fabricate a palmar-based wrist extension immobilization splint once the person regains function of the MCP extensors. The wrist splint allows the person to engage in functional activities.

In addition to the information the therapist obtains from a thorough evaluation, other factors dictate splint choice. To determine the most efficient and effective splint choice, the therapist must consider the physician's orders, the diagnosis, the therapist's judgment, the reimbursement source, and the person's function.

Physician's Orders

Physicians often predetermine the splint-application approach on the basis of their training, surgical technique, and restriction/torque transmission splint with the ring and little fingers in the anticlaw position of MCP flexion (ring-small finger MP extension restriction/ring-small finger IP extension torque transmission splint, ASHT, 1992). However, a spring wire splint to hold the MCPs in flexion may be ordered if that is the physician's preference. Sometimes the therapist may apply clinical reasoning to determine a different splint design or material than what was ordered. In that case, the therapist calls the physician.

Diagnosis

Frequently, the diagnosis mandates the approach to splint design. The diagnosis determines the number of joints the therapist must splint. The least number of joints possible should be restricted while allowing the splint to accomplish its purpose. Diagnosis also determines positioning and whether the splint should be of the mobilization or immobilization type. For example, using an early mobilization protocol for a flexor tendon repair, the therapist places the base of the splint on the dorsum of the forearm and hand to protect the tendon and to allow for rubber band traction. The wrist and MCPs should be in a flexed position (alternatively, some physicians now prefer a neutral position to block extension). These splints protect the repair and allow early tendon glide. In this example, the repaired structures and the need to begin tendon gliding guide the approach. (See Chapter 11 for more information on mobilization splint fabrication with tendon repairs.)

Therapist's Judgment

The therapist can also determine the splint design and type on the basis of knowledge and experience. For example, when dealing with elective carpal tunnel release the therapist can place a wrist immobilization splint dorsally or volarly directly over the surgical site. As an advocate of early scar management, the therapist chooses a palmar splint and adds silicone elastomer or Otoform to the splint.

Person's Function

The person's primary task responsibilities may influence splint choice. A construction worker's wrist has different demands placed on it than the wrist of a computer operator with the same diagnosis. Not only does the therapist choose different materials for each client but the design approach may be different. A thumb-hole volar wrist immobilization splint decreases the risk of the splint migrating up the arm during the construction worker's activities, as it tightly conforms to the hand. The computer operator may prefer a dorsal wrist immobilization splint to allow adequate sensory feedback and unimpeded flexibility of the digits during keyboard use. (See Chapter 7 for patterns of wrist splints.)

Table 6-2 outlines a variety of positioning choices for splint design. However, therapists should not view these suggestions as strict rules. For example, a skin condition may necessitate that a mobilization extension splint be volarly based rather than dorsally based.

Clinical Reasoning Considerations for Designing and Planning the Splint

The splint designing and planning process involves many clinical decisions about materials and techniques the therapist can use. (Refer to chapters throughout this book for more specifics on materials and techniques.) Initial considerations are often related to infection control procedures.

Infection-Control Procedures

The therapist considers whether dressing changes are necessary. If so, the therapist follows universal precautions and maintains a sterile environment. The therapist should be aware that skin maceration under a splint can more easily occur in the presence of a draining wound. In this situation the therapist first carefully applies a dressing that will absorb the fluid.

Splint fabrication should take place over the dressing, and the therapist should instruct the person in how to apply new dressings at appropriate intervals [Skotak and Stockdell 1988]. Before the application of the splinting material, the

Table 6-2 Common Positioning Choices in Splint Design

SPLINT	VOLAR	DORSAL	RADIAL	ULNAR
Hand immobilization hand splint	X	X		
Wrist immobilization splint	X	X		X
Thumb splint	X	X	X	
Ulnar nerve splint (anticlaw)		X		X
Radial nerve splint		X		
Median nerve splint (thumb CMC palmar abduction mobilization splint)	X	X	X	
Elbow positioning splint	X	X		
Mobilization hand extension splint		X		
Mobilization hand flexion splint	X			

therapist can place a stockinette over the person's bandages. This action prevents the thermoplastic material from sticking to the bandages.

If the person has a draining or infected wound, the therapist does not use regular strapping material to hold the splint in place. Strapping material can absorb bacteria. Instead, the therapist uses gauze bandages that are replaced at each dressing change. If a person is unwilling or unable to change a dressing, the therapist can instruct a family member or friend to do so. If this is not possible, the person may need to visit the therapist more frequently.

Time Allotment for Splint Fabrication and Person and Nursing or Caregiver Education

The therapist also considers the time required for splint fabrication and education. Splint fabrication time varies according to splint complexity and the person's ability to comply with the splinting process. For example, squirmy babies and people with spasticity are more difficult to splint and require more time. In these cases, it may be beneficial to have additional staff or a caregiver to help position the person.

Splint fabrication time is also dependent on the therapist's experience. If possible, a beginning therapist should schedule a large block of time for splint fabrication. As therapists gain clinical experience, they require less time to fabricate splints. With any splint application, the therapist should allow enough time for educating the person, family, and caregiver about the wear schedule, precautions, and their responsibility in the rehabilitation process. As discussed, education helps with compliance.

Batteson [1997] found that in an institutional setting a nurse training program developed by the occupational therapist that addressed splinting was very helpful in increasing compliance with a splint-wearing schedule. This program included splint rationale, common splint care questions, and familiarization with splinting materials. A nurse liaison was identified to deal specifically with the client's splint concerns. In addition, a splint resource file developed by the therapist was made available to the nurses.

Post-fabrication Monitoring

The therapist uses clinical reasoning skills to thoroughly evaluate and monitor the fabricated splint. In particular, the therapist must be aware of pressure areas and edema.

Monitoring Pressure

Regardless of its purpose or design, the splint requires monitoring to determine its effect on the skin. The therapist must remember that a person wearing a splint is superimposing a hard lever system on an existing lever system that is covered by skin, a living tissue that requires an adequate blood supply. The therapist must therefore follow mechanical principles during splint fabrication to avoid excessive pressure on the skin. With fabrication, therapists have to weigh the pros and cons of the amount of splint coverage. With minimal coverage from a splint, there is increased mobility. Increased coverage by a splint allows for more protection and better pressure distribution. To reduce pressure, the therapist should design a splint that covers a larger surface area [Fess et al. 2005]. Warning signs of an ill-fitting splint are red marks and ulcerations on the skin.

A well-fitting splint, after its removal, may leave a red area on the person's skin. This normal response to the pressure of the splint disappears within seconds. When a splint has applied too much pressure on one area, which usually occurs over a bony prominence, the redness may last longer. For persons with dark skin, in whom redness is not easily visible, the therapist may lightly touch the skin to determine the presence of hot spots or warmer skin. Another way to check skin temperature is with a thermometer. With any splint, the therapist checks the skin after 20 to 30 minutes of wearing time before the person leaves the clinic. If red areas are present after 20 to 30 minutes of wearing the splint, adjustments need to be made.

A person with intact sensibility who has an ill-fitting splint usually requests an adjustment or simply discards the splint because it is not comfortable. For a condition in which sensation is absent, vigorous splint monitoring is critical [Brand and Hollister 1993, Fess et al. 2005]. The therapist teaches the person and the family to remove the splint every one to two hours to check the skin so as to avoid skin breakdown.

Monitoring for Skin Maceration

Wet, white, macerated skin can occur when the skin under a splint holds too much moisture. This can occur for many reasons, such as a child drooling on a splint. When this happens to a person with intact skin who has simply forgotten to remove the splint, the therapist can easily correct the problem by washing and drying the area. Educating the person about proper care of the hand and providing a polypropylene stockinette to absorb moisture should resolve this situation.

Monitoring Edema

A therapist frequently needs to splint an edematous extremity. Edema is often present after surgery, in the presence of infection, with severe trauma (e.g., from a burn), or with vascular or lymphatic compromise. A well-designed, well-fitting splint can reduce edema and prevent the sequelae of tissue damage and joint contracture. A poorly designed or ill-fitting splint can contribute to the damaging results of persistent edema. Generally, the design and fit principles already discussed in this text apply.

The therapist also considers the method used to hold the splint in place. Soft, wide straps accommodate increases in edema and are better able to distribute pressure than rigid, non-yielding Velcro straps [Cannon et al. 1985]. When too tight, strapping can contribute to pitting edema as a result of hampered lymphatic flow [Colditz 2002]. For severe edema, the therapist may gently apply a wide elastic wrap to keep the splint in place. The continuous contact of the wrap helps reduce edema [Colditz 2002]. Therapists should be cautioned that straps applied at intervals may further restrict circulation and cause "windowpane" edema distally and between the straps. When using Ace wraps or compressive gauze, the therapist must apply them in a figure-of-eight pattern and use gradient distal-to-proximal pressure. The therapist must properly monitor the splint and wrap to ensure that the wrap does not roll or bunch [Mackin et al. 2002]. Pressure created by rolling or bunching could cause constriction and further edema and stiffness.

If the lymphatic system is not damaged, edema reduction usually begins relatively quickly with appropriate wound healing (i.e., no infection), proper elevation, and gentle active exercises as permitted. As edema resolves, the therapist remolds the splint to fit the new configuration of the extremity. The therapist asks the person with severe edema to return to the clinic daily for monitoring and treatment. When the edema appears to be within the normal postoperative range, the therapist asks the person to return to the clinic in three to five days for a splint check. Helping the person understand the frequency and purpose of the splint adjustments is also important. Again, education is an important part of the edema-reduction regimen [Mackin et al. 2002].

Monitoring Physical and Functional Status

When a person's physical or functional status changes, a splint adjustment is often necessary. If a person is receiving treatment for a specific injury and it is effective, the splint requires adjustments in conjunction with improvement. For example, if a person has a median nerve injury in which the thumb has an adduction contracture the therapist fabricates a thumb CMC palmar abduction mobilization splint [ASHT 1992] to gradually widen the tight web space. As treatment progresses and thumb motions increase, the therapist adjusts the splint to accommodate the gains in motion [Reynolds 1995].

Evaluation and Adjustment of Splints

After fabricating the splint, the splintmaker carefully evaluates the design to determine fit and necessary adjustments. The therapist looks carefully at the splint when the person is and is not wearing it and considers whether the splint serves its purpose. The splint should be functional for the person and should accomplish the goals for which it was intended. It should also have a design that uses correct biomechanical principles and should be cosmetically appealing. (Refer to specific chapters in this book for hints and splint-evaluation forms.)

Therapists learn from self-reflection before, during, and after each splint is made. This helps fine-tune professional thinking skills. The following are reflective questions the therapist can consider after splint fabrication.

- Did the splint accomplish the purpose for which it was intended?
- Is it correctly fitted according to biomechanical principles?
- Did I select the best materials for the splint?
- Did I take into consideration fluctuating edema?
- Is it cosmetically appealing?
- Is it comfortable for the person and free of pressure areas?
- Have I addressed how splinting impacts the person's valued occupations?
- Have I addressed functional considerations?
- What would I do differently if I were to refabricate this splint?

If major adjustments are required, the therapist should avoid using a heat gun except to smooth splint edges. If the therapist has selected the appropriate simple splint design and has used a thermoplastic product that is easily reheatable and remoldable, the water-immersion method is the best way to adjust the splint. Years of experience demonstrate that reheating the entire splint in water and reshaping it is more efficient than spot heating. The activity of the therapist reheating and adjusting one spot often affects the adjacent area, thereby producing another area requiring adjustment. This cycle may not end until the splint is useless. When possible, the therapist should use a splint product that is reheatable in water and easily reshapable to obtain a proper fit for the client.

Splint-Wearing Schedule Factors

Development of a splint-wearing schedule for a person is sometimes extremely frustrating for a beginning splintmaker because there are no magic numbers or formulas for each type of splint or diagnostic population. The therapist tailors and customizes the wearing schedule to the individual and exercises clinical judgment. Only general guidelines for splint-wearing schedules exist.

In the case of joint limitation, the therapist increases the wearing frequency and time as much as the person can tolerate. Alternatively, the therapist adjusts the treatment plan to try a different splint. If motion is increasing steadily, the therapist may decrease the splint-wearing time, allowing the person to engage in function by using the limited joint or joints. If the splint improves function or the extremity requires protection, the person wears the splint when necessary. The following are questions to consider when determining a wearing schedule.

- What is the purpose of the splint?
- Does the therapist anticipate that the person will be compliant with a splint-wearing schedule?
- Does the person have any medical contraindications or precautions for removing the splint?
- Which variables may affect the person's tolerance of the splint?
- Does the person need assistance to apply or remove the splint?
- Is the splint for day or night use, or both?
- Does the person need to apply or remove the splint for any functions?
- How often does the person need to perform exercises and hygiene tasks?

Answers to these questions should guide the development of a wearing schedule. The therapist should keep in mind that the wearing schedule may require adjustment as the person's condition progresses. In any situation, the therapist should discuss the wearing schedule with the person and caregiver. Box 6-5 shows a sample wearing schedule the therapist can post in a person's room or give to the person to take home.

Box 6-5 Sample Wearing Schedule

Person's name:
Name of splint:
The purpose of this splint is to maintain the hand in a functional position.
Prescribed wearing schedule:
8 AM-12 PM On*
12 PM -2 PM Off Provide PROM
2 PM -6 PM On*
6 PM -8 PM Off Provide PROM
8 PM -12 AM On*
12 AM -2 AM Off Provide PROM
2 AM -6 AM On*
6 AM -8 AM Off Provide PROM
Wear the splint on the right upper extremity. Please contact J. Smith at [phone number] in the Occupational Therapy Department if any of the following occur:

- Pink or reddened areas
- Complaints of increased pain because of the splint
- Increased swelling with splint wear
- Skin rash
- Complaints of decreased sensation because of the splint

*Skin check to be performed.
PROM (passive range of motion).

Discontinuation of a Splint

No distinct rules exist concerning a splint's discontinuation. Sometimes the physician makes the decision to discontinue a splint. Other times the physician defers to the clinical judgment of the therapist to determine when a splint is no longer beneficial. Sometimes specific protocols, such as for a flexor tendon repair, indicate when a splint should be discontinued. In such cases, the therapist should contact the physician for a splint-discharge order. Sometimes physicians order a splint to be discontinued "cold turkey." If the therapist clinically reasons that the person would benefit from being weaned off the splint, the physician should be contacted. The therapist should communicate the rationale for the weaning and ask for approval. The following are questions to consider when making the clinical decision to discontinue a splint.

- Have the person and the caregivers been compliant with the splint-wearing schedule? If not, why?
- What are the original objectives for the splint's provision, and has the person accomplished them?
- Will the same objectives be compromised or accomplished without a splint?

The compliance of the person and the caregiver is essential for success with a splint-wearing regimen. If the person is not wearing the splint, the therapist first uses clinical reasoning to identify the reasons for noncompliance. For example, the noncompliance of an older person in an institutional setting could be the result of one or more of the following factors: (1) poor communication among the staff about the splint-wearing schedule, (2) poor staff follow-through with the splint-wearing schedule, (3) the elder's lack of understanding about the splint's purpose, (4) discomfort of the splint, (5) the elder's fear of hidden costs associated with the splint, and (6) the elder's dislike of the splint's cosmetic appearance. Reasons for noncompliance could be beyond this list and it would be up to the therapist to ascertain the problem. After identifying the reason or reasons for noncompliance, the therapist can work on possible solutions.

An important factor in determining when to discontinue the splint is a careful review of the splint's objectives. For example, a therapist fabricates a mobilization splint for a person who has a proximal interphalangeal (PIP) soft-tissue flexion contracture of the middle finger. The splint's objective is mobilization of the PIP joint to help correct the flexion deformity. Gradually, the splint lengthens the restricting structures and extension is restored. By monitoring range of motion (ROM) and evaluating the splint's line of pull, the therapist determines that the splint has maximally helped the person and that the original treatment objectives were accomplished. At this time, the therapist calls the physician for an order to discontinue the splint.

The therapist must consider whether accomplishment of the objectives is possible without the splint. Timely discontinuation of any splint is important. The therapist should keep in mind that inappropriately provided or poorly fabricated splints can restrict movement, make postural compromises by causing atrophy in one muscle group and overuse in another, and injure other parts of the anatomy. In addition, preventing the person's dependence on a splint is important. When the person has the functional capabilities, the therapist should adjust the splint-wearing schedule to gradually wean the person away from the splint [Pascarelli and Quilter 1994].

Cost and Reimbursement Issues

Two issues exist regarding the cost of splints. First, how does the therapist arrive at the price of a splint? Second, how does the therapist receive payment for a splint? To calculate the price of a splint, the therapist totals the direct and indirect costs. Direct costs include such items as the thermoplastic material, strapping material, stockinette, rivets, shipping cost, tax, and so on. A hospital or clinic purchases supplies at wholesale cost. However, a percentage markup may appear on the cost. (This assists with replenishing the inventory.) Indirect costs include nondisposable supplies such as scissors and fry pans, the time required for the average therapist to make the splint, and overhead costs such as rent and electricity. See Table 6-3 for examples of how to figure out direct and indirect costs.

As a result of tighter control of the health-care dollar in managed care and prospective payment systems, many therapists are finding that reimbursement for splints is becoming increasingly difficult. It is important that when necessary the therapist take an active role in the outcome of a reimbursement policy of an insurance plan regarding splints. This may help obtain reimbursement for the splint. For example, knowing that a splint is reimbursed from a health maintenance organization (HMO), the therapist gets preauthorization to qualify the fabrication of a splint. The therapist will also get precertification to observe the person for a specified amount of time.

The therapist must remember, however, that the plan belongs to the person, not to the therapist. If a particular insurance plan reimburses costs partially or not at all, the therapist should inform the client of the responsibility for paying the balance of the cost. Some facilities make accommodations for people who are uninsured or underinsured and need splint provision, or there might be a pro-bono clinic available in the area. In addition, the therapist should provide specific documentation to insurance companies about the affected extremity and the type of splint and purpose of the splint [personal communication, R. B. Evans, February 7, 1995].

It is important that therapists know how to effectively navigate the system to receive reimbursement for splint

Table 6-3 Hints for Determining Direct and Indirect Costs

Indirect Costs

Items

- Lighting, space, fry pan, hydrocollator, scissors, heat gun, shipping, handling, and storage charges for materials.
- Indirect costs are usually figured in a percentage mark-up of the direct costs of a splint (for example, a 10% mark-up cost).

Direct Costs

Thermoplastic Material

- Know cost of sheet
- Estimate how much of the sheet you used
- Determine cost (¼ sheet used)

Strapping

- Know cost per inch
- Charge for number of inches used

Padding

- Know cost per square inch
- Charge for number of square inches used

Chemicals (cold spray, glue, solvent, and so on)

- Usually a small set amount is charged whenever chemicals are used

Other materials (finger loops, outrigger kit, D-rings, and so on)

- Charge the purchase amount

Time

- Know cost per unit of time
- Charge for number of units used to make the splint

fabrication. If a splint is ordered, it needs to be made. The therapist and the client should work out financial aspects with the facility. Communication with the appropriate persons in the facility.

For some persons with upper extremity problems that occurred on the job, rehabilitation is reimbursed from the Worker's Compensation System. Therapists must keep in mind that in every state the Worker's Compensation law is interpreted differently. Therefore, it is important to familiarize oneself with the state guidelines. Most state worker compensation plans cover medical costs related to the injury, such as medical care (including receiving a splint), vocational rehabilitation, and temporary disability (the amount varies from state to state) [Bailey 1998]. Many states have adopted a managed care system. If case managers are involved in the person's care, the therapist should provide consistent and clear communication about the person's progress.

Some insurance companies simply refuse to pay for splints, and others ask for so much documentation that more time is required to prepare the bill than to make the splint. For example, some insurance companies ask therapists for original invoices for the purchase of thermoplastic and strapping materials. Developing outcome studies or finding outcome data in the literature may help with reimbursement from insurers, especially managed care organizations (MCOs). Giving these outcomes to insurers will increase their understanding of the importance of splinting in its relation to function. The American Society of Hand Therapists (1992) published *Splint Classification Systems*, a book on naming and designing splints. This book helps with terminology becoming more uniform [American Society of Hand Therapists 1992].

Policy Regulations: The Health Insurance Portability and Accountability Act

This broad health legislation enacted in 1996 covers many areas with Title II, or *Administrative Simplification*, influencing therapy practice. Title II includes three main parts: *Transaction Rule*, *Privacy Rule*, and *Security Rule*.

The first part, *Transaction Rule*, affects billing procedures. It mandates uniform national requirements for formats and codes for electronic transmission [Wilson 2004].

Privacy Rule is another major component of *Administrative Simplification* and directly influences clinical practice. These rules involve protection of client-identifying or confidential information and client rights about their health information. It regulates how protected health information (PHI) or any client-identifying information is presented in written, verbal, or electronic format [U.S. Department of Health and Human Services 2003]. Therapists should obtain the client's consent prior to using PHI for treatment, payment, or health care operations. However, if a client objects or fails to provide consent therapists are permitted to use PHI for treatment, payment, or health care operations without the client's consent. In most other circumstances, with very few exceptions, therapists may not disclose PHI without the client's written authorization to do so [U.S. Department of Health and Human Services 2004].

Numerous privacy rights with respect to the client's health information are written into the regulations. For example, clients have a right to request to see their medical record. See Box 6-6 for a listing of client protections. Therapy clinics should have policies in place to protect the privacy of client information. Requiring working charts to be kept in a locked cabinet with the documents shredded after treatment completion is an example of an internal policy protecting privacy [Costa and Whitehouse 2003]. Some areas of client information are excluded from the law, such as allowing clients to sign in for treatment, calling out a client's name to go into the splint fabrication room, or sharing information with another health professional about the splint [Costa and Whitehouse 2003, Sullivan 2004]. However, reasonable efforts to avoid these types of disclosures should be taken. For instance, instead of calling out "Mr. Edward Jones, the therapist will see you now to customize your resting hand splint," a better approach would be "Edward, the therapist will see you now."

Incidental disclosures (information that is heard with reasonable efforts to not be overheard) or sharing information that is limited are not considered in violation of the HIPAA law [Sullivan 2004]. An example of an *incidental disclosure* is an occupational therapist discussing information about a splint bill with the secretary in the waiting room. These disclosures are not considered liable under the law as long as there are no other reasonable options (i.e., no other area for

Box 6-6 Client Protections

The following are key client protections with a brief description. For more complete information, go to *http://www.hhs.gov/news/facts/privacy.html*.

- *Access to medical records:* See or obtain copies of medical records and ask for corrections of errors.
- *Notice of privacy practice:* Covered providers must provide information on how personal medical information will be used and patient rights under HIPPA regulations.
- *Limits on use of personal medical information:* Sets guidelines on minimal standards of health care information sharing.
- *Prohibition on marketing:* Sets guidelines on disclosing of client information for marketing purposes.
- *Stronger state laws:* State laws that are stronger than HIPAA are followed.
- *Confidential communications:* Clients can request that confidentiality be kept (e.g., asking the therapist to call his or her work instead of home).
- *Complaints:* Clients have a right to file a formal complaint.

individual privacy to discuss the bill) [personal communication, J. M. Sullivan, October 12, 2004]. Because therapy often takes place in an open area with several people involved in conversations, some of which potentially involve sharing of PHI, it needs to be clear in the consent form about the clinic setup [Murer 2002].

Therapists working in such clinics can employ simple strategies to allow more privacy, such as partitioning off a private area or using a private room available for treatment, communicating with lower voices, and being careful with leaving sensitive messages on answering machines [York 2003]. As York [2003, p. 45] states, "creating a culture of privacy and maintaining good rapport with patients will go a long way to preventing HIPAA complaints as well as other types of legal problems."

The third main part of *Administrative Simplification*, the *Security Rule*, involves the policies and procedures a facility has in place to protect the PHI through "administrative, technical and physical safeguards" [Wilson 2004, p. 132]. It mainly focuses on "electronic protected health information" [Wilson 2004, p. 133] such as who has access to computer data in a clinic. Finally, therapists must keep abreast of their state privacy laws. If they are stricter, they take priority over the HIPAA regulations [York 2003].

Documentation

Splint application must be well documented. Documentation assists in third-party reimbursement and communication with other health care providers, helps ascertain the medical-legal necessity, and demonstrates the efficacy of the intervention.

Splint documentation should be specific and should include several elements, such as the onset of the medical condition that warrants a splint; the medical necessity for the splint; the level of function before the splint; the person's rehabilitation potential with the splint; and type, purpose, and anatomical location of the splint. Therapists should also document that they have communicated with the person an oral and written schedule and have had discussions about precautions. Any input the person provides to the treatment plan, such as mutual goal setting, should be documented.

Splint documentation, including goal setting, should be related to function. It is not sufficient to document that a person's ROM has improved to a certain level as a result of wearing a splint. The therapist should specifically document how the improved ROM has helped the person perform specific functional activities. For example, the therapist may document that because of improved wrist motion from wearing a splint the person is able to write at work.

As with any documentation, the therapist should consider legal implications. Documentation should be thorough, complete, and objective. The therapist should always remember, "If it wasn't documented it didn't happen." For example, the therapist should document the specific measurements by which the hand is splinted for a person who has de Quervain's tenosynovitis. Also for example, if the person has a reddened area as a result of wearing a splint the specific location and size of the reddened area as well as any splint adjustments made should be documented. Any communication or advice about the splint from the physician should be documented, with the time and date of the call [Ekelman-Ranke 1998].

Documentation for follow-up visits should include the date and time the person is supposed to return and a notation that the date and time had been discussed with the person. This helps protect the therapist if there are claims of negligence with follow-up care [Ekelman-Ranke 1998]. Documentation for follow-up visits should also include any changes in the splint's design and wearing schedule. In addition, the therapist should note whether problems with compliance are apparent. Documenting evidence of compliance includes documenting instructions provided and objective person's or caregiver's behavior that contradicts instructions. For example, the therapist might document that the person stated that he or she did not follow the splint-wearing schedule.

Also for example, for a person in a skilled nursing facility the therapist bases documentation on objective observations of dates and times the splint-wearing schedule is not being followed. The therapist in this case may then further educate the caregivers and note when and what type of education was completed. If the caregivers still do not properly follow the schedule, the therapist should come up with another plan and involve the caregivers in the decision-making process to ensure compliance. Another objective observation for a person followed in any setting is notation of signs of wear, such as scratching, light soil, or strap wear. In documentation, it is inappropriate to criticize other health care professionals, such as documenting that contractures developed in a person as a result of the nursing staff's not having applied a splint [Ekelman-Ranke 1998].

The therapist should perform splint reassessments regularly until completion of the person's weaning from the splint or discharge from services. Documentation after the reassessments should be timely and based on guidelines from the insurer [Ekelman-Ranke 1998]. Finally, the therapist should keep in mind that different facilities use different methods to document, and the therapist should be familiar with the routine method of the facility. (See Examples 6-1 and 6-2 for illustrations, respectively, of a narrative and a SOAP note for a splint.)

Splinting Error and Client Safety Issues

Splinting errors occur in occupational therapy [Scheirton et al. 2003]. Examples of these errors include fabricating the wrong type of splint for the condition or failure to follow through with the splint-wearing schedule. Either of these errors could cause client harm such as severe pain or breakdown of the skin. Although many errors are the direct result of individual failure, most errors are caused by system problems. System errors may occur due to diagnostic error, equipment/product failure, or miscommunication of medical orders, to name a few. Splinting errors can easily result from incorrect or inadequate communication. A physician, for example, may order a right hand splint when it is meant for the left hand. If the therapist fails to question the physician order, a splint may be fabricated for the wrong site.

According to data collected by the Joint Commission on Accreditation of Healthcare Organizations (JCAHO), team miscommunication is at the root of a great proportion of all errors made in health care [Joint Commission on Accreditation of Healthcare Organizations 2005a, 2005b]. Occupational therapists often lack assertiveness when communicating with physicians, and this failure to adequately communicate can result in patient harm [Lohman et al. 2004]. Understanding the nature of hierarchic organizational structures and the need for coordination of care through "interdisciplinary care management" and "coordinated communication" are vital to client safety [Joint Commission on Accreditation of Healthcare Organizations 2005a, p. 161].

To create this culture of safety, occupational therapists must debunk or dispel the myth of performance perfection. To err is human! After all, health care delivery is a very complex system. In complex systems, errors are inevitable regardless of how well trained, well intentioned, or ultra-careful the individual therapist may be. In the case of the therapist acting on the physician's wrong order, it would be unjust to simply require the last treating practitioner to be fully accountable for the error. In this situation, blaming and sanctioning would only encourage the therapist and/or physician to hide the error rather than disclose and report it.

Today's undisclosed near miss or minor error can become tomorrow's egregiously harmful error. Only by acknowledging error can we individually and collectively learn from that error and make individual and system practice changes to prevent errors in the future. Furthermore, truthful disclosure of error to clients by the therapist or a disclosure team is not only an ethical obligation but is now dictated by JCAHO standards as well as varied institutional policies [Joint Commission on Accreditation of Healthcare Organizations 2001, Minneapolis Children's Hospital and Clinics 2001, Dana-Farber Cancer Institute 2004]. Ultimately, creating an environment where practitioners are encouraged and supported for promoting safety and reporting errors and disclosing them to clients is everyone's goal. This practice safety goal for practice should always be a guidepost for clinical reasoning when splint fabrication failures occur.

EXAMPLE 6-1

The following is an initial progress note (IPN) following splint fabrication. Abbreviations used in the narrative are as follows: AROM = active range of motion, BUE = bilateral upper extremities, Hx = history, L = left, LTG = long-term goal, MMT = manual muscle testing, OT = occupational therapy, Pt. = patient, R = right, RUE = right upper extremity, STG = short-term goal, TAM = total active motion, and WNL = within normal limits.

February 24, 20__, 4:00 pm

This 42-year-old female was seen by an occupational therapist for fabrication of a right wrist immobilization splint on the dominant right upper-extremity. Client has a history of carpal tunnel syndrome since August this year. Client reports being independent in activities of daily living (ADL), work, and leisure tasks before condition developed. Client displays problems related to carpal tunnel syndrome including decreased R grip strength, R hand swelling at end of day, pain, tingling, decreased sensation in the area of the median nerve, and a positive Phalen's sign (refer to the summary report of the Semmes-Weinstein Monofilament testing). Client displays problems with cooking meals and typing on computer at work. Client currently requires help from her daughter for such tasks as opening cans and jars and cutting food with a knife. Client is employed as a secretary, and job demands primarily involve computer work. At work, client tolerates 20 minutes of typing on computer before pain and tingling develop in the R hand. Client stated, "It is difficult for me to type on the computer and cook a meal." BUE AROM was WNL except for the following motions RUE:

- Thumb: opposition to ring finger-unable to oppose little finger
- R Finger TAM: (normal = 250-265 degrees)
  - Index = 230 degrees
  - Middle = 230 degrees
  - Ring = 240 degrees
  - Little = 270 degrees
- R Wrist:
  - Flexion = 0-50 degrees (norm = 0-80 degrees)
  - Wrist Extension (WNL)
  - Radial Deviation = 0-15 degrees (norm = 0-20 degrees)
  - Ulnar Deviation (WNL)

Grip strength was tested with Jamar dynamometer. R grip strength = 30 pounds (10th percentile for age and gender) and L grip strength = 64 pounds (norm = 75th percentile for age and gender). MMT results as follows:

- R abductor pollicis = 3 (fair)/5, L = 5 (normal)/5
- Opponens pollicis: R = 3 (fair)/5, L = 5 (normal)/5

A R volar-based, neutral wrist immobilization splint was fabricated. Client presented with no pressure marks or rash after splint application. Client was evaluated for functional hand motions while wearing the splint. The splint does not restrict finger and thumb motions. Client received verbal and written instructions about splint wearing schedule and a form to document wearing compliance. Client was able to independently don and doff her splint. Client received verbal and written instructions for a home exercise program, splint precautions, and ergonomic adaptations for home and work environments. Client's understanding of all instructions appeared to be good. Client will be followed two more times per physician order to monitor splint and program and ergonomic adaptations.

OT Goals:

LTGs: Client will report a decrease in R hand pain and tingling so as to complete home and work activities independently by (date).

STGs:

- Client will independently complete computer tasks at work while wearing R wrist splint for 3 hours daily and taking hourly exercise breaks by (date).
- Client will independently cook a meal while wearing R wrist splint and report reduced pain by (date).
- Client will properly position BUEs during computer work activities and utilize ergonomic office equipment by (date).
- Client will comply with splint wearing schedule 90% of the time as evidenced by the splint wearing schedule compliance sheet by (date).

EXAMPLE 6-2

The following is an OT SOAP note. Abbreviations used in the SOAP note are as follows: AROM = active range of motion, BUE = bilateral upper extremities, Hx = history, L = left, LTG = long-term goal, OT = occupational therapy, Pt. = patient, R = right, RUE = right upper extremity, STG = short-term goal, TAM = total active motion, and WNL = within normal limits.

John Smith, OTR/L

February 24, 20__, 4:00 PM

S (subjective): "My right hand tingles and hurts all the time." Client also reports difficulty cooking meals and typing on the computer while at work.

O (objective): Client presents with an Hx of carpal tunnel symptoms in her dominant, R, hand since August of this year. Client reports being independent in activities of daily living (ADL), work, and leisure tasks before condition developed. Client displays a positive R Phalen's sign with decreased sensation in the R median nerve distribution area (refer to Semmes-Weinstein Monofilament summary sheet). BUE AROM was WNL, except for the following motions:

- R thumb opposition to ring finger-unable to oppose little finger
- R finger TAMs (normal = 250-265 degrees):
  - Index = 230 degrees
  - Middle = 230 degrees
  - Ring = 240 degrees
  - Little = 270 degrees
- R wrist: Flexion = 0-50 degrees (norm = 0-80 degrees)
- Wrist Extension (WNL)
- Radial Deviation = 0-15 degrees (norm = 0-20 degrees)
- Ulnar Deviation (WNL)

Grip strength was tested with Jamar dynamometer. R grip strength = 30 pounds (10th percentile for age and gender). L grip strength = 64 pounds (75th percentile for age and gender). MMT results as follows:

- Abductor pollicis: R = 3 (fair)/5, L = 5 (normal)/5
- Opponens pollicis: R = 3 (fair)/5, L = 5 (normal)/5

Client displays problems related to carpal tunnel syndrome including decreased R grip strength, R hand swelling at end of day, and problems with cooking meals and typing on computer at work. Client currently requires help from her daughter for such tasks as opening cans and jars and cutting food with a knife. At work, client tolerates 20 minutes of typing on computer before pain and tingling develop in the R hand.

A R volar-based, neutral wrist immobilization splint was fabricated. Client presented with no pressure marks or rash after splint application. Client was evaluated for functional hand motions while wearing the splint. The splint does not restrict finger and thumb motions. Client received verbal and written instructions about splint wearing schedule and a form to document wearing compliance. Client was able to independently don and doff her splint. Client received verbal and written instructions for a home exercise program, splint precautions, and ergonomic adaptations for home and work environments. Client's understanding of all instructions appeared to be good.

A (assessment): Client seems to have a good rehabilitation potential as she reports motivation to comply with OT treatment. Client is able to complete functional activities while wearing the R wrist immobilization splint. Symptoms may decrease with splint wear and with implementation of the home exercise program and ergonomic home and work adaptations.

P (plan): Client will be followed two more times per physician order to monitor splint and program and ergonomic adaptations.

OT Goals:

LTGs: Client will report a decrease in R hand pain and tingling so as to complete home and work activities independently by (date).

STGs:

- Client will independently complete computer tasks at work while wearing R wrist splint for 3 hours daily and taking hourly exercise breaks by (date).
- Client will independently cook a meal while wearing R wrist splint and report reduced pain by (date).
- Client will properly position BUEs during computer work activities and utilize ergonomic office equipment by (date).
- Client will comply with splint wearing schedule 90% of the time as evidenced by the splint wearing schedule compliance sheet by (date).

(John Smith, OTR)

SELF-QUIZ 6-1*

Circle either true (T) or false (F) with regard to the following questions.

1. T F An infant can follow a splint-wearing program without extraordinary methods.
2. T F Determining a person's lifestyle needs for splint design and material is important.
3. T F Paramount to a person's cooperation is education about the medical necessity for wearing a splint.
4. T F If a person has a wound that requires dressing, the therapist should fabricate the splint over the dressing and instruct the person to apply new dressings at appropriate intervals.
5. T F The only sign of an ill-fitting splint is red marks.
6. T F A well-fitting splint, upon removal, may leave a red area on the person's skin.
7. T F In the presence of severe edema, the therapist should use circumferential straps.
8. T F The therapist should use a heat gun for all necessary adjustments.
9. T F If motion is decreased because of joint limitation, the therapist should decrease the frequency or time the person wears the splint.
10. T F When deciding to discontinue a splint, the therapist must consider the original objectives of the splint's fabrication.
11. T F To calculate the cost of a splint, the therapist should consider the direct and indirect costs.
12. T F If a person develops a reddened area because of wearing a splint, the therapist should just document that fact and note specifics about location or size of the affected area.
13. T F Calling out a person's name in a waiting room to go back into the splinting area is considered in violation of HIPAA.

*See Appendix A for the answer key

CASE STUDY 6-1

Read the following scenario and answer the questions based on information in this chapter.

Randy, a 46-year-old construction worker who has problems with alcohol consumption, awakened from a drinking binge after he fell asleep with his arm over the top of a chair to find that his right hand and wrist were limp. He showed his wife how he could no longer extend his wrist to do activities and stated, "Maybe I had a stroke." Hoping that his function would improve, he waited a few days and then decided to see his primary physician. Randy asserted to his physician that he thought he had a stroke and was concerned about his ability to do work. The physician examined Randy's arm and stated, "I can't say for certain whether it was a small stroke or a nerve injury. In the past with issues like this I have referred patients to an occupational therapist at an outpatient therapy clinic." Occupational therapy was ordered for treatment and splint fabrication. The order was vague as to what type of splint.

You are a new therapist at the outpatient clinic. Initial evaluation reveals decreased sensation in the pathway of the radial nerve, absent wrist extension, MCP finger extension, and thumb abduction and extension. Please refer to Chapter 2 for information on nerve injuries.

1. What injury do you assume Randy has sustained and how did he sustain it?

2. How do you clarify the physician's order if you are unsure about it?

3. As a new therapist unsure about which one, where would you find the information about an appropriate splint for this patient?

4. After completion of the splint, you send Randy home with a home program and instructions about splint wear. What type of education and splint-wearing schedule will you provide? Why?

5. Upon return to the clinic Randy states that he does not like wearing the splint because, as he states, "It does not fit with my macho image and it seems like it is taking forever to do any good." He reports minimal wear of the splint. How will you handle his noncompliance?

*See Appendix A for the answer key.

CASE STUDY 6-2

Read the following scenario and answer the questions based on information in this chapter.

Abbreviations used in the narrative are as follows: *FA* = forearm, *IP* = interphalangeal, *LTG* = long-term goal, *LUE* = left upper extremity, *MP* = metaphalangeal, *ROM* = range of motion, *RUE* = right upper extremity, *STG* = short-term goal, *WNL* = within normal limits.

Marie, a 57-year-old woman, is employed as a department store clerk. She works part-time, except for during the winter holiday season. She has been in good health with the exception of having diabetes, which is well regulated. Her job demands involve unloading boxes, stocking new merchandise, and operating a cash register. During the winter holiday season Marie worked 40-hour weeks. In addition, she was busy at home decorating and baking. One week prior to Christmas she noted pain radiating up her dominant right forearm and around the radial styloid.

Marie complained to her employer of pain when moving the thumb and when turning her forearm up. Marie was seen by the company physician, who diagnosed her condition as de Quervain's tenosynovitis. She was provided with a prefabricated thumb immobilization splint, which she did not wear due to its being uncomfortable and causing some chafing on the volar surface of the thumb IP joint. Two weeks later, when symptoms did not improve, the company physician ordered occupational therapy. The order read: "Fabricate an R thumb splint and provide a home program." The following initial therapy note purposely displays flawed documentation.

10-13

Client was followed on 10-13 for fabrication of a splint and to provide a home exercise program. Client was wearing a prefabricated splint. Reddened areas were noted on the thumb. Client was instructed in a home program, splint precautions, and a wearing schedule. It doesn't appear that the client will be compliant with wearing the splint.

Results of the evaluation are as follows:

ROM

All ROM was WNL except for the following:

THUMB: DIP FLEXION 0-50; MP FLEXION, 0-30; PALMAR ABDUCTION, 0-30;

Radial Abduction 0-30; Opposition: to ring finger

WRIST: FLEXION 0-50; EXTENSION 0-40; ULNAR DEVIATION, 0-15; RADIAL DEVIATION, 0-15

FA: SUPINATION, (0=45),

Strength:

Grasp Strength: RUE 35#s; LUE 52#s

Pinch Strength: Lateral, tip, and key pinch RUE: 5#s LUE 10#s

Edema Evaluation:

Edema noted around area of radial styloid. Circumferential measurement at that area RUES 10 cm. LUE 9 cm.

Volometer reading:

RUE 420, LUE 380

Circulation:

WNL for Allen's testing. Temperature: WNL

Sensory Evaluation:

WNL to Semmes Weinstein Monofilaments

Goals

LTG: Pt will follow provided splint-wearing schedule by discharge from therapy.

STG: Pt will show decreased symptoms from de Quervain's tenosynovitis.

To encourage clinical reasoning skills, answer the following questions about the case. See Chapter 8 for specifics about splints for de Quervain's tenosynovitis.

1. List a minimum of five areas of the documentation that could be improved by being more specific or more complete.

____

____

____

2. On the basis of the interactive clinical reasoning approach, what are two questions that will facilitate an understanding of the impact that having de Quervain's tenosynovitis and wearing a splint has on Marie's work and home life?

____

____

____

3. What are some concerns about compliance you may have based on Marie's history with her prefabricated splint? How will you approach any compliance concerns?

4. Considering that the referral came from work, what type of insurance might Marie have?

*See Appendix A for the answer key.

REVIEW QUESTIONS

1. How would a therapist apply the various clinical reasoning models to splint provision?
2. What does a splint referral include?
3. How can the therapist facilitate communication with the physician's office about the splint referral?
4. Why is knowing the person's age important to the therapist when fabricating a splint?
5. Which lifestyle needs of the person must the therapist consider with splint provision?
6. How can the therapist enhance the compliance of a person wearing a splint?
7. What are the infection-control procedures a therapist should follow with splint provision?
8. What should therapists monitor when providing a splint for a person during the following conditions: pressure, edema, and physical status of a person?
9. What are the four directions of splint design?
10. What are some helpful hints for making adjustments after splint fabrication?
11. What are the factors the therapist should consider when establishing a person on a splint-wearing schedule?
12. What are the factors a therapist should consider for splint discontinuation?
13. What are the cost and reimbursement issues the therapist must keep in mind?
14. How might the HIPAA influence communication with clients about splints in a clinical setting?
15. What documentation issues should the therapist be aware of with splinting?

References

American Society of Hand Therapists (1992). *Splint Classification Systems*. Garner, NJ: The American Society of Hand Therapists.

Armstong J (2005). Splinting the pediatric patient. In EE Fess, KS Gettle, CA Philips, JR Janson (eds.), *Hand and Upper Extremity Splinting: Principles and Methods, Third Edition*. St. Louis: Elsevier Mosby, pp. 480-516.

Bailey DM (1998). Legislative and reimbursement influences on occupational therapy: Changing opportunities. In ME Neistadt, EB Crepeaau, *Willard & Spackman's Occupational Therapy, Ninth Edition*. Philadelphia: Lippincott, pp. 763-772.

Batteson R (1997). A strategy to improve nurse/occupational therapist communication for managing persons with splints. British Journal of Occupational Therapy 60:451-454.

Bower KA (1985). Compliance as a patient education issue. In KM Woldum, V Ryan-Morrell, MC Towson, KA Bower, K Zander (eds.), *Patient Education: Foundations of Practice*. Rockville, MD: Aspen Publications, pp. 45-111.

Brand PW, Hollister A (1993). *Clinical Mechanics of the Hand, Second Edition*. St. Louis: Mosby.

Callinan NJ, Mathiowetz V (1996). Soft versus hard resting hand splints in rheumatoid arthritis: Pain relief, preference, and compliance. American Journal of Occupational Therapy 50:347-354.

Cannon NM, Foltz RW, Koepfer JM, Lauck MR, Simpson DM, Bromley RS (1985). *Manual of Hand Splinting*. New York: Churchill Livingstone.

Colditz JC (2002). Therapist's management of the still hand. In EJ Mackin, AD Callahan, TM Skirven, LH Schneider, AL Osterman (eds.), *Rehabilitation of the Hand and Upper Extremity, Fifth Edition*. St. Louis: Mosby, pp. 1021-1049.

Costa DM, Whitehouse D (2003). HIPAA and fieldwork. OTPractice 8(17):23-24.

Dana Farber Cancer Institute (2004). Policy for disclosing medical errors to patients and families. Approved 7/12/01, reviewed 7/17/01 and 7/04.

Ekelman-Ranke BR (1998). Documentation in the age of litigation. OT Practice 3(3):20-24.

Fess EE, Gettle KS, Philips CA, Janson JR (2005). *Hand and Upper Extremity Splinting: Principles and Methods, Third Edition*. St. Louis: Elsevier Mosby.

Fleming MH (1994). Conditional reasoning: Creating meaningful experiences. In C Mattingly, MH Fleming (eds.), *Clinical Reasoning: Forms of Inquiry in a Therapeutic Practice*. Philadelphia: F. A. Davis, p. 197-235.

Fleming MH (1991). The therapists with the three-track mind. American Journal of Occupational Therapy 45:1007-1014.

Groth GN, Wilder DM (1994). The impact of compliance of rehabilitation of persons with mallet finger injuries. Journal of Hand Therapy 7(1):21-24.

Groth GN, Wulf MB (1995). Compliance with hand rehabilitation: Health beliefs and strategies. Journal of Hand Therapy 8:18-22.

Joint Commission on Accreditation of Healthcare Organizations (2001). Hospital Accreditation Standards RI.1.2.2, July 1.

Joint Commission on Accreditation of Health Care Organizations (2005a). *Patient Safety: Essentials for Healthcare, Third Edition*. Oakbrook, IL: Joint Commission Resources.

Joint Commission on Accreditation of Healthcare Organizations (2005b). *Sentinel Event Statistics*, 1995-2004, *http://www.jcaho.org/accredited+organizations/sentinel+events/sentinel+events+statistics.htm*.

Kirwan T, Tooth L, Harkin C (2002). Compliance with hand therapy programs: Therapists' and patients' perceptions. Journal of Hand Therapy 15(1):31-40.

Law M, Baptiste S, Carswell A, McCall MA, Polatajko H, Pollock N (1998). *Canadian Occupational Performance Measure, Third Edition*. Ottawa, ON: CAOT Publications.

Lohman H, Mu K, Scheirton L (2004). Occupational therapists perspectives on practice errors in geriatric settings. Physical and Occupational Therapy in Geriatrics 21(4).

Mackin EJ, Callahan AD, Skirven TM, Schneider LH, Osterman AL (eds.) (2002), *Rehabilitation of the Hand and Upper Extremity, Fifth Edition*. St. Louis: Mosby.

Malick MH (1972). *Manual on Static Splinting*. Hamarville, PA: Harmarville Rehabilitation Center.

Mattingly C (1991). The narrative nature of clinical reasoning. American Journal of Occupational Therapy 45:998-1005.

Mattingly C, Fleming MH (1994). *Clinical Reasoning: Forms of Inquiry in a Therapeutic Practice*. Philadelphia: F. A. Davis.

Minneapolis Children's Hospital and Clinics. Policy 703.00. Medical accidents, reporting, and disclosure, including sentinel events. Originally effective 28 July 1999, revised 1 October 2001.

Murer CG (2002). Trends and issues: Protecting patient privacy. Rehab Management 15(3):46-47.

Neistadt ME (1998). Teaching clinical reasoning as a thinking frame. American Journal of Occupational Therapy 52:211-229.

Parham D (1987). Towards professionalism: The reflective therapist. American Journal of Occupational Therapy 41:555-560.

Pascarelli E, Quilter D (1994). *Repetitive Strain Injury*. New York: John Wiley & Sons.

Reynolds CC (1995). Preoperative and postoperative management of tendon transfers after radial nerve injury. In JM Hunter, EJ Mackin, AD Callahan (eds.), *Rehabilitation of the Hand, Fourth Edition*. St. Louis: Mosby, pp. 753-763.

Scheirton LS, Mu K, Lohman H (2003). Occupational therapists' responses to practice errors in physical rehabilitation. American Journal of Occupational Therapy 57(3).

Schell BA, Cervero RM (1993). Clinical reasoning in occupational therapy: An integrated review. American Journal of Occupational Therapy 47:605-610.

Schon DA (1987). *Educating the Reflective Practitioner*. San Francisco: Jossey-Bass.

Skotak CH, Stockdell SM (1988). Wound management in hand therapy. In FS Cromwell, J Bear-Lehman (eds.), *Hand Rehabilitation in Occupational Therapy*. Binghamton, NY: Haworth Press, pp. 17-35.

Southam MA, Dunbar JM (1987). Integration of adherence problems. In D Meichenbaum, DC Turk (eds.), *Facilitating Treatment Adherence*. New York: Plenum Publishing.

Stern EB, Ytterberg SR, Krug HE, Larson LM, Portoghese CP, Kratz WNR, et al. (1997). Commercial wrist extensor orthoses: A descriptive study of use and preference in patients with rheumatoid arthritis. Arthritis Care and Research 10:27-35.

Sullivan JM (2004). *The OT's Guide to HIPAA: The Impact of Privacy Laws on the Practice of Occupational Therapy*. Minneapolis, MN: The American Occupational Therapy Association.

Trombly C (1993). Anticipating the future: Assessment of occupational function. American Journal of Occupational Therapy 47:253-257.

United States Department of Health and Human Services (2003). *Fact sheet: Protecting the privacy of patients' health information. http://www.hhs.gov/news/facts/privacy.html*.

United States Department of Health and Human Services (2004). *What is the difference between "consent" and "authorization" under the HIPAA Privacy Rule?* Retrieved on October 12, 2004, from *http://answers.hhs.gov/cgi-bin/hhs.cfg/php/enduser/std*.

Wilson HP (2004). HIPAA: The big picture for home care and hospice. Home-Health-Care-Mangement-and Practice 16(2):127-137.

Wright HH, Rettig A (2005). Management of common sports injuries. In EJ Mackin, AD Callahan, TM Skirven, LH Schneider (eds.), *Rehabilitation of the Hand and Upper Extremity, Fifth Edition*. St. Louis: Mosby, pp. 2076-2109.

York AM (2003). HIPAA smarts: Top 10 privacy musts. Rehab Management 16(2):44-45.

UNIT **TWO**

Splinting for Conditions and Populations

CHAPTER 7

Splints Acting on the Wrist

Helene Lohman, MA, OTD, OTR/L

Key Terms

Carpal tunnel syndrome
Circumferential
Complex regional pain syndrome I
Dorsal
Forearm trough
Hypothenar bar
Metacarpal bar
Radial nerve injuries
Rheumatoid arthritis
Tendonitis/tenosynovitis
Ulnar
Volar

Chapter Objectives

1. Discuss diagnostic indications for wrist immobilization splints.
2. Identify reasons to serial splint with a wrist immobilization splint.
3. Identify major features of wrist immobilization splints.
4. Understand the fabrication process for a volar or dorsal wrist splint.
5. Relate hints for a proper fit to a wrist immobilization splint.
6. Review precautions for wrist immobilization splinting.
7. Use clinical reasoning to evaluate a problematic wrist immobilization splint.
8. Use clinical reasoning to evaluate a fabricated wrist immobilization splint.
9. Apply knowledge about the application of wrist immobilization splints to a case study.
10. Understand the importance of evidenced-based practice with wrist splint provision.
11. Describe the appropriate use of prefabricated wrist splints.

Maintaining the wrist in proper alignment is important because the wrist is key to the health and balance of the entire hand. During functional activities, the wrist is positioned in extension for grasp and prehension. Therefore, the wrist extension immobilization type O splint [American Society of Hand Therapists 1992] or the wrist cock-up splint is the most common splint used in clinical practice. Wrist immobilization splints usually maintain the wrist in either a neutral or a mildly extended position, depending on the protocol for a particular diagnostic condition and the person's treatment goals. A wrist immobilization splint immobilizes the wrist while allowing full metacarpophalangeal (MCP) flexion and thumb mobility. Thus, the person can continue to perform functional activities with the added support and proper positioning of the wrist the splint provides. Positioning the wrist in a splint in 0 to 30 degrees of wrist extension promotes functional hand patterns for completing functional activities [Palmer et al. 1985, Melvin 1989].

Therapists fabricate wrist immobilization splints to provide volar, dorsal, ulnar, circumferential forearm, wrist, hand, and (infrequently) radial support (see Figures 7-1 through 7-4). Therapists can also use wrist immobilization splints as bases for mobilization and static progressive splinting (see Chapter 11). Although some wrist immobilization splints are commercially available, they cannot provide the exact fit of custom-made splints. However, commercially available splints made from soft material may be more comfortable in certain situations, especially in a work or sports setting. Commercially available splints are not as restrictive and allow more functional hand use [Stern et al. 1994]. Some people with rheumatoid arthritis may also prefer the comfort of a soft wrist splint due to its ability to reduce pain and provide stability during functional activities [Nordenskiold 1990, Stern et al. 1997, Biese 2002].

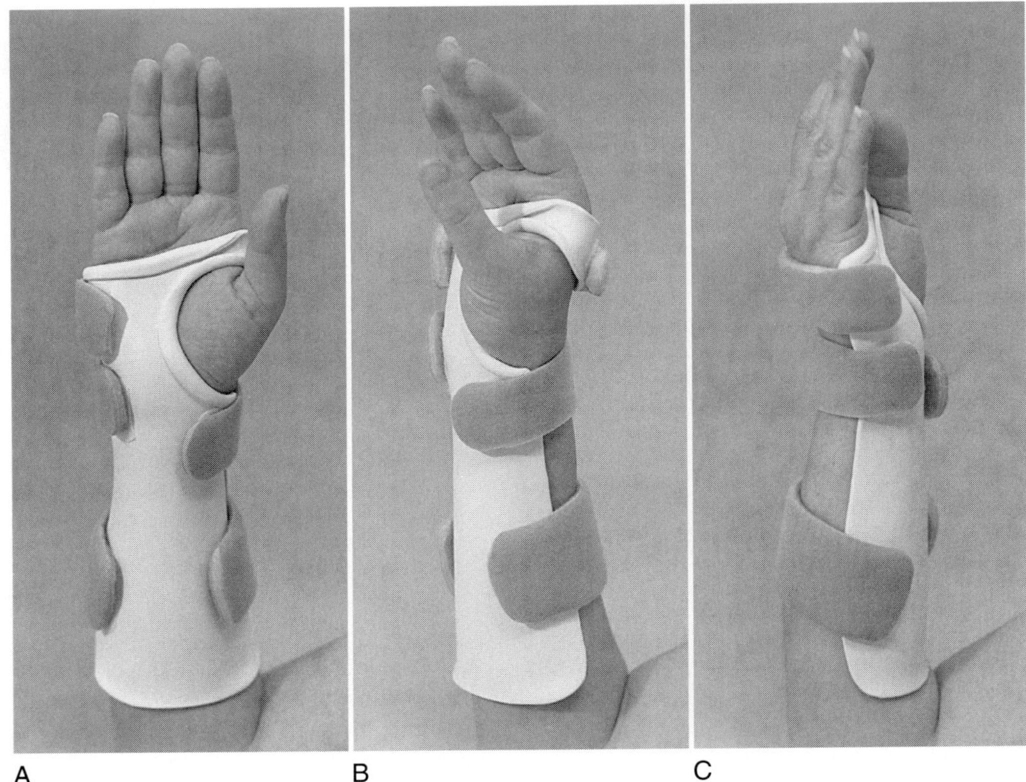

Figure 7-1 A volar wrist immobilization splint.

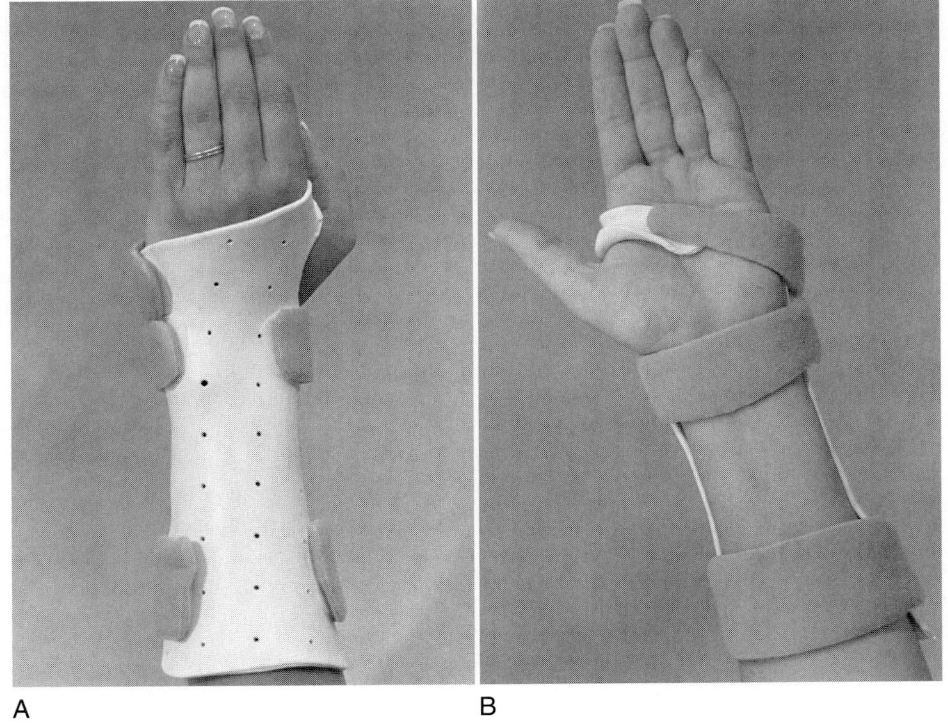

Figure 7-2 A dorsal wrist immobilization splint.

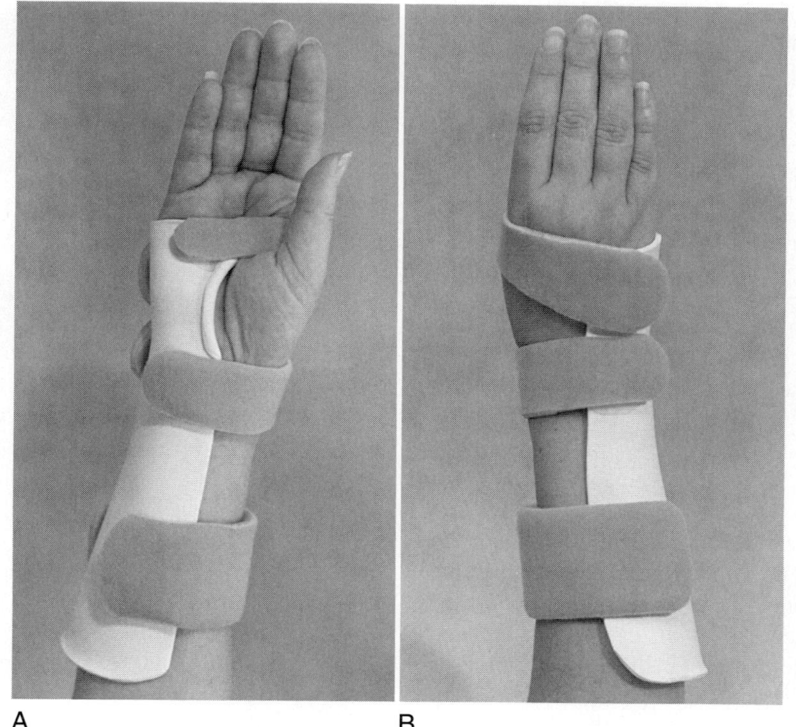

Figure 7-3 An ulnar wrist immobilization splint.

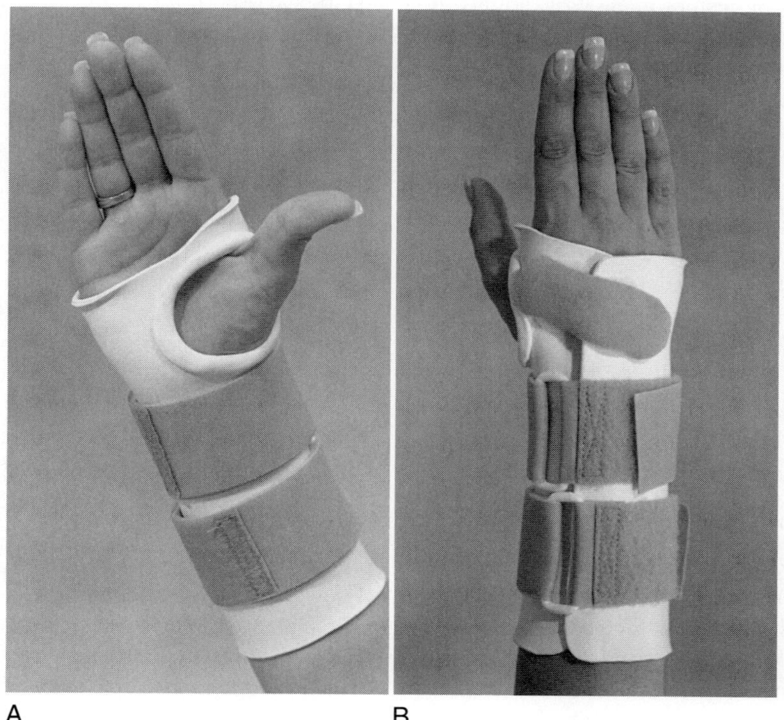

Figure 7-4 A circumferential wrist immobilization splint.

This chapter primarily overviews wrist immobilization splints according to type, features, and diagnoses. The chapter also explores technical tips, trouble shooting, the use of prefabricated splints, the impact on occupations, and the application of a wrist mobilization and serial static approach.

Volar, Dorsal, Ulnar, and Circumferential Wrist Immobilization Splints

In clinical practice the therapist must decide whether to fabricate a volar, dorsal, ulnar, or circumferential wrist immobilization splint. Each has advantages and disadvantages [Colditz 2002].

Volar

The volar wrist immobilization splint (Figure 7-1) depends on a dorsal wrist strap to hold the wrist in extension in the splint. An appropriate design furnishes adequate support for the weight of the wrist and hand. In cases in which the weight of the hand (flaccidity) must be held by the splint or in which the person is pulling against it (spasticity), the strap is not adequate to hold the wrist in the splint. However, a well-designed volar wrist splint with a properly placed wide wrist strap will support a flaccid wrist [personal communication, K. Schultz-Johnson, April 6, 2006]. The volar design is best suited for circumstances that require rest or immobilization of the wrist when the person still has muscle control of the wrist [Colditz 2002].

In one study [Stern 1991], the volar wrist splint allowed the hand the best dexterity of custom-made wrist splints. A volar wrist splint's greatest disadvantage is interference with tactile sensibility on the palmar surface of the hand and the loss of the hand's ability to conform around objects [personal communication, K. Schultz-Johnson, April 6, 2006]. In the presence of edema, one must use this design carefully because the dorsal strap can impede lymphatic and venous flow [Colditz 2002]. To address the presence of edema, a strap adaptation can be made by fabricating a continuous strap. The therapist applies self-adhesive Velcro hooks along the radial and ulnar borders of the splint, which are attached by a flexible fabric to create a soft dorsal shell.

Dorsal

Some therapists fabricate dorsal splints with a large palmar bar that supports the entire hand. This large palmar bar tends to distribute pressure well and is necessary for the comfort and function of the splint. However, a large palmar bar does not free up the palmar surface as much for sensory input as a dorsal splint fabricated with a thinner palmar bar (Figure 7-2). Dorsal wrist splints designed with a standard strap configuration can be better tolerated by persons who have edematous hands because of the pressure distribution. Either the volar or the dorsal design may be used as a base for mobilization (dynamic) splinting. However, these designs can sometimes lead to splint migration and suboptimal splint performance.

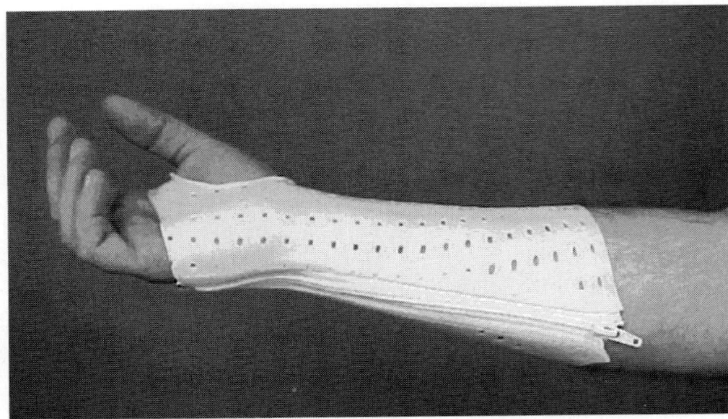

Figure 7-5 A "zipper" splint option for circumferential splinting (Sammons Preston & Rolyan). [From Bednar JM, Von Lersner-Benson C (2002). Wrist reconstruction: Salvage procedures. In EJ Mackin, AD Callahan, TM Shirven, LH Schneider, AL Osterman (eds.), *Rehabilitation of the Hand and Upper Extremity, Fifth Edition*. St. Louis: Mosby, p. 1200.]

Ulnar

The ulnar wrist splint is easy to don and doff and can be applied if the person warrants more protection on the ulnar side of the hand, such as with sports injuries (Figure 7-3). This splint design is sometimes used for a person who has carpal tunnel syndrome (CTS) or for ulnar wrist pain [LaStayo 2002]. It can also be used as a base for mobilization splinting.

Circumferential

A circumferential splint is helpful in preventing migration, especially when used as a base for mobilization splints. It also provides good forearm support, controls edema, provides good pressure distribution, and avoids edge pressure [personal communication, K. Schultz-Johnson, April 1999]. Some people may feel more confined in a circumferential splint. When fabricating a circumferential splint, the therapist is conscious of a possible pressure area over the distal ulna and checks that the fingers and thumb have full motion [Laseter 2002] (Figure 7-4). One among many circumferential splint options is a "zipper" splint made out of perforated thermoplastic material (Figure 7-5).

Features of the Wrist Immobilization Splint

Understanding the features of a wrist immobilization splint helps therapists splint appropriately. Whether fabricating a volar, dorsal, ulnar, or circumferential wrist splint, the therapist must be aware of certain features of the various components of the wrist immobilization splint—such as a

SELF-QUIZ 7-1*

In regard to the following questions, circle either true (T) or false (F).

1. T F Wrist immobilization splints can be volar, dorsal, ulnar, or circumferential.
2. T F A wrist immobilization splint usually decreases wrist pain or inflammation, provides support, enhances digital function, and prevents wrist deformity.
3. T F Most prefabricated splints are made to correctly fit someone who has CTS.
4. T F Some research suggests the value of early conservative intervention with splinting.
5. T F After removal of a cast for a Colles' fracture, if motion is limited in the wrist the therapist may consider serial splinting.
6. T F The therapist must follow standard treatment protocols exactly for any diagnosis that requires a wrist immobilization splint application.
7. T F With a wrist immobilization splint, the therapist usually splints the wrist in extreme extension, which promotes functional movement.
8. T F The hypothenar bar on a wrist immobilization splint helps to position the hand in a neutral resting position by preventing extreme ulnar deviation.
9. T F The therapist should position the volar wrist immobilization splint distal to the distal palmar crease.
10. T F If a mistake is made during fabrication of a volar wrist immobilization splint, in getting the correct wrist extension the therapist should spot heat the wrist area to make an adjustment.
11. T F People with CTS should be encouraged to perform strong finger flexion within their splints to allow for finger mobility.

*See Appendix A for the answer key.

forearm trough, metacarpal bar, and hypothenar bar [Fess et al. 2005] (Figures 7-6 and 7-7). With a volar or dorsal immobilization splint the forearm trough should be two-thirds the length of the forearm and one-half the circumference of the forearm to allow for appropriate pressure distribution. It is sometimes necessary to notch the area near the distal ulna on the forearm trough to avoid a pressure point.

The hypothenar bar helps to place the hand in a neutral resting position by preventing extreme ulnar deviation. The hypothenar bar should not inhibit MCP flexion of the ring and little fingers. The metacarpal (MP) bar supports the transverse metacarpal arch. When supporting the palmar surface of the hand, the MP bar is sometimes called a palmar bar. With a volar wrist immobilization splint, the therapist positions this bar proximal to the distal palmar crease and distal and ulnar to the thenar crease to ensure full MCP flexion. On the ulnar side of the hand, it is especially important that the MP bar be positioned proximal from the distal palmar crease to allow full little finger MP flexion.

On the radial side, it is important to note the position of the MP bar below the distal palmar crease and distal to the thenar crease to allow adequate index and middle MCP flexion and thumb motions. On a dorsal wrist immobilization splint, the therapist positions this bar slightly proximal to the MCP heads on the dorsal surface of the hand when it winds around to the palmar surface. The same principles apply when positioning the MP bar on the volar surface of the hand (proximal to the distal palmar crease, and distal and ulnar to the thenar crease).

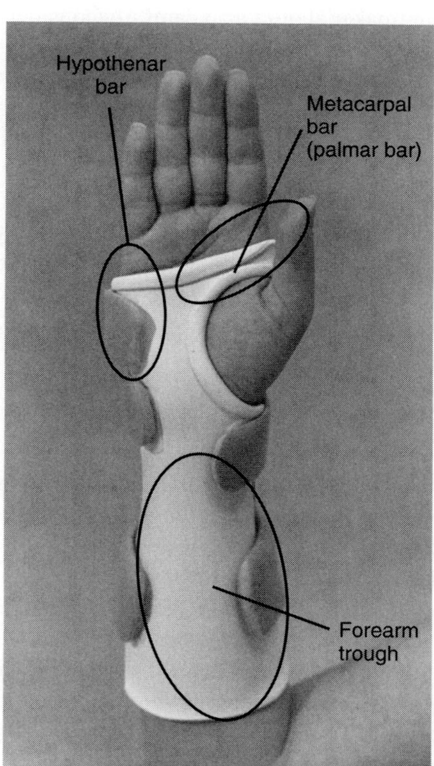

Figure 7-6 A volar wrist immobilization splint with identified components.*

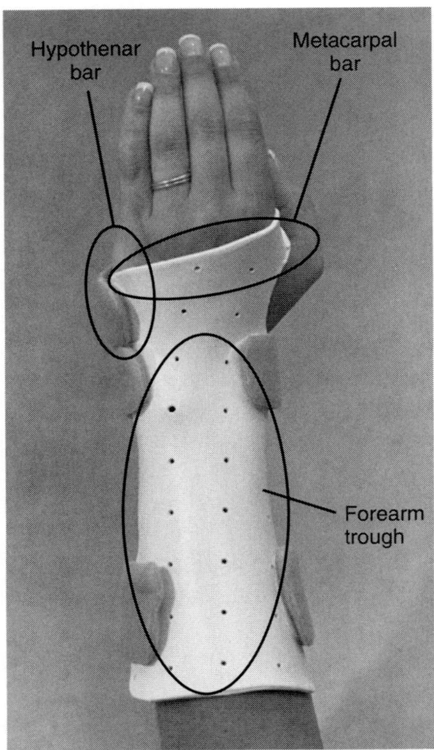

Figure 7-7 A dorsal wrist immobilization splint with identified components.

The splintmaker should also carefully consider the application of straps to the wrist splint. The therapist applies straps at the level of the MP bar, exactly at the wrist level, and at the proximal end of the splint. The straps attach to the splint with pieces of self-adhesive Velcro hook. The therapist should note that the larger the piece of self-adhesive hook Velcro, the larger the interface between it and the splint thermoplastic material. This larger interface helps ensure that it will remain in place and not peel off. With the identification of the potential for pressure or shear problems, the therapist applies padding to the splint (see Figures 7-1, 7-6, 7-14, 7-15, 7-16).

Diagnostic Indications

The clinical indications for the wrist immobilization splint vary according to the diagnosis. The therapist can apply the wrist immobilization splint for any upper extremity condition that requires the wrist to be in a static position. Application of this splint can work for a variety of goals, depending on the client's treatment needs. These goals include decreasing wrist pain or inflammation, providing support, enhancing digital function, preventing wrist deformity, minimizing pressure on the median nerve, and minimizing tension on involved structures.

In some cases a wrist mobilization splint serial static approach is used to increase passive range of motion. Specific diagnostic conditions that may require a wrist immobilization splint can include, but are not limited to, tendonitis, distal radius or ulna fracture, wrist sprain, radial nerve palsy, carpal ganglion, stable wrist fracture, wrist arthroplasty, complex regional pain syndrome I (reflex sympathetic dystrophy), and nerve compression at the wrist.

The specific wrist positioning depends on the diagnostic protocol, physician referral, and person's treatment goals. When the goal is functional hand use during splint wear, the therapist must avoid extreme wrist flexion or extension because either position disrupts the normal functional position of the hand. These positions can contribute to the development of CTS [Gelberman et al. 1981, Fess et al. 2005]. An exception to this rule is when the splint goal is to increase passive range of motion (PROM). In that case, an extreme position may be indicated. However, extreme positions may preclude function. The therapist must judge whether the trade-off is worth the loss of function [personal communication, K. Schultz-Johnson, April 1999].

The therapist performs a thorough hand evaluation before fitting a person with a wrist immobilization splint and provides the person with a wearing schedule, instructions about splint maintenance and precautions, and an exercise program based on particular needs. Physicians and experienced therapists may have detailed guidelines for positioning and wearing schedules. Every hand is slightly different, and thus splint positioning and wearing protocols vary. Table 7-1 lists suggested wearing schedules and positioning protocols of common hand conditions that may require wrist immobilization splints.

Wrist Splinting for Carpal Tunnel Syndrome

For CTS, splinting the wrist as close as possible to 0 degrees (neutral) helps avoid added pressure on the median nerve [Gelberman et al. 1981, Weiss et al. 1995, Kulick 1996]. One study using sonography to determine the best wrist position for splinting CTS found that the majority of subjects benefited from a neutral position. However, a few subjects improved from splinting in either a wrist position of 15 degrees extension or 15 degrees flexion [Kuo et al. 2001]. This suggests better front-end diagnostic procedures to determine the most accurate splinting position.

One must be careful when applying prefabricated wrist immobilization splints for CTS because some splints place the wrist in a functional position of 20 to 30 degrees of extension [Weiss et al. 1995, Osterman et al. 2002]. Therefore, if it is possible to adjust the wrist angle of the splint it should be modified to a neutral position. Some of the prefabricated splints have a compartment in which a metal or thermoplastic insert is placed, and the insert allows adjustments for wrist position. However, prefabricated splints that have their angles adjusted may become looser, less rigid, and less comfortable than a custom molded splint [Walker et al. 2000].

Generally, custom splints are recommended for CTS because they provide better support, positioning

Table 7-1 Conditions That May Require a Wrist Immobilization Splint

HAND CONDITION	SUGGESTED WEARING SCHEDULE	TYPE OF SPLINT AND WRIST POSITION
Nerve Compression		
Carpal tunnel syndrome (CTS) (median nerve compression)	There is no consistent protocol for splint provision with CTS. Some therapists determine the wear schedule based on what activities are irritating the person. For example, if activities during the day are irritating the person the splint should be worn during the day. Some therapists start with wear during sleep and increase the time if the splint does not decrease symptoms. Often during an acute flare-up the person wears the wrist immobilization splint continuously for 4 to 6 weeks with removal for hygiene and range-of-motion (ROM) exercises. The splint-wearing schedule gradually decreases. If the person undergoes steroid injection, the splint is worn continuously (except when removed for hygiene).	Volar, dorsal, or ulnar gutter splint with the wrist in a neutral position.
Carpal tunnel release surgery	There is no consistent protocol for splint provision with carpal tunnel release surgery. Some physicians have the splint fabricated preoperatively, and some are fabricated immediately postoperatively. Some physicians do not prescribe splints at all. Others may recommend a wrist immobilization splint 1 week after surgery, with the therapist providing instructions for a splint-wearing schedule (which includes splint application during sleep, during strenuous activities, and for support throughout the healing phase). Splint is weaned when appropriate to prevent adhesion formation.	A volar splint with the wrist in a neutral or slightly extended position.
Radial nerve palsy	Some physicians may advocate a wrist immobilization splint that maintains the wrist in a functional position and substitutes for the loss of the radial nerve by placing the wrist in extension.*	Volar or dorsal, 15 to 30 degrees of wrist extension.
Tendinitis/Tenosynovitis		
Any inflammation or degradation of the tendon and tendon sheath within the wrist	The person wears a wrist immobilization splint continuously, with removal for hygiene and ROM exercises followed by gradual weaning off the splint.	Volar or dorsal, 20 to 30 degrees of wrist extension.
Wrist synovitis	The person wears a wrist immobilization splint continuously during acute flare-ups, with removal for hygiene and ROM exercises.	Volar, 0 to 15 degrees of extension.
Rheumatoid Arthritis		
Periods of swelling, wrist subluxation, and joint inflammation	The person wears continuously a wrist immobilization splint with established periods for ROM exercises and hygiene during the splint-wearing schedule. If metacarpophalangeal (MCP) joints are developing an ulnar drift and interphalangeal (IP) joints are not involved, the therapist may fabricate a wrist splint that includes the MCP joints.	Volar in extension up to 30 degrees based on person's comfort level. During the early stage of the development of an ulnar drift, splint close to neutral.
Wrist fractures	After removal of the cast and healing of the fracture, the therapist fabricates a wrist immobilization splint. Usually the therapist discontinues the splint use as soon as possible to encourage functional movement. Sometimes the therapist may need to serially splint the wrist if there is not enough functional extension.	Dorsal, volar, or circumferential (if more support is needed) maximum passive extension the person can tolerate up to 30 degrees.

*The diagnosis may require additional types of splinting.

Continued

Table 7-1 Conditions That May Require a Wrist Immobilization Splint—cont'd

HAND CONDITION	SUGGESTED WEARING SCHEDULE	TYPE OF SPLINT AND WRIST POSITION
Wrist Sprain		
Any grade I or mild grade II tear of ligament	The person wears a wrist immobilization splint continuously for 3 to 6 weeks. The physician may allow removal during bathing, depending on severity.	Choose approach as needed for function. Location of ligament may help dictate position. The splint should remove stress (tension from ligament).
Other		
Complex regional pain syndrome I	The person wears a wrist immobilization splint during functional activities.	Volar, in extension as person tolerates. A circumferential wrist splint might also be used, as it helps avoid pressure on the edges and problems with edema.

[McClure 2003], and more constant allocation of pressure over the carpal tunnel than prefabricated splints—especially those that are incorrectly fitted [Hayes et al. 2002]. If a person does not tolerate a custom-made splint, the therapist may need to consider providing a prefabricated splint [personal communication, Lynn, 2003].

Another consideration with the wrist immobilization splint provision is the amount of finger flexion allowed. Recent research evidence suggests that finger flexion affects carpal tunnel pressure, especially if fingers fully flex to form a fist [Apfel et al. 2002]. That is because the lumbrical muscles may sometimes enter the carpal tunnel with finger flexion [Cobb et al. 1995, Seigel et al. 1995]. When splints are provided to clients with CTS, they should be instructed to not flex their fingers "beyond 75% of a full fist" [Apfel et al. 2002, p. 333]. Therefore, therapists should check finger position with splint provision. Osterman et al. [2002] advised therapists to fabricate a volar wrist splint with a metacarpal block to decrease finger flexion if CTS symptoms are not improving.

When fabricating a splint for a person who has CTS, the therapist considers home and occupational demands carefully, keeping in mind that the wrist contributes to the overall function of the hand [Schultz-Johnson 1996]. If a splint is worn at work, durability of the splint and the ability to wash it may be salient. Some people may benefit from the fabrication of two splints (one for work and one for home), especially if their job demands are in an unclean environment. Many computer operators tolerate a splint that supports the wrist position in the plane of flexion and extension but allows 10 to 20 degrees of radial and ulnar deviation for effective typing. Fabricating a slightly wider metacarpal bar on a custom-made wrist splint allows for a small area of mobility on the radial and ulnar sides of the hand [Sailer 1996]. Finally, the therapist simulates work and home tasks with the wrist immobilization splint on the person to check for functional fit [Sailer 1996].

Therapists also take into account splint-wearing schedules. Options that can be prescribed are nighttime wear only, wear during activities that irritate the condition, a combination of the latter two schedules, or constant wear. In one study, subjects were found to benefit most from full-time wear of the splint, but wearing compliance was an issue [Walker et al. 2000]. This study further validated improvements in clients who wore a neutral position wrist splint for six weeks. Nevertheless, it is important to consider nighttime wear of splints because some people maintain extreme wrist flexion or extension postures during sleep [Sailer 1996].

An exercise program issued with a splint may be an effective conservative treatment [Rozmaryn et al. 1998]. In one study (n = 197), a conservative treatment program for CTS that combined nerve and tendon gliding exercises with wrist immobilization splinting was found to be more effective in helping people avoid surgery than splint wear alone. It is hypothesized that these exercises help improve the excursion of the median nerve and flexor tendons because the exercises may contribute to the remodeling of the adhered tenosynovium [Rozmaryn et al. 1998]. Akalin et al. [2002] (n = 28) also studied tendon and nerve gliding exercises with splinting compared to splinting alone. Ninety-three percent of the splinting and exercise group participants reported good to excellent results compared to 72% of the splint-only group participants. However, the researchers did not consider the results statistically significant. Both studies accentuate the value of early conservative intervention.

Other effective treatment measures for CTS are the modification of activities (so that the person does not make excessive wrist and forearm motions, especially wrist flexion). It is also important to avoid sustained pinch or grip activities and to use good posture whenever possible with all activities of daily living (ADL). Because CTS is generically a disease of decreased blood supply to the soft tissues. Nerves need blood supply and an environment that is cold will additionally deprive the nerve of blood. Thus, staying warm is an important part of CTS care and splints provide local warmth [personal communication, K. Schultz-Johnson, April 6, 2006]. When conservative measures are ineffective, surgery is an option.

The goals of wrist splinting after carpal tunnel release surgery are to minimize pressure on the median nerve, prevent bowstringing of the flexor tendons [Cook et al. 1995], provide support during stressful activities, maintain gains from exercise [Messer and Bankers 1995; personal communication, K. Schultz-Johnson, April 1999], and rest the extremity during the immediate healing phase. Some therapists do not apply a wrist immobilization splint postoperatively because of concerns about the impact of immobilization on joint stiffness and muscle shortening [Hayes et al. 2002]. Findings from one study [Cook et al. 1995] (n = 50) suggest that splinting post-surgery resulted in joint stiffness as well as delays with returning to work, recovering grip and pinch strength, and resuming ADL. These researchers concluded that if splinting is used it should be applied for one week only postoperatively to prevent tendon bowstringing and nerve entrapment.

Splinting postoperatively is recommended to prevent extreme nighttime wrist postures (flexion and extension) or to manage inflammation [Hayes et al. 2002]. Therapists instruct the person to gradually wean away from the splint (when the splint is no longer meeting the person's therapeutic goals) in order to prevent stiffness and allow the person to return to work and ADL more quickly. Weaning is often done over the course one week, gradually decreasing the hours of splint wear [personal communication, K. Schultz-Johnson, April 6, 2006].

A series of recent studies were conducted to examine splinting compared to other treatments, such as surgery or steroid injections (see Table 7-2, which outlines the research evidence). The majority of studies comparing splinting to surgery favored surgery as the most effective treatment for CTS [Gerritsen et. al 2002, Verdugo et al. 2004]. Splinting did show some promising results, but was not as strong in efficacy as surgery. For example, with the Gerristen et al. [2002] study (n = 178) after 18 months 75% of the subjects improved with splint wear as compared to 90% of the surgery group. The researchers recommended that splinting is beneficial while waiting for surgery, or if a client does not desire surgery. When considering the results of this study, therapists should recognize that 75% improvement with splinting is a high success rate and is less risky than having surgery. Some people do not want therapy, splinting, and activity modification and therefore may best benefit from a surgical approach [personal communication, K. Schultz-Johnson, April 6, 2006].

Therapists need to critically examine such studies for limitations when making an informed decision for clients. McClure [2003], in an article on evidenced-based practice, considered limitations of studies about splinting with CTS. For example, he questioned the results of the Verdugo et al. [2004] study. He queried whether the same results would have occurred with mild CTS symptoms and that the study was done with "only one small randomized trial" [McClure 2003, p. 259]. McClure [2003] also considered the limitations of the Gerritsen et al. [2002] study. He mentioned that information regarding the splint-wearing schedule, other treatments, how clients were classified, and symptom severity were missing from the study [McClure 2003].

Other researchers examined the effect of splinting and nonsteroidal anti-inflammatory drugs (n = 33 hands) [Celiker et al. 2002, Graham et al. 2004]. Celiker et al. [2002] (n = 99 hands) found that splinting along with steroid injections for clients who had symptoms less than nine months resulted in significant improvement. In another study, steroid injections and wrist splinting for three weeks was found to be effective in clients who had symptoms of less than three months duration and no residual sensory impairments [Graham et al. 2004]. Using only splints for CTS was also studied (n = 66 subjects), with significant improvement after four weeks reported [O'Connor et al. 2003]. Gerritsen et al. [2003] (n = 89 subjects) reported that the shorter duration of complaints and the severity of nocturnal parasthesias were positively related to splinting success.

Therapists and physicians must be aware of current studies because these can influence treatment approaches. Therapists need to critically question how the studies were performed and be aware of limitations. As McClure [2003, p. 261] stated, "these details are important in deciding whether my patient is similar enough to those in the study to use these results with her." Awareness of current research also points to the fact that many of these studies emphasize the importance of splinting with early intervention because splints are less beneficial with ongoing parasthesia [Burke et al. 2003].

Wrist Splinting for Radial Nerve Injuries

Radial nerve injuries most commonly occur from fractures of the humeral shaft, fractures and dislocation of the elbow, or compressions of nerve [Skirven 1992]. Other reasons for radial nerve injuries include lacerations, gunshot wounds, explosions, and amputations. The classic picture of a radial nerve injury is a wrist drop position whereby the wrist and MCP joints are unable to actively extend. If the wrist is involved, sometimes a physician may order a wrist splint to place the wrist in a more functional position. The exact wrist positioning is highly subjective, and it is up to the therapist and the client to decide on the amount of extension that maximizes function.

Table 7-2 Research Efficacy on Wrist Splinting

AUTHOR'S CITATION	DESIGN	# OF PARTICIPANTS	DESCRIPTION	RESULTS	LIMITATIONS
Werner, R.A., Franzblau, A., Gell, N. (2005). Randomized controlled trial of nocturnal splinting for active workers with symptoms of carpal tunnel syndrome. *Archives of Physical Medicine and Rehabilitation,* 86: 1-7.	Randomized controlled trial	112 participants	Study performed in a Midwest auto plant. Workers with carpal tunnel syndrome (CTS) symptoms were included in the study. The treatment group was instructed to wear a customized wrist splint in a neutral posture at night for 6 weeks. Both groups viewed a video on workplace ergonomics and repetitive strain injuries. Outcome measures were assessed at 3, 6, and 12 months.	The 6-week trial of wrist splinting reduced discomfort scores, showed a trend in improvement of the Levine symptom severity scores among the participants in the treatment group and effects lasted throughout the 12-month assessment period.	This study included several limitations that could have affected the interpretation of the results. CTS was not diagnosed in participants before inclusion in the study. The sample size was small. The lack of complete data at 3 and 6 month appointments limited the interpretation of the outcomes. The loss of study subjects by the 3-month mark when optimal effects would have been expected may have confounded the analysis. Missing data in the regression model may have biased the analysis.
Gerritsen A.A., Korthals-de Bos I.B., Laboyrie P.M., de Vet H.C., Scholten R.J., Bouter L.M. (2003). Splinting for carpal tunnel syndrome: Prognostic indicators of success. *J Neurol Neurosurg Psychiatry,* 74: 1342-1344.	Randomized controlled trial	89 patients were randomized to the treatment group	Participants in the randomized treatment group were instructed to wear a neutral wrist splint at night for 6 weeks. Eighty-three participants attended follow-up sessions at 12 months after the initial intervention. Those patients (n = 33) who sought other types of treatment were not considered in the study's results.	Predicted probabilities of success of splinting at 12 months follow-up *Duration of complaints* / *Severity of paraesthesia at night* / *Predicted probability of success at 12 months* / *Actual success at 12 months* > 1 year / >6 / 5% / 13% (2/16) > 1 year / ≤6 / 19% / 12% (2/17) ≤ 1 year / >6 / 28% / 23% (6/26) ≤ 1 year / ≤6 / 62% / 67% (16/24)	The small number of participants involved in this study may have decreased detection of associations between the outcome and certain potential prognostic indicators. Authors cited this study as exploratory in nature.
Walker, W.C., Metzler, M., Cifu, D.X., Swartz, Z. (2000). Neutral wrist splinting in carpal tunnel syndrome: A comparison of night-only versus full-time wear instructions. *Archives of Physical Medicine and Rehabilitation,* 81 (4): 424-429.	Randomized clinical trial	21 patients participated, 17 completed the study	Subjects were randomly assigned to one of two groups: night-only wear or full-time wear. Participants were instructed to wear a custom-made thermoplastic neutral-positioned wrist splint. A self-administered questionnaire assessed symptom severity and functional deficits in CTS (Levine).	Six weeks of neutral wrist splinting in this study was associated with improved: symptoms, functional, and median nerve impairments. Despite a small sample size, there was a greater physiologic outcome in full-time splint wearers. More frequent wear lessened median nerve impairment.	This study was performed using a participant sample from the Veterans Administration consisting of predominantly male subjects (16 to 1). CTS appears more frequently in females, possibly decreasing the ability to generalize findings from the study. This study also lacked a nonintervention control group due to ethical considerations. This study could have benefited from a longer study period and larger sample size.

Celiker, R., Arslan, S., Inanici, F. (2002). Corticosteroid injection vs. nonsteroidal anti-inflammatory drug and splinting in carpal tunnel syndrome. *Phys Med Rehabil,* 81(3): 182-186.	Prospective, unblinded, randomized clinical trial	37 hands of 23 patients (none had thenar-atrophy)	Subjects were randomly assigned to either group A or group B. Group A was treated with a custom-made neutral wrist splint for night use only and acemetacine (120 mg/day). Intervention with group B included (40 mg methyl-prednisolone acetate) injected locally into the area of the carpal tunnel. Pre- and post-treatment measures included: VAS, Symptom Severity Scale, median nerve conduction studies, and Phalen's and Tinel tests.	Before treatment, Phalen's test was positive in 13 (81.3%) hands in group A and 14 (66.6%) hands in group B. Following treatment, Phalen's test was negative for all hands in group A and positive in three (14.3%) hands in group B. These findings were not statistically significant between groups. Scores from the VAS were not statistically significant between groups. Evaluation with the Symptom Severity Scale showed statistically significant improvement for both groups. Nerve conduction studies were statistically significant in improvement for both groups. In patients with symptom duration less than 9 months, splinting and steroid injection resulted in significant improvement in median nerve motor and sensory distal latencies. However, changes in conduction studies were not significant in clients with symptoms lasting more than 9 months.	Because of the short duration (8 weeks) of the study, long-term effects of the two treatment groups cannot be predicted. Results are derived from almost exclusively males and may not generalize beyond that population. This study also may not apply to those with severe CTS because patients with thenar atrophy were excluded from the study.
Graham, R.G., Hudson, D.A., Solomons, M., Singer, M. (2004). A prospective study to assess the outcome of steroid injections and wrist splinting for the treatment of carpal tunnel syndrome. *Plastic and Reconstructive Surgery,* 113(2): 550-556.	Prospective outcome study	75 patients with 99 affected hands were involved in the study	The protocol used in this study combined steroid injection with splinting for CTS. Each patient involved in the study received up to three betamethasone injections depending on the severity of their symptoms and wore a neutral wrist splint continuously for 9 weeks. Following the intervention, patients still experiencing symptoms received an open carpal tunnel release. Those who were asymptomatic received follow-up visits for 1 year. Patients who experienced a relapse after conservative treatment were scheduled for surgery.	In the conservative treatment group, only seven patients with 10 affected hands remained asymptomatic one year after the start of the study. Of the original treatment group, 10.1% of patients' symptoms were alleviated on a long-term basis using steroid injection and splinting alone. Of those patients that improved using conservative methods, most had shorter symptom duration (2.9 months versus 8.5 months) and less sensory involvement than those who did not improve with conservative methods. The researchers suggest that patients presenting with CTS receive one steroid injection and wear a neutral wrist splint for 3 weeks to determine whether or not a conservative approach might work for them or if they are good candidates for surgery.	One limitation of the study was the fluctuation of participants from beginning to end. Also, only patients experiencing symptoms for longer than 6 weeks were entered in the study. If patients with shorter symptom duration were included in the study, splinting may have shown greater efficacy.

Commonly, 30 degrees of extension is considered a position of function because it facilitates optimum grip and pinch [Cannon 1985]. Although a wrist splint is one option that can be fabricated for this condition, there are many other options therapists should critically consider. These include the location of splinting (volar versus dorsal), type of splint (e.g., wrist immobilization, tendodesis, or a splint with static elastic tension), and whether to fabricate one or two splints. More details about these other types of splinting options for a radial nerve injury are discussed in Chapter 13.

Wrist Splinting for Tendinitis and Tenosynovitis

Tendinitis (inflammation of the tendon), tenosynovitis (inflammation of the tendon and its surrounding synovial sheath), and tendinosis (a non-inflammatory tendon condition that involves collagen degeneration and disorganization of blood flow) [Khan et al. 2000] are painful conditions that benefit from conservative management, including wrist splinting. These conditions commonly occur because of cumulative and repetitive motions in work, home, and leisure activities. Tendinosis is more chronic in nature than tendonitis or tenosynovitis and usually impacts the lateral and medial elbow and rotator cuff tendons of the upper extremity [Khan et al. 2000]. Having tendonitis and tenosynovitis can result in an overuse cycle. The overuse cycle begins with friction, microscopic tears, pain, and limitations in motion, followed by resting the involved area, avoidance of use, and development of weakness. When activities resume, the cycle repeats itself [Kasch 2002]. Tendinitis or tenosynovitis can occur in many of the muscles on the volar (flexor muscles) and dorsal (extensor muscles) surfaces of the forearm.

These conditions often lead to substitution patterns and muscle imbalance [Kasch 2002]. Resting the hand in a splint helps to take tension off the muscle-tendon unit. Splinting for tendinitis or tenosynovitis minimizes tendon excursion and thus decreases friction at the insertion of the muscles. Splinting can serve as a reminder to decrease engagement in painful activities. It is beneficial to ask clients to pay attention to those activities that are limited by a splint because they are often aggravating factors for tendonitis. Clients should become more cognizant of aggravating activities and modify them so as not to enhance the condition [personal communication, K. Schultz-Johnson, April 6, 2006]. Clients should also be cautioned not to tense their muscles and thus fight against the splint when wearing it or it may aggravate the tendonitis. Rather, the muscles should be relaxed. Splints provided for tendonitis or tenosynovitis during acute flare-ups are worn continuously, with removal for hygiene and range-of-motion (ROM) exercises followed by gradual weaning.

Generally, when splinting for flexor carpi radialis (FCR) tenosynovitis it is recommended that the person's wrist be splinted at neutral to rest the tendons [Idler 1997]. Wrist extensor tendinitis can be splinted in 20 to 30 degrees of wrist extension, as this normal resting position provides a balance between the flexors and extensors.

Wrist Splinting for Rheumatoid Arthritis

For some conditions—such as rheumatoid arthritis (RA)—therapists fabricate wrist immobilization splints in functional positions of 0 to 30 degrees of wrist extension, thus promoting synergistic wrist-extension and finger-flexion patterns. This position allows the greatest level of function with grip ADL [Palmer et al. 1985, Melvin 1989].

Wearing a wrist splint may be used to control pain during activities [Kozin and Michlovitz 2000], and doing so is especially helpful in protecting the wrist during demanding tasks [Stern et al. 1997]. For people with radiocarpal or mid carpal arthritis, a wrist splint fabricated out of thin 1/16-inch thermoplastic material is recommended [Kozin and Michlovitz 2000]. For a total wrist arthrodesis, a volar wrist splint is provided when the cast is removed (usually about week 6 to 8). This volar wrist splint is worn full-time for 8 to 12 weeks [Bednar and Von Lersner-Benson 2002].

Wrist splinting for someone with RA can be quite challenging because of the tendency for the carpal structures of the rheumatoid arthritic wrist to sublux volarly and ulnarly [Dell and Dell 1996]. In addition, there can be related digital involvement to consider, such as MCP ulnar drift. In the early stages of this ulnar drift, the wrist joint should be positioned as close to neutral with respect to radial and ulnar deviation as can be comfortably tolerated. With consistent access to the person, the therapist can progress the wrist into neutral on successive visits. This position helps eliminate the development of a zigzag deformity. The zigzag deformity develops when the carpal bones deviate ulnarly and the metacarpals deviate radially, which exacerbates the ulnar deviation of the MCP joints [Dell and Dell 1996].

If the MCP joints but not the interphalangeal (IP) joints are involved, the therapist may consider fabricating a wrist splint in a neutral position that extends beyond the distal palmar crease and ends proximal to the proximal interphalangeal (PIP) crease. This splint supports the MCP joints (Figure 7-8) [Philips 1995]. Another recommendation for splinting someone with a zigzag deformity is to splint the entire hand (see Chapter 9).

When fabricating a wrist splint for a person with RA, the therapist uses a thermoplastic material with a high degree of conformability and drapability to help prevent pressure areas. However, when additional assistance is not available the long working time that highly rubber-based thermoplastic materials provide will help the therapist create a more cosmetic and well-fitting splint [personal communication, K. Schultz-Johnson, April 6, 2006]. The therapist carefully monitors for the development of pressure areas over many of the small bones of the hand and wrist, as shown in Figure 7-9 [Dell and Dell 1996]. Finally, some people with RA may prefer a prefabricated splint that is easy to apply and is perceived to be more comfortable than a fabricated splint because it is made out of softer material and has more flexibility. Further discussion later in this chapter addresses the functional implications of commercial wrist splints with RA.

Wrist Splinting for Fractures

The initial goal of rehabilitation after a fracture of the distal radius is to regain functional wrist extension [Laseter and Carter 1996]. To achieve this goal, splinting of the wrist in slight extension is beneficial while the person is receiving therapy. Wrist splinting post-fracture provides "protection and low load stress." It is best to fabricate a custom splint because prefabricated splints may not fit comfortably and may block range of motion of the fingers and thumb [Laseter 2002]. Sometimes serial static splinting may be necessary to regain PROM. (See the discussion later in this chapter for more details about serial static splinting).

The therapist fabricates a well-designed custom dorsal or volar splint. Laseter [2002] recommends fabricating a dorsal wrist splint because it helps control edema and allows for functional motions of the finger joints. If the person needs more support, a circumferential wrist splint may be considered [Laster 2002]. Circumferential splinting is highly supportive and very comfortable. It tends to limit forearm rotation more than a volar or dorsal wrist splint does [personal communication, K. Schultz-Johnson, April 1999]. The client should be weaned away from any splint as soon as possible [Laseter and Carter 1996, Laseter 2002]. To encourage regaining function, Weinstock [1999] recommended that the splint be part of treatment until 30 degrees to 45 degrees of active extension is obtained. For minimally displaced Colles' fractures, one researcher suggested that when a prefabricated Futuro splint was worn continuously for two weeks (with removal for hygiene) over a 6-week period subjects regained function faster than casted subjects [Mullett et al. 2003].

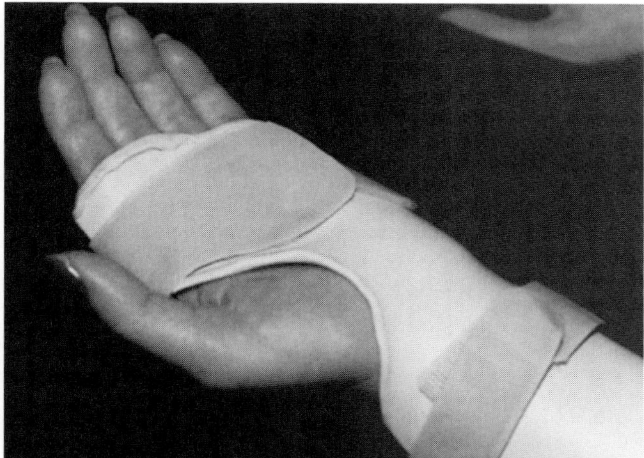

Figure 7-8 A splint for a zigzag deformity. [From Philips CA (1995). Therapist's management of patients with rheumatoid arthritis. In JM Hunter, EJ Mackin, AD Callahan (eds.), *Rehabilitation of the Hand, Fourth Edition*. St. Louis: Mosby, pp. 1345-1350.]

Wrist Splinting for Sprains

A grade I sprain results in a substance tear with minimal fiber disruption and no obvious tear of the fibers. A mild grade II sprain results in tearing of the ligament fibers. Persons with grade I and II sprains may benefit from wearing a wrist immobilization splint. With grade I sprains, the person will likely wear the splint for 3 weeks. For grade II sprains, 6 weeks of wear may be indicated. This wrist

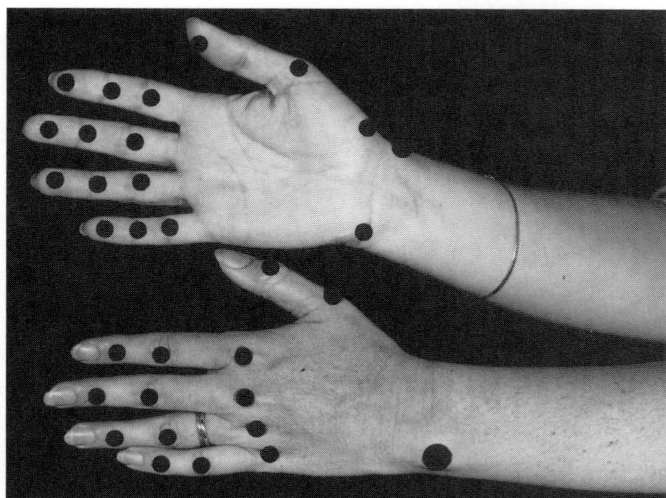

A

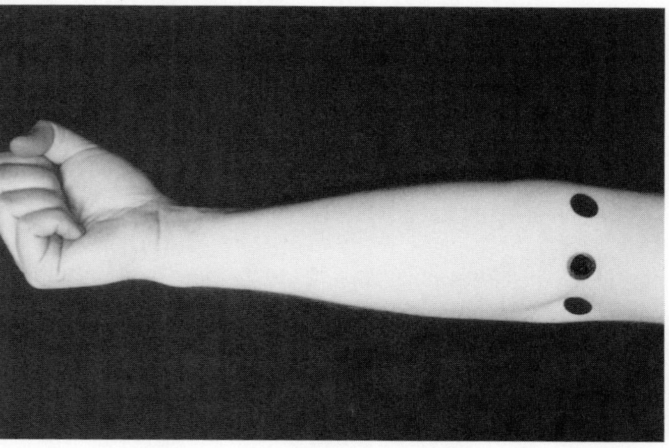

B

Figure 7-9 Potential areas of fingers, hand, wrist, and forearm include: dorsal MCP joints, thumb webspace, ulnar styloid, radial styloid, thumb CMC joint, center of palm (especially with flexion wrist contractures), proximal edge of splint. From Fess EE, Gettle KS, Phillips CA, et al: Hand and Upper Extremity Rehabilitation: Principles and Methods, ed 3, St. Louis, 2005, Mosby.

splint helps rest the hand during the acute healing phase and removes stress from the healing ligament.

Wrist Splinting for Complex Regional Pain Syndrome Type I (Reflex Sympathetic Dystrophy)

Complex regional pain syndrome (CRPS) describes a complex grouping of symptoms impacting an extremity and characterized by extreme pain, diffuse edema, stiffness, trophic skin changes, and discoloration [Taylor-Mullins 1992, Lankford 1995]. CRPS type I is a newer term coined by the World Health Organization to distinguish between sympathetically mediated and non-sympathetically mediated pain. CRPS type I is a sympathetically mediated pain [Mersky and Bogduk 1994, Phillips 2005]. CRPS type I refers to pain from a minor injury that lasts longer and hurts more than is anticipated. Type II refers to pain related to a nerve injury. Symptoms are similar for both types of pain [Phillips 2005].

Splinting is an important part of the rehabilitation program. The therapist applies clinical reasoning skills to determine which splint will meet the various therapeutic goals. (See the discussion on the use of resting hand splints with this condition in Chapter 11). The purposes for providing wrist immobilization splints include pain relief, muscle spasm relief, and regaining a functional resting wrist position [Lankford 1995, Saidoff and McDonough 1997, Walsh and Muntzer 2002]. Getting back to a functional resting hand position is important for normal hand motions and for the prevention of deforming forces as a result of muscle imbalance. To increase wrist extension to a more functional position, the therapist may need to provide serial wrist splints.

Wrist Joint Contracture: Serial Splinting with a Wrist Splint

When a wrist is not properly moving, as after removal of a cast for a Colles' fracture, the therapist may consider serial wrist splinting [Reiss 1995]. With serial splinting, the therapist intermittently remolds the splint to help increase wrist extension (Figure 7-10). The splint is first applied with the wrist positioned at the maximal amount of extension the current soft-tissue length allows and the person can tolerate. The person is instructed to wear the splint for long periods of time, with periodic removal for exercise and hygiene, until the wrist is able to move beyond that amount of extension.

The splint is readjusted to position the soft tissues at their maximum length [Colditz 2002]. Positioning living tissue at

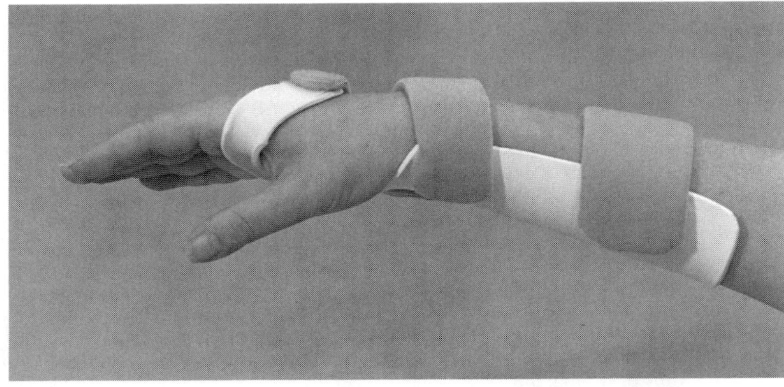

A

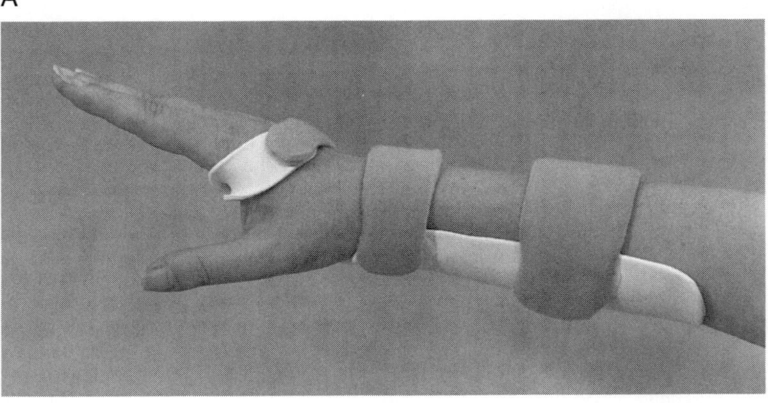

B

Figure 7-10 (A and B) Serial wrist splinting.

maximum length causes the tissue to remodel to a longer length [Schultz-Johnson 1996]. This process is repeated until optimal wrist extension is regained. Thus, serial splinting is beneficial for PROM limitations because it provides long periods of low load stress at or near the end of the soft-tissue length [Schultz-Johnson 1996]. Serial wrist splinting is only one splinting approach that can improve wrist PROM. Other approaches include fabricating a static progressive splint and an elastic tension splint (see Chapter 11).

Fabrication of a Wrist Immobilization Splint

The initial step in the fabrication of a wrist immobilization splint (after evaluation of the person's hand) is the drawing of a pattern. Pattern making is important in customizing a splint because every person's hand is different in shape and size. Pattern making also saves time and minimizes waste of materials.

A common mistake of a beginning splintmaker during fabrication of a wrist immobilization pattern is drawing the forearm trough narrower than the natural curve of the forearm muscle-bulk contour. This mistake can occur with anyone but especially with a person who has a large forearm. If the forearm trough is not one-half the circumference of the forearm, the splint does not provide adequate support. In addition, the therapist must follow the natural angle of the MCP heads with the pattern.

A volar wrist immobilization pattern presents another splinting option (Figure 7-11A). It is sometimes called a thumb-hole wrist splint [Stein 1991]. The therapist constructs the splint by punching a hole with a leather punch in the heated thermoplastic material and pushing the thumb through the hole. The therapist rolls the material away from the thumb and thenar eminence far enough that it does not interfere with functional thumb movement and yet allows adequate wrist support (Figure 7-11B). This thumb-hole wrist splint was found to be the most restrictive of wrist motion and slowest with dexterity performance compared with volar and dorsal wrist splints with metacarpal bars [Stein 1991, p. 47]. Figure 7-12A shows a pattern for a dorsal wrist immobilization splint. Figure 7-12B shows a pattern for an ulnar wrist immobilization splint. Figure 7-12C shows a pattern for a circumferential wrist immobilization splint.

Beginning splintmakers may learn to fabricate splint patterns by following detailed written instructions and looking at pictures of patterns. As therapists gain experience, they can easily draw patterns without copying from pictures. (See Figures 7-1, 7-2, 7-3, and 7-4 for pictures of completed splint products.) The following instructions are for construction of a volar wrist immobilization splint (Figures 7-6 and 7-13) and are similar to instructions for a dorsal wrist immobilization splint (Figures 7-7 and 7-12A).

1. Position the person's hand palm down on a piece of paper. The wrist should be as neutral as possible with respect to radial and ulnar deviation. The fingers should be in a natural resting position and slightly abducted. Draw an outline of the hand and forearm to the elbow.
2. While the person's hand is still on the paper, mark an *A* at the radial styloid and a *B* at the ulnar styloid. Mark the second and fifth metacarpal heads *C* and *D*, respectively. Mark the olecranon process of the elbow *E*. Remove the hand from the pattern. Mark two-thirds the length of the forearm on each side with an *X*. Place another *X* on each side of the pattern about 1 to 1-½ inches outside and parallel to the two previous *X* markings for two-thirds the length of the forearm and label each *F*. *These markings are to accommodate for the side of the forearm trough.*
3. Draw an angled line connecting the marks of the second and fifth metacarpal heads (*C* to *D*). Extend this line approximately 1 to 1-½ inches from the ulnar side of the hand and mark it *G*. On the radial side of the hand, extend the line straight out approximately 2 inches and mark it *H*.
4. On the ulnar side of the splint, extend the metacarpal line from the *G* down the hand and forearm of the splint pattern, making sure the pattern follows the person's forearm muscle bulk. End this line at *F*.

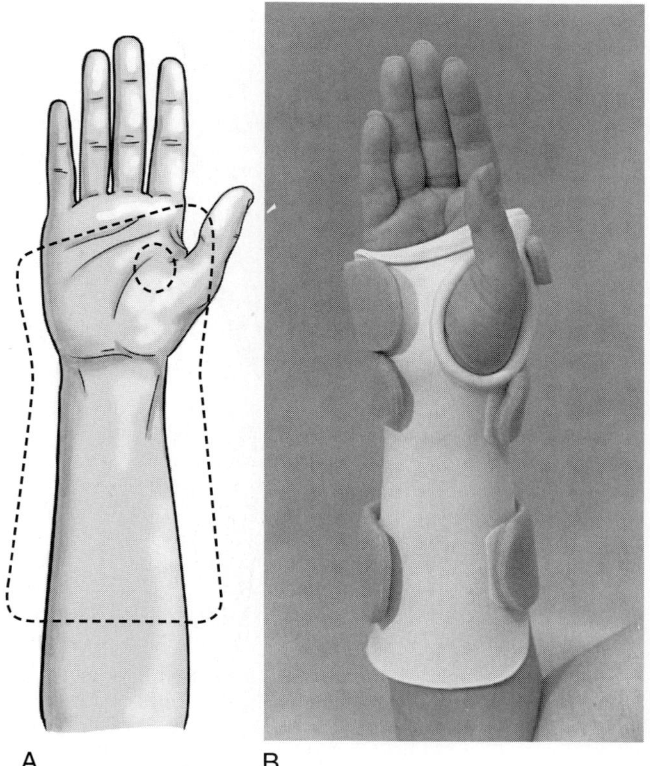

Figure 7-11 (A) A volar wrist immobilization pattern for a thumb-hole splint. (B) A volar wrist immobilization thumb-hole splint.

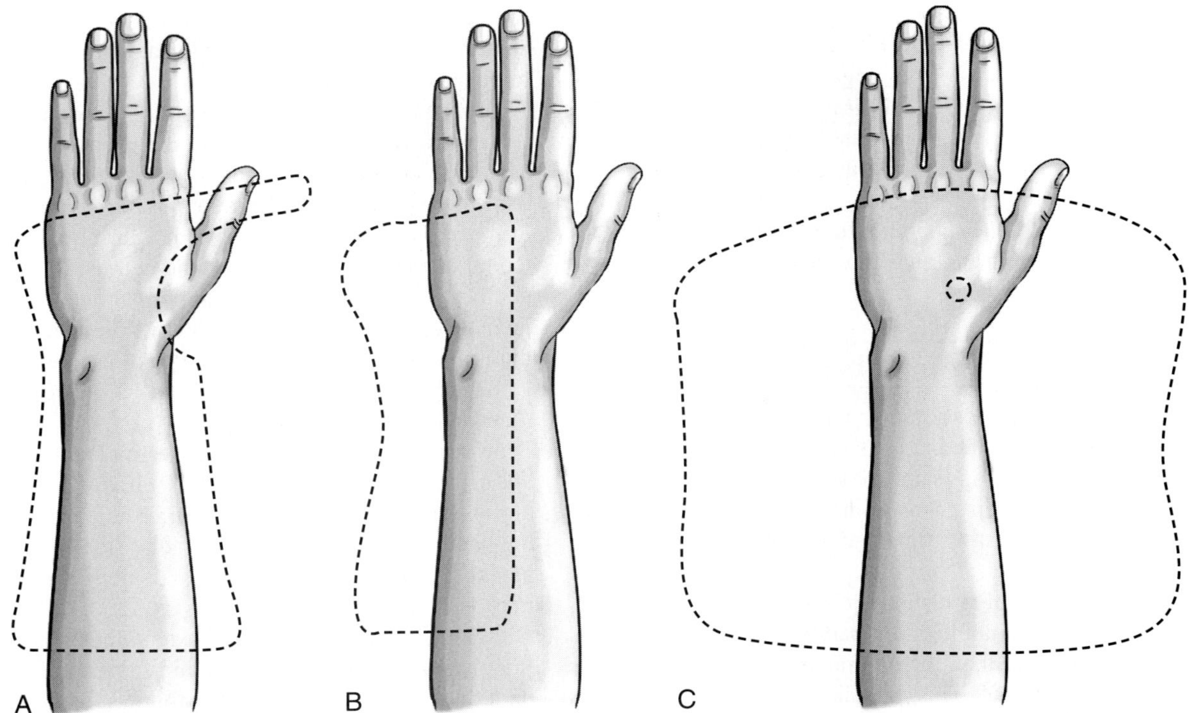

Figure 7-12 (A) A dorsal wrist immobilization pattern. (B) An ulnar wrist immobilization pattern. (C) A circumferential wrist immobilization pattern.

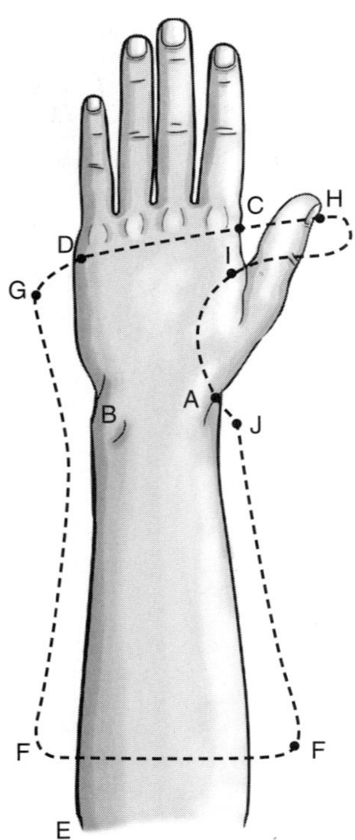

Figure 7-13 A detailed pattern for a volar wrist immobilization splint.

5. Measure and place an *I* approximately ¾ inch below the mark for the head of the index finger (*C*). Extend a line parallel from *I* to the line between *C* and *H*. Curve this line to meet *H*. This area represents the extension of the MP bar and usually measures approximately ¾ inch down from *C* to the outline on the other side of the MP bar. Draw a curved line that simulates the thenar crease from *I* to *A*. Extend the line past *A* about 1 inch and mark it *J*.
6. Draw a line from *J* down the radial side of the forearm, making sure the line follows the increasing size of the forearm. To ensure that the splint is two-thirds the length of the forearm, end the line at *F*.
7. For the bottom of the splint, draw a straight line connecting both *F* marks.
8. Make sure the pattern lines are rounded at *H*, *G*, *J*, and the two *F*s.
9. Cut out the pattern.
10. Position the person's upper extremity with the elbow resting on a pad (folded towel or foam wedge) on the table and the forearm in a neutral position rather than in supination or pronation, which results in a poorly fitted splint. Make sure the fingers are relaxed and the thumb is lightly touching the index finger. Place the wrist immobilization pattern on the person as shown in Figure 7-14A. Check that the wrist has adequate

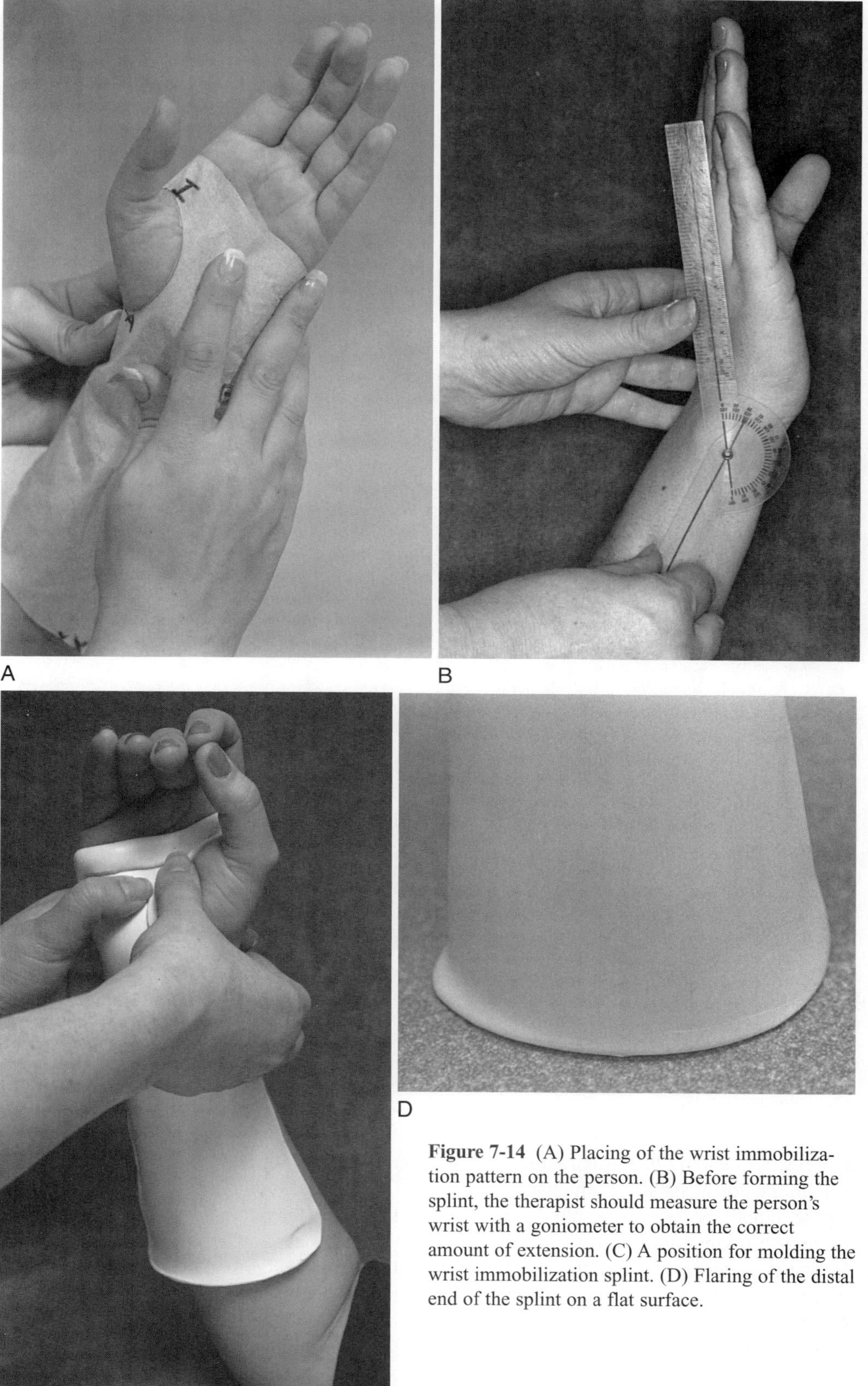

Figure 7-14 (A) Placing of the wrist immobilization pattern on the person. (B) Before forming the splint, the therapist should measure the person's wrist with a goniometer to obtain the correct amount of extension. (C) A position for molding the wrist immobilization splint. (D) Flaring of the distal end of the splint on a flat surface.

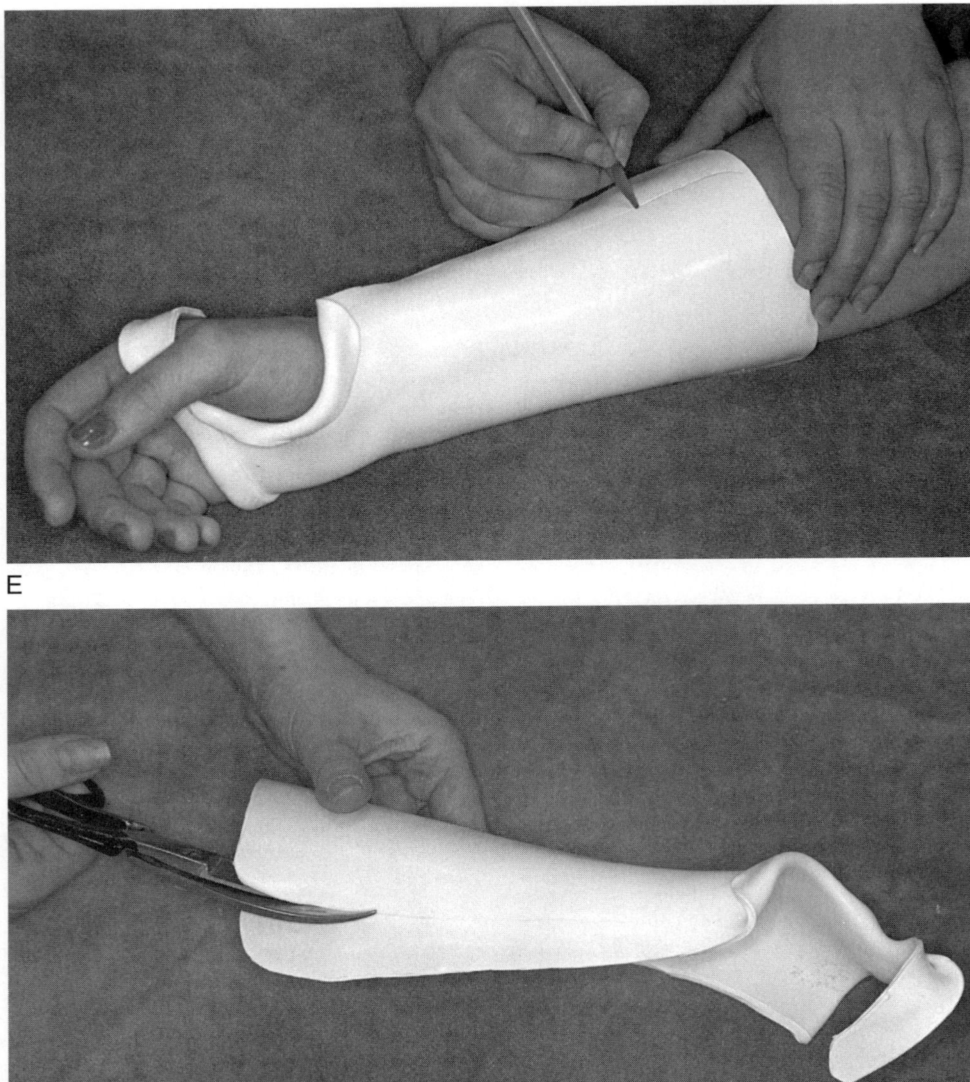

Figure 7-14, cont'd (E) Marking of the splint to make an adjustment. (F) Cutting off excess thermoplastic material to make an adjustment.

support, with the pattern ending just proximal to the MCP joint. On the dorsal surface of the hand, check whether the hypothenar bar on the ulnar side of the hand ends just proximal to the fifth metacarpal head. The metacarpal bar on the radial side of the hand should point to the triquetrum or distal ulna bone after it wraps through the first web space. On the volar surface of the hand, check below the thumb CMC joint to determine whether the pattern provides enough support at the wrist joint. Make sure the forearm trough is two-thirds the length and one-half the width of the forearm. Make necessary adjustments (i.e., additions or deletions) on the pattern.

11. Trace the pattern onto the sheet of thermoplastic material.
12. Heat the thermoplastic material.
13. Cut the pattern out of the thermoplastic material.
14. Measure the person's wrist using a goniometer to determine whether the wrist has been placed in the correct position. The therapist should instruct and practice with the person maintaining the correct position (Figure 7-14B).
15. Reheat the thermoplastic material.

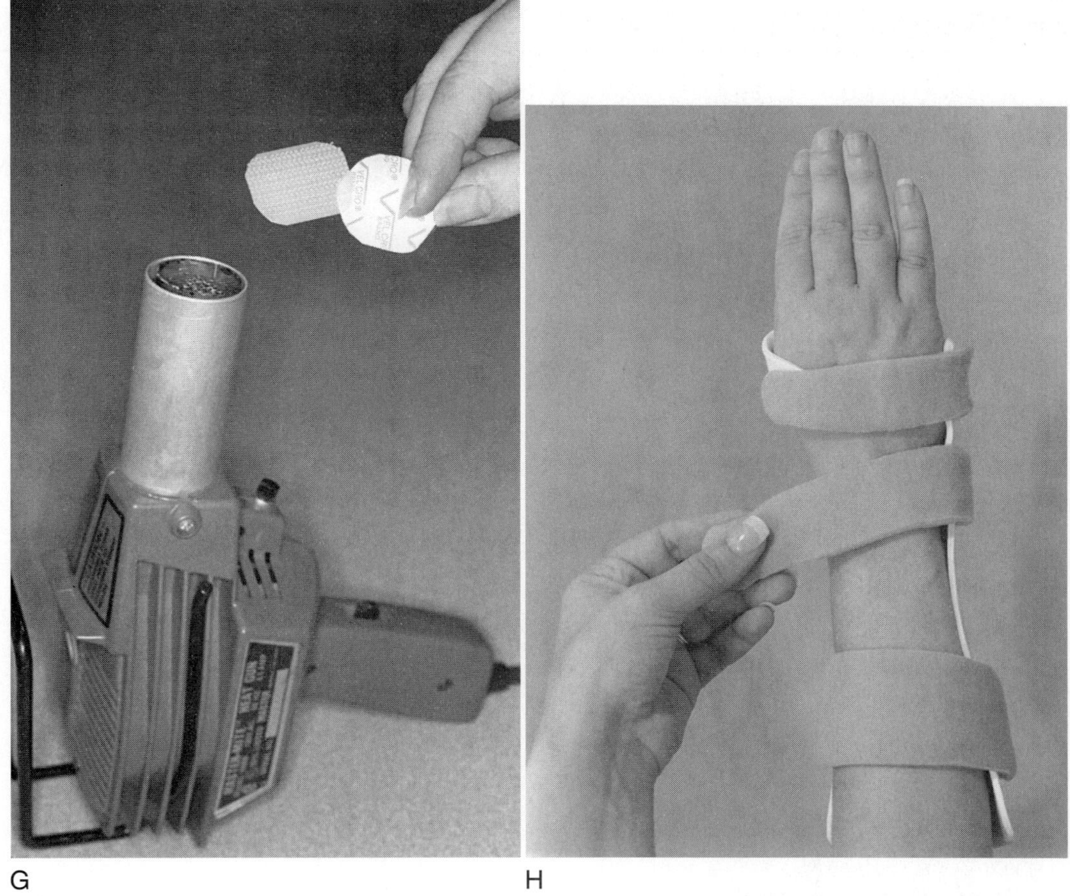

G H

Figure 7-14, cont'd (G) Heating of the Velcro tabs with a heat gun to help them adhere to the splint. (H) The therapist should place two straps on the forearm trough with one at the wrist level and one strap on the dorsal surface of the hand that connects the metacarpal bar to the hypothenar bar.

16. Mold the form onto the person's hand. To fit the splint on the person, place the person's elbow in a resting position on a pad on the table with the forearm in a neutral position. Make sure the fingers are relaxed and the thumb is lightly touching the index finger (Figure 7-14C). The advantage of this approach is that the therapist can better monitor the wrist position visually during splint formation.
17. Make sure the wrist remains correctly positioned as the thermoplastic material hardens. During the formation phase, roll the metacarpal bar just proximal to the distal palmar crease and roll the thermoplastic material toward the thenar crease. Flair the distal end of the splint on a flat surface (Figure 7-14D).
18. Make necessary adjustments on the splint (Figures 7-14E and 7-14F).
19. Cut the Velcro into approximately ½-inch oval shaped pieces for the MP bar area and 1-½- inch oval pieces for the forearm trough. Heat the adhesive with a heat gun to encourage adherence before putting them on the splint. Using a solvent on the thermoplastic material, scratch the thermoplastic material to remove some of the non-stick coating to help with adherence of the Velcro pieces (Figure 7-14G). For an adult, add two 2-inch straps on the forearm trough and one narrower strap on the dorsal surface of the hand, thus connecting the MP bar on the radial side to the hypothenar bar on the ulnar side of the hand. A child's splint will require straps that are narrower than an adult's. The strap placed at the wrist is located exactly at the wrist joint and not proximal to it to ensure a good fit (Figure 7-14H).

Laboratory Exercise 7-1

1. Practice making a wrist cock-up splint pattern on another person. Use the detailed instructions provided to draw the pattern.
2. Using the outline for the left and right hand following, draw a wrist immobilization pattern without the detailed instructions.

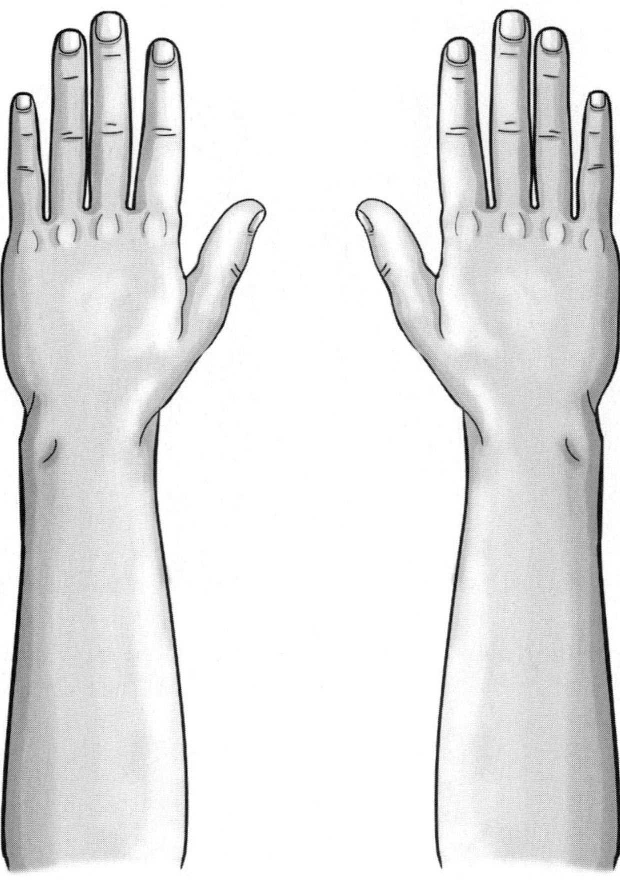

Technical Tips for a Proper Fit

- Choose a thermoplastic splinting material that has a high degree of conformability to allow a close fit and to prevent migration. Some therapists may prefer a rubber-based moderate drape thermoplastic material.
- Use caution when cutting a pattern out of thermoplastic material that stretches easily. Leave stretchable thermoplastic material flat on the table when cutting to prevent the material from stretching and the splint from losing the original shape of the pattern.
- Be sure the person's forearm is in neutral when forming the splint. Avoid splinting the forearm in a fully supinated or pronated position.
- It helps to mold the splint sequentially. For a volar wrist immobilization splint, form the hypothenar bar (Figure 7-15A), wrap the metacarpal bar around the palm to the dorsal side of the hand (Figure 7-15B), roll

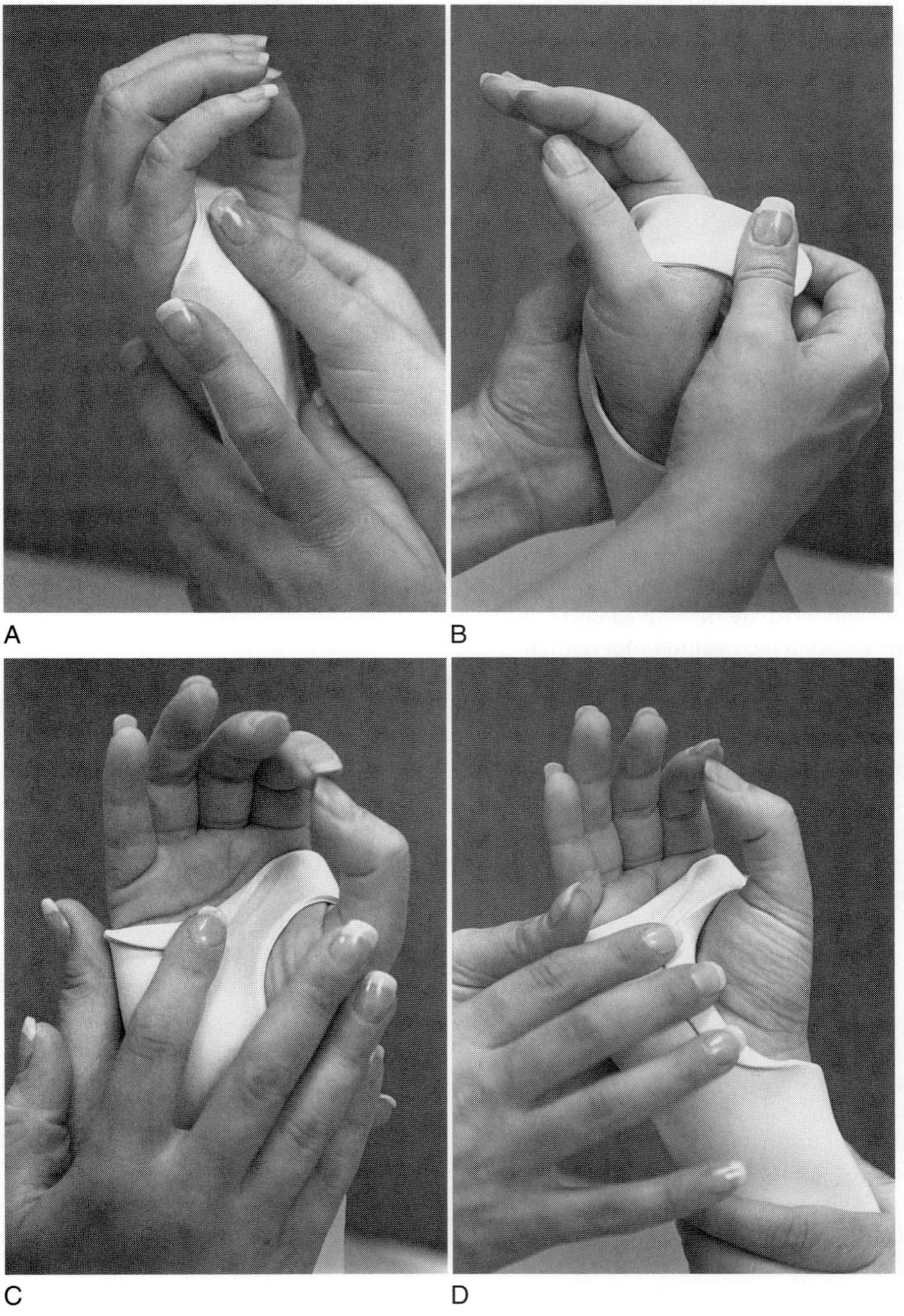

Figure 7-15 (A) The formation of the hypothenar bar. (B) Wrapping the metacarpal bar around the palm. (C) Rolling the metacarpal bar. (D) Forming the thenar area.

down the metacarpal bar (Figure 7-15C), and then form the thenar area (Figure 7-15D). See the specific comments in this section for hints about each of these areas.

- As the splint is being formed, be sure to follow the natural curves of the longitudinal, distal, and proximal arches. Having the person lightly touch the thumb to the index finger during molding will help conform the splint to the arches of the hand (Figure 7-14C). Mold the thermoplastic material to conform naturally to the center of the palm. Be careful not to flatten the transverse arch, which could cause metacarpal contractures. However, overemphasizing the transverse carpal arch can create a focal pressure point in the central palm that will be intolerable for the person.
- For a volar wrist immobilization splint, position the metacarpal bar on the volar surface just proximal to the distal palmar crease. This position allows adequate wrist support and full MCP flexion. In addition, make sure the metacarpal bar follows the natural angle of the distal transverse arch (Figure 7-15B). On the dorsal surface, position the metacarpal bar just proximal to the natural angle of the MCP heads. A correctly conformed dorsal metacarpal bar helps to hold the wrist in the correct position. If the metacarpal bar does not conform and there is a gap, the wrist will be mobile.
- Always determine whether the person has full finger flexion when wearing the splint by having him or her flex the MCP joints. If any areas of the metacarpal bar are too high, the therapist makes adjustments.
- Make sure the hand and wrist are positioned correctly by taking into consideration the position of a normal resting hand. On volar and dorsal wrist immobilization splints, the metacarpal bar (which wraps around the radial side of the hand) and the hypothenar bar (on the ulnar side) help position and hold the wrist (Figure 7-16). If adequate support is lacking on either side, the wrist may be in an incorrect position.
- A frequent fabrication mistake is to allow the wrist to deviate radially or ulnarly. This mistake can occur because of a lack of careful monitoring of the person's wrist position as the thermoplastic material is cooling. The therapist should closely monitor the wrist position in any splint that positions the wrist in neutral, because it is easy for the wrist to move in slight flexion. A quick spot check before the thermoplastic material is completely cool can address this problem.
- If a mistake occurs with a splint material that easily stretches, be extremely careful with adjustments to avoid further compromising of wrist position. For splinting material with memory, remold the entire splint rather than spot heating the wrist area because doing the latter tends to cause the material to buckle. Sometimes adjustments can be done by heating the entire splint made from material without memory.

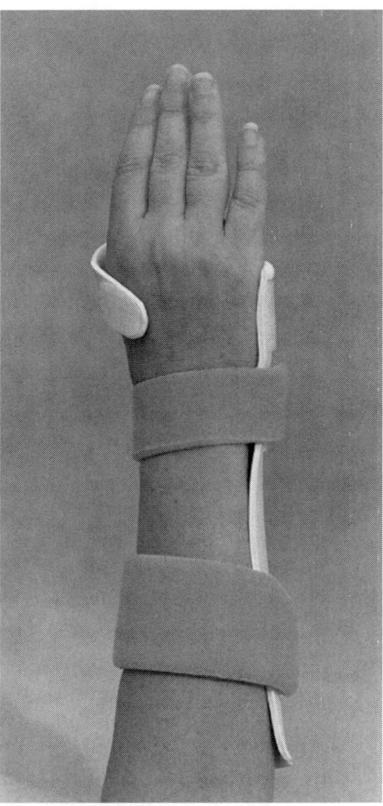

Figure 7-16 The metacarpal bar and hypothenar bar help position and hold the wrist.

- After the formation of the palmar and wrist part of the splint is complete, the therapist can begin to work on other areas of the splint, such as the forearm trough. A problem that can easily be corrected just before the thermoplastic material is cooled is twisting of the forearm trough. If this problem is not corrected, the splint will end up with one edge of the forearm trough higher than the other (Figure 7-17).
- After the thermoplastic material has cooled, determine whether the person can fully oppose the thumb to all fingers. The thenar eminence should not be restricted or flattened. Wrist support should be adequate to maintain the angle of the wrist. To check whether the thenar eminence area is rolled enough, have the person move the thumb in opposition to the little finger and sustain the hold while evaluating the roll. Also observe that the thenar crease is visible, to allow for full thumb mobility. Adjustments should be made to allow complete thumb excursion. Otherwise, there is a potential for a pressure sore to develop (Figure 7-18).
- Sometimes after the thermoplastic material is cooled the therapist will note areas that are too tight in the forearm trough, which can potentially result in pressure sores.

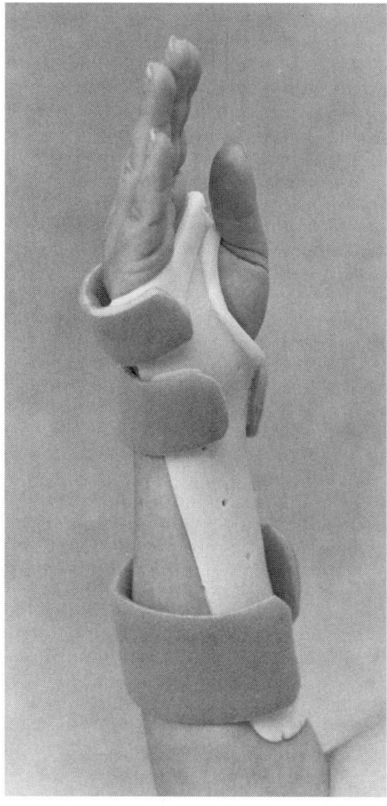

Figure 7-17 This forearm trough was twisted.

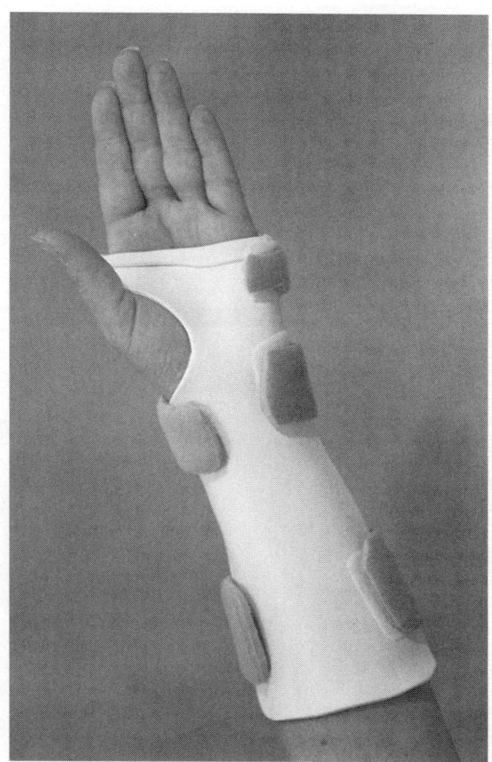

Figure 7-18 This thenar web space was not rolled enough to allow full thumb excursion.

To easily correct this problem, the therapist pulls apart the sides of the forearm trough.

Trouble Shooting Wrist Immobilization Splints

A careful splintmaker must continuously think of precautions, such as checking for pressure areas. Precautions for making a wrist immobilization splint include the following.

- Be aware of and make adjustments for potential pressure points on the radial styloid, on the ulnar styloid, at the first web space, and over the dorsal aspects of the metacarpals. The thumb web space is a prime area for skin irritation because it is so tender. Some people cannot tolerate plastic in the first web space, and it must be cut back and replaced with soft strapping. Others can tolerate the plastic if it is rolled and extremely thin [personal communication, K. Schultz-Johnson, April 1999]. Instruct the person to monitor the skin for reddened areas and to communicate immediately about any irritation that occurs.
- Try to control edema before splint provision. For persons with sustained edema, avoid using constricting wrist splints. Instead, fabricate a wider forearm trough with wide strapping material [Cannon et al. 1985]. Dorsal splints are better for edematous hands [Colditz 2002, Laseter 2002]. Carefully monitor persons who have the potential for edematous hands and make necessary splint adjustments. As discussed earlier, a "continuous strap" made out of flexible fabric is a good strapping option to help manage edema.
- For persons with little subcutaneous tissue and thin skin, carefully monitor the skin for pressure areas. Lining the splint with padding may help, but several adjustments may be necessary for a proper fit. Sometimes fabricating the splint over a thick splint liner or a QuickCast liner helps prevent skin irritation during splint fabrication.
- Make sure the splint provides adequate support for functional activities.
- Wrist immobilization splints are contraindicated for persons with active MCP synovitis and PIP synovitis [Melvin 1989]. These conditions often occur in hands with rheumatoid arthritis and may require wrist and hand splinting.

Laboratory Exercise 7-2 Splint A

1. What problems can you identify regarding this splint?

2. What problems may arise from continual splint wear?

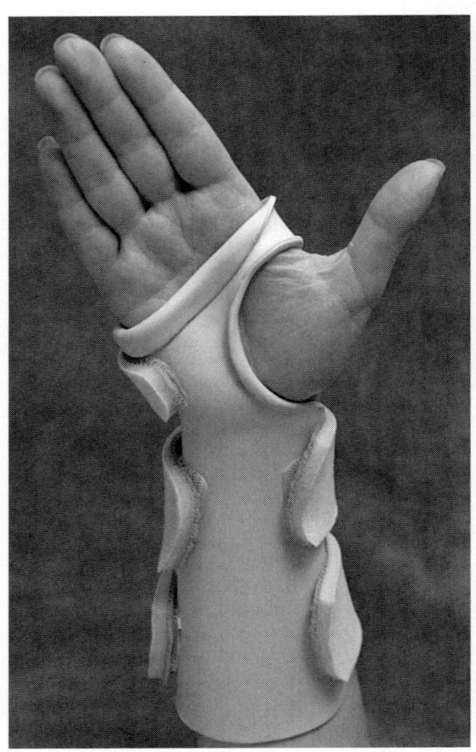

Laboratory Exercise 7-2 Splint B

You are supervising a student in clinical practice. You ask the student to practice making a wrist immobilization splint before actually fabricating a splint on a person. Splint B is a picture of the student's splint.

1. What problems should you address with the student regarding the splint?

____

____

____

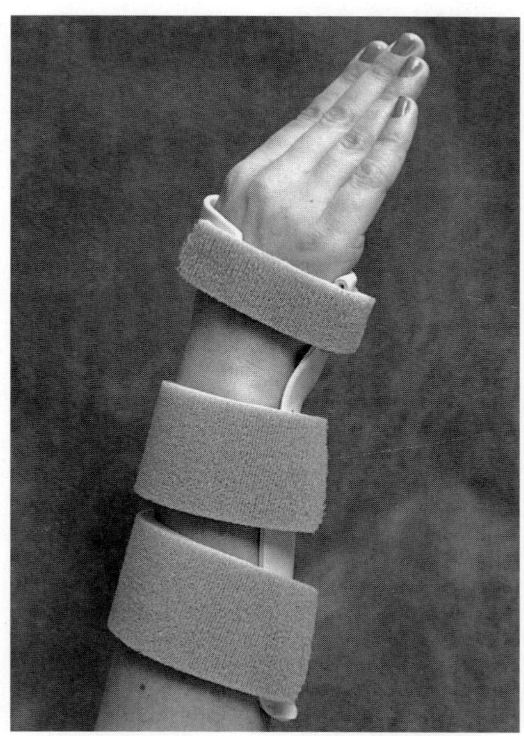

Laboratory Exercise 7-2 Splint C

Splint C was made for a 54-year-old man working as a bus driver. The person works full-time and has wrist extensor tendinitis.

1. What problems can you identify regarding this splint?

___

___

___

2. What problems may arise from continual splint wear?

___

___

___

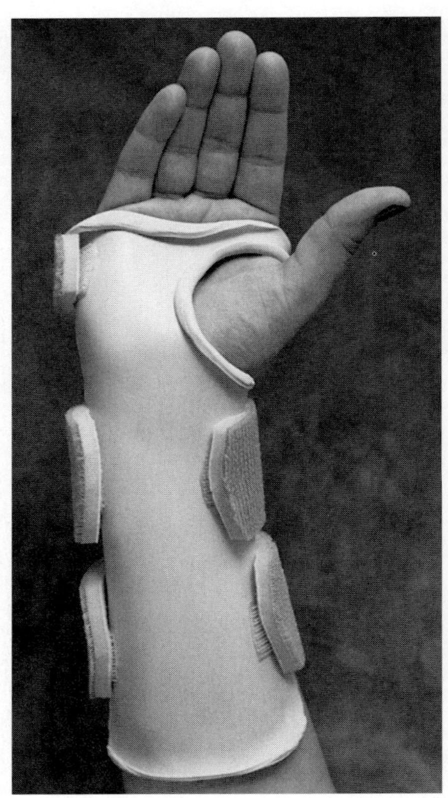

Laboratory Exercise 7-3

Practice fabricating a wrist immobilization splint on a partner. Before starting, determine the correct position for your partner's hand. Measure the angle of wrist extension with a goniometer to ensure a correct position. After fitting your splint and making all adjustments, use Form 7-1 as a self-evaluation of the wrist immobilization splint, and use Grading Sheet 7-1 as a classroom grading sheet.

FORM 7-1 Wrist immobilization splint

Name: ____________________

Date: ____________________

Type of cone wrist and hand splint:

Volar platform ❍ Dorsal platform ❍

Wrist position: ____________________

After the person wears the splint for 30 minutes, answer the following questions. (Mark *NA* for nonapplicable situations.) Discuss possible splint adjustments or changes you should make based on the self-evaluation. (What would you do differently next time?)

____

____

____

____

____

____

____

____

Evaluation Areas and Comments

Design

1. The wrist position is at the correct angle.	Yes ❍	No ❍	NA ❍
2. The wrist has adequate support.	Yes ❍	No ❍	NA ❍
3. The sides of the thenar and hypothenar eminences have support in the correct position.	Yes ❍	No ❍	NA ❍
4. The thenar and hypothenar eminences are not restricted or flattened.	Yes ❍	No ❍	NA ❍
5. The splint is two-thirds the length of the forearm.	Yes ❍	No ❍	NA ❍
6. The splint is one-half the width of the forearm.	Yes ❍	No ❍	NA ❍

Function

1. The splint allows full thumb motions.	Yes ❍	No ❍	NA ❍
2. The splint allows full MCP joint flexion of the fingers.	Yes ❍	No ❍	NA ❍
3. The splint provides wrist support that allows functional activities.	Yes ❍	No ❍	NA ❍

Straps

1. The straps are secure and rounded.	Yes ❍	No ❍	NA ❍

Comfort

1. The splint edges are smooth with rounded corners.	Yes ❍	No ❍	NA ❍
2. The proximal end is flared.	Yes ❍	No ❍	NA ❍
3. The splint does not cause impingements or pressure sores.	Yes ❍	No ❍	NA ❍
4. The splint does not irritate bony prominences.	Yes ❍	No ❍	NA ❍

Continued

FORM 7-1 Wrist immobilization splint—cont'd

Cosmetic Appearance

1. The splint is free of fingerprints, dirt, and pencil and pen marks. Yes ❍ No ❍ NA ❍
2. The splinting material is not buckled. Yes ❍ No ❍ NA ❍

Therapeutic Regimen

1. The person has been instructed in a wearing schedule. Yes ❍ No ❍ NA ❍
2. The person has been provided splint precautions. Yes ❍ No ❍ NA ❍
3. The person demonstrates understanding of the education. Yes ❍ No ❍ NA ❍
4. Client/caregiver knows how to clean the splint. Yes ❍ No ❍ NA ❍

GRADING SHEET 7-1* Wrist immobilization splint

Name: ______________________

Date: ______________________

Type of wrist immobilization splint:

Volar ❍ Dorsal ❍

Wrist position: ______________________

Grade:__________

1 = beyond improvement, not acceptable
2 = requires maximal improvement
3 = requires moderate improvement
4 = requires minimal improvement
5 = requires no improvement

Evaluation Areas						Comments
Design						
1. The wrist position is at the correct angle.	1	2	3	4	5	
2. The wrist has adequate support.	1	2	3	4	5	
3. The sides of the thenar and hypothenar eminences have support in the correct position.	1	2	3	4	5	
4. The splint is one-half the width of the forearm.	1	2	3	4	5	
5. The thenar and hypothenar eminences are not restricted or flattened.	1	2	3	4	5	
6. The splint is two-thirds the length of the forearm.	1	2	3	4	5	
Function						
1. The splint allows full thumb motion.	1	2	3	4	5	
2. The splint allows full MCP joint flexion of the fingers.	1	2	3	4	5	
3. The splint provides wrist support that allows functional activities.	1	2	3	4	5	
Straps						
1. The straps are secure and rounded.	1	2	3	4	5	
Comfort						
1. The splint edges are smooth with rounded corners.	1	2	3	4	5	
2. The proximal end is flared.	1	2	3	4	5	
3. The splint does not cause impingements or pressure sores.	1	2	3	4	5	
4. The splint does not irritate bony prominences.	1	2	3	4	5	
Cosmetic Appearance						
1. The splint is free of fingerprints, dirt, and pencil and pen marks.	1	2	3	4	5	
2. The splinting material is not buckled.	1	2	3	4	5	

*See Appendix C for a perforated copy of this grading sheet.

Prefabricated Splints

Prefabricated wrist splints are commonly used in the treatment of CTS and RA [Dell and Dell 1996, Stern et al. 1997, Williams 1992]. A variety of prefabricated wrist splints are available, as shown in Table 7-3.

As discussed, conservative management of CTS includes positioning the wrist as close to neutral as possible to maximize the space in the carpal tunnel. The supportive metal or thermoplastic stay in most prefabricated wrist splints positions the wrist in extension. Therefore, an adjustment must be made to position the wrist in the desired neutral position. However, care must be taken when adjustments are made to ensure that the splint adequately fits and supports the hand.

Several options for prefabricated wrist splints are marketed for CTS. Options for the work environment include padding to reduce trauma from vibration, leather for added durability, and metal internal pieces that act to position the wrist. Prefabricated wrist immobilization splints are also effective for symptoms of CTS during pregnancy [Courts 1995]. (See Figure 7-19.)

Splinting a person who has RA is most effective in the early stages and incorporates positioning, immobilization, and the assumed comfort of neutral warmth from a soft splint. The effects of RA can result in decreased joint stability, leading to decreased grip strength and the more obvious finger deformities [Dell and Dell 1996]. When persons with RA wear elastic wrist orthoses, they help decrease pain during ADL [Stern et al. 1996]. Prefabricated wrist splints marketed for persons with RA are designed for easy application and to decrease ulnar deviation. Some splints include correction or protection for finger joints as well as for the wrist joint.

Therapists need to determine whether or not to fabricate a custom wrist splint or to use a commercial prefabricated wrist splint. There are many factors to consider with this decision, such as the impact of the prefabricated or custom splint on hand function, pain reduction, and degrees of immobilization the splint provides [Stern et al. 1996a, 1996b; Pagnotta et al. 1998; Collier and Thomas 2002]. Research helps therapists select the best splint for their clients. Collier and Thomas [2002, p. 182] studied the degree of immobilization of a custom volar wrist splint as compared to three commercial prefabricated wrist splints. They found that the custom wrist splint allowed "significantly less palmar flexion and significantly more dorsi flexion" than the commercial splints. Thus, custom thermoplastic splints may block wrist motion better than prefabricated splints, which are more flexible.

Other studies considered the effect of commercial prefabricated splints on grip and dexterity [Stern 1996; Stern et al. 1996a, 1996b; Burtner et. al 2003], work performance [Pagnotta et al. 1998], and proximal musculature [Bulthaup et al. 1999]. See Table 7-2 for more details about the efficacy of these studies. Continued research needs to be done to analyze the efficacy of commercial splints, especially as newer ones are developed. Furthermore, as Stern et al. [1997] found, no single type of wrist splint will be appropriate for all clients and that satisfaction with a prefabricated splint is often associated with therapeutic benefits, comfort, and utility. Therefore, it benefits therapists to stock a variety of prefabricated splint options in the clinic [Stern et al. 1997]. Box 7-1 provides some questions for therapists to contemplate when considering a prefabricated wrist splint or custom-made wrist splint.

Impact on Occupations

Supporting the wrist to allow finger and thumb motions enables people with the discussed diagnoses in this chapter to continue their life occupations. For example, a person with CTS wears a wrist splint to avoid extreme wrist positions when working and doing other occupations. A person with arthritis obtains support and pain relief from wearing a wrist splint while doing functional activities. A person with a Colles' fracture after being serial splinted to decrease stiffness will eventually be able to better perform meaningful occupations. Wrist splints can help many people maintain or eventually improve their functional abilities.

Table 7-3 Prefabricated Wrist Splint Examples

THERAPEUTIC OBJECTIVE	DESCRIPTION
Positions the wrist in neutral, extension, or slight flexion to support and rest the wrist joint during functional tasks	Circumferential wrist splints are available in a variety of sizes. Some wrist splints have a metal or thermoplastic stay, which usually can be adjusted to position the wrist in neutral, extension, or slight flexion. Options available include D-ring straps (Figure 7-19A) and wrist support with laces (Figure 7-19B). Another wrist splinting option is this lightweight splint for CTS (Figure 7-19C). Splints are available in such materials as cloth, thermoplastic, neoprene (Figure 7-19D), elastic, and polyester/cotton laminates.

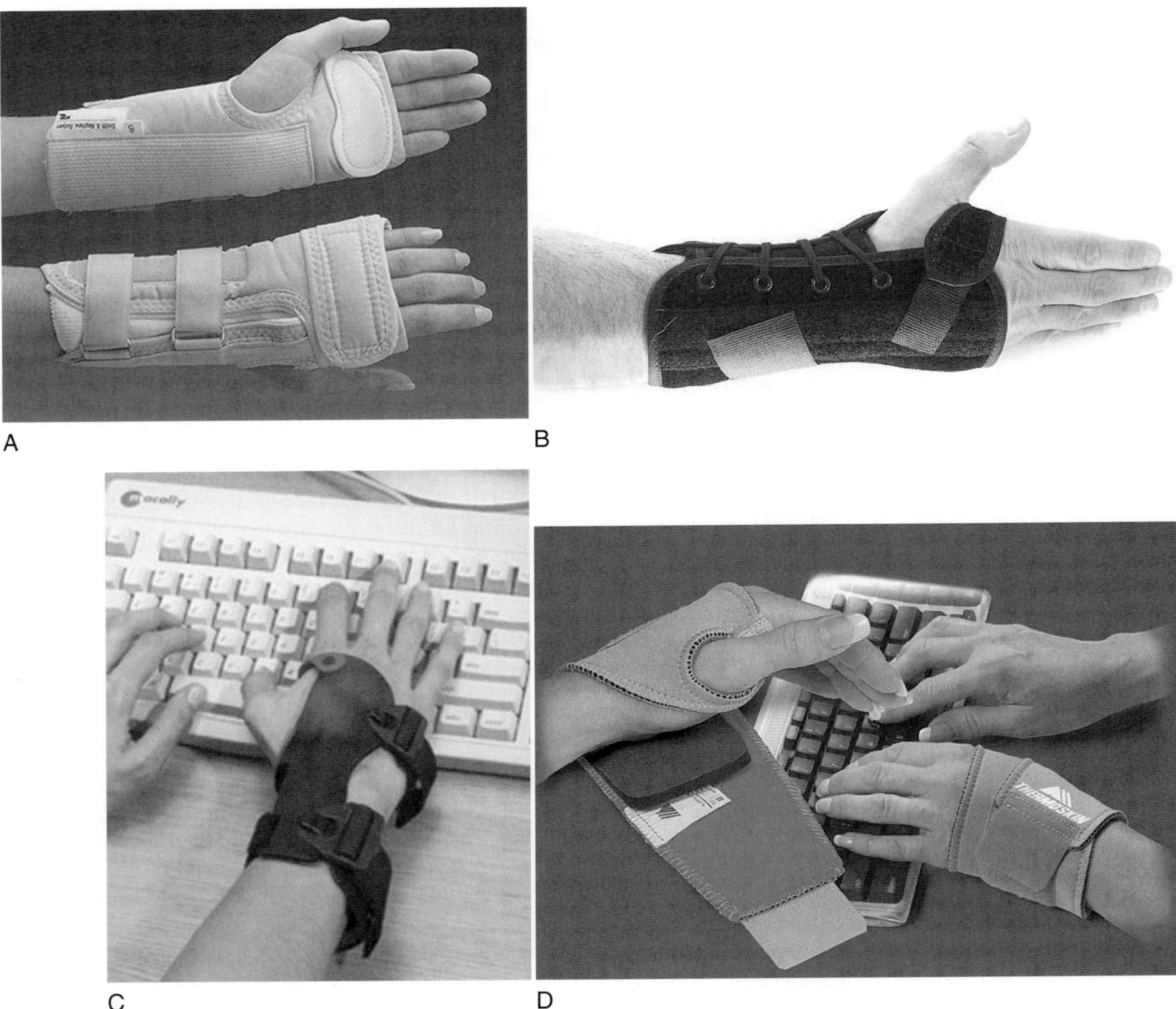

Figure 7-19 (A) This wrist splint has D-ring straps (Rolyan D-Ring Wrist Brace). (B) This wrist splint has a unique strapping system with laces (Sammons Preston Rolyan Laced Wrist Support). (C) This light weight splint can be used for carpal tunnel and other repetitive injuries (Exolite Wrist Brace). (D) This splint is made of a neoprene blend, which allows circulation to the skin (Termoskin Wrist Brace). [Courtesy of Sammons Preston Rolyan, Bolingbrook, IL.]

Box 7-1 Questions to Determine Use of Custom-made Versus Prefabricated Wrist Splint

Is time a factor? (Consider providing prefabricated splints, although with experience a custom splint can be made in a short time period.)
Is cost a factor? (Consider costs with custom splints versus prefabricated splints.)
Is fit a factor? (Consider whether the prefabricated splint is restricting too much motion, such as thumb opposition, or chafes the hand [Stern et al. 1996]. Or consider whether it is really doing what it is supposed to do, such as keeping the hand in neutral with carpal tunnel syndrome [Walker et al. 2000].)
Is only wrist support required? (Consider a prefabricated splint.)
Is restriction of motion a factor? (Consider a custom splint.)
Does the person need the splint only for pain relief, such as with arthritis? (Consider a prefabricated splint or a custom-made splint with padding.)
Is the person involved in sports? (Consider a soft prefabricated splint to avert injury to other people [Bell-Krotoski and Berger-Stanton 2002].)
Is wrist and hand edema a factor? (Consider fabricating a custom dorsal wrist splint, taking edema into consideration.)
Is the weight of the splint a factor? (Consider custom fabricated splints made of lighter thermoplastic material [1/16 inch] or lightweight prefabricated splints.)
What are the occupational demands of the person? (Consider custom fabrication if heavy labor is part of the person's life or a prefabricated splint if demands are minimal [Kozin and Michlovitz 2000]. Consider the material out of which the prefabricated splint is fabricated. A prefabricated splint out of leather may provide adequate durability, support, protection, and comfort for job demands.)
Have I accessed any research on the splints I am considering?

Summary

As this chapter content reflects, appropriate wrist alignment is very important to maintaining a functional hand. A well-fitted splint can be a key element to assist with recovery from many conditions. Therefore, therapists should be aware of diagnostic indications, types, parts, and appropriate fabrication for wrist splinting. As always in clinical practice, the therapist will need to apply clinical reasoning, as each case will be different. Finally, therapists should consider the person's occupations when providing a wrist splint.

CASE STUDY 7-1*

Read the following scenario and use your clinical reasoning skills to answer the questions based on information in this chapter.

Mrs B., a pharmacist working in research, found that when she was six months pregnant she developed nocturnal pain and numbness, grasp weakness, clumsiness, stiff hand, and parastheias over the median distribution in her left dominant hand. These symptoms tended to be intermittent. However, over time as she continued to use her left upper extremity the symptoms got worse. Mrs. B. went to her family physician, whose nurse provided her with a prefabricated wrist splint. Not being familiar with the correct wrist positioning for CTS, the nurse did not adjust the prefabricated splint and left it in 20 degrees of wrist extension.

Mrs. B. felt that the splint was uncomfortable as it migrated distally on her forearm, limiting thumb and finger motions. She dutifully wore the splint. Mrs. B. later remarked that because she was in the medical field she felt that it was important to correctly follow medical regimens. After pitting and canning 5 gallons of cherries, her symptoms intensified. She returned to her family physician. This time he referred her to a neurologist, who diagnosed her with CTS, provided a cortisone shot, and referred her to occupational therapy. The occupational therapist removed the prefabricated splint and requested an order for a custom splint. At that point, Mrs. B. had doubts about wearing any splint. She asked for valid reasons for the custom splint. She stated in frustration, "Why don't I just go ahead and have surgery after the birth!"

1. Provide two reasons the prefabricated splint was not the best choice.

____

____

____

____

2. Describe the correct position for Mrs. B.'s wrist.

____

____

3. What would be the suggested wearing schedule?

____

____

____

4. What precautions are important with splint wear?

____

____

____

____

5. How should the therapist address Mrs. B.'s concerns about getting a custom splint and surgery?

____

____

____

____

*See Appendix A for the answer key.

CASE STUDY 7-2*

Read the following scenario and use your clinical reasoning skills to answer the questions based on information from this chapter.

Mrs P., a 73-year-old woman, had gone out to a restaurant with her husband. At dusk, when they walked out of the building Mrs. P. tripped and fell with her right dominant outstretched hand onto a cement and metal surface. She underwent open reduction and internal fixation of the wrist for Colles' fracture. After her cast was removed, the physician ordered therapy for edema and pain control, ROM, and fabrication of a wrist splint for the right upper extremity.

1. Mrs. P. presents with her right wrist in 15 degrees flexion. Her wrist can be passively extended to neutral. Describe the splinting position for her right hand and the rationale for the position.
____
____
____

2. As Mrs. P.'s range of motion improves what will you do with splinting?
____
____
____

3. At what point would you discontinue wrist splinting?
____
____
____

*See Appendix A for the answer key.

REVIEW QUESTIONS

1. What are three main indications for use of a wrist immobilization splint?
2. When fabricating a wrist splint for a person with RA, what are some of the common deformities that can influence splinting?
3. When might a therapist consider serial splinting with a wrist immobilization splint?
4. What are the goals of wrist splinting with a Colles' fracture?
5. What is the advantage of a volar wrist immobilization splint?
6. What is a disadvantage of a dorsal wrist immobilization splint?
7. What purpose does the hypothenar bar serve on a wrist immobilization splint?
8. What are two positions the therapist can use for molding a static wrist splint, and what are the advantages of each?
9. Which precautions are unique to static wrist immobilization splints?
10. What are four questions therapists could consider when deciding on a prefabricated wrist splint versus a custom fabricated wrist splint?

References

Alakin E, El O, Peker O, Senocak O, Tamaci S, Gulbahar S, et al. (2002). Treatment of carpal tunnel syndrome with nerve and tendon gliding exercises. The American Journal of Physical Medicine and Rehabilitation 81:108-113.

American Society of Hand Therapists (1992). *Splint Classification System*. Chicago: American Society of Hand Therapists.

Apfel E, Johnson M, Abrams R (2002). Comparison of range-of-motion constraints provided by prefabricated splints used in the treatment of carpal tunnel syndrome: A pilot study. Journal of Hand Therapy 15(3):226-233.

Bednar JM, Von Lersner-Benson C (2002). Wrist reconstruction: Salvage procedures. In EJ Mackin, AD Callahan, TM Skirven, LH Schneider (eds.), *Rehabilitation of the Hand and Upper Extremity, Fifth Edition*. St. Louis: Mosby, pp. 1195-1202.

Bell-Krotoski JA, Breger-Stanton DE (2002). Biomechanics and evaluation of the hand. In EJ Mackin, AD Callahan, TM Skirven, LH Schneider (eds.), *Rehabilitation of the Hand and Upper Extremity, Fifth Edition*. St. Louis: Mosby, pp. 240-262.

Biese J (2002). Therapist's evaluation and conservative management of rheumatoid arthritis in the hand and wrist. In EJ Mackin, AD Callahan, TM Skirven, LH Schneider (eds.), *Rehabilitation of the Hand and Upper Extremity, Fifth Edition*. St. Louis: Mosby, pp. 1569-1582.

Bulthaup S, Cipriani DJ, Thomas JJ (1999). An electromyography study of wrist extension orthoses and upper extremity function. American Journal of Occupational Therapy 53(5):434-444.

Burke FD, Ellis J, McKenna H, Bradley MJ (2003). Primary care management of carpal tunnel syndrome. Postgraduate Medical Journal 79(934):433-437.

Burtner PA, Anderson JB, Marcum ML, Poole JL, Qualls C, Picchiarini MS (2003). A comparison of static and dynamic wrist splints using electromyography in individuals with rheumatoid arthritis. Journal of Hand Therapy 16(4):320-325.

Cannon NM (1985). *Manual of Hand Splinting*. New York: Churchill Livingstone.

Celiker R, Arslan S, Inanici F (2002). Corticosteroid injection vs. nonsteriodal antiinflammatory drug and splinting in carpal tunnel syndrome. American Journal of Physical Medicine and Rehabilitation 81(3):182-186.

Cobb TK, An KN, Cooney WP (1995). Effect of lumbrical muscle incursion within the carpal tunnel on carpal tunnel pressure: A cadaveric study. Journal of Hand Surgery 20A(2):186-192.

Colditz JC (2002). Therapist's management of the stiff hand. In EJ Mackin, AD Callahan, TM Skirven, LH Schneider (eds.), *Rehabilitation of the Hand and Upper Extremity, Fifth Edition*. St. Louis: Mosby, pp. 1021-1049.

Collier SE, Thomas JJ (2002). Range of motion at the wrist: A comparison study of four wrist extension orthoses and the free hand. American Journal of Occupational Therapy 56(2):180-184.

Cook AC, Szabo RM, Birkholz SW, King EF (1995). Early mobilization following carpal tunnel release: A prospective randomized study. Journal of Hand Surgery 20B:228-230.

Courts RB (1995). Splinting for symptoms of carpal tunnel syndrome during pregnancy. Journal of Hand Therapy 8:31-34.

Dell PC, Dell RB (1996). Management of rheumatoid arthritis of the wrist. Journal of Hand Therapy 9(2):157-164.

Fess EE, Gettle KS, Philips CA, Janson JR (2005). *Hand Splinting Principles and Methods, Third Edition*. St. Louis: Elsevier Mosby.

Gelberman RH, Hergenroeder PT, Hargens AR, Lundborg GN, Akeson WH (1981). The carpal tunnel syndrome: A study of carpal canal pressures. Journal of Bone and Joint Surgery American 63(3): 380-383.

Gerritsen AA, de Vet HC, Scholten RJ, Bertelsmann FW, de Krom MC, Bouter LM (2002). Splinting vs surgery in the treatment of carpal tunnel syndrome: A randomized controlled trial. JAMA 288(10):1245-1251.

Gerritsen AA, Korthals-de Bos IB, Laboyrie PM, de Vet HC, Scholten RJ, Bouter (2003). Splinting for carpal tunnel syndrome: Prognostic indicators of success. Journal of Neurology Neurosurgery and Psychiatry 74(9):1342-1344.

Graham RG, Hudson DA, Solomons M, Singer M (2004). A prospective study to assess the outcome of steroid injections and wrist splinting for the treatment of carpal tunnel syndrome. Plastic and Reconstructive Surgery 113(2):550-556.

Hayes EP, Carney K, Mariatis Wolf J, Smith J, Akelman E (2002). Carpal tunnel syndrome. In EJ Mackin, AD Callahan, TM Skirven, LH Schneider (eds.), *Rehabilitation of the Hand and Upper Extremity, Fifth Edition*. St. Louis: Mosby, pp. 643-659.

Idler RS (1997). Helping the patient who has wrist or hand tenosynovitis. Part 2: Managing trigger finger, de Quervain's disease. Journal of Musculoskeletal Medicine 14(2):62-65, 68, 74-75.

Kasch MC (2002). Therapist's evaluation and treatment of upper extremity cumulative-trauma disorders. In EJ Mackin, AD Callahan, TM Skirven, LH Schneider (eds.), *Rehabilitation of the Hand and Upper Extremity, Fifth Edition*. St. Louis: Mosby, pp. 1005-1018.

Khan KM, Cook JL, Taunton JE, Bonar F (2000). Overuse tendinosis, not tendonitis. Part 1: A new paradigm for a difficult clinical problem. Phys Sportsmed 28(5):38-48.

Kozin SH, Michlovitz SL (2000). Traumatic arthritis and osteoarthritis of the wrist. Journal of Hand Therapy 13(2):124-135.

Kulick RG (1996). Carpal tunnel syndrome. Orthopedic Clinics of North America 27(2):345-354.

Kuo MH, Leong CP, Cheng YF, Chang HW (2001). Static wrist position associated with least median nerve compression: Sonographic evaluation. Archives of Physical Medicine and Rehabilitation 80(4):256-260.

Lankford LL (1995). Reflex sympathetic dystrophy. In JM Hunter, EJ Mackin, AD Callahan (eds.), *Rehabilitation of the Hand: Surgery and Therapy, Fourth Edition*. St. Louis: Mosby, pp. 779-815.

Laseter GF (2002). Therapist's management of distal radius fractures. In EJ Mackin, AD Callahan, TM Skirven, LH Schneider (eds.), *Rehabilitation of the Hand and Upper Extremity, Fifth Edition*. St.Louis: Mosby, pp. 1136-1155.

Laseter GF, Carter PR (1996). Management of distal radius fractures. Journal of Hand Therapy 9(2):114-128.

LaStayo P (2002). Ulnar wrist pain and impairment: A therapist's algorithmic approach to the triangular fibrocartilage complex. In EJ Mackin, AD Callahan, TM Skirven, LH Schneider (eds.), *Rehabilitation of the Hand and Upper Extremity, Fifth Edition*. St.Louis: Mosby, pp. 1156-1170.

McClure P (2003). Evidence-based practice: An example related to the use of splinting in a patient with carpal tunnel syndrome. Journal of Hand Therapy 16(3):256-263.

Melvin JL (1989). *Rheumatic Disease in the Adult and Child: Occupational Therapy and Rehabilitation, Third Edition*. Philadelphia: F. A. Davis.

Mersky H, Bogduk N (1994). *Classification of Chronic Pain: Descriptions of Chronic Pain Syndromes and Definitions of Pain Terms, Second Edition*. Seattle: IASP Press.

Messer RS, Bankers RM (1995). Evaluating and treating common upper extremity nerve compression and tendonitis syndromes ... without becoming cumulatively traumatized. Nurse Practitioner Forum 6(3):152-166.

Nordenskiold U (1990). Elastic wrist orthoses: Reduction of pain and increase in grip force for women with rheumatoid arthritis. Arthritis Care and Research 3(3):158-162.

O'Connor D, Mullett H, Doyle M, Mofidl A, Kutty S, O'Sullivan M (2003). Minimally displaced Colles' fractures: A prospective randomized trial of treatment with a wrist splint or a plaster cast. Journal of Hand Surgery 28B(1):50-53.

Osterman AL, Whitman M, Porta LD (2002). Nonoperative carpal tunnel syndrome treatment. Hand Clinics 18(2):279-289.

Pagnotta A, Baron M, Korner-Bitensky N (1998). The effect of a static wrist orthosis on hand function in individuals with rheumatoid arthritis. Journal of Rheumatology 25(5):879-885.

Palmer AK, Werner FW, Murphy D, Glisson R (1985). Functional wrist motion: A biomechanical study. Journal of Hand Surgery American 10(1):39-46.

Philips CA (1995). Therapist's management of patients with rheumatoid arthritis. In JM Hunter, EJ Mackin, AD Callahan (eds.), *Rehabilitation of the Hand: Surgery and Therapy, Fourth Edition*. St. Louis: Mosby, pp. 1345-1350.

Phillips D (2005). FAQ: What is the difference between CRPS Type I and CRPS Type II? Retrieved on February 10, 2005, from *http://www.rsdalert.co.uk/FAQ/witdifference.htm*.

Reiss B (1995). Therapist's management of distal radial fractures. In JM Hunter, EJ Mackin, AD Callahan (eds.), *Rehabilitation of the Hand: Surgery and Therapy, Fourth Edition*. St. Louis: Mosby, pp. 337-351.

Rozmaryn LM, Dovelle S, Rothman ER, Gorman K, Olvey KM, Bartko JJ (1998). Nerve and tendon gliding exercises and the conservative management of carpal tunnel syndrome. Journal of Hand Therapy 11(3):171-179.

Saidoff DC, McDonough AL (1997). *Critical Pathways in Therapeutic Intervention: Upper Extremity*. St. Louis: Mosby.

Sailer SM (1996). The role of splinting and rehabilitation in the treatment of carpal and cubital tunnel syndromes. Hand Clinics 12(2):223-241.

Schultz-Johnson K (1996). Splinting the wrist: Mobilization and protection. Journal of Hand Therapy 9(2):165-176.

Siegel DB, Kuzma G, Eakins D (1995). Anatomic investigation the role of the lumbrical muscles in carpal tunnel syndrome. Journal of Hand Surgery 20A(5):860-863.

Skirven T (1992). Nerve injuries. In BG Stanley, SM Tribuzi (eds.), *Concepts in Hand Rehabilitation*. Philadelphia: F. A. Davis, pp. 323-352.

Stein CM, Svoren B, Davis P, Blankenberg B (1991). A prospective analysis of patients with rheumatic diseases attending referral hospitals in Harare, Zimbabwe. The Journal of Rheumatology 18(12):1841-1844.

Stern EB (1996). Grip strength and finger dexterity across five styles of commercial wrist orthoses. American Journal of Occupational Therapy 50(1):32-38.

Stern EB, Sines B, Teague TR (1994). Commercial wrist extensor orthoses: Hand function, comfort, and interference across five styles. Journal of Hand Therapy 7(4):237-244.

Stern EB, Ytterberg SR, Krug HE, Larson LM, Portoghese CP, Kratz WN, et al. (1997). Commercial wrist extensor orthoses: A descriptive study of use and preference in patients with rheumatoid arthritis. Arthritis Care and Research 10(1):27-35.

Stern EB, Ytterberg SR, Krug HE, Mahowald ML (1996a). Finger dexterity and hand function: Effect of three commercial wrist extensor orthoses on patients with rheumatoid arthritis. Arthritis Care and Research 9(3):197-205.

Stern EB, Ytterberg SR, Krug HE, Mullin GT, Mahowald ML (1996b). Immediate and short-term effects of three commercial wrist extensor orthoses on grip strength and function in patients with rheumatoid arthritis. Arthritis Care and Research 9(1):42-50.

Taylor-Mullins PA (1992). Reflex sympathetic dystrophy. In BG Stanley, SM Tribuzi (eds.), *Concepts in Hand Rehabilitation*. Philadelphia: F. A. Davis, pp. 446-471.

Verdugo RJ, Salinas RS, Castillo J, Cea JG. (2004). Surgical versus non-surgical treatment for carpal tunnel syndrome (Cochrane Review). In The Cochrane Library, Issue 2. Chichester, UK: John Wiley & Sons.

Walker WC, Metzler M, Cifu DX, Swartz Z (2000). Neutral wrist splinting in carpal tunnel syndrome: A comparison of night-only versus full-time wear instructions. Archives of Physical Medicine and Rehabilitation 81(4):424-429.

Walsh MT, Muntzer E (2002). Therapist's management of complex regional pain syndrome (reflex sympathetic dystrophy). In EJ Mackin, AD Callahan, TM Skirven, LH Schneider (eds.), *Rehabilitation of the Hand and Upper Extremity, Fifth Edition*. St. Louis: Mosby, pp. 1707-1724.

Weinstock TB (1999). Management of fractures of the distal radius: Therapists commentary. Journal of Hand Therapy 12(2):99-102.

Weiss ND, Gordon L, Bloom T, So Y, Rempel DM (1995). Position of the wrist associated with the lowest carpal-tunnel pressure: Implications for splint design. Journal of Bone and Joint Surgery American 77(11):1695-1699.

Williams K (1992). Carpal tunnel syndrome captivates American industry. Advance for Directors of Rehabilitation 12:13-18.

CHAPTER 8

Thumb Immobilization Splints

Helene Lohman, MA, OTD, OTR/L

Key Terms

de Quervain's tenosynovitis
Hypertonicity
Osteoarthritis
Rheumatoid arthritis
Scaphoid fracture
Ulnar collateral ligament injury (gamekeeper's thumb)

Chapter Objectives

1. Discuss important functional and anatomic considerations for splinting the thumb.
2. List appropriate thumb and wrist positions in a thumb immobilization splint.
3. Identify the three components of a thumb immobilization splint.
4. Describe the reasons for supporting the joints of the thumb.
5. Discuss the diagnostic indications for a thumb immobilization splint.
6. Discuss the process of pattern making and splint fabrication for a thumb immobilization splint.
7. Describe elements of a proper fit of a thumb immobilization splint.
8. List general and specific precautions for a thumb immobilization splint.
9. Use clinical reasoning to evaluate fit problems of a thumb immobilization splint.
10. Use clinical reasoning to evaluate a fabricated thumb immobilization splint.
11. Apply knowledge about thumb immobilization splinting to a case study.
12. Understand the importance of evidenced-based practice with thumb immobilization splint provision.
13. Describe the appropriate use of prefabricated thumb splints.

A commonly prescribed splint in clinical practice is the thumb palmar abduction immobilization splint [American Society of Hand Therapists 1992]. Other names for this splint are the *thumb spica splint*, the *short or long opponens splint* [Tenney and Lisak 1986], and the *thumb gauntlet splint*. The purpose of this splint is to immobilize, protect, rest, and position one or all of the thumb carpometacarpal (CMC), metacarpophalangeal (MCP), and interphalangeal (IP) joints while allowing the other digits to be free. Thumb immobilization splints can be divided into two broad categories: (1) forearm based and (2) hand based. Forearm-based thumb splints stabilize the wrist as well as the thumb. Stabilizing the wrist is beneficial for a painful wrist as the splint provides support. The hand-based immobilization splints provide stabilization for the thumb while allowing for wrist mobility.

Forearm-based or hand-based thumb immobilization splints are often used to help manage different conditions that affect the thumb's CMC, MP, or IP joints. For people who have de Quervain's tenosynovitis a forearm-based thumb splint provides rest, support, and protection of the tendons that course along the radial side of the wrist into the thumb joints. The therapist also applies a forearm-based thumb immobilization splint to splint postoperatively for control of motion in persons with rheumatoid arthritis after a joint arthrodesis or replacement. With the resulting muscle imbalance from a median nerve injury, the therapist may apply a hand-based thumb immobilization splint to keep the thumb web space adequately open. (Refer to Chapter 13 for more information on nerve injury). In addition, the thumb immobilization splint can position the thumb before surgery [Geisser 1984]. The splint provides support and positioning after traumatic thumb injuries, such as sprains, joint dislocations, ligament injuries, and scaphoid fractures. Frequently a hand-based thumb immobilization splint is applied to persons with gamekeeper's thumb, which involves the ulnar collateral ligament of the thumb MCP joint. For hypertonicity a thumb splint sometimes called a *figure-of-eight thumb wrap* or *thumb loop splint* facilitates hand use by decreasing the palm-in-thumb posture or palmar adduction that is often associated with this condition. Therefore, because this splint is so commonly prescribed it is important that therapists become familiar with its application and fabrication.

Functional and Anatomic Considerations for Splinting the Thumb

The thumb is essential for hand functions because of its overall importance to grip, pinch, and fine manipulation. The thumb's exceptional mobility results from the unique shape of its saddle joint, the arrangement of its ligaments, and its intrinsic musculature [Belkin and English 1996, Tubiana et al. 1996, Colditz 2002]. The thumb provides stability for grip, pinch, and mobility because it opposes the fingers for fine manipulations [Wilton 1997]. Sensory input to the tip of the thumb is important for functional grasp and pinch.

A thorough understanding of the anatomy and functional movements of the thumb is necessary before the therapist attempts to splint the thumb. The therapist must understand that the most crucial aspect of the thumb immobilization splint design is the position of the CMC joint [Wilton 1997]. Positioning of the thumb in a thumb post allows for palmar abduction and some opposition, which are critical motions for functional prehension. See Chapter 4 for a review of the anatomy and functional movements of the thumb.

Features of the Thumb Immobilization Splint

The thumb immobilization splint prevents motion of one, two, or all of the thumb joints [Fess et al. 2005]. The splint has numerous design variations. It can be a volar (Figure 8-1), dorsal (Figure 8-2), or radial gutter (Figure 8-3). The splint may be hand based or wrist based, depending on the person's diagnosis, the anatomic structures involved, and the associated pain at the wrist. If the wrist is included, the wrist position will vary according to the diagnosis. For example, with de Quervain's tenosynovitis the wrist is commonly positioned in 15 degrees of extension to take the pressure off the tendons.

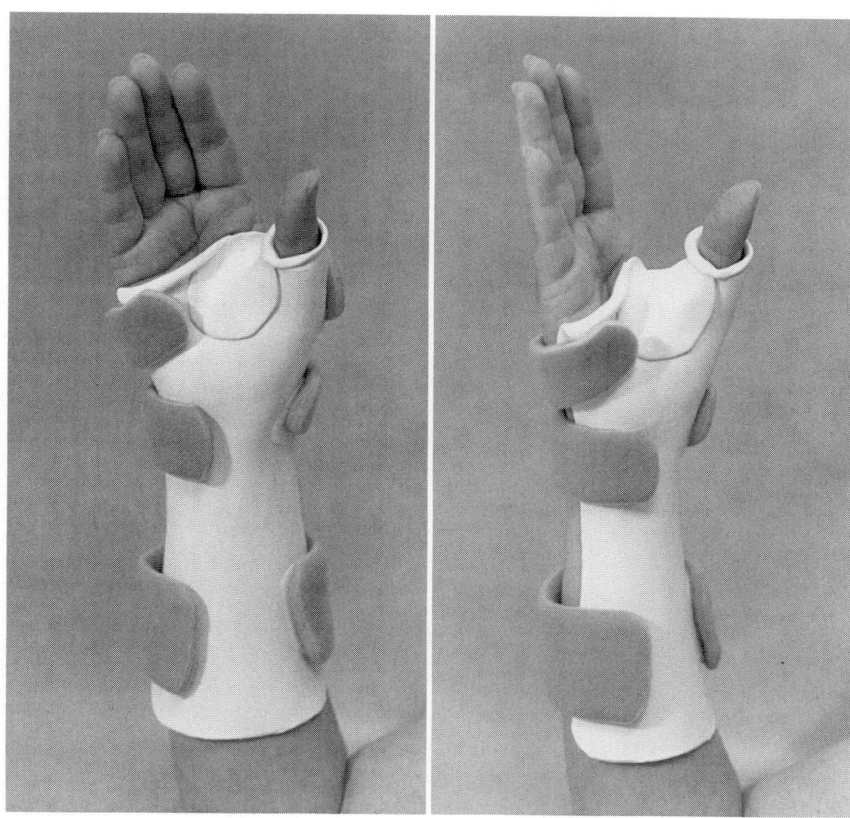

Figure 8-1 A volar thumb immobilization splint.

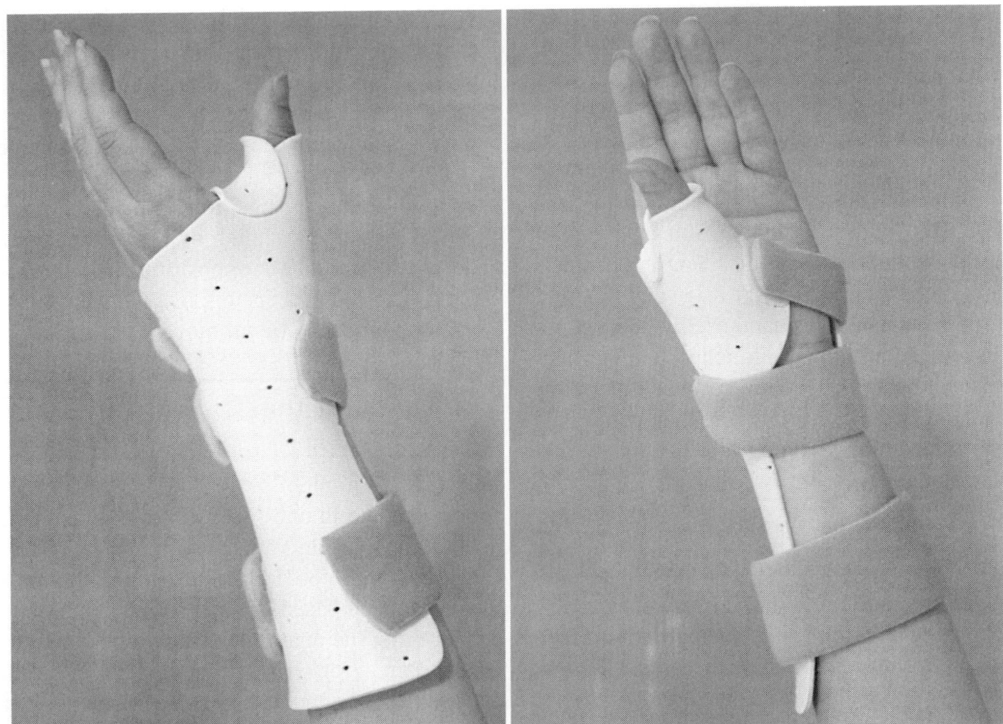

Figure 8-2 A dorsal thumb immobilization splint.

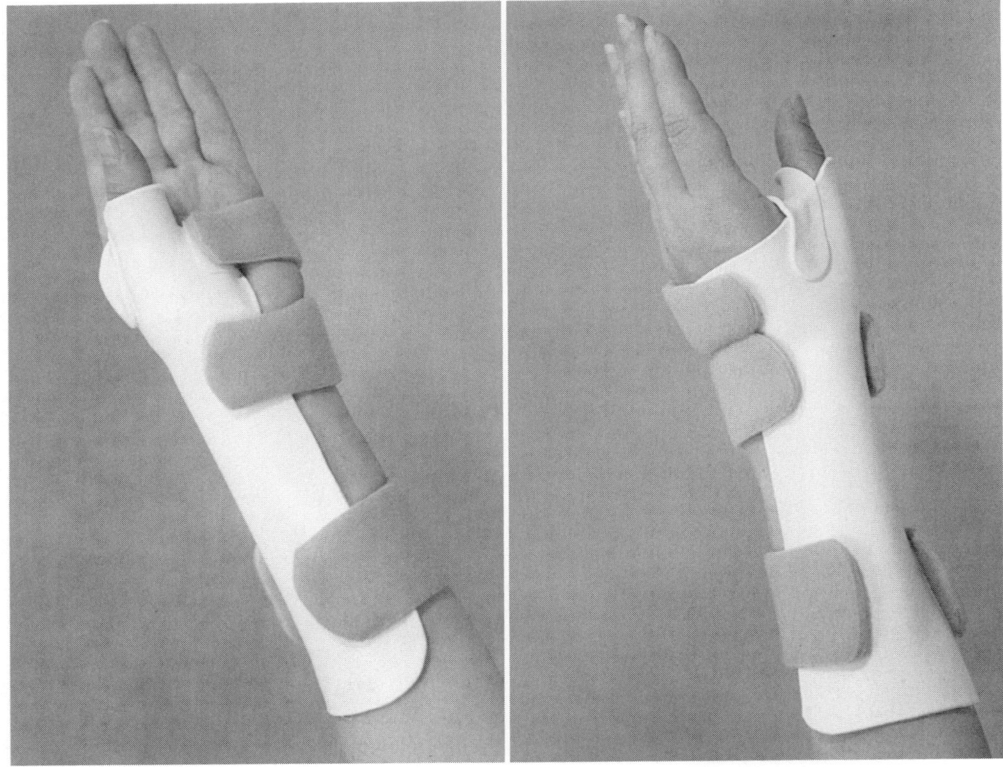

Figure 8-3 A radial gutter thumb immobilization splint.

The splint components fabricated in the final product will vary according to the thumb joints that are included. The final splint product will be formed based on the therapeutic goals for the client. The therapist should have a good understanding of the purpose and the fabrication process for the various splinting components. Central to most thumb immobilization splints are the opponens bar, C bar, and thumb post (Figure 8-4) [Fess et al. 2005]. The opponens bar and C bar position the thumb, usually in some degree of palmar abduction. The thumb post, which is an extension of the C bar, immobilizes the MP only or both the MP and IP joints.

The position of the thumb in a splint varies from palmar abduction to radial abduction, depending on the person's diagnosis. With some conditions, such as arthritis, the therapist can assist prehension by stabilizing the thumb CMC joint in palmar abduction and opposition. Certain diagnostic protocols—such as those for extensor pollicis longus (EPL) repairs, tendon transfers for thumb extension, and extensor tenolysis of the thumb—require the thumb to have an extension and a radial abducted position [Cannon et al. 1985].

The thumb immobilization splint may do one of the following: (1) stabilize only the CMC joint; (2) include the CMC and MP joints; or (3) encompass the CMC, MCP, and IP joints. The physician's order may specify which thumb joints to immobilize in the splint. In some situations, the therapist may be responsible for determining which joints the splint should stabilize. The therapist uses diagnostic protocols and an assessment of the person's pain to make this decision. If the therapist deems it necessary to limit thumb motion and to protect the thumb, the IP may be immobilized. Certain diagnostic protocols (such as those for thumb replantations, tendon transfers, and tendon repairs) often require the inclusion of the IP joint in the splint [Tenney and Lisak 1986]. Overall the therapist should fabricate a splint that is the most supportive and least restrictive in movement.

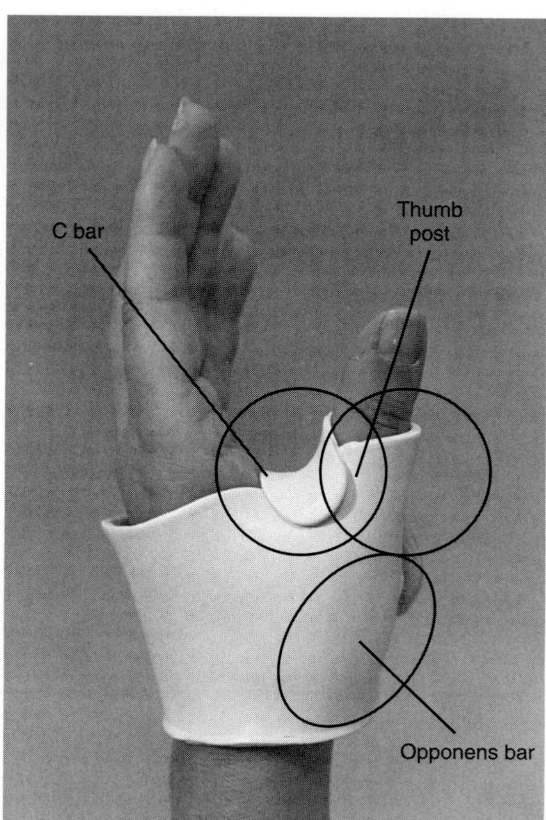

Figure 8-4 The opponens bar in conjunction with a C bar and a thumb pad.

Diagnostic Indications

Therapists fabricate thumb immobilization splints in general and specialized hand therapy practices. Specific diagnostic conditions that require a thumb immobilization splint include, but are not limited to, the following: scaphoid fractures, stable fractures of the proximal phalanx of the first metacarpal, tendon transfers, radial or ulnar collateral ligament strains, repair of MCP joint collateral ligaments, rheumatoid arthritis, osteoarthritis, de Quervain's tenosynovitis, median nerve injuries, MCP joint dislocations, capsular tightness of the MCP and IP joints after trauma, post-traumatic adduction contracture, extrinsic flexor or extensor muscle contracture, flexor pollicis longus (FPL) repair, uncomplicated EPL repairs, hypertonicity, and congenital adduction deformity of the thumb.

Treatment of many of these conditions may require the expertise of experienced hand therapists. In general clinical practice, therapists commonly treat persons who have de Quervain's tenosynovitis, rheumatoid arthritis, osteoarthritis, fractures, and ligament injuries. (Table 8-1 contains guidelines for these hand conditions.) The novice therapist should keep in mind that physicians and experienced therapists may have their own guidelines for positioning and splint-wearing schedules. The therapist should also be aware that thumb palmar abduction may be uncomfortable for some persons. Therefore, the thumb may be positioned midway between radial and palmar abduction.

Splinting for de Quervain's Tenosynovitis

De Quervain's tenosynovitis, which results from repetitive thumb motions and wrist ulnar deviation, is a form of tenosynovitis affecting the abductor pollicis longus (APL) and the extensor pollicis brevis (EPB) in the first dorsal compartment. Those persons whose occupations involve repetitive wrist deviation and thumb motions (such as the home construction tasks of painting, scraping, wall papering, and hammering) are prone to this condition [Idler 1997]. De Quervain's tenosynovitis is the most commonly diagnosed wrist tendonitis in athletes [Rettig 2001], such as with golfers [McCarroll 2001]. It may be recognized by pain over the radial styloid, edema in the first dorsal compartment, and positive results from the Finkelstein's test.

During the acute phase of this condition, conservative therapeutic management involves immobilization of the thumb

Table 8-1 Conditions That May Require a Thumb Immobilization Splint

HAND CONDITION	SUGGESTED WEARING SCHEDULE	TYPE OF SPLINT, WRIST POSITION
	SOFT TISSUE INFLAMMATION	
de Quervain's tenosynovitis	During an acute flare-up, the therapist fabricates a thumb immobilization splint (wrist extension, thumb carpometacarpal (CMC) palmar abduction, and MP flexion immobilization splint, [ASHT 1992]) which the person wears continuously, with removal for hygiene and exercise. The interphalangeal (IP) joint is included the person is overusing the thumb or fights if the splint, causing more pain.	Long forearm-based or radial gutter splint—the wrist in 15 degrees of extension, the thumb CMC joint palmarly abducted 40 to 45 degrees, and the thumb metacarpophalangeal (MCP) joint in 5 to 10 degrees of flexion. To allow slack for inflamed tendons, the thumb CMC joint is sometimes positioned in radial abduction and extension instead of palmar abduction.
	RHEUMATOID ARTHRITIS	
Periods of pain and inflammation in the thumb joints	The therapist provides a thumb immobilization splint (wrist extension, thumb CMC palmar abduction, and MP flexion immobilization splint) for the person to wear continuously during periods of pain and inflammation. The person removes the splint for exercise and hygiene. The therapist adjusts the wearing schedule according to the person's pain and inflammation levels.	Long forearm-based thumb immobilization splint—the wrist in 20 to 30 degrees of extension, the thumb CMC joint palmarly abducted 45 degrees, or midway between radial and palmar abduction, depending on person's tolerance; and the MCP joint (if included) in 5 degrees of flexion. Other specific splints for arthritic deformities are listed in the chapter.
	OSTEOARTHRITIS	
CMC joint of the thumb	The person wears a thumb immobilization splint (CMC palmar abduction immobilization splint) continuously during an acute flare-up, with removal for range of motion (ROM) and hygiene. Once edema has decreased, the splint can be worn during activities that stress the thumb joints.	Hand-based thumb immobilization splint—the MCP joint is immobilized or free, depending on the protocol. The thumb CMC joint is palmarly abducted to a position that the person can tolerate. Or, a hand-based splint that frees the thumb MCP joint for motion and stabilizes the first metacarpal (CMC) joint in extension.
	TRAUMATIC INJURIES OF THE THUMB	
Gamekeeper's thumb (ulnar collateral ligament injury)	**Grade I** The person wears a hand-based thumb splint (MP radial and ulnar deviation restriction splint, ASHT, 1992) during activities that are stressful and during sleep. The person wears a thumb immobilization splint continuously for 3 to 4 weeks, with removal for hygiene. **Grade II** The person wears a hand-based thumb immobilization splint continuously for 4 to 5 weeks. **Grade III** After immobilization in a cast, the person is provided with a hand-based thumb immobilization splint and follows the same protocol described previously.	Hand-based thumb immobilization splint with the MCP joint immobilized and the thumb CMC joint palmarly abducted 30 to 40 degrees and MCP joint in neutral to slight flexion. (It is important to position the thumb CMC joint in a position of comfort and may not be exactly the suggested degrees.)

Table 8-1 Conditions That May Require a Thumb Immobilization Splint—cont'd

HAND CONDITION	SUGGESTED WEARING SCHEDULE	TYPE OF SPLINT, WRIST POSITION
Scaphoid fracture (stable and non-displaced)	The therapist provides a forearm volar thumb immobilization splint (thumb CMC palmar abduction and MP flexion immobilization splint) or dorsal/volar thumb splint (wrist extension, thumb CMC palmar abduction, and MP flexion immobilization splint). The wear schedule will vary widely depending on the time after injury, the bone status, the physician preference, and the location of the fracture on the scaphoid. If the client has undergone a long course of casting and the doctor is worried about bony union (this is often the case), initially, the splint will be prescribed for continuous wear with perhaps removal for hygiene and definitely to check the skin.	Volar forearm thumb immobilization splint, with the thumb in palmar abduction, MCP joint in 0 to 10 degrees flexion and the wrist in slight flexion and radial deviation or neutral depending on the physician preference [Fess et al. 2005]
Hypertonicity	Wearing schedule varies according to the person's therapeutic needs. Splint should be removed and skin carefully monitored at periodic intervals.	The therapist provides a thumb loop splint or a figure-of-eight thumb wrap splint, which can be customized out of thermoplastic or soft material. A prefabricated splint can also be used. With a prefabricated splint, a neoprene strip is wrapped around the thumb web space and the hand to provide radial or palmar abduction while pulling the wrist into extension and radial deviation. Purchased thumb loops are available in sizes to fit premature infants to adults.

and wrist for symptom control [Lee et al. 2002]. This splint is classified by the American Society of Hand Therapists (ASHT) as a wrist extension, thumb CMC palmar abduction and MP flexion immobilization splint [ASHT 1992]. It may cover the volar or dorsal forearm or the radial aspect of the forearm and hand. The therapist positions the wrist in 15 degrees of extension, neutral wrist deviation, 40 to 45 degrees of palmar abduction of the thumb CMC joint, and 5 to 10 degrees of flexion in the MCP joint [Idler 1997]. Usually the therapist allows the IP joint to be free for functional activities and includes the joint in the splint if the person is overusing the thumb or fights the splint, causing even more pain.

The splint is worn continuously, with removal for hygiene and exercise within a pain-free range [Lee et al. 2002]. A prefabricated splint is recommend after the person's pain subsides [Lee et al. 2002] for work and sports activities [Fess et al. 2005], or if the person does not want to wear a custom splint [Biese 2002]. Post-surgical management of de Quervain's tenosynovitis also involves splinting, usually for 7 to 10 days [Rettig 2001].

Few studies have considered the efficacy of thumb splinting for de Quervain's tenosynovitis and results have been variable (see Table 8-2). Lane et al. [2001] studied 300 subjects and compared splinting with oral nonsteroidal anti-inflammatory drugs (NSAIDs) and steroid injections over a 2- to 4-week time period. Subjects were splinted in a custom thumb immobilization splint with the wrist in neutral and the thumb in 30 degrees between palmar and radial abduction. Subjects were placed in three groups based on symptoms (minimal, mild, moderate/severe). Those subjects who had mild symptoms responded well to splinting with NSAIDs. Limitations of this study included no control group for the mild symptom group, small numbers in the mild group, the subjective nature of classifying subjects, and no mention of a splint-wearing schedule.

Weiss et al. [1994] (n = 93) compared splinting to steroid injection or combined in treatment with steroid injections. They did not find strong benefits for thumb splinting. Witt et al. [1991] (n = 95) also studied the provision of a long thumb immobilization splint including the wrist (which was worn continuously for 3 weeks, along with steroid injection) and had a good success rate. Avci et al. [2002] focused their research on conservative treatment of 19 pregnant women with de Quervain's tenosynovitis. One group received cortisone injections and the other group received

Table 8-2 Efficacy Studies About Thumb Splinting

AUTHOR'S CITATION	DESIGN	# OF PARTICIPANTS	DESCRIPTION	RESULTS	LIMITATIONS
Berggren M, Joost-Davidsson A, Lindstrand J, Nylander G, Povlsen B (2001). Reduction in the need for operation after conservative treatment of osteoarthritis of the first carpometacarpal joint: A seven year prospective study. Scand J Plast Reconstr Hand Surg 35: 415-417.	Prospective study	33 clients randomized into three groups	A hand therapist met with each participant to discuss how to avoid loading the joint through the use of splints or accessories and how to modify their work environment. These subjects, awaiting surgery for carpometacarpal (CMC) joint replacement, were started on a regimen. Group 1 received technical accessories (ergonomically designed assistive devices). Group 2 received accessories and a textile splint. Group 3 received accessories and a leather splint. All groups were advised on how to accommodate activities of daily living (ADL) to reduce pain and decrease the need for surgery. A hand therapist treated each subject for 3 individual sessions over a 7-month period. Adjustments were made to the technical accessories or splints as needed. A surgeon assessed all subjects at the end of 7 months to determine the need for surgery. The surgeon acted as a blind reviewer.	Of the 33 clients, 23 (70%) avoided surgery. The clients 7 reassessed after seven years. Only 2 clients required surgery. The authors recommended a 6-month period of conservative treatment before determining a client's need for surgery.	There was a significant difference in age between clients electing to have surgery (mean age of 59) and those declining surgery (mean age of 65). Older participants may be less likely to elect to have surgery if their lifestyle does not require the same functional outcome as that of a younger individual. The mean age of participants in this study was 63 years of age and may have played a role in the number of participants choosing to have surgery at the conclusion of the study.
Day CS, Gelberman R, Patel AA, Vogt MT, Ditsios K, Boyer MI (2004). Basal joint osteoarthritis of the thumb: A prospective trial of steroid	Prospective study	30 clients (30 thumbs)	The purpose was to evaluate the effectiveness of a single steroid injection and use of a thumb spica splint for individuals with osteoarthritis in Eaton stages 1 to 4. The clients had trapeziometacarpal (TM) pain. The participants were at varying stages in the disease process, and the researchers hypothesized that this conservative approach would provide temporary relief no matter the stage of osteoarthritis	13 of the 30 clients experienced a mean improvement in pain intensity of 5.5 points up to 4 weeks following the injection. The remaining 17 clients did not experience relief. Of the 13 clients experiencing pain relief, 12 demonstrated increased function and	It is difficult to say whether the steroid injection or the splinting was the more effective method in decreasing pain intensity of individuals with TM osteoarthritis.7 of the 30 clients declined follow-up. There was some speculation that the injection did not

injection and splinting. J Hand Surg, 49, 247-251.			present. The participants were asked to answer the Disability of the Arm, Shoulder and Hand (DASH) questionnaire and rate their pain level initially, at 6 weeks and at 18 to 31 weeks after the intervention.	decreased pain. Such effects lasted throughout the final follow-up (an average of 21 months). There was an increase in the DASH daily activities ratings (severely difficult to minimally difficult). The clients showing the most improvement were those in the early stages of TM osteoarthritis (Eaton stages 1, 2 and 3). Those clients who did not experience pain relief had the option of surgery.	accurately get into the TM joint.
Lane LB, Boretz RS, and Stuchin SA (2001). Treatment of de Quervain's disease: Role of conservative management, Journal of Hand Surgery *26*, 256-260.	Retrospective study	319 wrists in 300 clients	The purpose of the study was to compare two methods used to treat de Quervain's disease including radial gutter thumb spica splints with nonsteroidal anti-inflammatory drugs (NSAIDs) and steroid injections. Records of 300 clients presenting with de Quervain's disease between 1980 through 1986 were reviewed. Participants were followed up through a physical exam, telephonecall, or written questionnaire. Clients wereclassified into three groups. Group 1 (n = 17) had minimal symptoms (discomfort overall the radial side of the wrist during a few ADL and no pain at rest). Group 2 (n = 45) had pain over the radial side of the wrist and mild interference with ADLs. Group 3 (n = 257) had moderate to severe tenderness, a positive Finkelstein's test, and swelling. Client improvement was categorized as having complete resolution of symptoms, having improvement or having no improvement of symptoms. If their symptoms were not relieved, the treatment was determined to be unsuccessful and they were offered a steroid injection. If a client received steroid injection(s), they were categorized in the steroid group.	15 of the 17 clients in group 1 reported complete symptom relief with splinting and NSAID treatment. In group 2, 20 or 45 clients refused steroid injections and were treated with NSAIDS and splints. No one received surgery from Group 2. In Group 3, 2 of 8 clients were treated with splints and NSAIDs and experienced improvement in symptoms. 189 of the 249 wrists had complete symptom relief, and 17 had improvement with injections. The researchers concluded that splinting and NSAID treatment is effective for a small number of persons with de Quervain's in the early stages. Findings show efficacy of steroid injection for clients with de Quervain's for whom splinting and NSAID treatment is not effective.	It is difficult to distinguish between minimal, mild, moderate symptoms of de Quervain's disease. Splinting was not tested alone as a treatment option. There was not a control group for Group 1.

Continued

Table 8-2 Efficacy Studies About Thumb Splinting—cont'd

AUTHOR'S CITATION	DESIGN	# OF PARTICIPANTS	DESCRIPTION	RESULTS	LIMITATIONS
Swigart CR, Eaton RG, Glickel SZ, Johnson C (1999). Splinting in the treatment of arthritis of the first carpometacarpal joint. J Hand Surg 24, 86-91.	Retrospective study	114 clients (130 thumbs)	The purpose of the study was to determine the effectiveness of a splinting protocol for CMC arthritis and its effect on daily activities. 114 clients with pain and disability associated with CMC arthritis were treated with a long opponens splint for 3 to 4 weeks followed by a 3 to 4 week "weaning" period. The splint was designed to eliminate wrist movement, but not to correct any previous deformities. Through a mail survey, clients self-reported their percentage of perceived improvement in symptoms. Clients choose from 0, 25, 50, 75, or 100% improvement immediately after the splint was worn and 6 months thereafter. Clients were categorized into two groups, A and B depending on the extent of joint disease present. Group A (57 thumbs) were in stage 1 or 2 of the disease. Group B (69 thumbs) were in stage 3 or 4. 4 thumbs were excluded from the study.	74 of 85 clients responded to the survey. Of the clients that responded, 53 thumbs (67%) experienced some relief with splinting. Those who experienced relief rated their improvement at 60% initially and 59% 6 months later. Between groups A and B, clients in group A (stage 1 and 2) showed greater improvement than those in group B. This supports the researchers' hypothesis that conservative methods of treatment such as splinting are most effective early on in the disease process. 22% of clients in group A who failed to experience improvements with splinting elected to have surgery. In group B, 61% of clients elected to have first CMC surgery. Many clients who did not experience pain reduction through splinting and decided against surgery chose to modify their activities to reduce stress on the thumb.	Similar to many retrospective studies, this one had a relatively low response rate (33%). With any self report design, there is a potential for misperception and personal bias in respondents answers.

thumb splints. The group receiving cortisone injections had complete pain relief compared to partial relief from the splint-wearing group. The splint-wearing group experienced pain relief only when wearing the splint. Finally, the researchers pointed out that pregnancy-related de Quervain's disease is self-limiting (with cessation of symptoms after breast feeding is terminated). Much more research needs to be completed to truly determine the efficacy of thumb splinting with de Quervain's tenosynovitis. It is helpful for therapists to review these studies because these also provide information about the effectiveness of physician treatments, such as steroid injections, their clients are receiving.

Splinting for Rheumatoid Arthritis and Osteoarthritis

Rheumatoid arthritis often affects the thumb joints, particularly the MCP and CMC joints. Splinting for rheumatoid arthritis can reduce pain, slow deformity, and stabilize the thumb joints [Ouellette 1991]. The disease includes three stages, each of which has a different splinting approach, even though the therapist may apply the same thumb immobilization splint.

The first stage involves an inflammatory process. The goal of splinting at this stage is to rest the joints and reduce inflammation. The person wears the thumb immobilization splint continuously during periods of inflammation and periodically thereafter for pain control as necessary. When the disease progresses in the second stage, the hand requires mechanical support because the joints are less stable and are painful with use. The person wears a thumb immobilization splint for support while doing daily activities and perhaps at night for pain relief. In the third stage, pain is usually not a factor, but the joints may be grossly deformed and unstable. In lieu of surgical stabilization, a thumb immobilization splint may provide support to increase function during certain activities. At this stage, splinting is rarely helpful for the person at night unless to help manage pain [personal communication, J. C. Colditz, April 1995]. Another treatment approach is to provide the person who has arthritis with a rigid and a soft splint along with education for the benefits and activity usages of each type [personal communication, K. Schultz-Johnson, June 2006].

Common thumb deformities from the arthritic process are boutonnière's deformity (type I, MP joint flexion and IP joint extension) and swan neck deformity (type 3, MP extension or hyperextension and IP flexion) [Nalebuff 1968, Colditz 2002]. During the beginning stages of boutonnière's deformity a circumferential neoprene splint is applied to support the MCP joint with the IP joint free to move [Colditz 2002]. To address progression of MCP joint deformity, Colditz [2002] suggested a carefully fabricated thermoplastic splint to stabilize the joint to eliminate volar subluxation and to allow for CMC motion (Figure 8-5).

For early stages of swan neck deformity, a small custom-fitted dorsal thermoplastic splint over the MCP joint prevents

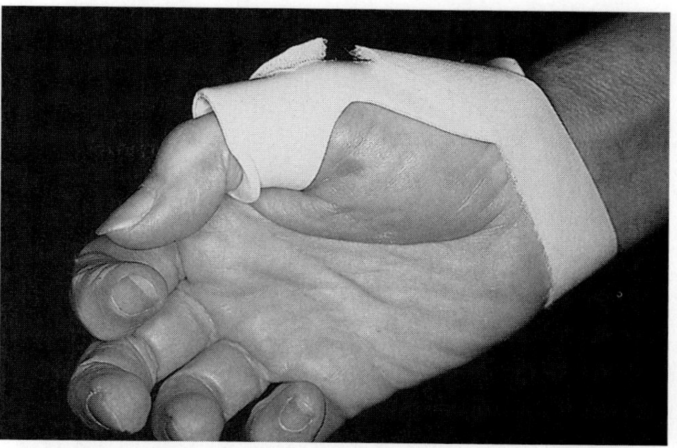

Figure 8-5 This splint stabilizes the MCP joint. [From Colditz JC (2002). Anatomic considerations for splinting the thumb. In EJ Mackin, AD Callahan, TM Skirven, LH Schneider, AL Osterman (eds.), *Rehabilitation of the Hand and Upper Extremity, Fifth Edition*. St. Louis: Mosby, pp. 1858-1874.]

MCP hyperextension [Colditz 2002]. Later dorsal and radial subluxation at the CMC joint causes CMC joint adduction, MCP hyperextension, and IP flexion [Colditz 2002]. For this deformity, Colditz [2002] suggested fabricating a hand-based thumb immobilization splint that blocks MCP hyperextension (Figure 8-6). With rheumatoid arthritis, laxity of the ulnar collateral ligament at the IP and MCP joint can also develop. Figure 8-7 shows a functional splint, which can also be used with rheumatoid arthritis or osteoarthritis for lateral instability of the thumb IP joint.

One approach to splinting a hand with arthritis is to immobilize the thumb in a forearm-based, thumb immobilization splint with the wrist in 20 to 30 degrees of extension, the CMC joint in 45 degrees of palmar abduction (if tolerated), and the MCP joint in 0 to 5 degrees of flexion [Tenney and Lisak 1986]. This splint is classified by ASHT as a wrist extension, thumb CMC palmar abduction and MP extension immobilization splint [ASHT 1992]. Resting the hand in this position is extremely beneficial during periods of inflammation, or if the thumb is unstable at the CMC joint [Marx 1992]. Incorporating the wrist in a forearm-based thumb splint is appropriate when the client's wrist is painful or if there is also arthritis involvement.

Some persons with rheumatoid arthritis affecting the CMC joint benefit from a hand-based thumb immobilization splint (thumb CMC palmar abduction immobilization splint) [ASHT 1992], as shown in Figure 8-8 [Melvin 1989, Colditz 1990]. Positioning the thumb in enough palmar abduction for functional activities is important. With a hand-based thumb immobilization splint, if the IP joint is painful and inflamed the therapist should incorporate the IP joint into the splint. However, putting any material (especially plastic) over the thumb pad will virtually eliminate thumb and hand function. The person wears this splint constantly for a minimum of 2 to 3 weeks, with removal for

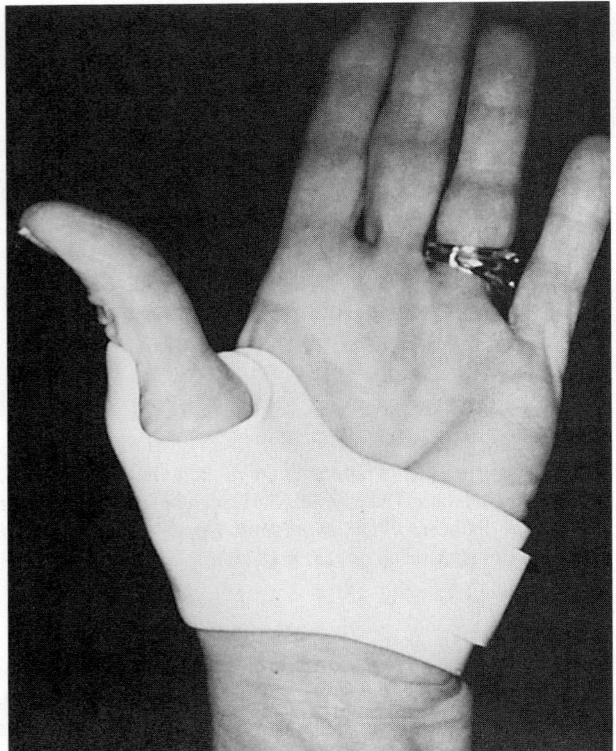

Figure 8-6 This splint, which blocks MCP hyperextension, is applied for advanced swan neck deformity. [From Colditz JC (2002). Anatomic considerations for splinting the thumb. In EJ Mackin, AD Callahan, TM Skirven, LH Schneider, AL Osterman (eds.), *Rehabilitation of the Hand and Upper Extremity, Fifth Edition*. St. Louis: Mosby, pp. 1858-1874.]

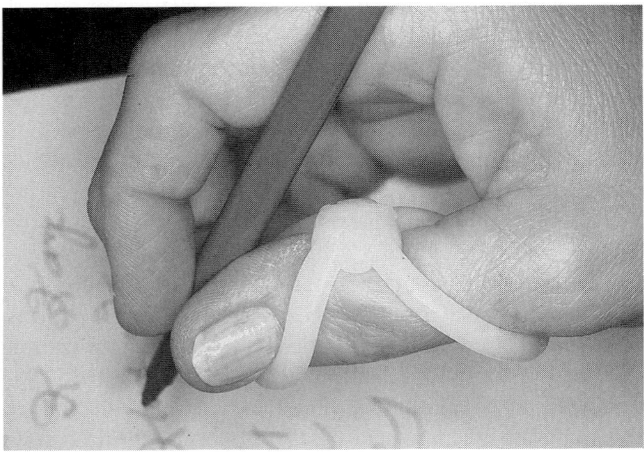

Figure 8-7 This small splint can help a person with arthritis who has lateral instability of the thumb IP joint. [From Colditz JC (2002). Anatomic considerations for splinting the thumb. In EJ Mackin, AD Callahan, TM Skirven, LH Schneider, AL Osterman (eds.), *Rehabilitation of the Hand and Upper Extremity, Fifth Edition*. St. Louis: Mosby, pp. 1858-1874.]

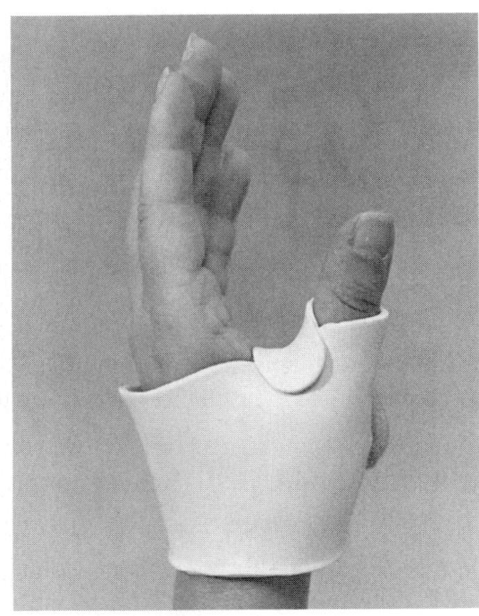

Figure 8-8 A hand-based thumb immobilization splint (thumb CMC palmar abduction immobilization splint).

hygiene and exercise. The therapist adjusts the wearing schedule according to the person's pain and inflammation levels.

On the other hand, some therapists stabilize the thumb CMC joint alone with a short splint that is properly molded and positioned (Figures 8-9 and 8-10). This splint works effectively on people who have CMC joint subluxation resulting in adduction of the first MP joint and anyone with CMC arthritis who can tolerate wearing a rigid splint. This splint can be also used for CMC osteoarthritis, discussed in more detail later in this chapter [Colditz 2000, 2002].

Often when a physician refers a person who has rheumatoid arthritis for splinting, deformities have already developed. If the therapist attempts to place the person's joints in the ideal position of 40 to 45 degrees of palmar abduction, excessive stress on the joints may result. The therapist should always splint a hand affected by arthritis in a position of comfort [Colditz 1984].

When fabricating a splint on a person who has rheumatoid arthritis, the therapist should be aware that the person may have fragile skin. The therapist should monitor all areas that can cause skin breakdown, including the ulnar head, Lister's tubercle, the radial styloid along the radial border, the CMC joint of the thumb, and the scaphoid and pisiform bones on the volar surface of the wrist [Dell and Dell 1996]. Padding the splint for comfort to prevent skin irritation may be necessary.

The selected splinting material should be easily adjustable to accommodate changes in swelling and repositioning as the disease progresses. Asking persons about their swelling patterns is important because splints fabricated during the day should allow enough room for nocturnal swelling. Thermoplastic material less than 1/8-inch thick is best for

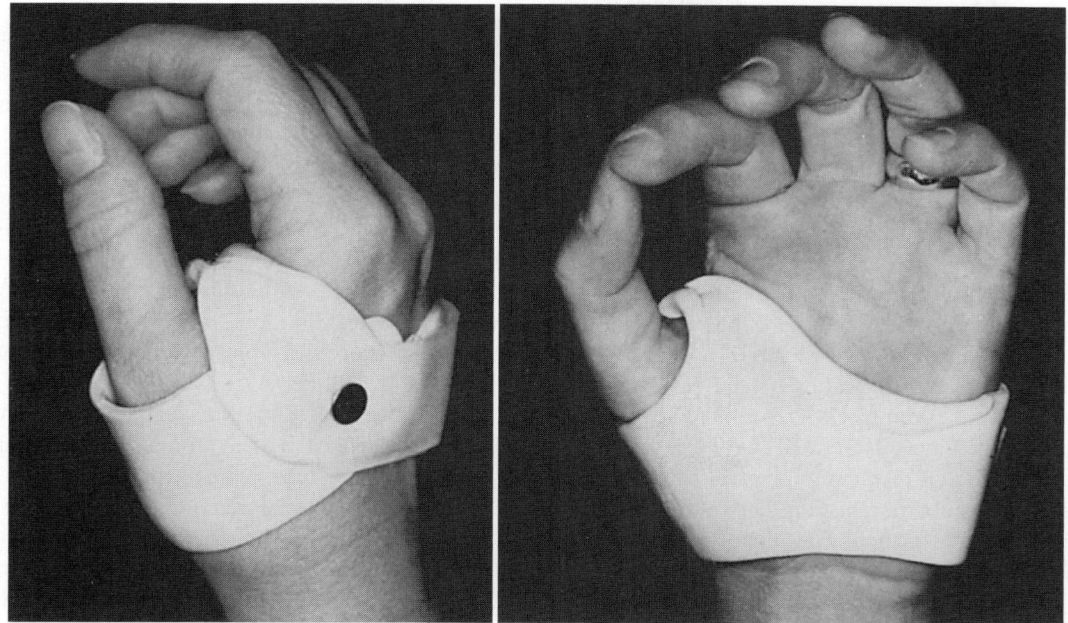

Figure 8-9 A splint for rheumatoid arthritis or osteoarthritis that stabilizes only the CMC joint. [From Colditz JC (2002). Anatomic considerations for splinting the thumb. In EJ Mackin, AD Callahan, TM Skirven, LH Schneider, AL Osterman (eds.), *Rehabilitation of the Hand and Upper Extremity, Fifth Edition*. St. Louis: Mosby, pp.1858-1874.]

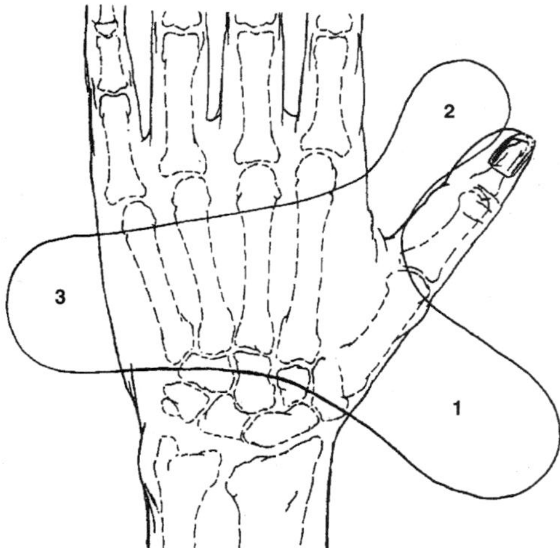

Figure 8-10 A pattern for a thumb cmc immobilization splint. [From Colditz JC (2000). The biomechanics of a thumb carpometacarpal immobilization splint: Design and fitting. Journal of Hand Therapy 13(3):228-235.]

small hand splints. Splints fabricated from heavier splinting material have the potential to irritate other joints [Melvin 1989]. Therapists must carefully evaluate all hand splints for potential stress on other joints and should instruct persons to wear the splints at night, periodically during the day, and during stressful daily activities. However, therapists should always tailor any splint-wearing regimen for each person's therapeutic needs.

CMC joint osteoarthritis is a common thumb condition, especially among women over 40 [Zelouf and Posner 1995, Melvin 1989]. Pain from osteoarthritis at the base of the thumb interferes with the person's ability to engage in normal functional activities as the CMC joint is the most critical joint of the thumb for function [Chaisson and McAlindon 1997, Neumann and Bielefeld 2003]. Precipitating factors include hypermobility, repetitive grasping, pinching, use of vibratory tools, and a family history of the condition [Winzeler and Rosenstein 1996, Melvin 1989].

Over time, the dorsal aspect of the CMC joint is stressed by repetitive pinching and the strong muscle pull of the adductor pollicis muscle and the short intrinsic thumb muscles. Altogether, these forces may cause the first CMC joint to sublux dorsally and radially. This typically results in the first metacarpal losing extension and becoming adducted. The MCP joint hyperextends to accommodate grasp [personal communication, J. C. Colditz, April 1995; Melvin 1989; personal communication, K. Schultz-Johnson, June 2006].

Splinting for CMC joint arthritis helps to manage pain, provides stability for intrinsic weakness of the capsular structures, and preserves the first web space. In addition, splinting helps with inflammation control, joint protection, and maintaining function [Poole and Pellegrini 2000, Neumann and Bielefeld 2003]. Static splinting is recommended for hypermobile or unstable joints but not for fixed joints [Neumann and Bielefeld 2003]. There are many options for splint design, ranging from forearm splints (with the CMC and MCP joints included) to hand-based splints (with the CMC and MCP joints included, or only the CMC joint included). With any selected design, the thumb is generally positioned in palmar abduction [Neumann and Bielefeld 2003]. Based on cadaver research, people with a hypermobile MCP joint who are positioned with the thumb in 30 degrees of flexion experience reduced pressure on the palmar part of the trapeziometacarpal joint, an area prone to deterioration [Moulton et al. 2001].

Melvin [1989] suggested fabricating a hand-based thumb immobilization splint (thumb CMC palmar abduction immobilization splint, Figure 8-8) [ASHT 1992], with the primary therapeutic goal of restricting the mobility of thumb joints to decrease pain and inflammation. The splint stabilizes the CMC and MCP joints in the maximal amount of palmar abduction that is comfortable for the person and allows for a functional pinch. Splinting both joints in a thumb post stabilizes the CMC joint in abduction so that the base of the MCP is stabilized. With the splint on, the person should continue to perform complete functional tasks, such as writing, comfortably. This thumb immobilization splint may be fabricated from a thin (1/16-inch) conforming thermoplastic material.

As discussed, another splinting option for CMC osteoarthritis designed by Colditz [2000] is a hand-based splint that allows for free motion of the thumb MCP joint and stabilizes the CMC joint to manage pain (Figures 8-9 and 8-10). The wrist is not included in the splint's design to allow for functional wrist motions. Colditz suggested an initial full-time wear of 2 to 3 weeks with removal for hygiene. Afterward, the splint should be worn during painful functional activities [Colditz 2000].

Therapists should fabricate this splint only on hands that have "a healthy MP joint" because the MP joint may sustain additional flexion pressure due to the controlled flexion position of the CMC joint [Melvin 2002, p. 1652]. Therapists must be attentive to wear on the MP joint [Neuman and Bielefeld 2003]. Prefabricated splints can also be considered for CMC osteoarthritis. However, prefabricated splints should be used with caution because positioning the thumb in abduction within the splint can increase MP joint extension, which can worsen a possible deformity [Biese 2002].

Given the variety of splinting options available, therapists critically analyze which splint to provide (forearm based or hand based) and which thumb joints to immobilize. Critical thinking considerations include presence of pain, need for stability, work, and functional demands. Researchers offer some guidance. Weiss et al. [2000] compared providing a long thumb immobilization splint with the MCP joint included to a hand-based splint with only the CMC joint included. In this 2-week study (n = 26), both splints were applied to individuals in grades 1 through 4 of CMC osteoarthritis as rated by Eaton and Littler [1973]. Both splints were found to be effective for pain control with all grades of the disease. However, the splints were only effective in reducing subluxation of the CMC joint for subjects in the earlier stages (grades 1 and 2) of the disease.

Subjects in the later stages of the disease (grades 3 and 4) preferred the short splint and reported pain relief with splint wear. Subjects in grades 1 and 2 slightly preferred the long splint (56%). Neither splint increased pinch strength nor changed pain levels when completing pinch strength measurements. Activities of daily living (ADL) improved with the short splint (93%) compared to (44%) with the long splint. Subjects reported that ADL were more difficult to complete with the long splint [Weiss et al. 2000].

Swigart et al. [1999] retrospectively researched (n = 114) the application of a custom long thumb immobilization splint with CMC osteoarthritis and found it to be a beneficial conservative treatment. Overall, subjects (regardless of disease stage) benefited from splinting (with a "60% improvement rate after splinting and 59% 6 months later" [Swigart et al. 1999, p. 90]). Some subjects were not able to tolerate the long splint because it felt too confining and uncomfortable. Day et al. [2004] studied splinting and steroid injections for people with thumb osteoarthritis and found that people in the earlier stages of the disease showed good improvement with conservative measures.

Splinting for Ulnar Collateral Ligament Injury

Acute or chronic injury to the ulnar collateral ligament (UCL), a condition also known as *gamekeeper's thumb* or *skier's thumb*, is a common injury that can occur at the MCP joint of the thumb [Landsman et al. 1995]. Gamekeeper's thumb was the original name of the injury because gamekeepers stressed this joint when they killed birds by twisting their necks [Colditz 2002].

The UCL helps stabilize the thumb by resisting radial stresses across the MCP joint [Winzeler and Rosenstein 1996]. The UCL can be injured if the thumb is forcibly abducted or hyperextended. This can occur from falling with an outstretched hand and the thumb in abduction, as during skiing [Winzeler and Rosenstein 1996]. It can also occur in basketball, gymnastics, rugby, volleyball, hockey, and football [Fess et al. 2005].

Treatment protocols depend on the extent of ligamental tear. There are protocols that involve immediate postoperative motion, and thus duration of casting postoperatively varies widely. Injuries are classified by the physician as grade I, II, or III [Wright and Rettig 1995]. The following is one of many suggested splinting protocols for each grade of injury. This splinting protocol is accompanied by hand therapy [Wright and Rettig 1995]. Grade I injuries, or those involving microscopic tears with no loss of ligament integrity, are positioned in a hand-based thumb immobilization splint with the CMC joint of the thumb in 40 degrees of palmar abduction (or in the most comfortable amount of palmar abduction).

This splint is also called a thumb MP radial and ulnar deviation restriction splint [ASHT 1992]. The purpose of this splint is to provide rest and protection during the healing phase. The person wears the splint continuously for 2 to 3 weeks, with removal for hygiene purposes. Grade II injuries involve a partial ligament tear, but the overall integrity of the ligament remains intact. The splinting protocol is the same as for grade I injuries, except that the thumb immobilization splint is worn for a longer time period (up to 4 or 5 weeks). Grade III injuries involve a completely torn ligament and usually require surgery.

After the person is casted, the cast is replaced by a thumb immobilization splint with the same protocol as described for grade I injuries. There is some recent evidence that a complete rupture may be managed conservatively with a thumb immobilization splint [Landsman et al. 1995]. If the UCL is still in an anatomic position, a thumb immobilization splint fabricated with the thumb in neutral with respect to flexion/extension and in maximum tolerated ulnar deviation worn consistently will heal the tear. The positioning will approximate the ends of the UCL and allow it to scar together. The physician and the therapist must assess whether the person is reliable enough to follow through with the splint. If there is any doubt, the person should be casted so that ligament protection is ensured [personal communication, K. Schultz-Johnson, 1999].

A unique "hybrid" splint was designed for athletes with a UCL injury who require splinting for protection during sports activities [Ford et al. 2004]. This splint design is a custom-made circumferential thermoplastic splint molded around the MCP joint, which is held in place by a fabricated neoprene wrap. The advantage of this splint design is that it provides MCP stability with the thermoplastic insert and allows for movement of other joints because of the neoprene stretch. In addition, this splint helps control pain and allows for activities involving grip and pinch (Figure 8-11). Therapists could either fabricate both parts of this splint or fabricate the circumferential splint and purchase a prefabricated neoprene thumb wrap. For those who return to skiing soon after a UCL injury, researchers suggest fabricating a small thermoplastic splint held in place with tape inside a ski glove [Alexy and De Carlo 1998].

Finally, as with any therapeutic intervention, success is dependent on many factors (such as carefully following therapeutic protocols and good surgery techniques). Zeman et al. [1998] (n = 58) found that a new suture technique for grade III (complete rupture) of the UCL combined with splinting post-surgery resulted in a high success rate of return to functional activities (98%), especially those activities difficult to perform pre-surgery.

A radial collateral ligament (RCL) injury (or "golfer's thumb") is an injury that occurs less commonly than UCL [Campbell and Wilson 2002] and requires a hand-based thumb immobilization splint. The splint is almost the same as for a UCL injury, except that the thumb is positioned in maximal comfortable radial deviation at the MCP joint. This splint helps remove stress to the healing ligament. The golfer who has injured a thumb and wants to return to the sport may find it difficult to play in a rigid splint. Rather than wearing a rigid splint during play, the person can be weaned from the splint in the same time as required for a UCL injury. The client learns how to wrap the thumb, which will be necessary for at least a year post injury [personal communication, K. Schultz-Johnson, 1999], or purchases a soft prefabricated splint.

Splinting for Scaphoid Fractures

Fracture of the scaphoid bone is the second most common wrist fracture [Cailliet 1994]. Similar to Colles' fracture,

SELF-QUIZ 8-1*

Please circle either true (T) or false (F).

1. T F One purpose of a thumb immobilization splint is to protect the thumb.
2. T F A therapist should apply a thumb immobilization splint only during the chronic phase to a person with de Quervain's tenosynovitis.
3. T F Fabricating either a long forearm thumb immobilization splint or a radial gutter thumb immobilization splint is best for a person who has de Quervain's tenosynovitis.
4. T F Splinting material more than 1/8-inch thick is best for splinting a rheumatoid arthritic hand because this material adds more support.
5. T F If a person with rheumatoid arthritis has pain in the wrist, the therapist includes the wrist in the thumb immobilization splint.
6. T F Splinting for grade I ulnar collateral thumb injuries requires that the person wear the splint continuously for 2 to 3 weeks, with removal only for hygiene.
7. T F The main purpose of splinting for an ulnar collateral thumb injury is to keep the web space open.
8. T F Fracture of the scaphoid bone requires splinting in a hand-based thumb immobilization splint.

*See Appendix A for the answer key.

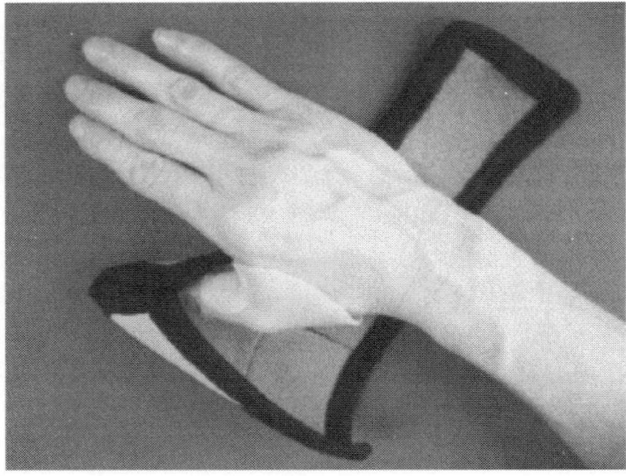

Figure 8-11 A protective splint for a UCL injury that combines a custom-made circumferential thermoplastic splint molded around the MCP joint, which is held in place by a fabricated neoprene wrap. [From Ford M, McKee P, Szilagyi M (2004). A hybrid thermoplastic and neoprene thumb metacarpophalangeal joint orthosis. Journal of Hand Therapy 17(1):64-68.]

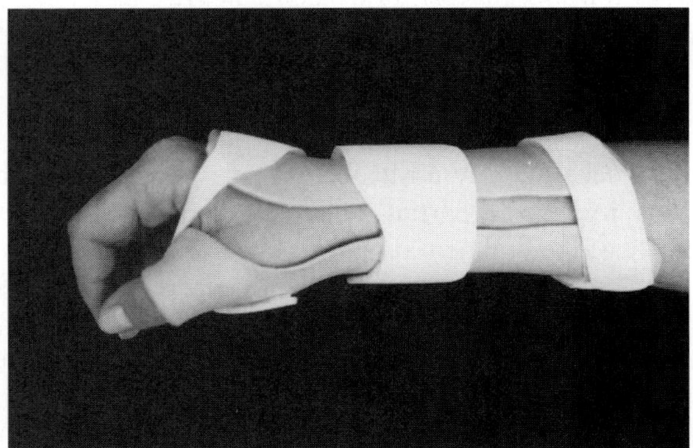

Figure 8-12 This combination volar and dorsal splint adds stability to the healing scaphoid fracture. [From Fess EE, Gettle KS, Philips CA, Janson JR (2005). *Hand and Upper Extremity Splinting: Principles and Methods, Third Edition.* St. Louis: Elsevier/Mosby.]

scaphoid fractures usually occur because of a fall on an outstretched hand with the wrist dorsiflexed more than 90 degrees [Geissler 2001] and are a consequence of strong forces to the wrist [Cooney 2003]. Scaphoid fractures happen with impact sports, such as basketball, football, and soccer [Riester et al. 1985, Werner and Plancher 1998, Geissler 2001]. Clinically, persons who have a scaphoid fracture present with painful wrist movements and tenderness on palpation of the scaphoid in the anatomical snuffbox between the EPL and the EPB [Cailliet 1994].

Physicians cast the arm and, after the immobilization stage, the hand may be positioned in a splint. This splint may be a volar forearm-based thumb immobilization splint [Cooney 2003] with the thumb in a position for function so that it lightly contacts the index and middle finger pads (0 to 10 degrees flexion) and with the wrist in neutral [Cannon 1991, Wright and Rettig 1995, Fess et al. 2005].

Some clients (especially those in noncontact competitive sports) may benefit from a combination dorsal/volar thumb splint for added stability, protection, and pain and edema control [Fess et al. 2005] (Figure 8-12). Therapists should educate clients that proximal scaphoid fractures take longer to heal, sometimes up to months, because of a poor vascular supply [Rettig et al. 1998, Fess et al. 2005]. For people who play sports and have a healing scaphoid fracture, a soft commercial thumb immobilization splint may also be recommended as a prevention measure [Geissler 2001].

Fabrication of a Thumb Immobilization Splint

There are many approaches to fabrication of a thumb immobilization splint. Figure 8-13 shows a detailed pattern that can be used for either a volar or dorsal thumb immobilization splint. The *thumb immobilization splint radial design* [ASHT 1992] provides support on the radial side of

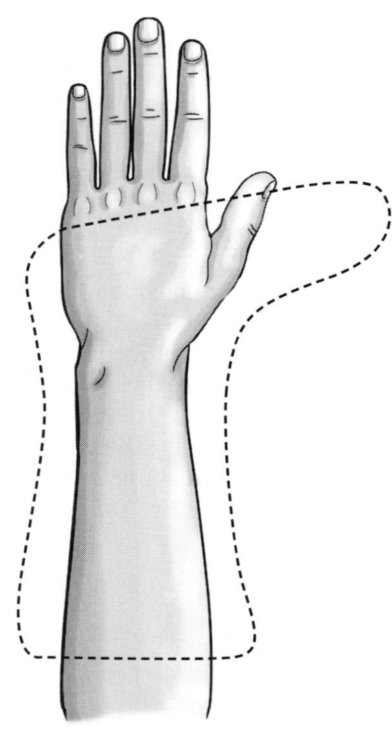

Figure 8-13 A detailed pattern for either a volar or a dorsal thumb immobilization splint.

the hand while stabilizing the thumb. This design allows some wrist flexion and extension but limits deviation [Melvin 1989]. The therapist usually places the thumb in a palmar abducted position so that the thumb pad can contact the index pad. The therapist leaves the IP joint free for functional movement but can adapt the splint pattern to include the IP joint if more support becomes necessary. The thumb can be placed in a position of comfort (i.e., out of the functional plane) if the client does not tolerate the thumb placed in the functional position or when the physician does not want the thumb to incur any stress.

Laboratory Exercise 8-1

These components are in various types of thumb immobilization splints. They are also part of other splints, such as the wrist cock-up and resting hand splint. Label the splinting components shown in the following figure.

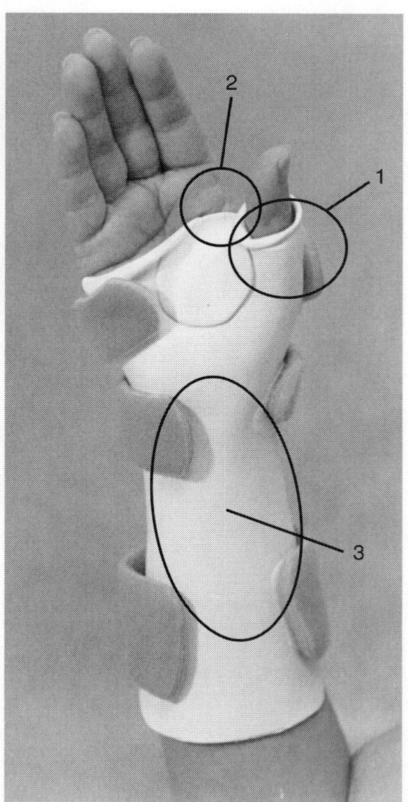

1. ______________________________
2. ______________________________
3. ______________________________

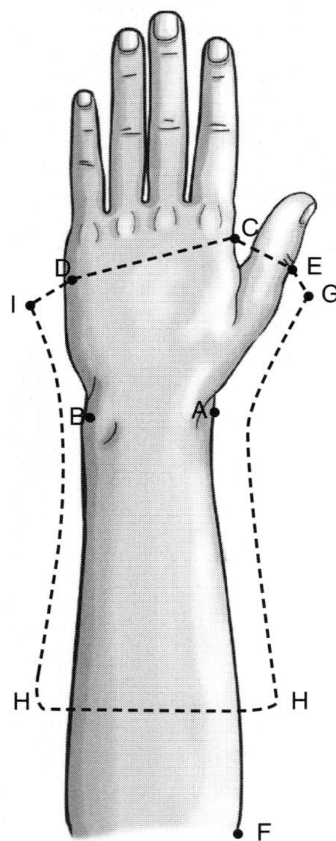

Figure 8-14 A detailed pattern for a radial gutter thumb immobilization splint.

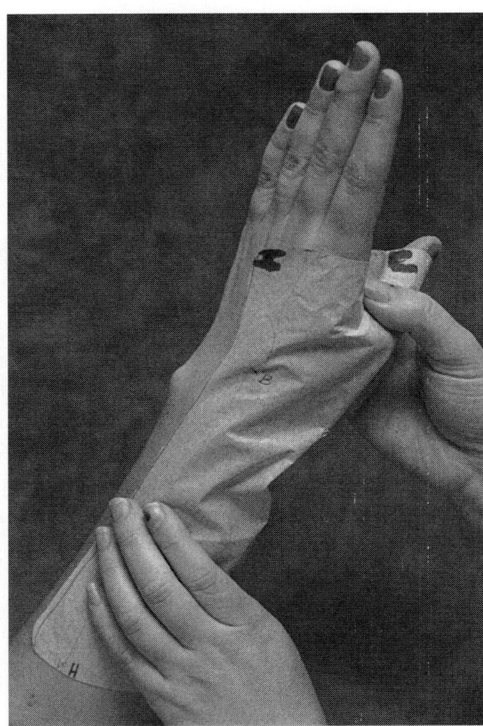

Figure 8-15 To ensure proper fit, place the paper pattern on the person.

Figure 8-14 shows a detailed radial gutter thumb immobilization pattern that excludes the IP joint. (See Figure 8-3 for a picture of the completed splint product.)

1. Position the forearm and hand palm down on a piece of paper. The fingers should be in a natural resting position and slightly abducted; the wrist should be neutral with respect to deviation. Draw an outline of the hand and forearm to the elbow. As you gain experience with pattern drawing, you will not need to draw the entire hand and forearm outline. The experienced therapist can estimate the placement of key points on the pattern.
2. While the person's hand is on the paper, mark an *A* at the radial styloid and a *B* at the ulnar styloid. Mark the second and fifth metacarpal heads *C* and *D*, respectively. Mark the IP joint of the thumb *E*, and mark the olecranon process of the elbow *F*. Then remove the person's hand from the paper pattern.
3. Place an *X* two-thirds the length of the forearm on each side. Place another *X* on each side of the pattern approximately 1 to 1-½ inches outside and parallel to the two *X* markings for two-thirds the length of the forearm. Mark these two *X*s *H*.
4. Draw an angled line connecting the second and fifth metacarpal heads (*C* to *D*). Extend this line approximately 1 to 1-½ inches to the ulnar side of the hand and mark it *I*.
5. Connect *C* to *E*. Extend this line approximately ½ to 1 inch. Mark the end of the line *G*.
6. Draw a line from *G* down the radial side of the forearm, making sure the line follows the size of the forearm. To ensure that the splint is two-thirds the length of the forearm, end the line at *H*.
7. Begin a line from *I* and extend it down the ulnar side of the forearm, making certain that the line follows the increasing size of the forearm. End the line at *H*.
8. For the proximal edge of the splint, draw a straight line that connects both *H*s.
9. Make sure the splint pattern lines are rounded at *G*, *I*, and the two *H*s.
10. Cut out the pattern.
11. Place the splint pattern on the person (Figure 8-15). Make certain the splint's edges end mid-forearm on the volar and dorsal surfaces of the person's hand and forearm. Check that the splint is two-thirds the forearm length and one-half the forearm circumference. Check the thumb position and make any necessary adjustments (e.g., additions, deletions) on the splint pattern.
12. Carefully trace with a pencil the thumb immobilization splint pattern on a sheet of thermoplastic material.
13. Heat the thermoplastic material.
14. Cut the pattern out of the thermoplastic material.
15. Reheat the material, mold the form onto the person's hand, and make necessary adjustments. Make sure the thumb is correctly positioned as the material hardens by having the person lightly touch the thumb tip to the pads of the index or middle fingers. Another approach is to provide light pressure over the plastic of the

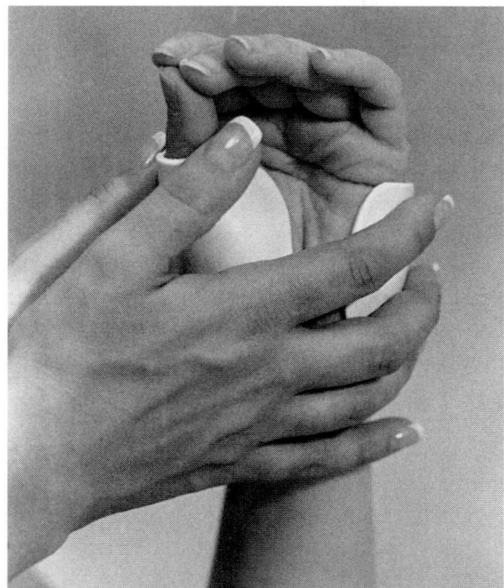

Figure 8-16 Have person lightly touch the thumb tip to the pads of the index and middle fingers to position the thumb in palmar abduction.

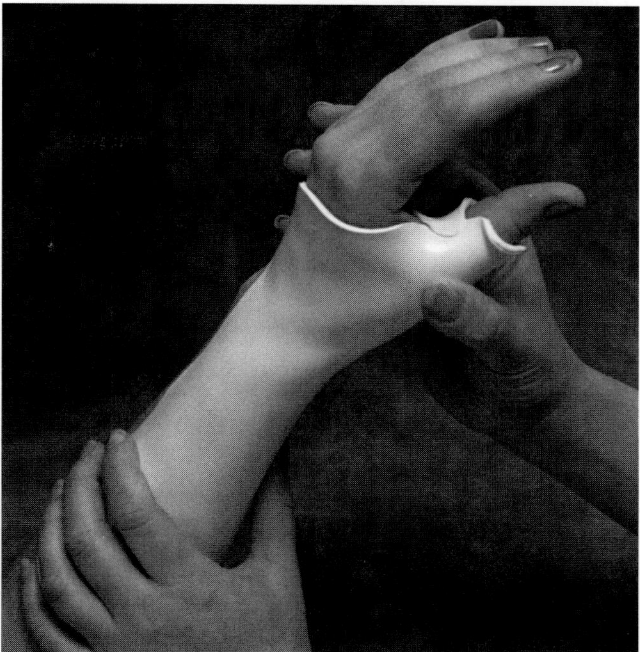

Figure 8-17 Although the actual movement comes from the CMC joint, provide light pressure on the thumb MCP joint to position the thumb correctly in palmar abduction.

thumb MCP joint to align it in palmar abduction (Figures 8-16 and 8-17).

16. Add three 2-inch straps (one at the wrist joint, one towards the proximal end of the forearm trough, and one across the dorsal aspect of the hand) connecting the hypothenar bar to the metacarpal bar.

Fabrication of a Hand-Based Thumb Immobilization Splint

Hand-based thumb immobilization splints can be fabricated for people who have the following diagnoses: low median nerve injury, ulnar or radial collateral ligament injury of the MCP joint, osteoarthritis, and the potential for a first web space contracture. Each of these diagnoses may require placement of the thumb post in a different degree of abduction, based on protocols. With this splint, the IP joint is usually left free for functional movement, unless there is extreme pain in that joint. However, if the IP joint is left free (especially during rigorous activity) it too can become vulnerable to stresses. This hand-based splint design is most appropriate for stabilizing the MP joint because the position of the CMC is irrelevant. Finally, because this hand-based splint design incorporates the dorsal aspect of the palm, the therapist may need to add padding since the dorsal skin has a minimal subcutaneous layer and the boniness of the dorsal palm can cause skin breakdown.

Figure 8-18 shows a detailed hand-based thumb immobilization pattern. (See Figure 8-8 for a picture of the completed splint product.)

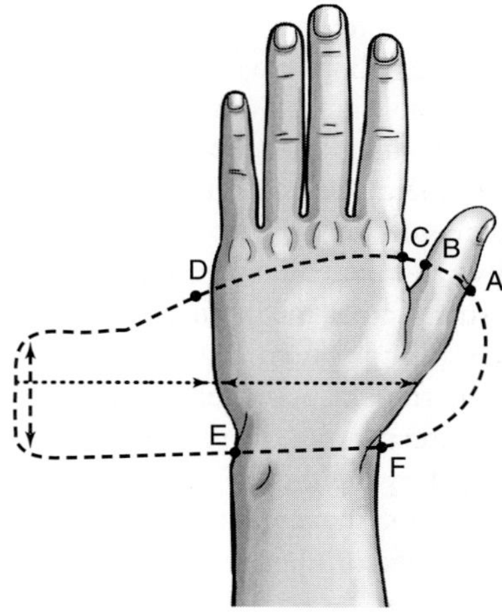

Figure 8-18 A detailed pattern for hand-based thumb immobilization splint.

1. Position the person's forearm and hand palm down on a piece of paper. Ensure that the client's thumb is radially abducted. The fingers should be in a natural resting position and slightly abducted. Draw an outline of the hand, including the wrist and a couple of inches of the forearm.
2. While the person's hand is on the paper, mark the IP joint of the thumb on both sides and label it *A* (radial side of thumb) and *B* (ulnar side of the thumb), respectively. Then mark the second and fifth metacarpal heads *C* and *D*, respectively. Mark the wrist joint on the ulnar side of the hand *E*, and mark *F* on the radial side of the wrist. Remove the hand from the pattern.

3. Draw an angled line connecting the marks of the second and fifth metacarpal heads (*D* to *C*). Then connect *C* to *B* and *B* to *A*. Curve the line around and angle it down to *F*. Connect *F* to *E*. Then extend the line out from *E* approximately equal to the length of the pattern on the hand. Go up vertically and curve the line around and connect it to *D*. Make sure that all edges on this pattern are rounded.
4. Cut out the pattern, check fit, and make any adjustments. Make sure the pattern allows enough room for an adequately fitting thumb post.
5. Position the person's upper extremity with the elbow resting on the table and the forearm in a neutral position.
6. Trace the pattern onto a sheet of thermoplastic material.
7. Heat the thermoplastic material.
8. Cut the pattern out of the thermoplastic material.
9. Measure the CMC joint to make sure it is in the correct position.
10. Reheat the thermoplastic material.
11. Mold the splint onto the person's hand. First form the thumb post around the thenar area. Make sure the thumb is correctly positioned as the material hardens. Allowances are made in the circumference of the thumb post to ensure that the client can move the thumb. This is particularly important when fabricating a splint from thermoplastic material that shrinks or has memory. Roll the volar part of the thumb post proximal to the thumb IP crease to allow adequate IP flexion. Then form the splint across the dorsal side of the hand from the thumb (radial side) to the ulnar side. Curving around the ulnar side, fit the splint material proximal to the distal palmar crease on the volar side of the hand. There will be just enough room between the thumb post and the end of the splint on the ulnar side to add a strap across the palm. Make sure the proximal end of the splint is flared.
12. After the thermoplastic material has hardened, check that the person can perform IP thumb flexion without impingement by the thumb post and that he or she can perform all wrist movements without interference by the proximal end of the splint. Make adjustments as necessary.
13. Add one strap across the palm.

Technical Tips for Proper Fit

1. Before molding the splint, place the person's elbow on a tabletop, positioned in 90 degrees of flexion and the forearm in a neutral position. Position the thumb and wrist according to diagnostic indications.
2. Monitor joint positions by measuring during and after splint fabrication. A common mistake when splinting is incorrect placement of the thumb in a midposition between palmar abduction and radial abduction when the diagnostic protocol calls for palmar abduction. The best way to position the thumb in palmar abduction for fabrication of a splint is to have the person lightly touch the thumb tip to the pad of the index or middle finger. However, there will be some persons (for example, a person who has rheumatoid arthritis) who will find the thumb post more comfortable between radial and palmar abduction.
3. Follow the natural curves of the longitudinal, distal, and proximal arches. Position the splint area that covers the thenar eminence just proximal to the proximal palmar crease. Be especially careful to check that the index finger has full flexion because of its close proximity to the opponens bar, C bar, and thumb post.
4. When molding the thumb post, overlap the splinting material into the thumb web space (Figure 8-19). Be certain the thumb IP joint remains in extension during molding to facilitate later splint application and removal. Be extremely careful in making adjustments with a heat gun on the thumb post, or the result may be an inappropriate fit.
5. When applying thermoplastic material that shrinks during cooling and because the thumb is circumferential in shape, allowances must be made to ensure easy application and removal of the splint. There are several options to address this issue. One is to have the person make very small thumb circles as the plastic cools because this motion allows for some extra room [personal communication, K. Schultz-Johnson, June 2006]. Another option is to gently flare the thumb post with a narrow pencil [McKee and Morgan 1998].
6. A thumb post can be fabricated with *overlapping material* that does not bond. This design method allows

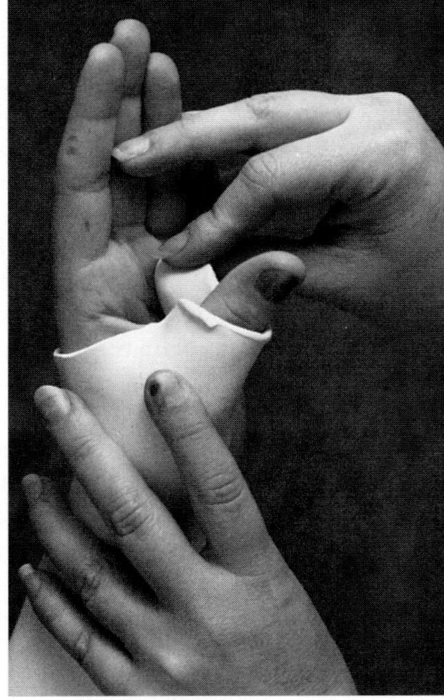

Figure 8-19 Overlap the extra splinting material into the thumb web space.

Laboratory Exercise 8-2

1. Practice making a pattern for a radial gutter thumb immobilization splint on another person. Use the detailed instructions on the previous pages to draw the pattern. Make necessary adjustments to the pattern after cutting it out.
2. Practice drawing a pattern for a radial gutter thumb immobilization splint on the following outlines of the hands without using detailed instructions. Label the landmarks.

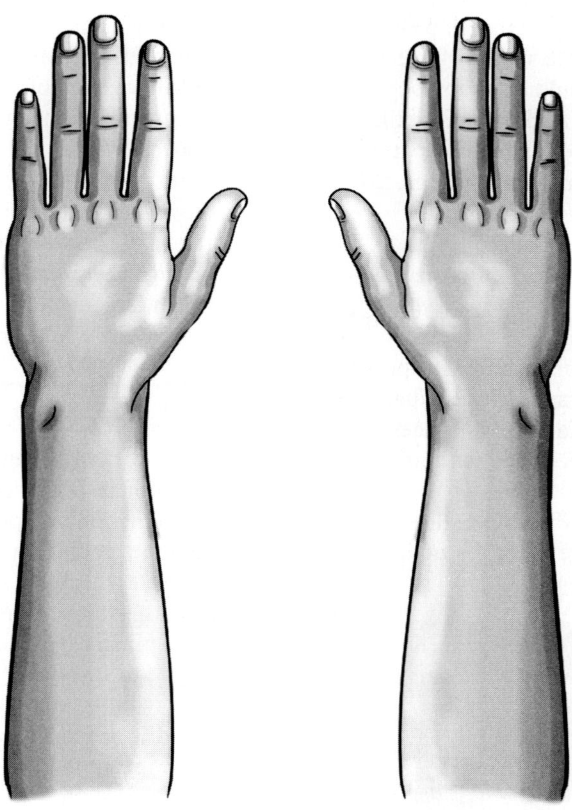

for adjustment to expand or contract the thumb post with the velcro straps that secure the post [personal communication, K. Schultz-Johnson, June 2006].

7. For a thumb immobilization splint that allows IP mobility, make sure the distal end of the thumb post on the volar surface has been rolled to allow full IP flexion (Figure 8-20).
8. Concentrate during splint fabrication on the thenar area. Note several areas prior to hardening of the thermoplastic material. Check that the thumb post is not too loose and provides adequate support for the thumb joints. The thumb post should also provide enough room for ease of donning and doffing of the splint. Check that the distal end of the thumb post is just proximal to the MP joint and has not migrated lower. Check that the forearm trough is correctly placed in mid-forearm. Make sure that the splint does not interfere with functional hand movements.

Precautions for a Thumb Immobilization Splint

The cautious splintmaker checks for areas of skin pressure over the distal ulna, the superficial branch of the radial nerve at the radial styloid, and the volar and dorsal surfaces of the thumb MCP joint. Specific precautions for the molding of the splint include the following:

- If the thumb post extends too far distally on the volar surface of the IP joint, the result is restriction of the IP joint flexion and a likely area for skin irritation.
- Because of its close proximity to the opponens bar, C bar, and thumb post, the radial base of the first metacarpal and first web space has a potential for skin irritation.
- With a radial gutter splint, monitor the splint for a pressure area at the midline of the forearm on the volar and dorsal surfaces. Pull the sides of the forearm trough apart if it is too tight.
- Be careful to fabricate a thumb splint that is supportive and not too constrictive. Constriction results in decreased circulation and possible skin breakdown. Make allowances for edema when fabricating the thumb post.
- If using a thermoplastic material that has memory properties, be aware that the material shrinks when cooling. Therefore, the thumb post opening must remain large enough for comfortable application and removal of the splint.

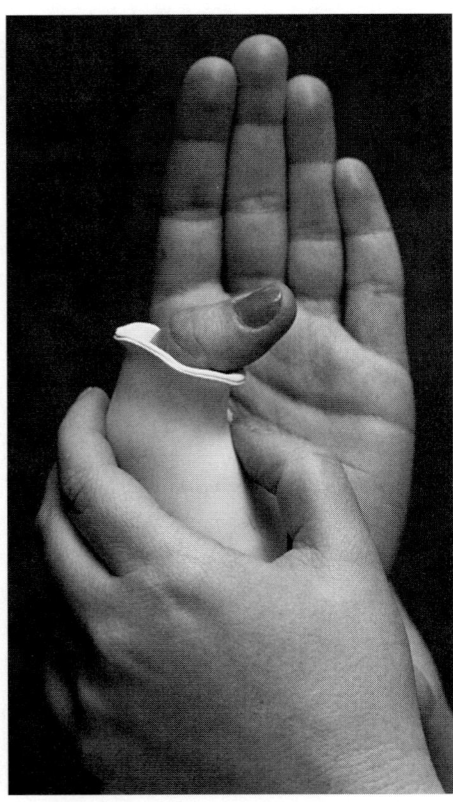

Figure 8-20 Roll the distal end of the thumb post to allow full IP flexion.

Impact on Occupations

Having a workable thumb for grasp and pinch is paramount for functional activities. Research findings support the thumb's functional importance. Swigart et al. [1999] established that people with CMC arthritis had decreased involvement in crafts and changed their athletic involvement. With gamekeeper's thumb, lack of thenar strength and adequate pinch can impact daily functional activities such as turning a key or opening a jar [Zeman et al. 1998].

Even with the stability provided by a splint, some people may find it more difficult to perform meaningful occupations. For example, Weiss et al. [2000] found in their study (n = 25) that with some subjects, the long thumb immobilization splint inhibited function and was more than necessary to meet therapeutic goals. Therefore, the goal of splinting is to improve function. It is intended that with the benefits of splint wear and a therapeutic program the person will return to meaningful activities [Zeman et al. 1998].

Prefabricated Splints

Deciding to furnish a prefabricated thumb splint requires careful reflection. Therapists should critically consider the condition, for which the splint is being provided, materials that the splint is made out of as well as design and comfort factors. Furthermore, therapists should review the literature to determine whether a custom thumb splint is preferable over a prefabricated thumb splint to treat a condition.

Conditions

Prefabricated thumb splints are manufactured for a variety of conditions, including arthritis, thumb MP collateral ligament injuries, de Quervain's tenosynovitis, and hypertonicity.

Splint types and positions for all these conditions have been discussed in this chapter (see Table 8-1).

Materials

Therapists should be aware of the characteristics of the wide variety of materials available for prefabricated thumb splints. Material firmness varies from soft to rigid. Soft materials are often used with thumb splinting because they can be easier to apply and provide a more comfortable fit for a client with a painful and edematous thumb IP joint than a rigid splint. A commonly used soft material with prefabricated splints is neoprene. It has the advantage of providing *hugging* support with flexibility for function, but it has the disadvantage of retaining moisture next to the skin. Another soft material used in prefabricated splints is leather. Splints made of leather absorb perspiration and are pliable; however, they often become odiferous and soiled. Some splints are lined with moisture wicking material or are fabricated from perforated material to address this issue.

Examples of prefabricated splints made out of rigid materials are those fabricated out of thermoplastic, vinyl, or adjustable polypropylene materials.

An awareness of the splint's function, condition for which it is being used, and the client's occupational demands can help the therapist critically determine the degree of material firmness to use. A prefabricated splint made out of a rigid material might be very appropriate to supply to a client for sports, heavier work activities, or for any condition that requires a higher amount of support and protection. Finally, people who are allergic to latex will require splints made from latex-free materials.

Design and Comfort

Similar to fabricated thumb splints prefabricated splints are either hand based or forearm based. The hand-based thumb immobilization designs provide support to the thumb joints through the circumferential thumb post component, thermoplastic material, or optional stays. The forearm-based immobilization designs derive some of their support from a longer lever arm. Prefabricated forearm-based splints contain many features which should be critically considered for client usage. Examples of these features are adjustable or additional straps and adjustable thumb stays to provide optimal support and fit. Some designs for both the forearm- and hand-based splints are hybrid designs. These splints usually have a softer outer layer with removable and adjustable inserts made out of thermoplastic material to customize the fit of the splint.

Another consideration is the comfort of the prefabricated thumb splint. Factors to think about are adjustability, temperature, bulkiness, and padding of the possible splint selection. When adjusting the splint therapists should take into account the number and location of strap and types of strapping material to obtain an appropriate fit. For example, with a long thumb splint the therapist should consider whether the wrist straps provide adequate support. With temperature the type of splinting material that is used for the prefabricated splint is taken into account as some materials are more breathable than others. Thumb splints made out of neoprene or other soft materials are usually more breathable than rigid splinting materials. A prefabricated splint made out of a breathable material might be a consideration for a person living or working in a hot environment. A person with arthritis might prefer a thumb splint that provides warmth. Padding may be an essential consideration with a person who has a tendency towards skin breakdown. Thumb immobilization splints may chafe the web space, so the therapist must monitor for fit and consider padding in that area. Some prefabricated thumb immobilization designs include added features, such as a gel pad for scar control or leather for added durability. Figures 8-2 A through F outline prefabricated thumb splint options.

Summary

Thumb splinting is commonly provided in clinical practice. Applying a critical analysis approach will help with thumb splinting. It behooves therapists to be aware of the appropriate splints (whether fabricated or prefarbricated) to provide clients splints based on conditions and occupational needs.

THERAPEUTIC OBJECTIVE	DESCRIPTION
Prefabricated thumb immobilization splints provide rest to inflamed, injured, and painful thumb joints.	Thumb immobilization splints are available in low-temperature thermoplastic and soft materials (leather, neoprene) to support thumb joints (Figure 8-21, A through C. Some thumb splints contain extra layers, which can add warmth (Figure 8-21D). Others can be customized for the client (Figure 8-21E). Thumb loops can be used for hypertonicity (Figure 8-21F). Pre-thumb immobilization splints are available in different sizes, hand or forearm bases, radial or palmar based, and provide radial or palmar thumb abduction.

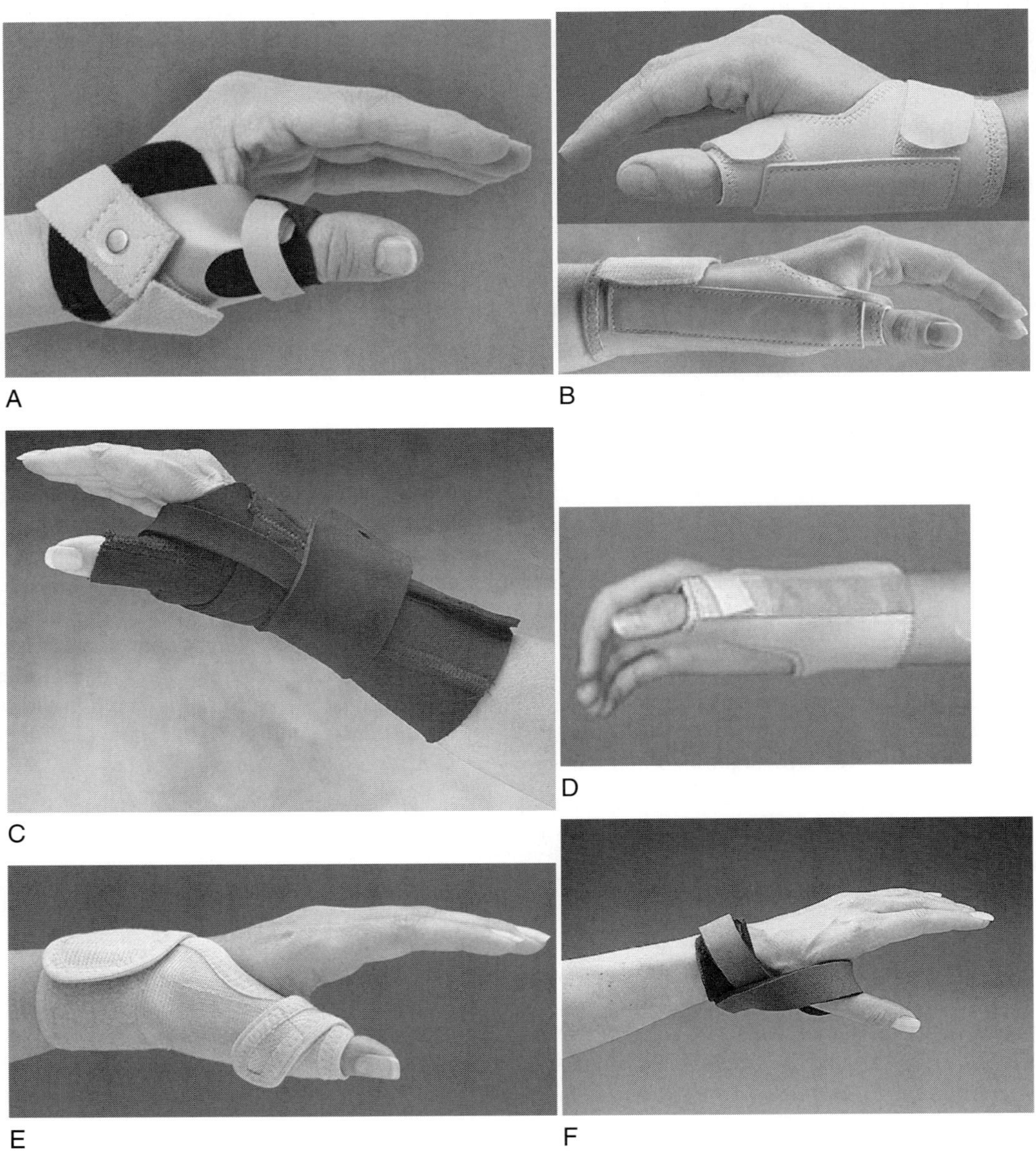

Figure 8-21 (A) This thermoplastic splint supports the MP and CMC joints. [ThumSaver MP; courtesy 3-Point Products, Stevensville, Maryland.] (B) Thumb splint is made from leather. [Collum CMC Thumb Brace; courtesy Adaptive Abilities, Oroville, WA.] (C) This Comfort Cool Wrist and Thumb CMC Restriction Splint is made out of perforated neoprene, which keeps the extremity cool. It has additional strapping at the wrist to allow for extra support. [Courtesy Sammons Preston Rolyan, Bollington, IL.] (D) This Rolyan Preferred 1st thumb splint can be used with a person who has arthritis as it contains extra layers to help wick moisture from the skin, retain body warmth, and provide heat. [Courtesy Sammons Preston Rolyan, Bollington, IL.] (E) This Roylan Gel Shell thumb spica splint contains a gel shell Rolyan pad that helps with scar formation and hypersensitivity. It also contains a moldable thermoplastic stay that can be adjusted along the radial side of the hand. [Courtesy Sammons Preston Rolyan, Bollington, IL.] (F) This Rolyan thumb loop is latex free and positions the thumb to decrease tone and facilitate function. [Courtesy Sammons Preston Rolyan, Bollington, IL.]

Laboratory Exercise 8-3*

The following illustration shows a thumb immobilization splint for a 35-year-old woman working as a secretary. She has a long history of rheumatoid arthritis. Her physician ordered a thumb immobilization splint after she complained of pain and inflammation in the thumb MCP joint. Keeping in mind the diagnostic protocols for thumb immobilization splinting, identify two problems with the illustrated splint.

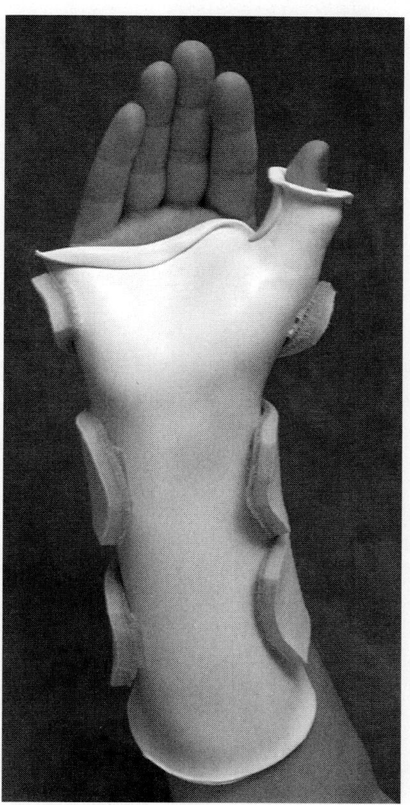

1. List two problems with this splint.

   a. ______________________________

   b. ______________________________

2. Which problems might arise from continual splint wear?

   ____

   ____

*See Appendix A for the answer key.

Laboratory Exercise 8-4

On a partner, practice fabricating a radial gutter thumb immobilization splint that does not immobilize the thumb IP joint. Before starting, use a goniometer to ensure that the wrist is in 15 degrees of extension, the CMC joint of the thumb in 45 degrees of palmar abduction, and the MCP joint of the thumb in 5 to 10 degrees of flexion. Check the finished product to ensure that full finger flexion and thumb IP flexion are possible after you fit the splint and make all adjustments. Use Form 8-1 as a check-off sheet for a self-evaluation of the thumb immobilization splint. Use Grading Sheet 8-1 as a classroom grading sheet.

FORM 8-1* Thumb immobilization splint

Name: ______________________________

Date: ______________________________

Type of thumb immobilization splint:

Volar ❍ Dorsal ❍ Radial gutter ❍ Hand based ❍

Thumb joint position: ______________________________

After the person wears the splint for 30 minutes, answer the following questions. (Mark *NA* for nonapplicable situations.)

Evaluation Areas				**Comments**
Design				
1. The wrist position is at the correct angle.	Yes ❍	No ❍	NA ❍	
2. The thumb position is at the correct angle.	Yes ❍	No ❍	NA ❍	
3. The thenar eminence is not restricted or flattened.	Yes ❍	No ❍	NA ❍	
4. The thumb post provides adequate support and is not constrictive.	Yes ❍	No ❍	NA ❍	
5. The splint is two-thirds the length of the forearm.	Yes ❍	No ❍	NA ❍	
6. The splint is one-half the width of the forearm.	Yes ❍	No ❍	NA ❍	
Function				
1. The splint allows full thumb IP flexion.	Yes ❍	No ❍	NA ❍	
2. The splint allows full MCP joint flexion of the fingers.	Yes ❍	No ❍	NA ❍	
3. The splint provides wrist support that allows functional activities.	Yes ❍	No ❍	NA ❍	
Straps				
1. The straps avoid bony prominences.	Yes ❍	No ❍	NA ❍	
2. The straps are secure and rounded.	Yes ❍	No ❍	NA ❍	
Comfort				
1. The splint edges are smooth with rounded corners.	Yes ❍	No ❍	NA ❍	
2. The proximal end is flared.	Yes ❍	No ❍	NA ❍	
3. The splint does not cause impingements or pressure sores.	Yes ❍	No ❍	NA ❍	
Cosmetic appearance				
1. The splint is free of fingerprints, dirt, and pencil and pen marks.	Yes ❍	No ❍	NA ❍	
2. The splint is smooth and free of buckles.	Yes ❍	No ❍	NA ❍	
Therapeutic regimen				
1. The person has been instructed in a wearing schedule.	Yes ❍	No ❍	NA ❍	
2. The person has been provided splint precautions.	Yes ❍	No ❍	NA ❍	
3. The person demonstrates understanding of the education.	Yes ❍	No ❍	NA ❍	
4. Client or caregiver knows how to clean the splint.	Yes ❍	No ❍	NA ❍	

Continued

FORM 8-1* Thumb immobilization splint—cont'd

Discuss possible splint adjustments or changes you should make based on the self-evaluation. (What would you do differently next time?)

____

____

____

____

____

____

____

____

____

*See Appendix B for a perforated copy of this form.

GRADING SHEET 8-1* Thumb immobilization splint

Name: ______________________________

Date: ______________________________

Type of thumb immobilization splint:

Volar ❍ Dorsal ❍ Radial gutter ❍ Hand based ❍

Thumb joint position: ______________________________

Grade: ____________________

1 = beyond improvement, not acceptable
2 = requires maximal improvement
3 = requires moderate improvement
4 = requires minimal improvement
5 = requires no improvement

Evaluation Areas

Design

1. The wrist position is at the correct angle. 1 2 3 4 5
2. The thumb position is at the correct angle. 1 2 3 4 5
3. The thenar eminence is not restricted or flattened. 1 2 3 4 5
4. The thumb post provides adequate support and is not constrictive. 1 2 3 4 5
5. The splint is two-thirds the length of the forearm. 1 2 3 4 5
6. The splint is one-half the width of the forearm. 1 2 3 4 5

Function

1. The splint allows full thumb motion. 1 2 3 4 5
2. The splint allows full MCP joint flexion of the fingers. 1 2 3 4 5
3. The splint provides wrist support that allows functional activities. 1 2 3 4 5

Straps

1. The straps avoid bony prominences. 1 2 3 4 5
2. The straps are secure and rounded. 1 2 3 4 5

Comfort

1. The splint edges are smooth with rounded corners. 1 2 3 4 5
2. The proximal end is flared. 1 2 3 4 5
3. The splint does not cause impingements or pressure sores. 1 2 3 4 5

Cosmetic appearance

1. The splint is free of fingerprints, dirt, and pencil and pen marks. 1 2 3 4 5
2. The splinting material is not buckled. 1 2 3 4 5

Comments:

____

____

____

____

____

*See Appendix C for a perforated copy of this sheet.

CASE STUDY 8-1*

Read the following scenario and use your clinical reasoning skills to answer the questions based on information in this chapter.

T J, a 21-year-old male, is a skier training to compete in the Olympics. During one training session he fell in a snow drift with an outstretched right dominant hand and the thumb positioned in abduction. His thumb became painful and edematous. The team physician diagnosed a partial tear of the ulnar collateral ligament (grade II) and casted the forearm, wrist, and thumb. After the cast was removed, therapy was ordered to fabricate a thumb splint.

1. What type of splint does the therapist fabricate, and in which position is the thumb splinted?

   ____

   ____

2. What is the purpose of the splint?

   ____

   ____

3. What would be a suggested wearing schedule?

   ____

   ____

4. Before the 4- to 5-week healing period is over, T J's physician releases him back to skiing with another order to fabricate a splint to allow him to continue involvement in skiing. What type of splint should the therapist fabricate?

   ____

   ____

   ____

   ____

*See Appendix A for the answer key.

CASE STUDY 8-2*

Read the following scenario and use your clinical reasoning skills to answer the questions based on information in this chapter.

S Y, a 58-year-old woman, went to her physician complaining of thumb pain at the CMC joint with her daily living activities. This pain had occurred for less than 1 year. She was particularly concerned about difficulty with knitting and doing her needlework. Clinical examination revealed no additional pain or symptoms in the wrist, fingers, or other joints of the thumb. S Y was diagnosed with osteoarthritis of the CMC joint. Her physician ordered therapy to fabricate a thumb splint. The order was not specific as to which joints to be splinted and what type of splint.

1. What type of splint should the therapist fabricate and which thumb joints should be splinted?

____

____

____

2. What is the purpose of the splint?

____

____

3. What would be a suggested wearing schedule?

____

____

____

4. S Y was discontinued from therapy and 3 years later her symptoms worsened due to continuing her hobby of needlework. S Y presented with pain in her wrist and the thumb MCP joint due to progression of the osteoarthritis. Describe a splint the therapist might consider fabricating.

____

____

____

5. What position should the therapist splint the thumb in the thumb post?

____

____

____

*See Appendix A for the answer key.

REVIEW QUESTIONS

1. What are the general reasons for provision of a thumb immobilization splint?
2. What are some of the clinical indications for including the IP joint of the thumb in a thumb immobilization splint?
3. What is a proper wearing schedule for a person with rheumatoid arthritis who wears a thumb immobilization splint?
4. What is the suggested position for a thumb splint for a person who has CMC joint arthritis? What joints are splinted?
5. Which type of thumb immobilization splint should a therapist fabricate for a person who has de Quervain's tenosynovitis?
6. What is some of the research evidence for splinting for de Quervain's tenosynovitis?
7. Which type of thumb immobilization splint should a therapist fabricate for an injury of the thumb ulnar collateral ligament?
8. What is the splint-wearing schedule for each grade of ulnar collateral ligament injury?

References

Alexy C, De Carlo M (1998). Rehabilitation and use of protective devices in hand and wrist injuries. Clinics in Sports Medicine 17(3):635-655.

American Society of Hand Therapists (1992). *Splint Classification System*. Garner, NC: American Society of Hand Therapists.

Avci S, Yilmaz C, Sayli U (2002). Comparision of nonsurgical treatment measures for de Quervain's disease of pregnancy and lactation. Journal of Hand Surgery 27A(2):322-324.

Belkin J, English C (1996). Hand splinting: Principles, practice, and decision making. In LW Pedretti (ed.), *Occupational Therapy: Practice Skills for Physical Dysfunction, Fourth Edition.* St. Louis: Mosby, pp. 319-343.

Biese J (2002). Short splints: Indications and techniques. In EJ Mackin, AD Callahan, TM Skirven, LH Schneider, AL Osterman (eds.), *Rehabilitation of the Hand and Upper Extremity, Fifth Edition.* St. Louis: Mosby, pp. 1846-1857.

Cailliet R (1994). *Hand Pain and Impairment*. Philadelphia: F. A. Davis.

Campbell PJ, Wilson RL (2002). Management of joint injuries and intraarticular fractures. In EJ Mackin, AD Callahan, TM Skirven, LH Schneider, AL Osterman (eds.), *Rehabilitation of the Hand and Upper Extremity, Fifth Edition*. St. Louis: Mosby, pp. 396-411.

Cannon NM (1991). *Diagnosis and Treatment Manual for Physicians and Therapists, Third Edition*. Indianapolis: The Hand Rehabilitation Center of Indiana.

Cannon NM, Foltz RW, Koepfer JM, Lauck MR, Simpson DM, Bromley RS (1985). *Manual of Hand Splinting*. New York: Churchill Livingstone.

Chaisson C, McAlindon TS (1997). Osteoarthritis of the hand: Clinical features and management. The Journal of Musculoskeletal Medicine 14:66-68, 71-74, 77.

Colditz JC (2002). Anatomic considerations for splinting the thumb. In EJ Mackin, AD Callahan, TM Skirven, LH Schneider, AL Osterman (eds.), *Rehabilitation of the Hand and Upper Extremity, Fifth Edition*. St. Louis: Mosby, pp. 1858-1874.

Colditz JC (1984). Arthritis. In MH Malick, MC Kasch (eds.), *Manual on Management of Specific Hand Problems*. Pittsburgh: AREN Publications, pp. 112-136.

Colditz JC (2000). The biomechanics of a thumb carpometacarpal immobilization splint: Design and fitting. Journal of Hand Therapy 13(3):228-235.

Cooney WP III (2003). Scaphoid fractures: Current treatments and techniques. Instructional Course Lectures 52:197-208.

Day CS, Gelberman R, Patel AA, Vogt MT, Ditsios K, Boyer MI (2004). Basal joint osteoarthritis of the thumb: A prospective trial of steroid injection and splinting. Journal of Hand Surgery 29A(2):247-251.

Dell PC, Dell RB (1996). Management of rheumatoid arthritis of the wrist. Journal of Hand Therapy 9(2):157-164.

Eaton RG, Littler W (1973). Ligament reconstruction for the painful thumb carpometacarpal joint. The Journal of Bone and Joint Surgery 55A:1655-1666.

Fess EE, Gettle KS, Philips CA, Janson JR (2005). *Hand Splinting Principles and Methods, Third Edition*. St. Louis: Elsevier/Mosby.

Ford M, McKee P, Szilagyi M (2004). A hybrid thermoplastic and neoprene thumb metacarpophalangeal joint orthosis. Journal of Hand Therapy 17(1):64-68.

Geisser RW (1984). Splinting the rheumatoid arthritic hand. In EM Ziegler (ed.), *Current Concepts in Orthosis*. Germantown, WI: Rolyan Medical Products, pp. 29-49.

Geissler WB (2001). Carpal fractures in athletes. Clinics in Sports Medicine 20(1):167-188.

Idler RS (1997). Helping the patient who has wrist or hand tenosynovitis. Part 2: Managing trigger finger and de Quervain's disease. The Journal of Musculoskeletal Medicine 14:62-65, 68, 74-75.

Landsman JC, Seitz WH, Froimson AI, Leb RB, Bachner EJ (1995). Splint immobilization of gamekeeper's thumb. Orthopedics 18(12): 1161-1165.

Lane LB, Boretz RS, Stuchin SA (2001). Treatment of de Quervain's disease: Role of conservative management. Journal of Hand Surgury (Br) 26(3):258-260.

Lee MP, Nasser-Sharif S, Zelouf DS (2002). Surgeon's and therapist's management of tendonopathies in the hand and wrist. In EJ Mackin, AD Callahan, TM Skirven, LH Schneider, AL Osterman (eds.), *Rehabilitation of the Hand and Upper Extremity, Fifth Edition.* St. Louis: Mosby, pp. 931-953.

Marx H (1992). Rheumatoid arthritis. In BG Stanley, SM Tribuzi (eds.), *Concepts in Hand Rehabilitation*. Philadelphia: F. A. Davis, pp. 395-418.

McCarroll JR (2001). Overuse injuries of the upper extremity in golf. Clinics in Sports Medicine 20(3):469-479.

McKee P, Morgan L (1998). *Orthotics and Rehabilitation: Splinting the Hand and Body*. Philadelphia: F. A. Davis.

Melvin JL (1989). *Rheumatic Disease in the Adult and Child, Third Edition*. Philadelphia: F. A. Davis.

Melvin JL (2002). Therapist's management of osteoarthritis in the hand. In EJ Mackin, AD Callahan, TM Skirven, LH Schneider, AL Osterman and JM Hunter (Eds). Rehabilitation of the hand and upper extremity, Fifth Edition. St. Louis: Mosby, 99. 1646-1663.

Moulton MJ, Parentis MA, Kelly MJ, Jacobs C, Naidu SH, Pellegrini VD Jr. (2001). Influence of metacarpophalangeal joint position on basal joint-loading in the thumb. Journal of Bone and Joint Surgery 83-A(5):709-716.

Nalebuff EA (1968). Diagnosis, classification and management of rheumatoid thumb deformities. Bulletin of the Hospital for Joint Diseases 2:119-137.

Neumann DA, Bielefeld T (2003). The carpometacarpal joint of the thumb: Stability, deformity, and therapeutic intervention. Journal of Orthopaedic & Sports Physical Therapy 33(7):386-399.

Ouellette E (1991). The rheumatoid hand: orthotics as preventive. Seminars in Arthritis and Rheumatism 21(2):65-72.

Poole JU, Pellegrini VD Jr. (2000). Arthritis of the thumb basal joint complex. Journal of Hand Therapy 13(2):91-107.

Rettig AC (2001). Wrist and hand overuse syndromes. Clinics in Sports Medicine 20(3):591-611.

Rettig ME, Dassa GL, Raskin KB, Melone CP Jr. (1998). Wrist fractures in the athlete: Distal radius and carpal fractures. Clinics in Sports Medicine 17(3):469-489.

Riester JN, Baker BE, Mosher JF, Lowe D (1985). A review of scaphoid fracture healing in competitive athletes. American Journal of Sports Medicine 13(3):159-161.

Swigart CR, Eaton RG, Glickel SZ, Johnson C (1999). Splinting in the treatment of arthritis of the first carpometacarpal joint. Journal of Hand Surgery 24A(1):86-91.

Tenney CG, Lisak JM (1986). *Atlas of Hand Splinting*. Boston/Toronto: Little, Brown & Co.

Tubiana R, Thomine JM, Mackin E (1996). *Examination of the Hand and Wrist*. St. Louis: Mosby.

Weiss AP, Akelman E, Tabatabai M (1994). Treatment of de Quervain's disease. Journal of Hand Surgery 19A(4):595-598.

Weiss S, LaStayo P, Mills A, Bramlet D (2000). Prospective analysis of splinting the first carpometacarpal joint: An objective, subjective and radiographic assessment. Journal of Hand Therapy 13(3):218-226.

Werner SL, Plancher KD (1998). Biomechanics of wrist injuries in sports. Clinics in Sports Medicine 17(3):407-420.

Wilton JC (1997). *Hand Splinting: Principles of Design and Fabrication*. London: W. B. Saunders.

Winzeler S, Rosenstein BD (1996). Occupational injury and illness of the thumb. American Association of Occupational Health Nurses Journal 44(10):487-492.

Witt J, Pess G, Gelberman RH (1991). Treatment of de Quervain tenosynovitis: A prospective study of the results of injection of steroids and immobilization in a splint. Journal of Bone and Joint Surgery 73-A(2):219-222.

Wright HH, Rettig AC (1995). Management of common sports injuries. In JM Hunter, EJ Mackin, AD Callahan (eds.), *Rehabilitation of the Hand, Fourth Edition*. St. Louis: Mosby, pp. 1809-1838.

Zelouf DS, Posner MA (1995). Hand and wrist disorders: How to manage pain and improve function. Geriatrics 50(3):22-26, 29-31.

Zeman C, Hunter RE, Freeman JR, Purnell ML, Mastrangelo J (1998). Acute skier's thumb repaired with a proximal phalanx suture anchor. American Journal of Sports Medicine 26(5):644-650.

CHAPTER 9

Hand Immobilization Splints

Brenda M. Coppard, PhD, OTR/L

Key Terms

Dupuytren's contracture
Complex regional pain syndrome
Functional position
Antideformity position

Chapter Objectives

1. List diagnoses that benefit from resting hand splints (hand immobilization splints).
2. Describe the functional or mid-joint position of the wrist, thumb, and digits.
3. Describe the antideformity or intrinsic-plus position of the wrist, thumb, and digits.
4. List the purposes of a resting hand splint (hand immobilization splint).
5. Identify the components of a resting hand splint (hand immobilization splint).
6. Explain the precautions to consider when fabricating a resting hand splint (hand immobilization splint).
7. Determine a resting hand (hand immobilization) splint-wearing schedule for different diagnostic indications.
8. Describe splint-cleaning techniques that address infection control.
9. Apply knowledge about the application of the resting hand splint (hand immobilization splint) to a case study.
10. Use clinical judgment to evaluate a fabricated resting hand splint (hand immobilization splint).

Physicians commonly order resting hand splints, also known as hand immobilization splints [American Society of Hand Therapists 1992] or resting pan splints. A resting hand splint is a static splint that immobilizes the fingers and wrist. The thumb may or may not be immobilized by the splint. Therapists fabricate custom resting hand splints or purchase them commercially. Some of the commercially sold resting hand splints are prefabricated, premolded, and ready to wear. Table 9-1 outlines prefabricated splints for the wrist and hand. Others are sold as *precut* resting hand splint kits that include the precut thermoplastic material and strapping mechanism. Each of these splints has advantages and disadvantages.

Premolded Hand Splints

Therapists can order premolded commercial splints according to hand size (i.e., small, medium, large, and extra large) for the right or left hand. An advantage of premade splints is their quick application (usually only straps require application). There is an advantage to ordering a premolded resting hand splint made from perforated material. The premolded splint has perforations only in the body of the splint. The edges are smooth because there are no perforations near the edges of the splint. However, if the perforated premolded or precut splint must be trimmed through the perforations a rough edge may result. Perforations at the edges of splints are undesirable because of the discomfort they often create.

Another disadvantage is that the commercial splint may not exactly fit each person. With premolded splints, the therapist has little control over positioning joints into particular therapeutic angles—which may be different from the angles already incorporated into the splint's design. The splints must be ordered for application on the right or left extremity, whereas the precut splint is universal for the right or left hand.

Precut Splint Kits

A resting hand splint kit typically contains strapping materials and precut thermoplastic material in the shape of a resting hand splint. Kits are available according to hand size (i.e., small, medium, large, and extra large). An advantage of

Table 9-1 Wrist/Hand Splint Examples

THERAPEUTIC OBJECTIVE	DESCRIPTION	
Resting hand splints immobilize the wrist, thumb, and metacarpophalangeal (MCP) joints to provide rest and reduce inflammation. The proximal interphalangeal (PIP) and distal interphalangeal (DIP) joints are free to move for functional tasks.	Similar to the resting hand splint design, splints can provide rest to the wrist, thumb, and MCP joints (Figure 9-1). Padding and strapping systems can help control deviation of the wrist and MCPs. Splints are available in different sizes for the right and left hands.	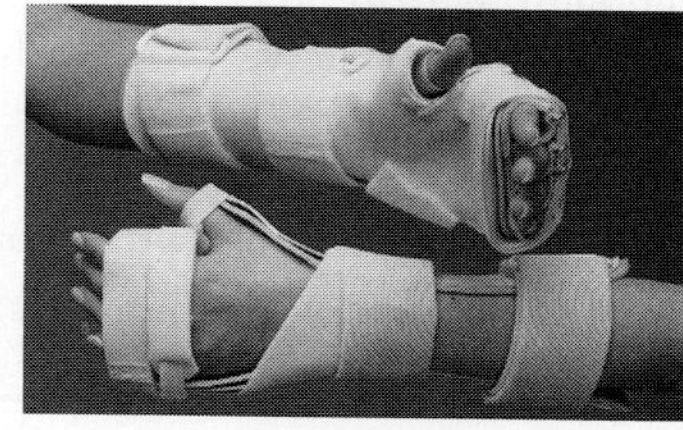 **Figure 9-1** This splint is based on a resting hand splint design and is often used for individuals with rheumatoid arthritis. *(Rolyan Arthritis Mitt splint; courtesy Rehabilitation Division of Smith & Nephew, Germantown, Wisconsin.)*
Design to optimally position the hand in an intrinsic-plus position after a burn injury.	Burn resting hand splints typically position the wrist in 20 to 30 degrees of extension, the MCP joints in 60 to 80 degrees of flexion, the PIP and DIP joints in full extension, and the thumb midway between radial and palmar abduction (Figure 9-2). 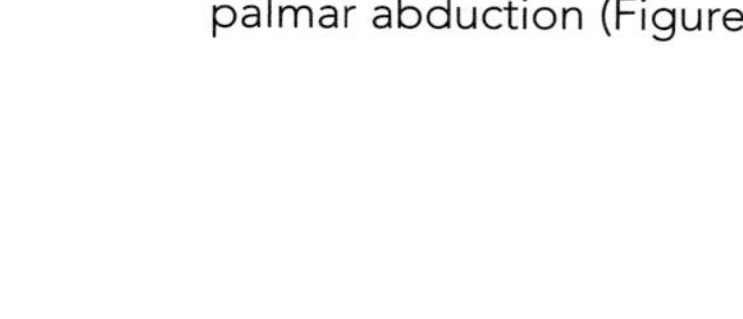	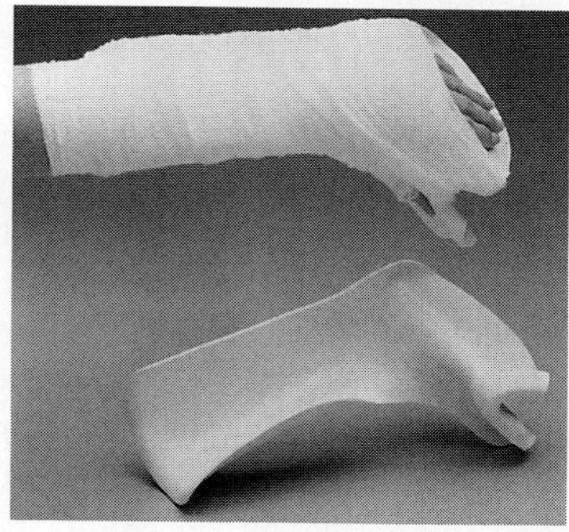 **Figure 9-2** This resting hand splint positions the hand in an antideformity position for individuals with hand burns. *(Rolyan Burn splint; courtesy Rehabilitation Division of Smith & Nephew, Germantown, Wisconsin.)*
Several splints are designed to reduce spasticity.	Ball splints implement a reflex-inhibiting posture by positioning the wrist in neutral (or slight extension) and the fingers in extension and abduction. Cone splints combine a hand cone and a forearm trough, which maintains the wrist in neutral, inhibits the long finger flexors, and maintains the web space (Figure 9-3). A resting hand splint positioning the hand in a functional position is also advocated for spasticity (Figure 9-4).	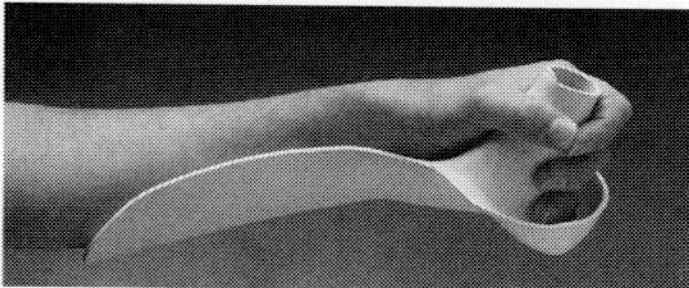 **Figure 9-3** This cone splint is often used to help manage tone abnormalities. *(Preformed Anti-Spasticity Hand Splint; courtesy North Coast Medical, Inc., Morgan Hill, California.)* 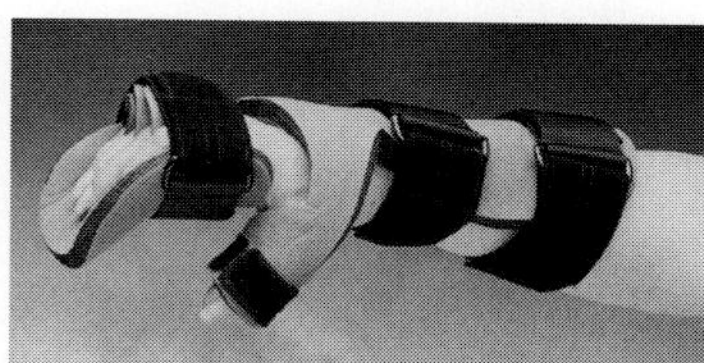 **Figure 9-4** This resting hand splint is fabricated of soft materials and includes a dorsal forearm base design. *(Progress Dorsal Anti-Spasticity splint; courtesy North Coast Medical, Inc., Morgan Hill, California.)*

using a kit is the time the therapist saves by elimination of pattern making and cutting of thermoplastic material. Similar to premolded splints, precuts from perforated materials contain perforations in only the body of the splint. Precuts are interchangeable for right or left extremity application. The therapist has control over joint positioning. A disadvantage is that the pattern is not customized to the person. Therefore, the precut splint may require many adjustments to obtain a proper fit.

Customized Splints

A therapist can customize a resting hand splint by making a pattern and fabricating the splint from thermoplastic material. The advantage is an exact fit for the person, which increases the splint's support and comfort. The therapist also has control over joint positioning. A disadvantage is that customization may require more of the therapist's time to complete the splint and may be more costly. In addition, when a resting hand splint pattern is cut out of perforated thermoplastic material it is difficult to obtain smooth edges because of the likelihood of needing to cut through the perforations (which causes a rough edge). Commercially available products such as the Rolyan Aquaplast UltraThin Edging Material can be applied over the rough edges to help create a smooth-edged reinforcement on splints fabricated from Aquaplast materials [Sammons Preston Rolyan 2005].

Therapists must make informed decisions about whether they will fabricate or purchase a splint. Many products are advertised to save time and to be effective, but few studies compare splinting materials when used by therapists with the same level of experience [Lau 1998]. Lau [1998] compared the fabrication of a resting hand splint with use of a precut splint, the QuickCast (fiberglass material) with Ezeform thermoplastic material. The study employed second-year occupational therapy students as splintmakers and first-year occupational therapy students as their clients.

The clients responded to a questionnaire addressing comfort, weight, and aesthetics. The splintmakers also responded to a questionnaire asking about measuring fit, edges, strap application, aesthetics, safety, and ease of positioning. The analysis of timed trials revealed no significant difference in time required for fabricating the precut QuickCast and the Ezeform thermoplastic material. The thermoplastic material was rated safer than the fiberglass material. Because of the small sample, these results should be cautiously interpreted—and further studies are warranted.

Purpose of the Resting Hand Splint

The resting hand splint has three purposes: to immobilize, to position in functional alignment, and to retard further deformity [Malick 1972, Ziegler 1984]. When inflammation and pain are present in the hand, the joints and surrounding structures become swollen and result in improper hand alignment. The resting hand splint may retard further deformity for some persons. The therapist may provide a splint for a person with arthritis who has early signs of ulnar drift by placing the hand in a comfortable neutral position with the joints in mid-position. Rest through immobilization reduces symptoms. Joints that are receptive to proper positioning may allow for optimal maintenance of range of motion (ROM) [Ziegler 1984].

The therapist must know the splint's components to make adjustments for a correct fit. Four main components comprise the resting hand splint: the forearm trough, the pan, the thumb trough, and the C bar (Figure 9-5) [Fess et al. 2005].

Forearm troughs can be volarly or dorsally based. The volarly based forearm trough at the proximal portion of the splint supports the weight of the forearm. Dorsally based forearm troughs are located on the dorsum of the forearm. The therapist should apply biomechanical principles to make the trough about two-thirds the length of the forearm to distribute pressure of the hand and to allow elbow flexion when appropriate. The width should be one-half the circumference

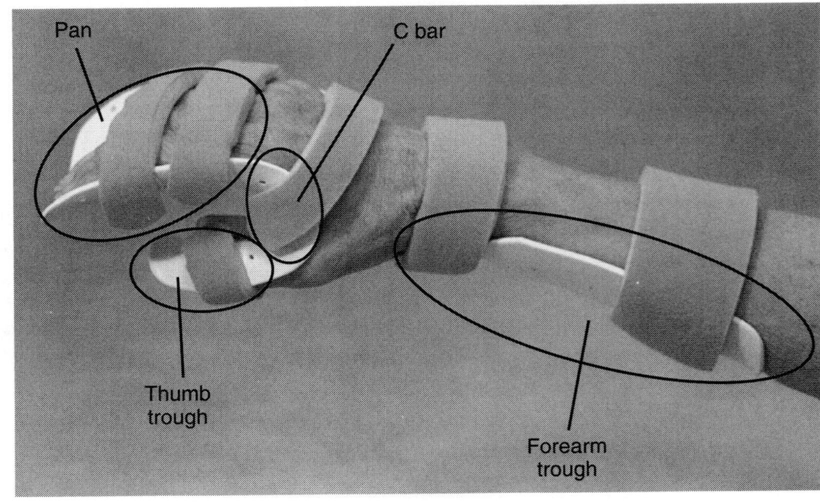

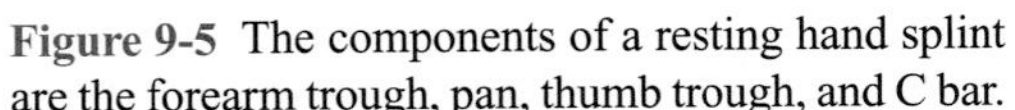
Figure 9-5 The components of a resting hand splint are the forearm trough, pan, thumb trough, and C bar.

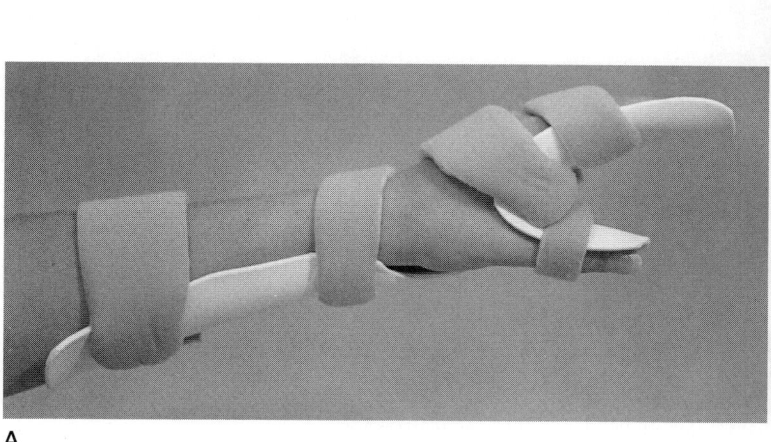

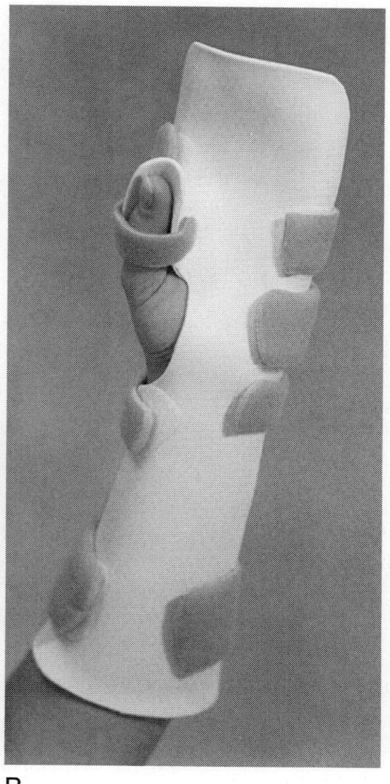

Figure 9-6 Volar-based resting hand splint: (A) side view, (B) volar view.

of the forearm. The proximal end of the trough should be flared or rolled to avoid a pressure area.

When a great amount of forearm support is desired, a volarly based forearm trough is the best design (Figure 9-6). When the volar surface of the forearm must be avoided because of sutures, sores, rashes, or intravenous needles, a dorsally based forearm trough design is frequently used (Figure 9-7). Dorsally based troughs can be a helpful design for applying a resting hand splint to a person with hypertonicity. The forearm trough can be used as a lever to extend the wrist in addition to extending the fingers.

The pan of the splint supports the fingers and the palm. The therapist conforms the pan to the arches of the hand, thus helping to maintain such hand functions as grasping and cupping motions. The pan should be wide enough to house the width of the index, middle, ring, and little fingers when they are in a slightly abducted position. The sides of the pan should be curved so that they measure approximately ½ inch in height. The curved sides add strength to the pan and ensure that the fingers do not slide radially or ulnarly off the sides of the pan. However, if the pan's edges are too high the positioning strap bridges over the fingers and fails to anchor them properly.

The thumb trough supports the thumb and should extend approximately ½ inch beyond the end of the thumb. This extension allows the entire thumb to rest in the trough. The width and depth of the thumb trough should be one-half the circumference of the thumb, which typically should be in a palmarly abducted position. The therapist should attempt to position the carpometacarpal (CMC) joint in 40 to 45 degrees of palmar abduction [Tenney and Lisak 1986] and extend the thumb's interphalangeal (IP) and metacarpal joints.

The C bar keeps the web space of the thumb positioned in palmar abduction. If the web space tightens, it inhibits cylindrical grasp and prevents the thumb from fully opposing the other digits. From the radial side of the splint, the thumb, the web space, and the digits should resemble a C (see Figure 9-6).

Resting Hand Splint Positioning

Generally, two types of positioning are accomplished by a resting hand splint: a functional (mid-joint) position and an antideformity (intrinsic-plus) position. Diagnostic indication determines the general position used.

Functional Position

To rest the wrist and hand joints, the resting hand splint positions the hand in a functional or mid-joint position [Colditz 1995] (Figure 9-8). According to Lau [1998, p. 47], "The exact specifications of the functional position of the hand in a resting hand splint and the recommended joint positions vary." One functional position that we suggest places the wrist in 20 to 30 degrees of extension, the thumb

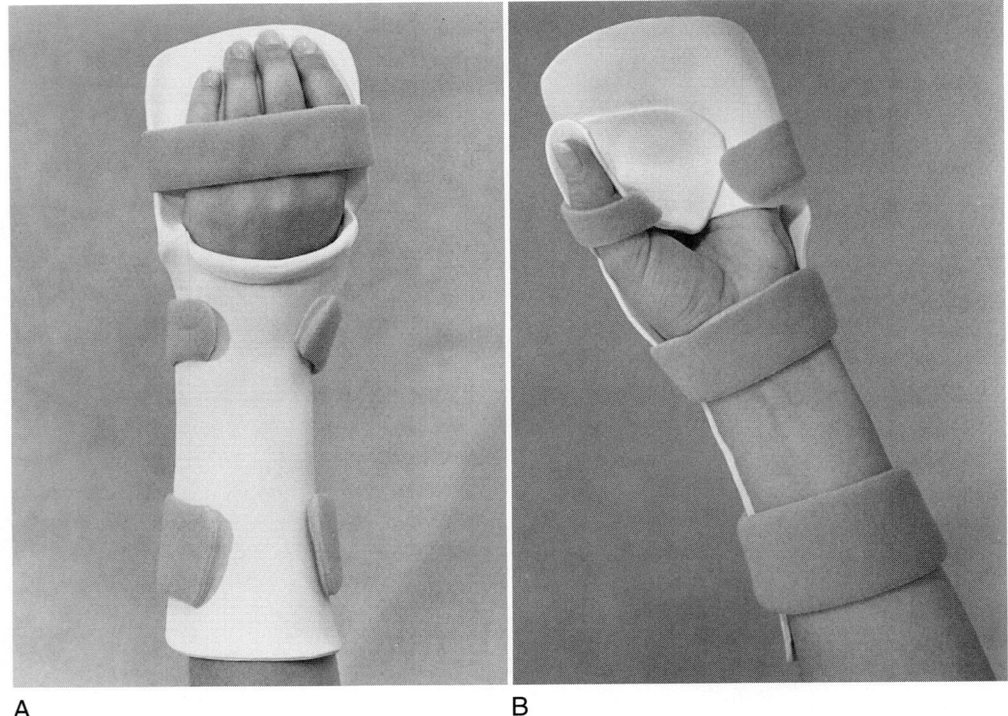

Figure 9-7 Dorsal-based resting hand splint: (A) dorsal view, (B) volar view.

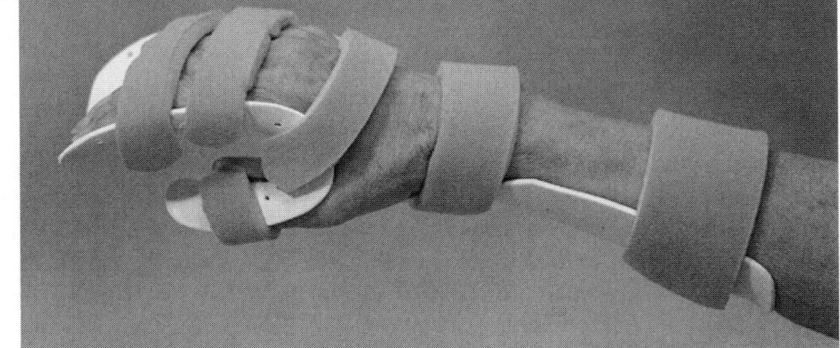

Figure 9-8 A resting hand splint with the hand in a functional (mid-joint) position.

in 45 degrees of palmar abduction, the metacarpophalangeal (MCP) joints in 35 to 45 degrees of flexion, and all proximal interphalangeal (PIP) and distal interphalangeal (DIP) joints in slight flexion.

Antideformity Position

The antideformity position is often used to place the hand in such a fashion as to maintain a tension/distraction of anatomic structures to avoid contracture and promote function. The antideformity position places the wrist in 30 to 40 degrees of extension, the thumb in 40 to 45 degrees of palmar abduction, the thumb IP joint in full extension, the MCPs at 70 to 90 degrees of flexion, and the PIPs and DIPs in full extension (Figure 9-9).

Diagnostic Indications

Several diagnostic categories may warrant the provision of a resting hand splint. Persons who require resting hand splints commonly have arthritis [Egan et al. 2001, Ouellette 1991]; postoperative Dupuytren's contracture release [Prosser and Conolly 1996]; burn injuries to the hand, tendinitis, hemiplegic hand [Pizzi et al. 2005]; and tenosynovitis [Richard et al. 1994].

The resting hand splint maintains the hand in a functional or antideformity position, preserves a balance between extrinsic and intrinsic muscles, and provides localized rest to the tissues of the fingers, thumb, and wrist [Tenney and Lisak 1986]. Although hand immobilization splints are commonly used, a paucity of literature exists on their efficacy.

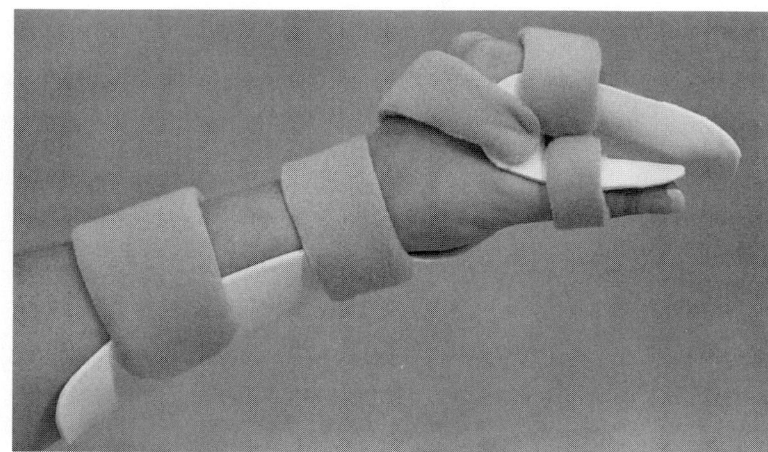

Figure 9-9 A resting hand splint with the hand in an antideformity (intrinsic-plus) position.

Thus, it is a ripe area for future research. Therapists should consider the resting hand splint as a legitimate intervention for appropriate conditions despite the lack of evidence.

Rheumatoid Arthritis

Therapists often provide resting hand splints for people with rheumatoid arthritis (RA) during periods of acute inflammation and pain [Biese 2002, Ziegler 1984] and when these people do not use their hands for activities but require support and immobilization [Leonard 1990]. The biomechanical rationale for splinting acutely inflamed joints is to reduce pain by relieving stress and muscle spasms. However, it may not additionally prevent deformity [Biese 2002, Falconer 1991].

Typical joint placement for splinting a person with RA positions the wrist in 10 degrees of extension, the thumb in palmar abduction, the MCP joints in 35 to 45 degrees of flexion, and all the PIP and DIP joints in slight flexion [Melvin 1989]. For a person who has severe deformities or exacerbations from arthritis, the resting hand splint may also position the wrist at neutral or slight extension and 5 to 10 degrees of ulnar deviation [Geisser 1984, Marx 1992]. The thumb may be positioned midway between radial and palmar abduction to increase comfort. These joint angles are ideal. Therapists use clinical judgment to determine what joint angles are positions of comfort for splinting.

Note that wrist extension varies from the typical 30 degrees of extension. When the wrist is in slight extension, the carpal tunnel is open—as opposed to being narrowed, with 30 degrees of extension [Melvin 1989]. Finger spacers may be used in the pan to provide comfort and to prevent finger slippage in the splint [Melvin 1989]. Melvin [1989] cautions that finger spacers should not be used to passively correct ulnar deformity because of the risk for pressure areas. In addition, once the splint is removed there is no evidence that splint wear alters the deformity. However, it may prevent further deformity.

Acute Rheumatoid Arthritis

In persons who have RA, the use of splints for purposes of rest during pain and inflammation is controversial [Egan et al. 2001]. Periods of rest (three weeks or less) seem to be beneficial, but longer periods may cause loss of motion [Ouellette 1991]. Phillips [1995] recommended that persons with acute exacerbations wear splints full-time except for short periods of gentle ROM exercise and hygiene. Biese [2002] recommended that persons wear splints at night and part-time during the day. In addition, persons may find it beneficial to wear splints at night for several weeks after the acute inflammation subsides [Boozer 1993].

Chronic Rheumatoid Arthritis

When splinting a joint with chronic RA, the rationale is often based on biomechanical factors. According to Falconer [1991, p. 83], "Theoretically, by realigning and redistributing the damaging internal and external forces acting on the joint, the splint may help to prevent deformity...or improve joint function and functional use of the extremity." Therapists who splint persons with chronic RA should be aware that prolonged use of a resting hand splint may also be harmful [Falconer 1991]. Studies on animals indicate that immobilization leads to decreased bone mass and strength, degeneration of cartilage, increase in joint capsule adhesions, weakness in tendon and ligament strength, and muscle atrophy [Falconer 1991].

In addition to splint intervention, persons with RA benefit from a combination of management of inflammation, education in joint protection, muscle strengthening, ROM maintenance, and pain reduction [Falconer 1991, Philips 1995]. Persons in late stages of RA who have skeletal collapse and deformity may benefit from the support of a splint during activities and at nighttime [Biese 2002, Callinan and Mathiowetz 1996].

Compliance of persons with RA in wearing resting hand splints has been estimated at approximately 50%

[Feinberg 1992]. The degree to which a person's compliance with a splint-wearing schedule affects the disease outcome is unknown. However, research indicates that some persons with RA who wore their splints only at times of symptom exacerbation did not demonstrate negative outcomes in relation to ROM or deformities [Feinberg 1992].

Hand Burns

For persons who have hand burns, therapists do not splint in the functional position. Instead, the therapist places the hand in the intrinsic-plus or antideformity position (see Figure 9-9). Richard et al. [1994] conducted an in-depth literature review to find a standard dorsal hand burn splint design. The literature cited 43 splints to position the dorsally burned hand joints. Twenty-six of these splints were labeled as antideformity splints and 17 were identified as having a position of function. Thus, a wide range of designs exists for splinting dorsal hand burns [Richard et al. 1994].

Positioning may vary, depending on the surface of the hand that is burned. In general, the goal of splinting in the antideformity position is to prevent deformity by keeping structures whose length allows motion from shortening. These structures are the collateral ligaments of the MCPs, the volar plates of the IPs, and the wrist capsule and ligaments. The dorsal skin of the hand will maintain its length in the antideformity position. The thumb web space is also vulnerable to remodeling in a shortened form in the presence of inflammation and in a situation in which tension of the structure is absent.

The antideformity position for a palmar or circumferential burn places the wrist in 30 to 40 degrees of extension and 0 degrees (i.e., neutral) for a dorsal hand burn. For dorsal and volar burns, the therapist should flex the MCPs into 70 to 90 degrees, fully extend the PIP joints and DIP joints, and palmarly abduct the thumb to the index and middle fingers with the thumb IP joint extended [Salisbury et al. 1990]. After a burn injury, the thumb web space is at risk for developing an adduction contracture [Torres-Gray et al. 1996]. Therefore, palmar abduction of the thumb is the position of choice for the thumb CMC joint.

These joint angles are ideal. Some persons with burns may not initially tolerate these joint positions. When tolerable, the resting hand splint for the person who has hand burns can be adjusted more closely to the ideal position. Stages of burn recovery should be considered with splinting. The phases of recovery are emergent, acute, skin grafting, and rehabilitation.

Emergent Phase

The emergent phase is the first 48 to 72 postburn hours [deLinde and Miles 1995]. During this time frame, dorsal edema occurs and encourages wrist flexion, MCP joint hyperextension, and IP joint flexion [deLinde and Miles 1995]. Static splinting is initiated during the emergent phase to support the hand and maintain the length of vulnerable structures [deLinde and Miles 1995]. Positioning to counteract the forces of edema includes placing the wrist in 15 to 20 degrees of extension, the MCP joints in 60 to 70 degrees of flexion, and the PIP and DIP joints in full extension, with the thumb positioned midway between palmar and radial abduction and with the IP joint slightly flexed [deLinde and Miles 1995].

For children with dorsal hand burns, during the emergent phase the MCP joints may not need to be flexed as far as 60 to 70 degrees. deLinde and Knothe [2002] suggested that for children under the age of three therapists may not need to splint unless it is determined that the wrist requires support. If a child is age three or older, splinting should be considered. Young children who have burned hands may not need splints because the bulky dressings applied to the burned hand may provide adequate support.

A prefabricated resting hand splint in an antideformity position can be applied if a therapist cannot immediately construct a custom-made splint [deLinde and Miles 1995]. deLinde and Miles [1995] suggested that prefabricated splints may be appropriate for superficial burns with edema for the first three to five days. For full-thickness burns with excessive edema, custom-made splints are necessary [deLinde and Miles 1995]. A splint applied in the first 72 hours after a burn may not fit the person 2 hours after application because of the significant edema that usually follows a burn injury.

The therapist should closely monitor the person to make necessary adjustments to the splint. When fabricating a custom splint for a person with excessive edema, a therapist should avoid forcing wrist and hand joints into the *ideal* position and risking ischemia from damaged capillaries [deLinde and Miles 1995]. With edema reduction, serial splinting may be necessary as ROM is gained to splint toward the ideal position. Serial resting hand splints for persons with burns should conform to the person, rather than conforming the person to the splints [deLinde and Miles 1995].

Persons with hand burns have bandages covering burn sites. According to Richard et al. [1994, p. 370], "As layers of bandage around the hand increase, accommodation for the increased bandage thickness must be accounted for in the splint's design, if it is to fit correctly." To correct for bandage thickness on a resting hand splint, the bend corresponding to MCP flexion in the pan should be formed more proximally [Richard et al. 1994].

The initial splint provision for a person with hand burns should be applied with gauze rather than straps. This reduces the risk of compromising circulation. Splints on adults should be removed for exercise, hygiene, and appropriate functional tasks. For children, splints are removed for exercise, hygiene, and play activities [deLinde and Miles 1995].

Acute Phase

The acute phase begins after the emergent phase and lasts until wound closure [deLinde and Miles 1995]. Once edema begins to decrease, serial adjustments should be made to the splint. Therefore, it is advantageous to use thermoplastic material with memory properties. During the acute phase, therapists monitor the direction of deforming forces and make adjustments in the existing splint or design an additional splint to "orient the collagen being deposited during the early stages of wound healing as well as maintain joint alignment" [deLinde and Knothe 2002, p. 1502].

Healing wounds are also monitored, and splints are evaluated for fit and for correct donning and doffing. As ROM is improved, the person can decrease wearing of the splint during the day. If the person is unwilling or uncooperative in participating in self-care and supervised activities, the splint should be worn continuously to prevent contractures. It is important for persons to wear splints at nighttime.

Skin Graft Phase

Before a skin graft, it is crucial to obtain full ROM. After the skin graft, the site needs to be immobilized for about 5 days postoperatively [deLinde and Miles 1995]. Usually an antideformity position resting hand splint is appropriate. The splint may have to be applied in the operating room to ensure immobilization of the graft.

Rehabilitation Phase

The rehabilitation phase occurs after wound closure or graft adherence until scar maturation [deLinde and Miles 1995]. Throughout the person's rehabilitation after a burn, splints may be donned over an extremity covered with a pressure garment. Splints may also be used in conjunction with materials that manage scar formation, including silicone gel sheeting or elastomer/elastomer putty inserts. During the rehabilitation phase, static and dynamic splinting may be needed. Plaster or synthetic material casting may also be considered [deLinde and Knothe 2002].

Dupuytren's Disease

Dupuytren's disease is characterized by the formation of finger flexion contracture(s) with a thickened band of palmar fascia [McFarlane 1995]. Nodules develop in the distal palmar crease, usually in line with the finger(s). Slowly the condition matures into a longitudinal cord that is readily distinguishable from a tendon [McFarlane 1995] (Figure 9-10). In addition, pain and decreased ROM are the primary symptoms that often lead to impaired functional performance [Kaye 1994]. Dupuytren's contractures are common and often severe in persons of Northern European origin. However, this disorder is not uncommon in most ethnic groups [McFarlane 1995]. Epilepsy, diabetes mellitus, and chronic alcoholism are associated with Dupuytren's contracture [Kaye 1994, McFarlane 1995, Swedler et al. 1995].

When a Dupuytren's contracture is apparent, stretching or splinting joints in extension does not delay the progression of the contracture [McFarlane 1995]. Surgery is performed to correct joint contractures and to prevent recurrences of the disease. Although surgery does not cure the disease, it is often indicated in the presence of painful nodules; uncomfortable induration; and MCP, PIP, or DIP joint contractures [McFarlane and MacDermid 1995]. Surgical procedures to treat Dupuytren's disease include fasciotomy, regional fasciectomy, and dermofasciectomy [McFarlane and MacDermid 1995, Prosser and Conolly 1996]. The surgical sites may be closed by Z-plasty or skin graft, or they may be left open to heal spontaneously. This open wound is frequently called the *open palm technique*. Other surgical techniques associated with a fasciectomy include a PIP or DIP joint release and amputation [Prosser and Conolly 1996].

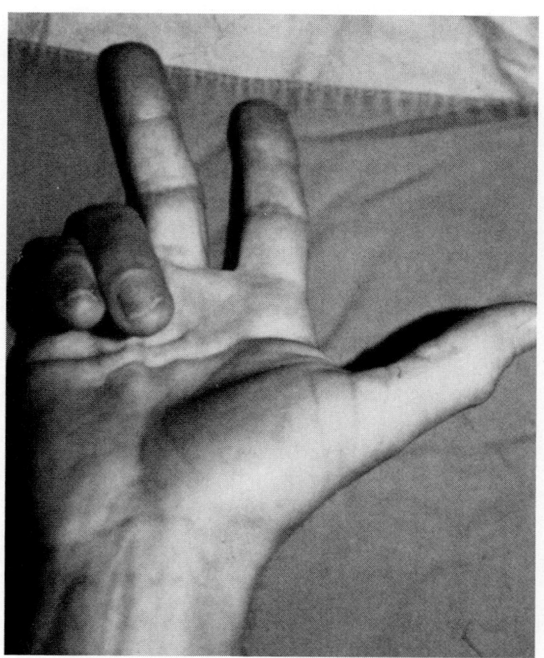

Figure 9-10 Dupuytren's contractures of ring and little fingers. [From Fietti VG, Mackin EJ (1995). Open-palm technique in Dupuytren's disease. In JM Hunter, EJ Mackin, AD Callahan (eds.), *Rehabilitation of the Hand, Fourth Edition*. St. Louis: Mosby, p. 996.]

The results of surgery may vary, depending on the affected joint [McFarlane 1995]. For example, the MCP joint has a single fascial cord that is relatively easy to release. The PIP joint has four fascial cords that are difficult to release. In addition, the soft tissue around the PIP joint may contract and pull the joint into flexion, and components of the extensor mechanism may adhere to surrounding structures. The PIP joint of the little finger is the most difficult to correct. Flexion contractures at the DIP joint are uncommon but are difficult to correct for the same reasons as the PIP joint contracture. Contractures of the web spaces may be present, limiting the motion of adjacent fingers. Web space contractures may also result in poor hygiene between the fingers.

Therapy and splinting begin immediately after surgery [McFarlane and MacDermid 1995]. Postoperative splinting

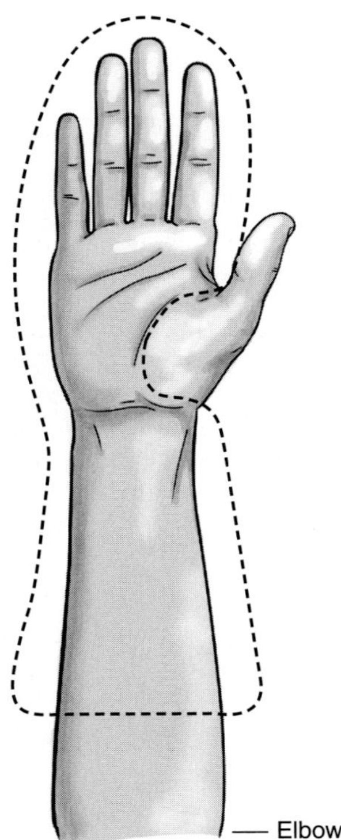

Figure 9-11 A pattern for a resting hand splint after surgical release of Dupuytren's contracture. Note that the thumb is not incorporated into the splint design.

may include a resting hand splint or a dorsal forearm-based static extension splint. Some therapists and physicians prefer a dorsal splint to reduce pressure over the surgical site. When a resting hand splint is used, the wrist is placed in a neutral or slightly flexed position [McFarlane and MacDermid 2002]. The MCP, PIP, and DIP joints are splinted in full extension. If the thumb is involved, it is incorporated into the splint. However, the uninvolved thumb usually does not need to be immobilized in the splint. Therefore, the splint will not have a thumb trough component (Figure 9-11). The thumb may be incorporated into the splint, particularly when the adjacent index finger has been released from a contracture.

Wearing schedules vary. The surgical procedure and the propensity of the person to lose ROM usually determine schedules. Persons should wear their splints until the wounds have healed, and longer if PIP joint contractures were corrected [McFarlane 1995]. Splints are removed for hygiene and exercise. Motion is initiated 1 to 2 days after surgery [McFarlane and MacDermid 1995], and the therapist focuses on regaining extension through the use of splinting and exercising. Exercise includes a tailored program of active and passive wrist, hand, and finger motions. McFarlane [1995] recommends that as long as composite finger flexion is possible when the splint is removed splint wear should continue. However, most persons eventually stop wearing their splints and accept some degree of PIP joint contracture. Removing the splint too soon without weaning the person from the splint typically results in loss of extension after surgery [McFarlane and McDermid 2002].

Therapists working with persons who undergo a Dupuytren's release must be aware of possible complications. Complications include excessive inflammation, wound infection, abnormal scar formation, joint contractures, stiffness, pain, and complex regional pain syndrome [Prosser and Conolly 1996].

Complex Regional Pain Syndrome (Reflex Sympathetic Dystrophy)

Complex regional pain syndrome (CRPS) is a chronic pain condition thought to be a result of impairment in the central or peripheral nerve systems. Outdated terms used to describe CRPS include reflex sympathetic dystrophy, causalgia, and shoulder-hand syndrome. Typical symptoms include [Koman et al. 2002] the following:

- *Pain:* Out of proportional intensity to the injury, burning, and skin sensitivity
- *Skin color changes:* Blotchy, purple, pale, or red
- *Skin temperature changes:* Warmer or cooler compared to contralateral side
- *Skin texture changes:* Thin, shiny, and sometimes excessively sweaty
- Swelling and stiffness
- Decreased ability to move the affected body part

There are two types of CRPS. CRPS I is usually triggered by tissue injury. The term applies to all persons with the symptoms listed previously, but with no underlying peripheral nerve injury. CRPS II is associated with the symptoms in the presence of a peripheral nerve injury.

The goal of rehabilitation for persons with CRPS is to eliminate one of the three etiologic factors: pain, diathesis, and abnormal sympathetic reflex [Lankford 1995]. This is accomplished by minimizing ROM and strength losses, managing edema, and providing pain management so that the therapist is able to maximize function and provide activities of daily living (ADL) and instrumental activities of daily living training for independence. The physician may be able to intervene with medications and nerve blocks.

As part of a comprehensive therapy regimen for CRPS, a resting hand splint may initially provide rest to the hand, reduce pain, and relieve muscle spasm [Lankford 1995]. Splinting during the presence of CRPS should be of a low force that does not exacerbate the pain or irritate the tissues [Walsh and Muntzer 2002]. Walsh and Muntzer [2002] recommend that the resting hand splint position for the person be in 20 degrees of wrist extension, palmar abduction of the thumb, 70 degrees of MCP joint flexion, and 0 to 10 degrees of PIP joint extension. This is an ideal position, which persons with CRPS may not tolerate. Above all, therapists working with persons who have CRPS should avoid causing pain. Therefore, they should be splinted in a position of comfort. Splints other than a resting hand splint may also be appropriate for this diagnostic population. (See Chapter 7 for a discussion of wrist splinting for CRPS.)

Hand Crush Injury

To splint a crushed hand the therapist can position the wrist in 0 to 30 degrees of extension, the MCPs in 60 to 80 degrees of flexion, the PIPs and DIPs in full extension, and the thumb in palmar abduction and extension [Colditz 1995]. Splinting a crushed hand into this position provides rest to the injured tissue and decreases pain, edema, and inflammation [Stanley and Tribuzi 1992].

Other Conditions

Resting hand splints are appropriate "for protecting tendons, joints, capsular and ligamentous structures" [Leonard 1990, p. 909]. These diagnoses usually require the expertise of experienced therapists and may warrant different splints for daytime wear and resting hand splints for nighttime use. (See Chapter 13 for splint interventions for nerve injuries.)

Therapists sometimes use resting hand splints to treat persons who experience a stroke and who are at risk for developing contractures because of increased tone or spasticity [Malick 1972]. (See Chapter 14 for more information on splinting an extremity that has increased tone or spasticity.) Table 9-2 lists common hand conditions that may require a resting hand splint and includes information regarding suggested hand positioning and splint-wearing schedules. Beginning therapists should remember that these are general guidelines and physicians and experienced therapists may have their own specific protocols for splint positioning and wearing.

Splint-Wearing Schedule

Wearing schedules for resting hand splints vary depending on the diagnostic condition, splint purpose, and physician order (see Table 9-2). Persons with RA often wear resting hand splints at night. A person who has RA may also wear a resting hand splint during the day for additional rest but should remove the splint *at least* once each day for hygiene and appropriate exercises. A person who has bilateral hand splints may choose to wear alternate splints each night.

Persons commonly wear resting hand splints during the healing stages of burns. After wounds heal, persons may wear day splints with pressure garments or elastomer molds to increase ROM and to control scarring. In addition to daytime splints, it is important for the person to wear a resting hand splint at night to maintain maximum elongation of the healing skin and provide rest and functional alignment.

After a surgical release of a Dupuytren's contracture, the person should wear the splint continuously during both day and night—with removal for hygiene and exercise. The splint should be worn until the wounds have completely healed, and should be worn longer if there has been a PIP contracture release. As the risk of losing ROM dissipates, the person may be weaned from the splint until its use is finally discontinued.

Resting hand splints provided to persons with CRPS should initially be worn at all times, with removal for therapy, hygiene, and (if possible) ADLs. As pain reduction and motion improvement occur, the amount of time the person wears the splint is decreased.

Fabrication of a Resting Hand Splint

The first step in the fabrication of a resting hand splint is drawing a pattern similar to that shown in Figure 9-12. Beginning splintmakers may learn to fabricate splint patterns by following detailed written instructions and by looking at pictures of splint patterns. As beginners gain more experience, they will be able to easily draw splint patterns without having to follow detailed instructions or pictures. The following are the detailed steps for fabricating a resting hand splint.

1. Place the person's hand flat and palm down, with the fingers slightly abducted, on a paper towel. Trace the outline of the upper extremity from one side of the elbow to the other.
2. While the person's hand is on the piece of paper, mark the following areas: (1) the radial styloid *A* and the ulnar styloid *B*, (2) the carpometacarpal joint of the thumb *C*, (3) the apex of the thumb web space *D*, (4) the web space between the second and third digits *E*, and (5) the olecranon process of the elbow *F*.
3. Remove the person's hand from the piece of paper. Draw a line across, indicating two-thirds of the length of the forearm. Then label this line *G*. After doing this, extend line *G* about 1 to 1-½ inches beyond each side of the outline of the arm. Then mark an *H* about 1 inch from the outline to the radial side of *A*. Mark an *I* about 1 inch from the outline to the ulnar side of *B*.
4. Draw a dotted vertical line from the web space of the second and third digits (*E*) proximally down the palm about 3 inches. Draw a dotted horizontal line from the bottom of the thumb web space (*D*) toward the ulnar side of the hand until the line intersects the dotted vertical line. Mark a *J* at the intersection of these two dotted lines. Mark an *N* about 1 inch from the outline to the radial side of *D*.
5. Draw a solid vertical line from *J* toward the wrist. Then curve this line so that it meets *C* on the pattern (see Figure 9-12). This part of the pattern is known as the thumb trough. After reaching *C*, curve the line upward until it reaches halfway between *N* and *D*.
6. Mark a *K* about 1 inch to the radial side of the index finger's PIP joint. Mark an *L* 1 inch from the top of the outline of the middle finger. Mark an *M* about 1 inch to the ulnar side of the little finger's PIP joint.
7. Draw the line that ends to the side of *N* through *K* and extend the line upward and around the corner through *L*.

From *L*, round the corner to connect the line with *M* and then pass it through *I*. Continue drawing the line and connect it with the end of *G*. Connect the radial end of *G* to pass through *H*. From *H*, extend the line toward *C*. Curve the line so that it connects to *C* (see Figure 9-12).
8. Cut out the pattern. Cut the solid lines of the thumb trough also. Do not cut the dotted lines.
9. Place the pattern on the person in the appropriate joint placement. Check the length of the pan, thumb trough, and forearm trough. Assess the fit of the *C* bar by forming the paper towel in the thumb web space. Make necessary adjustments (e.g., additions, deletions) on the pattern.
10. With a pencil, trace the splint pattern onto the sheet of thermoplastic material.
11. Heat the thermoplastic material.
12. Cut the pattern out of the thermoplastic material and reheat. Before placing the material on the person, think about the strategy you will employ during the molding process.

Table 9-2 Conditions That Require a Resting Hand Splint

HAND CONDITION	SUGGESTED WEARING SCHEDULE	POSITION
Rheumatoid Arthritis		
Acute exacerbation*	Fitted to maintain as close to a functional (mid-joint) position as possible until exacerbation is over. Removed for hygiene and exercise purposes, and worn during the day and at nighttime as necessary. Finger deformities must be taken into consideration if present.	Wrist: neutral or 20 to 30 degrees of extension depending on person's tolerance, 15 to 20 degrees of metacarpophalangeal (MCP) flexion, and 5 to 10 degrees of ulnar deviation. Thumb: position of comfort in between radial and palmar abduction.
Hand Burns		
Dorsal or volar hand burns*	Generally, worn immediately after the burn injury. Continuously worn until healing begins, and removed for dressing changes, hygiene, and exercises.	Wrist: volar or circumferential burn (30 to 40 degrees of extension), dorsal burn (0 degrees = neutral). MCPs: flexion of 70 to 90 degrees. Proximal interphalangeal (PIP) and distal interphalangeal (DIP): full extension. Thumb: palmar abduction and extension.
Acute phase	Initially, worn at all times except for therapy. Monitor fit for fluctuations in bandage bulk and edema. As range of motion (ROM) improves, decrease wearing time to allow for participation in activities.	Splint as close to the previously indicated position as possible.
Skin graft phase	Worn after skin graft at all times for 5 days or with physician's order for removal.	Position as close to antideformity position as possible.
Rehabilitation phase	Splint worn during nighttime to maintain ROM. Splint wear should be limited during daytime to allow for participation in activities.	Position joints to oppose deforming forces.
Dupuytren's Disease		
Contractures*	Worn after surgery and removed for hygiene and exercise. Worn at nighttime.	Wrist: neutral or slight extension. MCP, PIP, and DIPs: full extension.
Trauma		
Crush injuries of the hand	Fitted after the injury to reduce pain and edema and to prevent shortening of critical tissue and contracture formation. Worn at nighttime, and possibly worn as necessary during painful periods.	Wrist: extension of 0 to 30 degrees. MCPs: of 60 to 80 degrees. PIP and DIPs: full extension. Thumb: palmar abduction and extension.
Complex regional pain syndrome	Splint is worn at all times, initially with removal for therapy, hygiene, and activities of daily living (if possible). Person should be weaned from splint with pain reduction and improved motion.	Splint in position of comfort with the ideal position being wrist: 20 degrees of extension, thumb in palmar abduction. MCPs: 70 degrees of flexion. PIPs: 0 to 10 degrees of extension.

*Diagnosis may require additional types of splinting.

13. Instruct the person to rest the elbow on the table. The arm should be vertical and the hand relaxed. Although some thermoplastic materials in the vertical position may stretch during the molding process, the vertical position allows the best control of the wrist position. Mold the plastic form onto the person's hand and make necessary adjustments. Cold water or vapocoolant spray can be used to hasten the cooling time. However, this is not appropriate for persons with open wounds such as burns.
14. Add straps to the pan, the thumb trough, and the forearm trough (Figure 9-13). One pan strap is located across the PIP joints; the other is just proximal to the MCP joints. The strap across the thumb lies proximal to the IP joint. The forearm has two straps: one courses across the wrist and one is located across the proximal forearm trough. (See also Laboratory Exercise 9-1.)

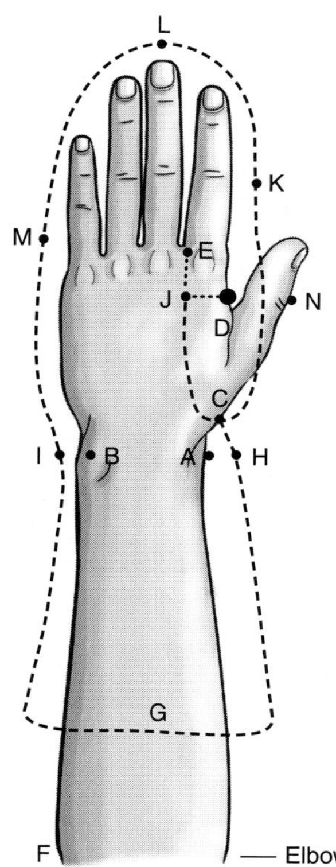

Figure 9-12 A detailed resting hand splint pattern.

Technical Tips for a Proper Fit

- For persons who have fleshier forearms, the splint pattern requires an allowance of more than 1 inch on each side. To be accurate, the therapist could measure the circumference of the person's forearm at several locations and make the splint pattern corresponding to the location of the measurements one-half of these measurements.
- Check pattern carefully to determine fit, particularly the length of the pan, thumb trough, and forearm trough and the conformity of the C bar. Moistening the paper towel pattern allows detailed assessment of pattern fit.
- Select a thermoplastic material with strength or rigidity. Avoid materials with excessive stretch characteristics. The splint material must be strong enough to support the entire hand, wrist, and forearm. A thermoplastic material with memory can be reheated several times and is beneficial if the splint requires serial adjustments. To make a splint more lightweight, select a thermoplastic material that is perforated or is thinner than 1/8 inch when splinting to manage conditions such as RA.
- Make sure the splint supports the wrist area well. If the thumb trough is cut beyond the radial styloid, the wrist support is compromised.

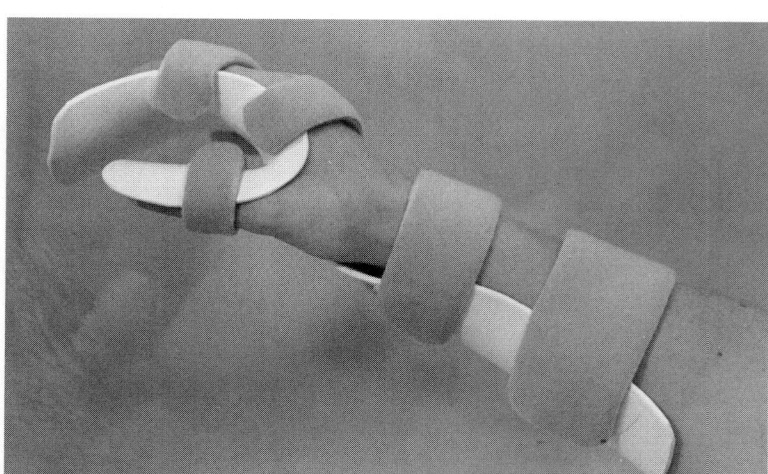
Figure 9-13 Strap placement for a resting hand splint.

Laboratory Exercise 9-1 Making a Hand Splint Pattern

1. Practice making a resting hand splint pattern on another person. Use the detailed instructions provided to draw the pattern. Cut out the pattern and make necessary adjustments.
2. Use the outline of the hands following to draw the resting hand splint pattern without using the detailed instructions.

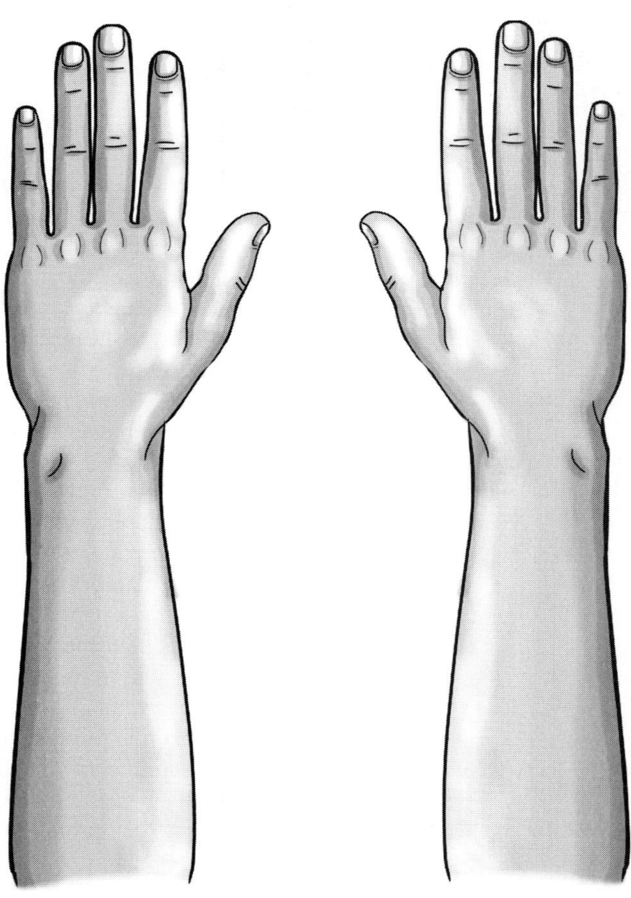

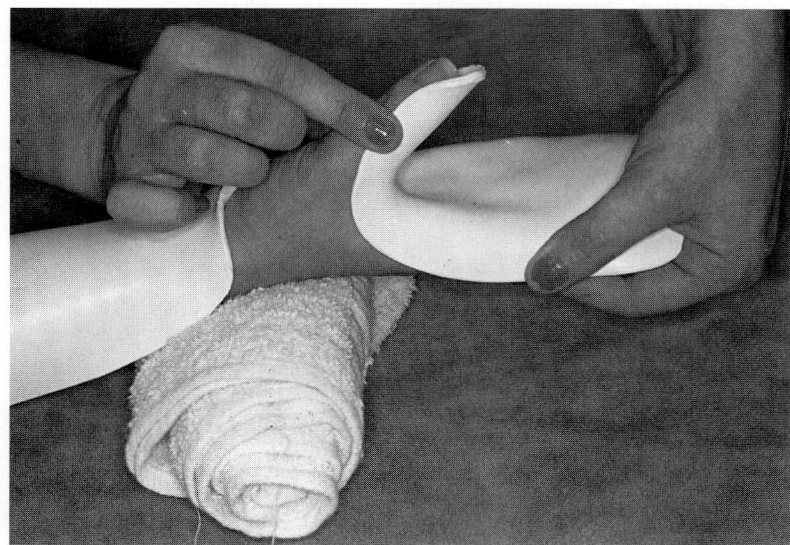

Figure 9-14 C bar conformity to the thumb web space on a resting hand splint.

- Measure the person's joints with a goniometer to ensure a correct therapeutic position before splinting. Be cautious of splinting the wrist in too much ulnar or radial deviation.
- When applying the straps, be sure the hand and forearm are securely fit into the splint. For maximal joint control, place straps across the PIPs, thumb IP, palm, wrist, and proximal forearm. Additional straps may be necessary, particularly for persons who have hypertonicity.
- Contour the splint's pan to the hand to preserve the hand's arches. The pan should be wide enough to comfortably support the width of the index, middle, ring, and little fingers.
- Make sure the C bar conforms to the thumb web space (Figure 9-14). The therapist may find it helpful to stretch the edge of the C bar and then conform it to the web space. Cut any extra material from the C bar as necessary.
- Verify that the thumb trough is long enough and wide enough. Stretch or trim the thumb trough as necessary.
- For fabrication of a dorsally based resting hand splint, the pattern remains the same—with the addition of a slit cut at the level of the MCP joints in the pan portion of the splint. The slit should begin and end about 1 inch from the ulnar and radial sides of the pan, as shown in Figure 9-15. When the splint is placed on the person, the person puts the hand through the slit in such a way so that the fingers rest on top of the pan portion and the forearm trough rests on the dorsal surface of the forearm. The edges of the slit require rolling or slight flaring away from the surface of the skin to prevent pressure areas. In addition, the thumb trough is a separate piece and must be attached to the pan and wrist portion of the splint. Thus, material with bonding or self-adherence characteristics is important. (See also Laboratory Exercise 9-2.)

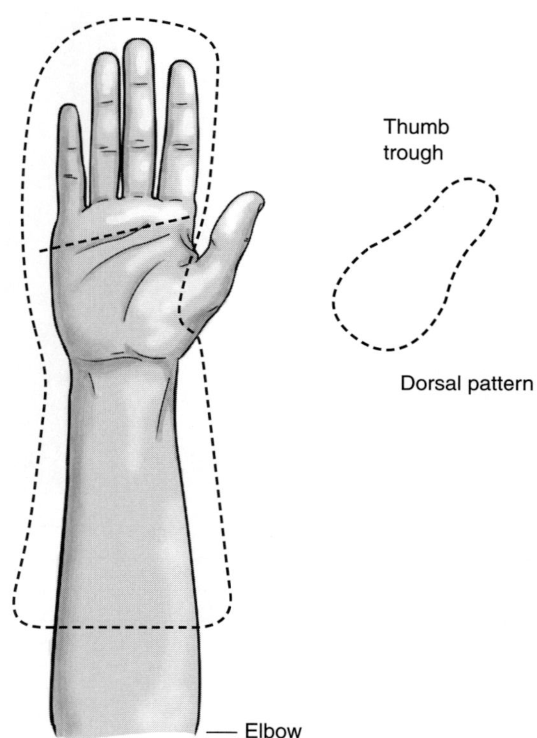

Figure 9-15 Pattern for a dorsal-based resting hand splint.

Precautions for a Resting Hand Splint

The therapist should take precautions when applying a splint to a person. If the diagnosis permits, the therapist should instruct the person to remove the splint for an ROM schedule to prevent stiffness and control edema.

- The therapist should monitor the person for pressure areas from the splint. With burns and other conditions resulting in open wounds, the therapist should make adjustments frequently as bandage bulk changes.

Laboratory Exercise 9-2* Identifying Problems with Splints

There are three persons who sustained burns on their hands. Their wounds have healed, and they must wear splints at night to prevent contractures. The therapist fabricated the following splints. Look at each picture and try to identify the problem with each.

1. What is the problem with this splint?

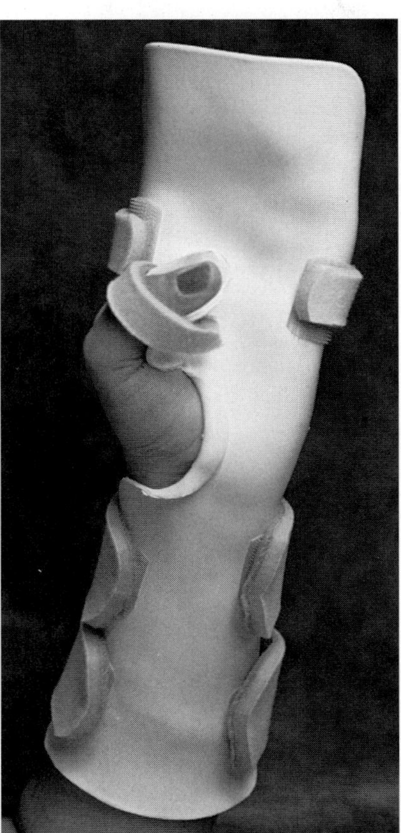

____

____

____

____

Continued

Laboratory Exercise 9-2 Identifying Problems with Splints—cont'd

2. What is the problem with this splint?

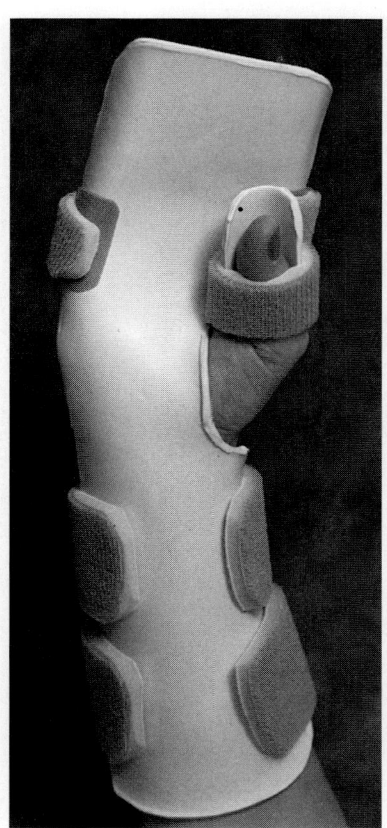

___

___

___

___

Laboratory Exercise 9-2 Identifying Problems with Splints—cont'd

3. What is the problem with this splint?

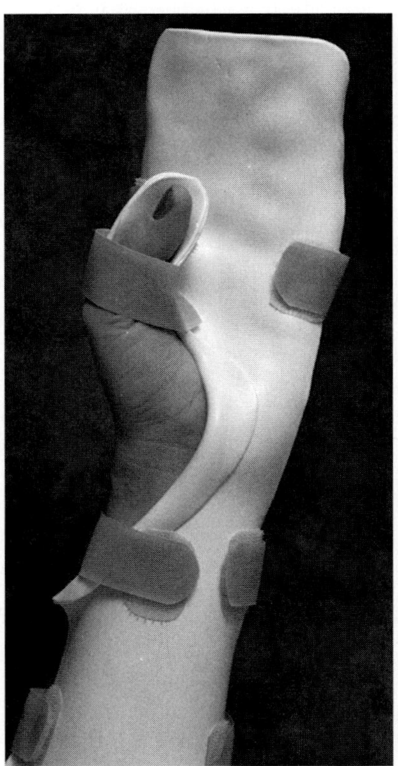

____

____

____

____

*See Appendix A for the answer key.

Box 9-1 Cleaning Techniques to Control Infection of Splints

During Splint Fabrication

1. After cutting pattern from the thermoplastic material, reimmerse the plastic in hot water.
2. Remove and spray with quaternary ammonia cleaning solution.
3. Place the splint between two clean cloths to maintain heat and reduce the microorganism contamination from handling the material.
4. Use gloves when molding the splint to the person. Latex gloves are recommended. Vinyl gloves adhere to the plastic.

Splint Donning in the Operating Room

Follow steps 1 through 4.

5. Clean splints after the fit evaluation is completed and place in a clean cloth during transportation.
6. Transport splint only when the person receiving the splint is in the operating room.
7. Keep splint in clean cloth until it is needed in the operating room. The splint in the cloth should be kept off of sterile surfaces in the operating room.
8. When the person leaves the operating room, all splints should be taken with him or her to the appropriate recovery room.

Data from Wright MP, Taddonio TE, Prasad JK, Thompson PD (1989). The microbiology and cleaning of thermoplastic splints in burn care. Journal of Burn Care & Rehabilitation 10(1):79-83.

- To prevent infection, the therapist must teach the person or caregiver to clean the splint when open wounds with exudate are present. After removing the splint, the person or caregiver can clean it with warm soapy water, hydrogen peroxide, or rubbing alcohol and dry it with a clean cloth (Box 9-1). Rubbing alcohol may be the most effective for removing skin cells, perspiration, dirt, and exudate.
- For a resting hand splint for a person in an intensive care unit (ICU), supplies and tools should be kept as sterile as possible. Careful planning about supply needs before going into the unit helps prevent repetitious trips. The splintmaker may enlist the help of a second person, aide, or therapist to assist with the splinting process. The therapist working in a sterile environment should follow the facility's protocol on universal precautions and body substance procedures. Prepackaged sterilized equipment can be used for splinting. Alternatively, any equipment that can withstand the heat from an autoclave can be used.
- Depending on facility regulations, various actions may be taken to ensure optimal wear and care of a splint. The therapist should consider hanging a wearing schedule in the person's room. This precaution is especially helpful if others are involved in applying and removing the splint. A photograph of the person wearing the splint posted in the room or in the person's care plan in the chart may help with correct splint application. The therapist should inform nursing staff members of the wearing schedule and care instruction.
- After splinting a person in the ICU, the therapist should follow up at least once after the splint's application regarding the fit and the person's tolerance of the splint. Splints on persons with burns require frequent adjustments. As the person recovers, the splint design may change several times.
- A person who has RA may benefit from a splint made from thinner thermoplastic (less than $^{1}/_{8}$ inch). This type of splint reduces the weight over affected joints [Melvin 1982].

Laboratory Exercise 9-3 Fabricating a Hand Splint

Practice fabricating a resting hand splint on a partner. Before starting, determine the position in which you should place your partner's hand. Use a goniometer to measure the angles of wrist extension, MCP flexion, and thumb palmar abduction to ensure a correct position. After fitting the splint and making all adjustments, use Form 9-1 as a self-evaluation check-off sheet. Use Grading Sheet 9-1 as a classroom grading sheet. (Grading Sheet 9-1 may also be used as a self-evaluation sheet.)

FORM 9-1* Resting Hand Splint

Name: ______________________

Date: ______________________

Position of resting hand splint:

Functional position ❍ (mid-joint)   Antideformity position ❍ (intrinsic plus)

Answer the following questions after the person wears the splint for 30 minutes. (Mark *NA* for nonapplicable situations.)

Evaluation Areas				**Comments**
Design				
1. The wrist position is at the correct angle.	Yes ❍	No ❍	NA ❍	
2. The MCPs are at the correct angle.	Yes ❍	No ❍	NA ❍	
3. The thumb is in the correct position.	Yes ❍	No ❍	NA ❍	
4. The wrist has adequate support.	Yes ❍	No ❍	NA ❍	
5. The pan is wide enough for all the fingers.	Yes ❍	No ❍	NA ❍	
6. The length of the pan and thumb trough is adequate.	Yes ❍	No ❍	NA ❍	
7. The splint is two-thirds the length of the forearm.	Yes ❍	No ❍	NA ❍	
8. The splint is half the width of the forearm.	Yes ❍	No ❍	NA ❍	
9. Arches of the hand are supported and maintained.	Yes ❍	No ❍	NA ❍	
Function				
1. The splint completely immobilizes the wrist, fingers, and thumb.	Yes ❍	No ❍	NA ❍	
2. The splint is easy to apply and remove.	Yes ❍	No ❍	NA ❍	
Straps				
1. The straps are rounded.	Yes ❍	No ❍	NA ❍	
2. Straps are placed to adequately secure the hand/arm to the splint.	Yes ❍	No ❍	NA ❍	
Comfort				
1. The edges are smooth with rounded corners.	Yes ❍	No ❍	NA ❍	
2. The proximal end is flared.	Yes ❍	No ❍	NA ❍	
3. The splint does not cause impingements or pressure areas.	Yes ❍	No ❍	NA ❍	
Cosmetic Appearance				
1. The splint is free of fingerprints, dirt, and pencil or pen marks.	Yes ❍	No ❍	NA ❍	
2. The splint is smooth and free of buckles.	Yes ❍	No ❍	NA ❍	
Therapeutic Regimen				
1. The person has been instructed in a wearing schedule.	Yes ❍	No ❍	NA ❍	
2. The person has been provided with splint precautions.	Yes ❍	No ❍	NA ❍	
3. The person demonstrates understanding of the education.	Yes ❍	No ❍	NA ❍	
4. Client/caregiver knows how to clean the splint.	Yes ❍	No ❍	NA ❍	

Continued

FORM 9-1 Resting Hand Splint—cont'd

Discuss adjustments or changes you would make based on the self-evaluation. What would you do differently next time?

____

____

____

____

____

____

____

____

*See Appendix B for a perforated copy of this form.

GRADING SHEET 9-1* Resting Hand Splint

Name: ______________________________

Date: ______________________________

Position of resting hand splint:

Functional position ❍ (mid-joint)   Antideformity position ❍ (intrinsic plus)

Grade: ______________

1 = beyond improvement, not acceptable
2 = requires maximal improvment
3 = requires moderate improvement
4 = requires minimal improvement
5 = requires no improvement

Evaluation Areas						**Comments**
Design						
1. The wrist position is at the correct angle.	1	2	3	4	5	
2. The MCPs are at the correct angle.	1	2	3	4	5	
3. The thumb is in the correct position.	1	2	3	4	5	
4. The wrist has adequate support.	1	2	3	4	5	
5. The pan is wide enough for all the fingers.	1	2	3	4	5	
6. The length of the pan and thumb trough is adequate.	1	2	3	4	5	
7. The splint is two-thirds the length of the forearm.	1	2	3	4	5	
8. The splint is half the width of the forearm.	1	2	3	4	5	
9. Arches of the hand are supported and maintained.	1	2	3	4	5	
Function						
1. The splint completely immobilizes the wrist, fingers, and thumb.	1	2	3	4	5	
2. The splint is easy to apply and remove.	1	2	3	4	5	
Straps						
1. The straps are rounded.	1	2	3	4	5	
2. Straps are placed to adequately secure the hand/arm to the splint.	1	2	3	4	5	
Comfort						
1. The edges are smooth with rounded corners.	1	2	3	4	5	
2. The proximal end is flared.	1	2	3	4	5	
3. The splint does not cause impingements or pressure areas.	1	2	3	4	5	
Cosmetic Appearance						
1. The splint is free of fingerprints, dirt, and pencil or pen marks.	1	2	3	4	5	
2. The splint is smooth and free of buckles.	1	2	3	4	5	

*See Appendix C for a perforated copy of this grading sheet.

CASE STUDY 9-1*

Read the following scenario and use your clinical reasoning skills to answer the questions based on information in this chapter.

Juan, a 39-year-old man with bilateral dorsal hand burns, has just been admitted to the ICU. Juan has second- and third-degree burns resulting from a torch exploding in his hands. He is receiving intravenous pain medication and is not alert. Approximately 14 hours have passed since his admission, and you have just received orders to fabricate bilateral hand splints.

1. Which type of splint is appropriate for dorsal hand burns?
   a. Bilateral resting hand splints with the hand in a functional (mid-joint) position
   b. Bilateral resting hand splints with the hand in an antideformity (intrinsic-plus) position
   c. Bilateral wrist cock-up splints
2. What is the appropriate wrist position?
   a. Neutral
   b. 30 degrees of flexion
   c. 30 degrees of extension
3. What is the appropriate MCP position?
   a. 70 to 90 degrees of extension
   b. 70 to 90 degrees of flexion
   c. Full extension
4. What is the appropriate thumb position?
   a. Radial abduction
   b. Palmar abduction
   c. Full flexion
5. Which of the following statements is false regarding the splint process for the previous scenario?
   a. The supplies should be sterile.
   b. An extremely stretchable material is necessary to fabricate the splints over the bandages.
   c. The therapist should give a splint-wearing schedule to the ICU nurse for inclusion in the treatment plan.

*See Appendix A for the answer key to this case study.

CASE STUDY 9-2*

Read the following scenario and use your clinical reasoning to answer the questions based on information from this chapter and previous chapters.

Shelly, a 45-year-old right-hand-dominant woman with diabetes mellitus and Dupuytren's disease, underwent an elective surgical procedure to release PIP flexion contractures in her right ring and little fingers. The physician used a Z-plasty open palm technique. Shelly returns from the surgical suite and you receive an order to "evaluate, treat, and splint." She is an accountant who is married with a 16-year-old son.

1. What diagnosis in Shelly's past medical history is associated with Dupuytren's disease?

2. What splint designs are appropriate for Shelly's condition?

3. What therapeutic position will be used in the splint design?

4. What wearing schedule will you give Shelly?

5. You notice that Shelly's bandage bulk is considerable. How will you design the splint to accommodate for bandage thickness? What type of thermoplastic material properties will you choose?

6. How frequently will Shelly require therapy?

7. What support systems may Shelly require for rehabilitation from this surgery?

*See Appendix A for the answer key to this case study.

REVIEW QUESTIONS

1. What are four common diagnostic conditions in which a therapist may provide a resting hand splint for intervention?
2. In what position should the therapist place the wrist, MCPs, and thumb for a functional resting hand splint?
3. For a resting hand splint, in what joint positions should a person with RA be placed?
4. When might a therapist choose to use a dorsally based resting hand splint rather than a volarly based splint?
5. In what position should the therapist place the wrist, MCPs, and thumb for an antideformity resting hand splint?
6. What are the three purposes for using a resting hand splint?
7. What are the four main components of a resting hand splint?
8. Which equipment must be sterile to make a resting hand splint in a burn unit?

References

American Society of Hand Therapists (1992). *Splint Classification System*. Garner, NC: American Society of Hand Therapists.

Biese J (2002). Therapist's evaluation and conservative management of rheumatoid arthritis in the hand and wrist. In EJ Mackin, AD Callahan, TM Skirven, LH Schneider, AL Osterman (eds.), *Rehabilitation of the Hand: Surgery and Therapy, Fifth Edition*. St. Louis: Mosby.

Boozer J (1993). Splinting the arthritic hand. Journal of Hand Therapy 6(1):46.

Callinan NJ, Mathiowetz V (1996). Soft versus hard resting hand splints in rheumatoid arthritis: Pain relief, preference and compliance. AJOT 50:347-353.

deLinde LG, Knothe B (2002). Therapist's management of the burned hand. In EJ Mackin, AD Callahan, TM Skirven, LH Schneider, AL Osterman (eds.), *Rehabilitation of the Hand: Surgery and Therapy, Fifth Edition*. St. Louis: Mosby.

deLinde LG, Miles WK (1995). Remodeling of scar tissue in the burned hand. In JM Hunter, EJ Mackin, AD Callahan (eds.), *Rehabilitation of the Hand: Surgery and Therapy, Fourth Edition*. St. Louis: Mosby.

Egan M, Brosseau L, Farmer M, Ouimet M, Rees S, Tugwell P, et al. (2001). Splints and orthoses for treating rheumatoid arthritis. Cochrane Database of Systematic Reviews, 4, Art. No. CD004018. DOI: 10.1002/14651858.CD004018.

Falconer J (1991). Hand splinting in rheumatoid arthritis. Journal of Hand Therapy 4(2):81-86.

Feinberg J (1992). Effect of the arthritis health professional on compliance with use of resting hand splints by persons with rheumatoid arthritis. Journal of Hand Therapy 5(1):17-23.

Fess EE, Philips CA (1987). *Hand Splinting Principles and Methods, Second Edition*. St. Louis: Mosby.

Geisser RW (1984). Splinting the rheumatoid arthritic hand. In EM Ziegler (ed.), *Current Concepts in Orthotics: A Diagnosis-related Approach to Splinting*. Germantown, WI: Rolyan Medical Products.

Kaye R (1994). Watching for and managing musculoskeletal problems in diabetes. The Journal of Musculoskeletal Medicine 11(9):25-37.

Koman LA, Smith BP, Smith TL (2002). Reflex sympathetic dystrophy (complex regional pain syndromes- types 1 and 2). In EJ Mackin, AD Callahan, TM Skirven, LH Schneider, AL Osterman (eds.), *Rehabilitation of the Hand: Surgery and Therapy, Fifth Edition*. St. Louis: Mosby.

Lankford LL (1995). Reflex sympathetic dystrophy. In JM Hunter, EJ Mackin, AD Callahan (eds.), *Rehabilitation of the Hand: Surgery and Therapy, Fourth Edition*. St. Louis: Mosby.

Lau C (1998). Comparison study of QuickCast versus a traditional thermoplastic in the fabrication of a resting hand splint. Journal of Hand Therapy 11:45-48.

Leonard J (1990). Joint protection for inflammatory disorders. In JM Hunter, LH Schneider, EJ Mackin, AD Callahan (eds.), *Rehabilitation of the Hand: Surgery and Therapy, Third Edition*. St. Louis: Mosby.

McFarlane RM (1995). The current status of Dupuytren's disease. Journal of Hand Therapy 8(3):181-184.

McFarlane RM, MacDermid JC (1995). Dupuytren's disease. In JM Hunter, EJ Mackin, AD Callahan (eds.), *Rehabilitation of the Hand: Surgery and Therapy, Fourth Edition*. St. Louis: Mosby.

McFarlane RM, MacDermid JC (2002). Dupuytren's disease. In EJ Mackin, AD Callahan, TM Skirven, LH Schneider, and AL Osterman (eds.), *Rehabilitation of the Hand: Surgery and Therapy, Fifth Edition*. St. Louis: Mosby.

Malick MH (1972). *Manual on Static Hand Splinting*. Pittsburgh: Hamarville Rehabilitation Center.

Marx H (1992). Rheumatoid arthritis. In BG Stanley, SM Tribuzi (eds.), *Concepts in Hand Rehabilitation*. Philadelphia: F. A. Davis.

Melvin JL (1982). *Rheumatic Disease: Occupational Therapy and Rehabilitation, Second Edition*. Philadelphia: F. A. Davis.

Melvin JL (1989). *Rheumatic Disease in the Adult and Child: Occupational Therapy and Rehabilitation*. Philadelphia: F. A. Davis.

Ouellette EA (1991). The rheumatoid hand: Orthotics as preventative. Seminars in Arthritis and Rheumatism 21:65-71.

Philips CA (1995). Therapist's management of persons with rheumatoid arthritis. In JM Hunter, EJ Mackin, AD Callahan (eds.), *Rehabilitation of the Hand: Surgery and Therapy, Fourth Edition*. St. Louis: Mosby.

Pizzi A, Carlucci G, Falsini C, Verdesca S, Grippo A (2005). Application of a volar static splinit in poststroke spasticity of the upper limb. Archives of Physical Medicine and Rehabilitation 86:1855-1859.

Prosser R, Conolly WB (1996). Complications following surgical treatment for Dupuytren's contracture. Journal of Hand Therapy 9(4):344-348.

Richard R, Schall S, Staley M, Miller S (1994a). Hand burn splint fabrication: Correction for bandage thickness. Journal of Burn Care and Rehabilitation 15(4):369-371.

Richard R, Staley M, Daugherty MB, Miller SF, Warden GD (1994b). The wide variety of designs for dorsal hand burn splints. Journal of Burn Care and Rehabilitation 15(3):275-280.

Salisbury RE, Reeves SU, Wright P (1990). Acute care and rehabilitation of the burned hand. In JM Hunter, LH Schneider, EJ Mackin, AD Callahan (eds.), *Rehabilitation of the Hand: Surgery and Therapy, Third Edition*. St. Louis: Mosby 831-840.

Sammons Preston Rolyan (SPR) (2005). Hand Rehab Catalog. Bolingbrook, IL: Sammons Preston Rolyan.

Stanley BG, Tribuzi SM (1992). *Concepts in Hand Rehabilitation*. Philadelphia: F. A. Davis.

Swedler WI, Baak S, Lazarevic MB, Skosey JL (1995). Rheumatic changes in diabetes: Shoulder, arm, and hand. The Journal of Musculoskeletal Medicine 12(8):45-52.

Tenney CG, Lisak JM (1986). *Atlas of Hand Splinting*. Boston: Little, Brown & Co.

Torres-Gray D, Johnson J, Mlakar J (1996). Rehabilitation of the burned hand: Questionnaire results. Journal of Burn Care and Rehabilitation 17(2):161-168.

Walsh MT, Muntzer E (2002). Therapist's management of complex regional pain syndrome (reflex sympathetic dystrophy). In EJ Mackin, AD Callahan, TM Skirven, LH Schneider, AL Osterman (eds.), *Rehabilitation of the Hand: Surgery and Therapy, Fifth Edition*. St. Louis: Mosby.

Ziegler EM. (1984). *Current Concepts in Orthotics: A Diagnostic-related Approach to Splinting*. Germantown, WI: Rolyan Medical Products.

CHAPTER 10

Elbow Immobilization Splints

Aviva Wolff, OTR/L, CHT

Key Terms

Olecranon process
Radial head
Medial and lateral epicondyle
Posterior elbow immobilization splint
Elbow arthroplasty
Elbow instability
Cubital tunnel syndrome

Chapter Objectives

1. Define anatomic and biomechanical considerations for splinting the elbow.
2. Discuss clinical/diagnostic indications for elbow immobilization splints.
3. Identify the components of elbow immobilization splints.
4. Describe the fabrication process for an anterior and posterior elbow splint.
5. Review precautions for elbow immobilization splinting.
6. Use clinical reasoning to evaluate a problematic elbow immobilization splint.
7. Use clinical reasoning to evaluate a fabricated elbow immobilization splint.
8. Apply knowledge about the application of elbow immobilization splints to a case study.

Anatomic and Biomechanical Considerations

The elbow joint consists of three bones: distal humerus, proximal ulna (olecranon process), and the head of the radius. The elbow joint is comprised of three complex articulations: ulna-humeral, radio-capitellar, and proximal radio-ulnar. Flexion and extension of the elbow occur at the ulnohumeral joint. Flexion, extension, and rotation occur at the radiohumeral joint. Forearm rotation occurs at the proximal and distal radioulnar joints along a longitudinal axis [Morrey 2000a].

The elbow is particularly prone to contracture and stiffness due to the high congruity, multiple articulations, and the close relationship of ligaments and muscle to the joint capsule [Hotchkiss 1996]. For this reason prolonged immobilization is to be avoided whenever possible. The bony prominences, lateral and medial epicondyle, radial and ulnar heads, and olecranon require protection and special consideration during splinting.

Clinical Indications and Common Diagnoses

Splints are commonly constructed for elbow fractures, elbow arthroplasty, elbow instability, biceps and triceps repair, and cubital tunnel syndrome (Table 10-1).

Splinting for Fractures

Elbow trauma can result in a simple one-bone fracture or a complex fracture/dislocation involving a combination of bones. These injuries vary by the bones and structures involved, and the extent of the injury. Elbow dislocations occur in isolation or along with a fracture. Both fractures and dislocations often include concomitant soft-tissue injury such as ligament, muscle, or nerve. Seven percent of all fractures are elbow fractures [Jupiter and Morrey 2000], and of this one-third involve the distal humerus. The mechanism of injury is a posterior force directed at the flexed elbow, often a fall to an outstretched hand, or axial loading of an extended elbow. Thirty-three percent of all elbow fractures occur in the radial head and neck by axial loading on a pronated forearm, with the elbow in more than 20 degrees of flexion [Morrey 2000c].

Radial head fractures are often associated with ligament injuries. Radial head fractures associated with interosseous membrane disruption and distal radial ulnar joint dislocation are termed Essex-Lopresti lesions. Twenty percent of elbow

Table 10-1 Conditions That Require an Elbow Immobilization Splint

CONDITION	SUGGESTED WEARING SCHEDULE	TYPE OF SPLINT AND POSITION
Elbow fractures	After removal of the postoperative dressing, the therapist fabricates an elbow immobilization splint. The splint is worn at all times, and removed for exercises and hygiene if permitted.	Posterior angle depends on which structures need to be protected.
Elbow arthroplasty	After removal of the postoperative dressing the therapist fabricates an elbow immobilization splint or fits the client for a brace. The splint is worn at all times, and removed for protected range-of-motion exercises until the joint is stable.	Posterior in 90 degrees of flexion, or Bledsoe brace or Mayo elbow brace in 90 degrees.
Elbow instability	After removal of the postoperative dressing a posterior elbow immobilization splint in 120 degrees of flexion is provided. Therapist-supervised protected range-of-motion exercises are performed until the joint become more stable. The client is not permitted to remove the splint unsupervised.	Posterior in 120 degrees of flexion or brace locked in 120 degrees.
Biceps/triceps repair	Splint is worn at all times and removed for protected range-of-motion exercises.	Posterior elbow splint immobilized in prescribed angle based on structures requiring protection. Splint is usually adjusted to increase the angle of immobilization by 10 to 15 degrees per week at 3 weeks postoperatively.
Cubital tunnel syndrome	A nighttime splint is provided for use while sleeping. Proper positioning during work and leisure activities is reviewed.	Volar splint elbow immobilized in 30 to 45 degrees extension or reverse elbcw pad.

fractures occur in the olecranon as a result of direct impact or of a hyperextension force [Cabanela and Morrey 2000]. When the radial head dislocates anteriorly along with an ulnar fracture, the result is a Monteggia fracture. Another common fracture location along the proximal ulna is the coronoid process [Regan and Morrey 2000]. Elbow fractures are managed conservatively with closed manipulation or immobilization and surgically with open reduction internal fixation (ORIF) or external fixation.

Healing structures are protected in a brace, cast, or custom-molded thermoplastic splint to maintain alignment and prevent deformity. Splint designs vary and are based on the surgeon's preference, therapist's experience, and the client's needs. The protective splint is worn for as long as 2 to 8 weeks postoperatively, depending on the stability of the fracture/joint and the severity of the injury. The position and angle of immobilization are based on the type of fracture. Distal humeral fractures are immobilized in 90 degrees of elbow flexion, with the forearm in neutral rotation (Figure 10-1A).

Olecranon and proximal ulna fractures often involve injury to the triceps tendon. To protect the injured tendon, the elbow is immobilized in 60 to 70 degrees of flexion, the forearm in neutral, and the wrist in slight extension (Figure 10-1B). Complex radial head fractures/dislocations and radial head replacements are immobilized in up to 120 degrees of flexion to stabilize the radial head (Figure 10-1C). The protective splint is worn continuously at first, and is removed only for protected exercises (when indicated) and for hygiene. Once the fracture/joint is considered stable, the splint is removed more frequently for exercises and light functional activities. The splint is gradually weaned during the day, and continues to be worn for sleep and protection until the fracture is completely stable [Barenholtz and Wolff 2001].

Splinting for Total Elbow Arthroplasty

Elbow arthroplasty refers to resurfacing or replacement of the joint. The primary goal of total elbow arthroplasty is pain relief with restoration of stability and functional motion (arc of 30 to 130 degrees). An elbow replacement is considered when the joint is painful, is restricted in motion, or has destroyed articular cartilage. Clients who are elderly or have low demands that present with rheumatoid arthritis, advanced post-traumatic arthritis, advanced degenerative arthritis, or nonunion and comminuted distal humeral fractures are good candidates for this surgery [Morrey 2000b]. Total elbow arthroplasty includes three types of implants: constrained, nonconstrained, and semiconstrained.

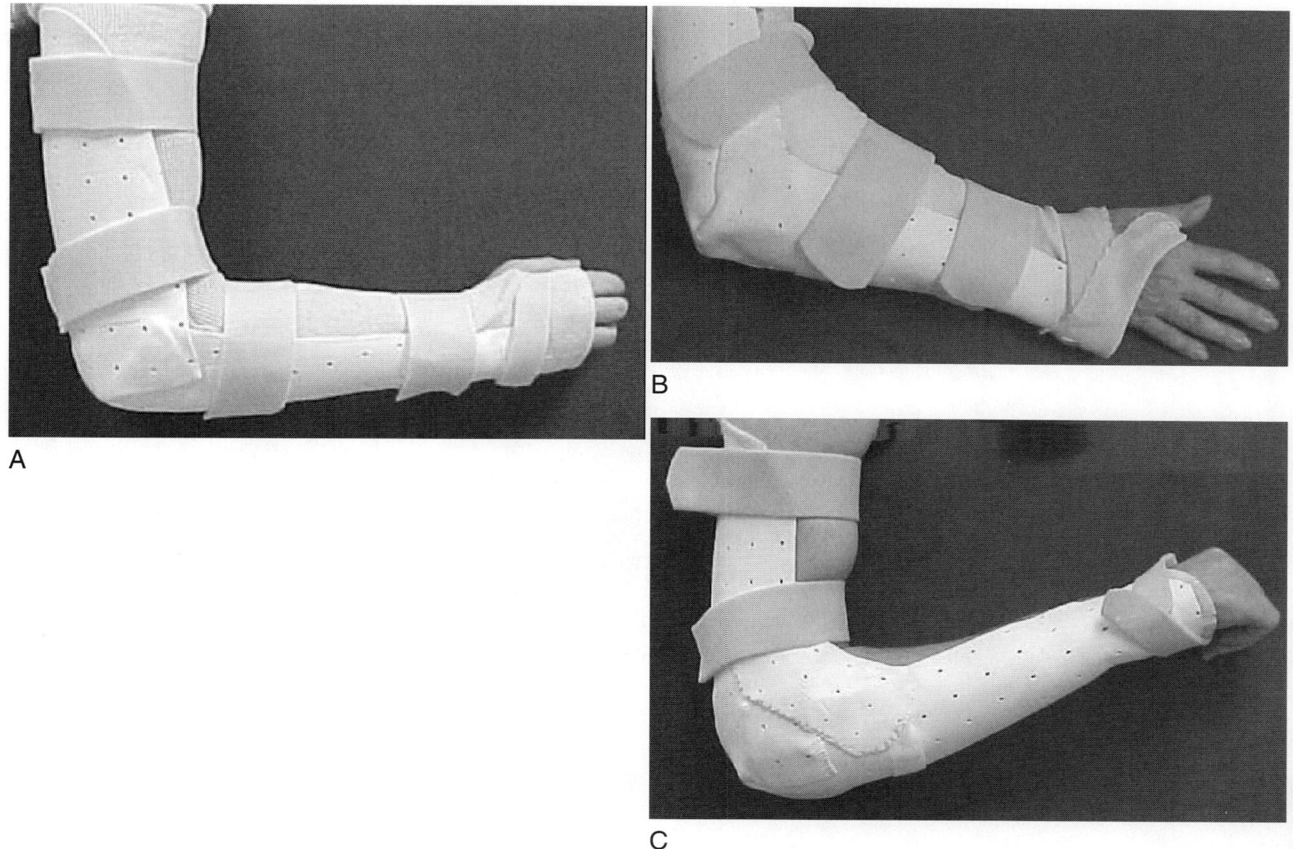

Figure 10-1 (A) A posterior elbow immobilization splint in 90 degrees of flexion. (B) A posterior elbow immobilization splint in 75 degrees of flexion. (C) A posterior elbow immobilization splint in 120 degrees of flexion.

The choice for a specific implant is based on the extent and cause of the disease, the specific needs of the client, and the surgeon's preference [Cooney 2000, Morrey et al. Wolff 2000].

An immobilization splint or brace is provided on the first postoperative visit. Several options are available based on the preference of the surgeon and the experience of the therapist. Some surgeons prefer a brace such as the Bledsoe brace (Bledsoe Brace Systems, Grand Prairie) (Figure 10-2A) or Mayo Elbow Universal Brace (Aircast, Summit, NJ) (Figure 10-2B). The brace provides medial and lateral stability while allowing flexion and extension of the elbow. The parameters of the brace are preset to limit end range in both flexion and extension. Extension is set to tolerance, and flexion is determined by the condition of the triceps muscle and surgical repair. Protected range of motion exercises are initiated with the brace on for 2 to 3 weeks.

Another common option is a posterior elbow immobilization splint (see Figure 10-1A), a custom-molded thermoplastic splint positioned in 80 to 90 degrees of flexion. The advantages of this splint are that it fits well by conforming to the client's elbow and that it can be remolded to accommodate changes in edema. Disadvantages of the splint include posterior pressure at the incision site and development of an elbow flexion contracture if the splint is not removed regularly for exercise. The splint is removed 3 to 4 times daily for the performance of protected range-of-motion exercises. In the presence of infection or instability, the splint is worn continuously and for a longer period of time. Many surgeons prefer no splint at all. Instead, the arm is wrapped lightly in an Ace bandage and positioned in a sling. This approach encourages early functional use and is comfortable and well tolerated. The rationale is that pain and postsurgical swelling will limit the end range of motion.

Splinting for Instability

Elbow instability results from a dislocation of the ulnohumeral joint and injury to the varus and valgus stabilizers of the elbow and the radial head [Hotchkiss 1996]. This injury often results from a forceful fall on an outstretched hand. The impact drives the head of the radius into the capitellum of the humerus [O'Driscoll 2000]. This may result in radial head and coronoid process fracture, medial collateral, and posterolateral and/or lateral collateral

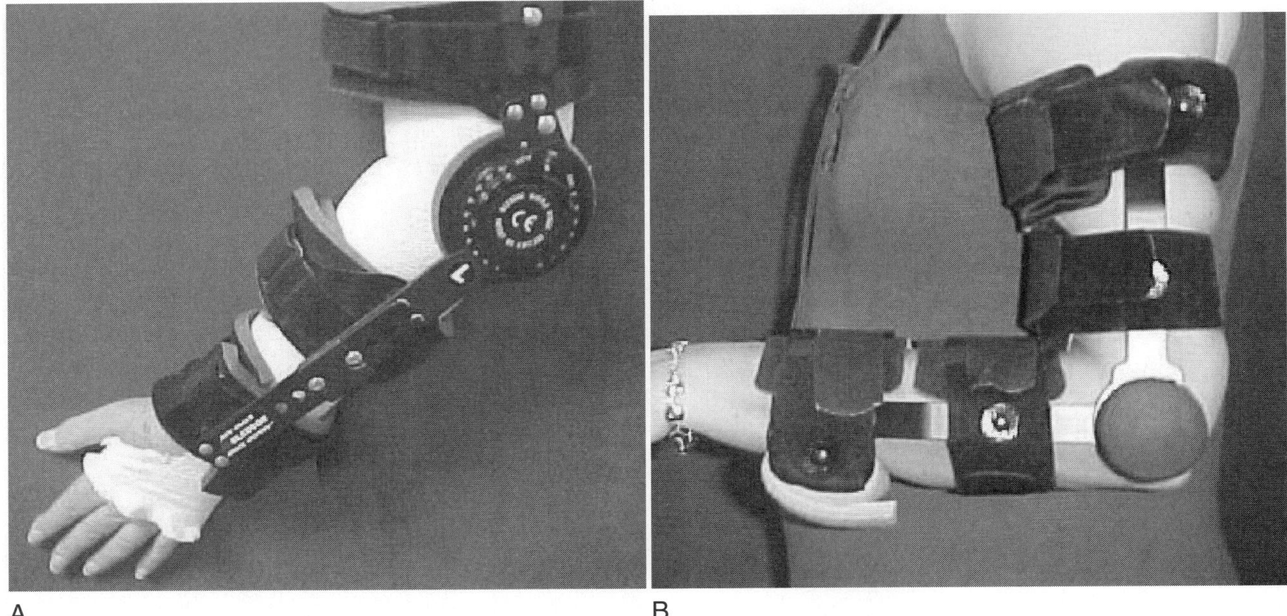

Figure 10-2 (A) A Bledsoe brace (Bledsoe Brace Systems, Grand Prairie, TX). (B) The Mayo elbow universal brace (Aircast, Summit, NJ).

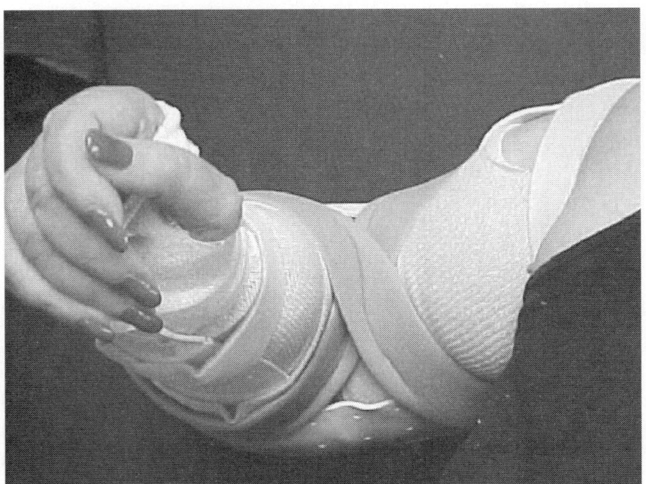

Figure 10-3 Figure-of-eight strap to stabilize the elbow within the splint.

ligament disruption. When all of these structures are injured, the condition is described as the "terrible triad" [Hotchkiss 1996].

The treatment plan begins with fabrication of a custom thermoplastic posterior elbow shell with the elbow positioned in 120 degrees or more of flexion and the forearm in full pronation (see Figure 10-1C). The wrist is included and splinted in neutral. A figure-of-eight strap may be added to further stabilize the elbow in 120 degrees for a larger-framed individual (Figure 10-3). The splint is worn at all times and removed 3 to 5 times daily for protected exercises. The elbow must be in 120 degrees or more of flexion to ensure approximation of the radial head.

If this is not achieved, an instability may occur. An alternative to the thermoplastic splint, and a preference of some surgeons is a Bledsoe brace (Bledsoe Brace Systems, Grand Prairie, TX) or the Mayo elbow universal brace (Aircast, Summit, NJ). The brace is locked in 120 degrees of elbow flexion and neutral foream rotation. The brace is worn at all times, and exercises are performed within protected range with the brace on. Some surgeons immobilize the elbow in 90 degrees of flexion if adequate stability was achieved intraoperatively.

Splinting for Biceps and Triceps Rupture

Distal biceps tendon rupture is uncommon and occurs more frequently in men than in women. The mechanism of injury is a strong extension force applied to the elbow in the flexed position, such as attempting to catch a heavy object with an outstretched hand [Kannus and Natri 1997]. Treatment varies from conservative management via immobilization to surgical repair via a one-incision or two-incision approach. The position and method of immobilization is determined by the preference of the surgeon. Common methods of immobilization include a brace or posterior elbow splint locked at 90 degrees of flexion and the forearm immobilized in pronation.

Some physicians prefer that the forearm be immobilized in neutral rotation, and yet others immobilize in supination. Elbow flexion is permitted as tolerated from the locked position of 90 degrees. Three weeks postoperatively elbow

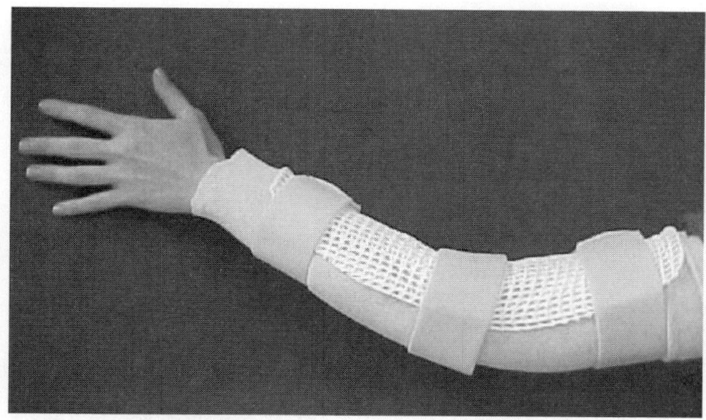

Figure 10-4 An anterior elbow immobilization splint in 30 degrees of extension.

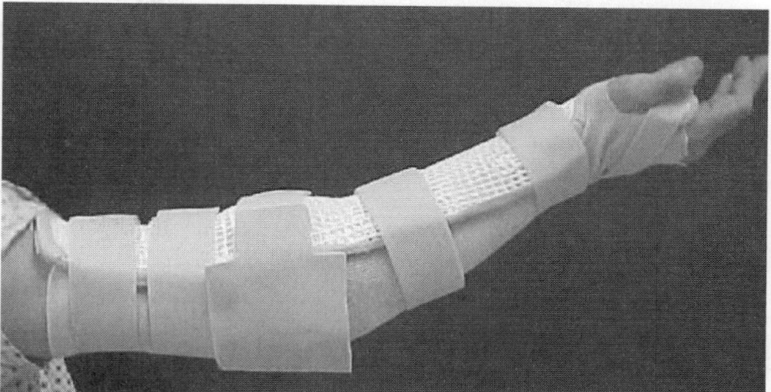

Figure 10-5 A serial static elbow extension splint.

extension is increased by 10 to 15 degrees per week. The brace is generally worn for a period of 6 to 8 weeks. The benefit of using a brace for biceps tendon repairs is that it is easily adjusted to accommodate the change in the angle of motion. A thermoplastic splint requires frequent readjustment and remolding that can be cumbersome and time consuming.

Triceps rupture is commonly seen in olecranon fractures. Following a triceps repair, the elbow is immobilized in a splint 70 to 90 degrees. The client is instructed to actively extend the elbow to tolerance and to flex to the parameters of the splint or brace. Either a posterior or anterior splint is appropriate, although a posterior splint may be required to protect the incision.

Splinting for Cubital Tunnel Syndrome

Cubital tunnel syndrome is the second most common site of nerve compression in the upper extremity following carpal tunnel [Blackmore 2002, Rayan 1992]. Anatomically, the ulnar nerve is susceptible to injury at the elbow. Injury to the nerve may occur as a result of trauma or prolonged or sustained motion that compresses the nerve over time [Fess et al. 2005]. Symptoms include pain and parasthesias (numbness, tingling) over the sensory distribution of the ulnar nerve, the ulnar two digits of the hand.

In advances stages, weakness and atrophy of the hypothenar muscles and thumb adductor may be seen. Conservative management focuses on avoiding postures and positions that aggravate the symptoms. Clients are instructed to avoid repetitive or sustained elbow flexion. For this purpose, a nighttime anterior elbow extension splint is fabricated with the elbow positioned in 30 to 45 degrees of extension (Figure 10-4). A commercial elbow pad is helpful to protect the ulnar nerve at the elbow. The pad can be reversed and worn anteriorly as an alternative to the splint to prevent elbow flexion.

Serial Static and Static Progressive Splinting of the Elbow

Serial static and static progressive splints are designed to increase motion in a stiff joint by providing a low-load and prolonged stretch [Flowers and LaStayo 1994]. Posttraumatic stiffness following elbow fractures and dislocations is the most common cause of elbow contracture. Other causes include osteoarthritis or inflammatory arthritis, congenital or developmental deformities, burns, and head injury. The elbow joint is prone to stiffness for several reasons. Anatomically, the joint is highly congruent. In most joints of the body, the *tendinous portions* of the muscles that act on the joint lie over the joint capsule. In the elbow, however, the brachialis muscle *belly* lies directly over the anterior joint capsule—making adhesion formation between the two structures inevitable following injury.

The elbow is often held in 70 to 90 degrees of flexion post-injury, as that is the position of greatest intracapsular volume for accommodation of edema. The thin joint capsule responds to trauma by thickening and becoming fibrotic, quickly adapting to this flexed position of the elbow. This results in a tethering of joint motion, particularly in the direction of extension [Wolff and Altman 2006]. Biomechanically, the strong (and often co-contracting) elbow flexors overpower the weaker elbow extensors—which challenges the ability to regain extension [Griffith 2002]. Last, the elbow joint is prone to heterotopic ossification following trauma and surgery.

For extension contractures of less than 45 degrees, an anterior thermoplastic serial static elbow extension splint (Figure 10-5) is fabricated for use at night. This provides low-load prolonged positioning at the end range of elbow extension [Gelinas et al. 2000]. It is remolded into greater extension as tolerated. For extension contractures of greater than 45 degrees, a static progressive elbow splint is either fabricated or provided. An effective design for a static progressive elbow extension splint is the turnbuckle splint (Figure 10-6). It should be noted that this splint requires experience, expertise, and time. A simpler alternative is the Mayo elbow universal brace (Aircast, Summit, NJ), described previously. The brace can be locked in position

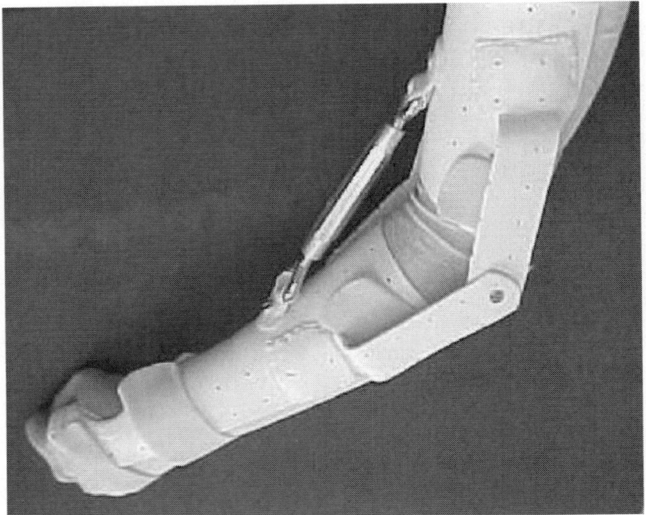

Figure 10-6 A static progressive turnbuckle elbow extension splint.

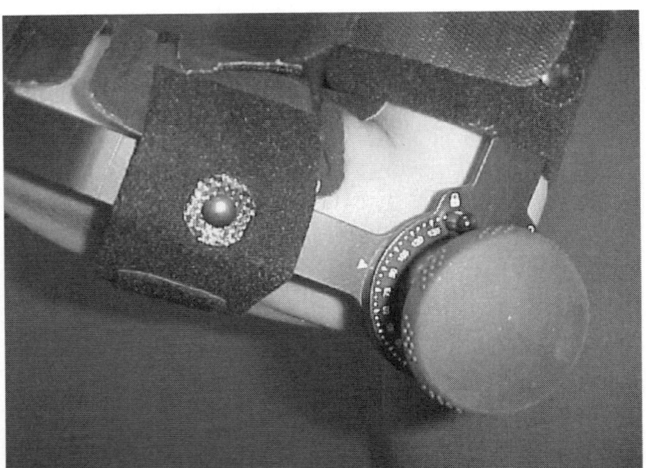

Figure 10-7 Static progressive component of Mayo elbow universal brace with dial shown up close. [Courtesy of Coleen Gately, DPT.]

and has a static progressive component that can be used to gain motion in both flexion and extension (Figure 10-7).

For a custom static progressive elbow flexion splint, the D-ring design (referred to as a "come-along" splint) is often used effectively (Figure 10-8). It is often necessary to fabricate multiple static splints for limitations in elbow motion and forearm rotation, depending on the range-of-motion deficits of the client. Clients are instructed to wear the splint for 2-hour intervals, for a total of 6 hours daily. At first, only short intervals are tolerated. The goal is to develop a tolerance for longer intervals. Clients are instructed to adjust the tension, to allow increased motion as tolerated.

When more than one splint is required, the client may alternate the splints during the day or wear one during the day and the other at night for sleeping. The splint regimen is highly individualized and tailored to meet the specific needs

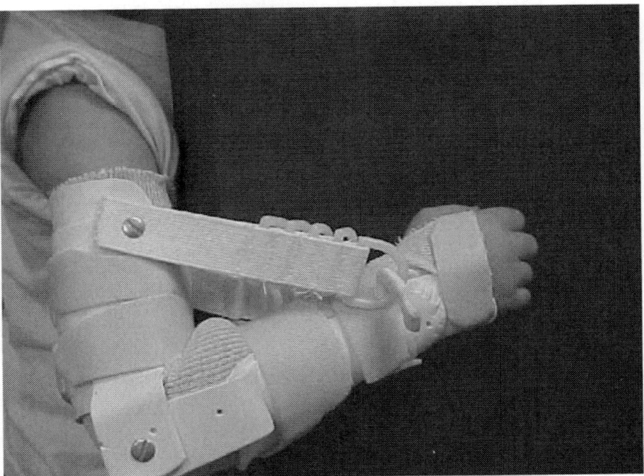

Figure 10-8 A static progressive elbow flexion "come-along" splint.

and limitations of each client. Dynamic splinting is often not well tolerated, and is not recommended. Off-the-shelf prefabricated static progressive flexion/extension splints are currently available and are effective in many cases. The shape of the client's arm, the degree of joint stiffness, and the firmness of joint end feel all impact the fit (and therefore effectiveness) of commercial splints.

Features of the Elbow Immobilization Splint

The elbow splint immobilizes the elbow joint from moving in flexion and extension. A splint that extends distally to include the wrist will partially immobilize the forearm. For forearm immobilization splinting to prevent forearm rotation, a better choice would be a sugar tong or Muenster-type splint (Figure 10-9). The exact angle of immobilization is dictated by the structures requiring protection. A strong rigid material that conforms well is required to properly immobilize the elbow joint.

The wrist is most often included to prevent wrist drop and hand edema. The wrist is splinted in a neutral position of 15 degrees of extension. Unless otherwise indicated, the forearm is positioned in neutral rotation. The proximal portion of the splint should extend as high as possible while allowing clearance of the axilla. It is important to maximize the length of the lever arm in order to stabilize the joint in the splint. Reinforcement is required at the joint to add strength to the splint and prevent buckling of the material. The distal portion extends beyond the wrist to the distal palmar crease to allow thumb and digit motion while providing wrist support (Figure 10-10).

Indications for Anterior Elbow Splinting

Anterior elbow splinting is indicated in situations where there is a posterior wound that cannot tolerate posterior pressure or contact. It is also used to prevent or correct

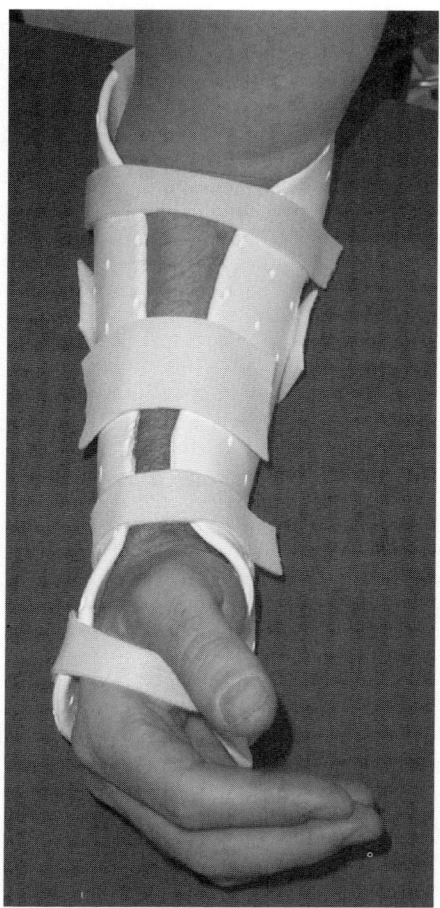

Figure 10-9 A forearm immobilization splint, sugar tong type.

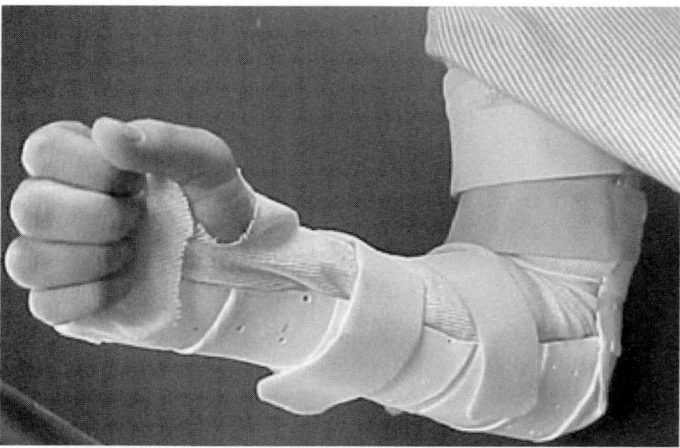

Figure 10-10 Distal component clears the distal palmar crease to allow full digital flexion.

elbow flexion contractures. Following a contracture release of a stiff elbow, an anterior elbow splint would be used as a serial static splint to slowly gain extension of the elbow over time by remolding the splint in increased extension at weekly intervals. In addition, the anterior design is effective in blocking elbow flexion such as with ulnar nerve compression neuropathies.

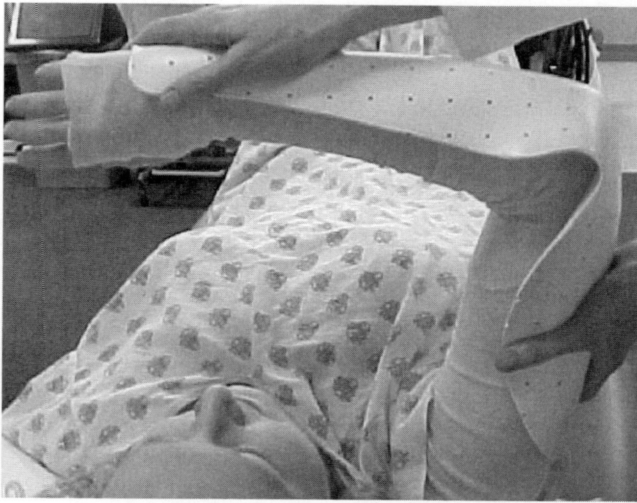

Figure 10-11 Supine position for molding posterior immobilization splint. [Courtesy of Carol Page, PT, CHT.]

Fabrication of an Elbow Immobilization Splint

The initial step in the fabrication of an elbow immobilization splint is the drawing of a pattern. Elbow splint patterns differ from hand patterns in that measurements of the client's arm, elbow, and forearm are taken and recorded. A pattern is drawn based on the recorded measurements. The following materials will be required to fabricate the splint: a strong rigid perforated thermoplastic material such as Ezeform (Northcoast), 3/8-inch open cell contour padding, 1/8-inch polycushion padding, 2-inch Velcro hook, 2-inch cushion strap, 2- or 3-inch stockinette, a tape measure, wax pencil, and scissors. It is important that a strong rigid material be used to support the elbow joint and weight of the arm, and to properly immobilize the joint.

The material must also be able to contour easily and should be of medium to low plasticity. Perforated material is chosen to provide ventilation and prevent moisture from accumulating in the splint. The following steps describe the fabrication process for a posterior elbow immobilization splint in 90 degrees of flexion. The angle of the splint is determined by the structures to be protected. For an anterior splint (see Figure 10-4), the same procedures are followed (additional clearance is required at the axilla) and the splint is applied to the volar surface of the arm.

1. The client is positioned in the position of immobilization, and the joint is prepared for splinting. The position of the client is dependent on the diagnosis and the client's tolerance. The easiest position for molding the splint is with the client supine, the shoulder in 90 degress of flexion, and the elbow in 90 degrees of flexion (Figure 10-11). Alternatively, the client may be seated with the shoulder slightly abducted.
2. A stockinette is applied to the arm.

3. The bony prominences are padded prior to measuring and fabricating the splint (Figure 10-12A). This includes the olecranon, lateral epicondyle and radial head, medial epicondyle, and ulnar head and styloid at the wrist. Polycushion padding (1/8 inch) is used to pad the prominences. The padding is then covered with an additional layer of stockinette to prevent the padding from adhering to the splint material (Figure 10-12B).
4. The following measurements are taken (Figure 10-13A through F):
   a. The length from level of axillary crease to olecranon process. One inch is added to provide sufficient proximal support (Figure 10-13A).
   b. The length from the olecranon process to the distal palmar crease on the ulnar aspect of the hand (Figure 10-13B).
   c. Two-thirds the circumference of the upper arm (Figure 10-13C).
   d. Two-thirds the circumference of the elbow (Figure 10-13D).
   e. Two-thirds the circumference of the mid-forearm (Figure 10-13E).
   f. Two-thirds the circumference of the hand at the distal palmar crease level (Figure 10-13F).
5. A pattern is drawn on paper towel (two pieces taped together will be needed) using the measurements taken (Figure 10-14).
6. The pattern is cut and measured on the client. The pattern should clear the axilla and extend laterally higher than the axilla to ensure proper support. The elbow portion must be wide enough to cover two-thirds of the circumference. A common error is to make the elbow portion too narrow. This compromises the stability of the splint, and does not provide adequate support. The distal portion extends to the distal palmar crease. The thenar eminence and distal palmar crease are cleared to allow full digit and thumb motion. Another common error is when the distal portion of the splint ends just distal to the wrist. The wrist is not sufficiently supported and is placed in an uncomfortable and often intolerable position. If errors are noted while the pattern is measured, adjustments are made or a new pattern is drawn.
7. Once it has been determined that the pattern is accurate, the pattern is traced with the wax pencil on the splint material and cut out (Figure 10-15).
8. The material is heated in a splint pan, removed, and patted dry.
9. The material is cut and reheated.
10. The material is dried and carefully draped over the arm in the proper position (Figure 10-16).
11. The sides at the elbow are pinched and folded, carefully checking the elbow position. A common error is for the client to extend the elbow slightly during the molding process, causing a loss of the flexion angle (Figure 10-17).
12. Light Ace wrap is used to position and mold the material, while continuing to support the arm in the correct position. Care should be taken to contour around the elbow and wrist joints (Figure 10-18A).
13. Once the splint has cooled off, the Ace wrap is removed. The padding and outer stockinette layer is removed.
14. The elbow seams are smoothed and a space for pressure relief over the olecranon is created by gently pushing the material out (Figure 10-19).
15. The padding is inserted in the splint (Figure 10-20).

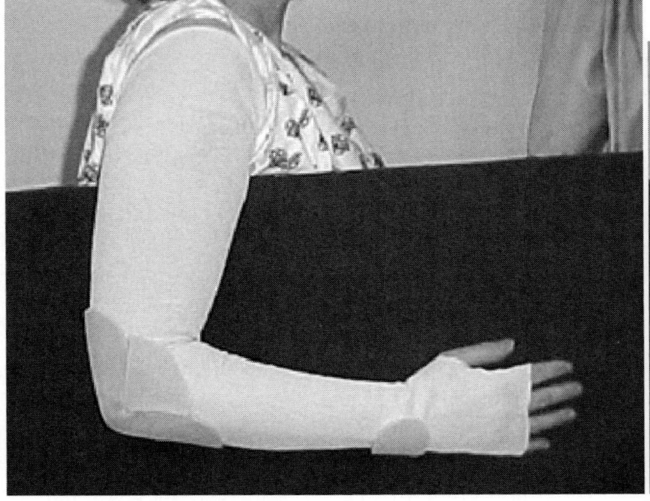
A

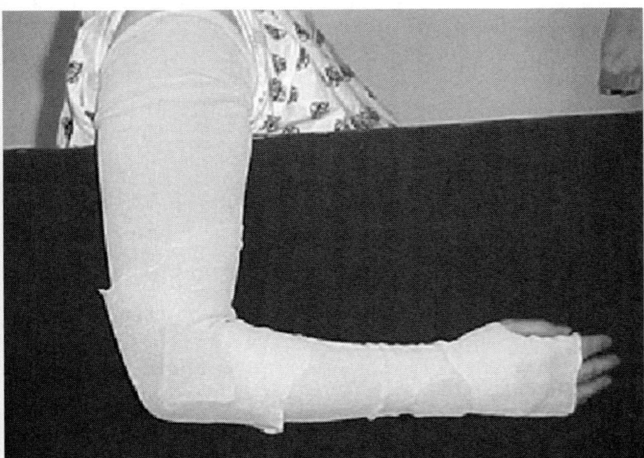
B

Figure 10-12 (A) Bony prominences are padded. (B) Padding is covered with additional layer of stockinette. [Courtesy of Carol Page, PT, CHT.]

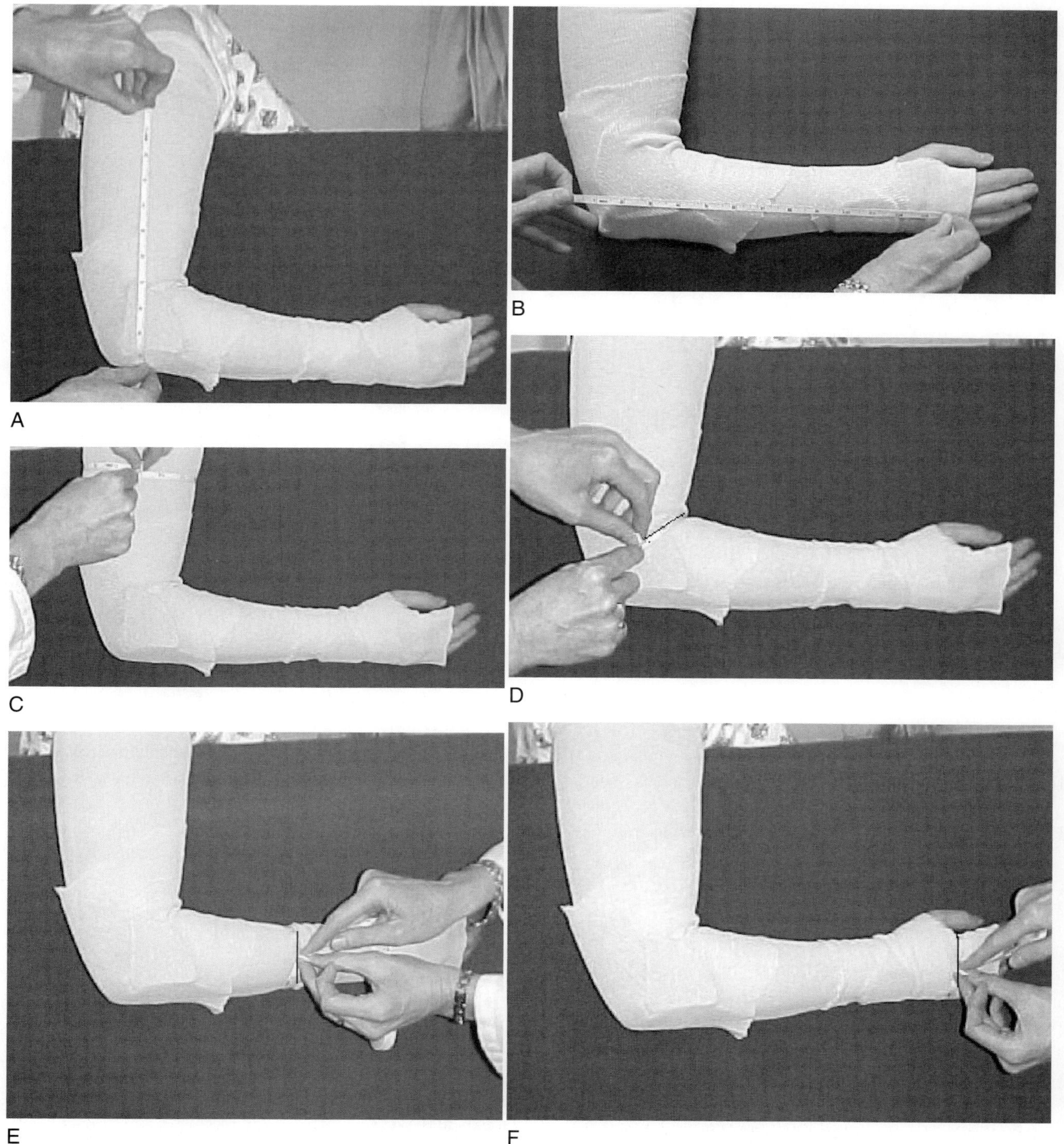

Figure 10-13 (A) Length of axillary crease to olecranon process. (B) Length from olecranon process to the distal palmar crease. (C) Two-thirds the circumference of the upper arm. (D) Two-thirds the circumference of the elbow. (E) Two-thirds the circumference of the mid-forearm. (F) Two-thirds the circumference of the hand at the distal palmar crease level. [Courtesy of Carol Page, PT, CHT.]

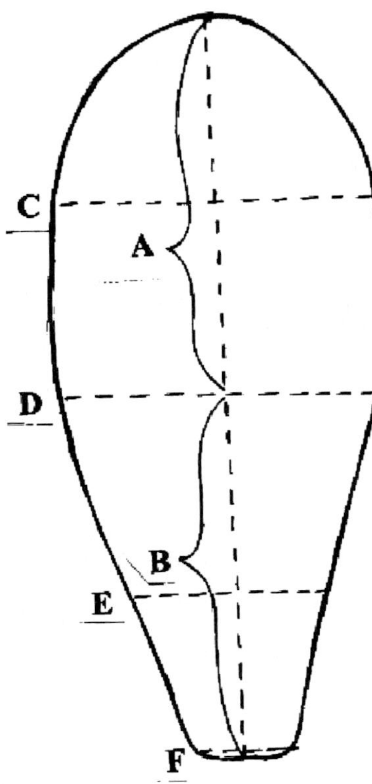

Figure 10-14 Pattern is drawn using the measurements taken. [Courtesy of Carol Page, PT, CHT.]

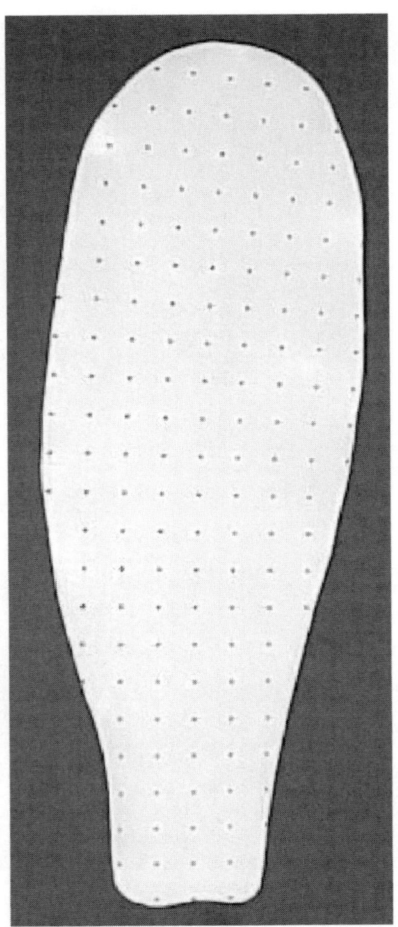

Figure 10-15 Pattern is traced on the splint material and cut. [Courtesy of Carol Page, PT, CHT.]

16. The fit is checked and adjustments are made as needed (Figure 10-21A).
17. Velcro straps are applied (Figure 10-21B) to the following:
    a. The proximal upper arm
    b. The distal upper arm, proximal to the elbow
    c. The proximal forearm
    d. Wrist
    e. Hand
    f. Extra straps if needed
18. The splint is applied and the fit rechecked (Figure 10-21C).
19. The client is educated in proper donning/doffing and wearing schedule.

Technical Tips for a Proper Fit

- Select a thermoplastic splinting material that is rigid enough to support the elbow yet conforms well to the arm and joint.
- Align the material along the arm. Make sure to properly position the material before you start molding.
- Use Ace wrap to position and hold the material in place. This will free up your hands to support the arm in the correct position and to contour around the elbow joint.

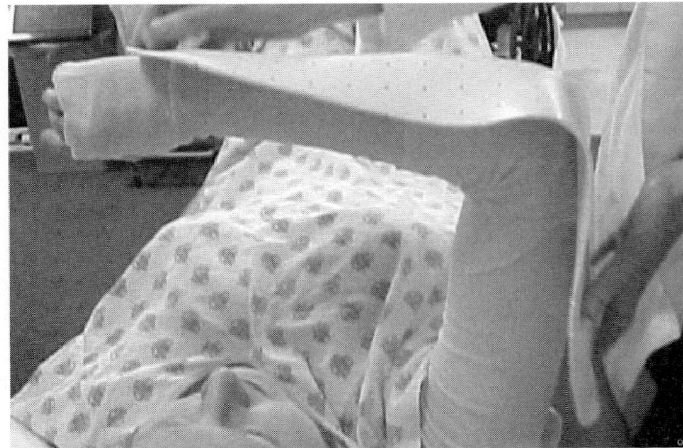

Figure 10-16 Material is draped over the arm in the proper position. [Courtesy of Carol Page, PT, CHT.]

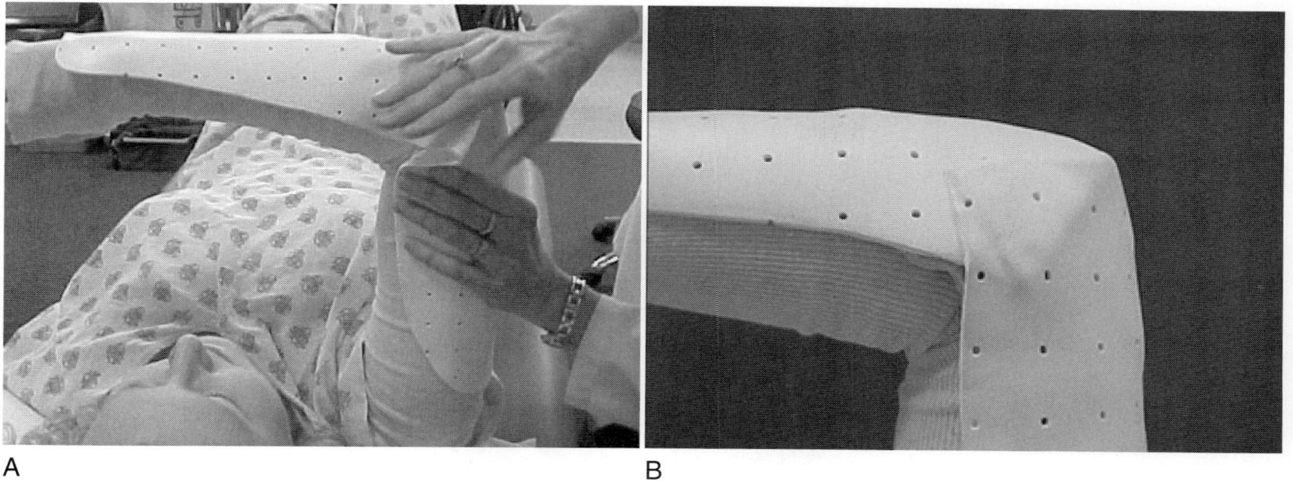

Figure 10-17 (A) The sides at the elbow are pinched. (B) The sides at the elbow are folded carefully. [Courtesy of Carol Page, PT, CHT.]

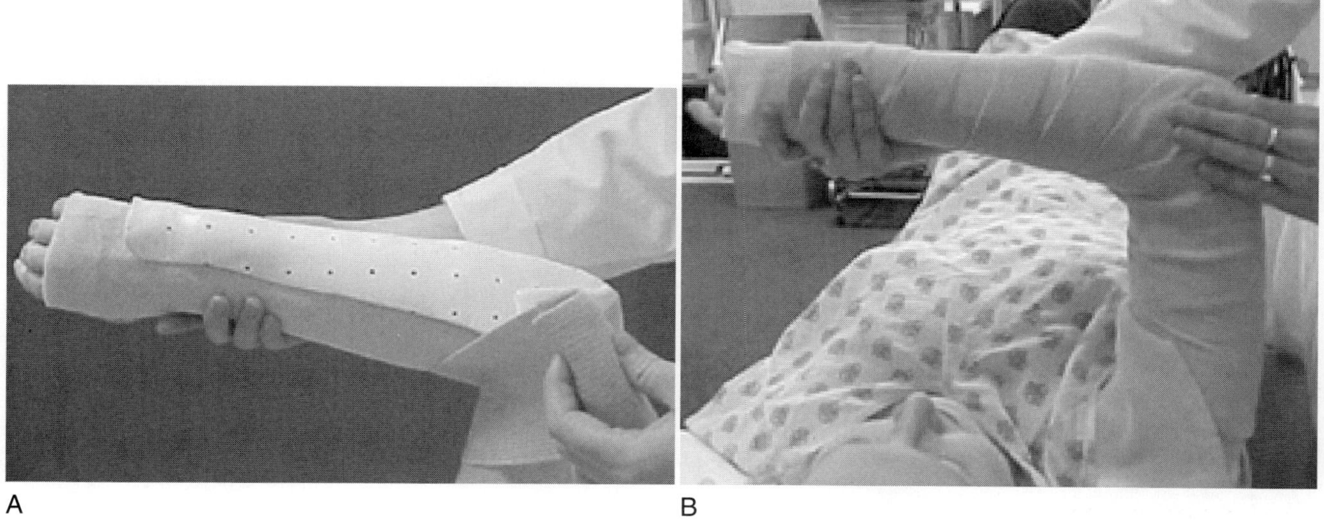

Figure 10-18 (A and B) A light Ace wrap is used to mold the material. [Courtesy of Carol Page, PT, CHT.]

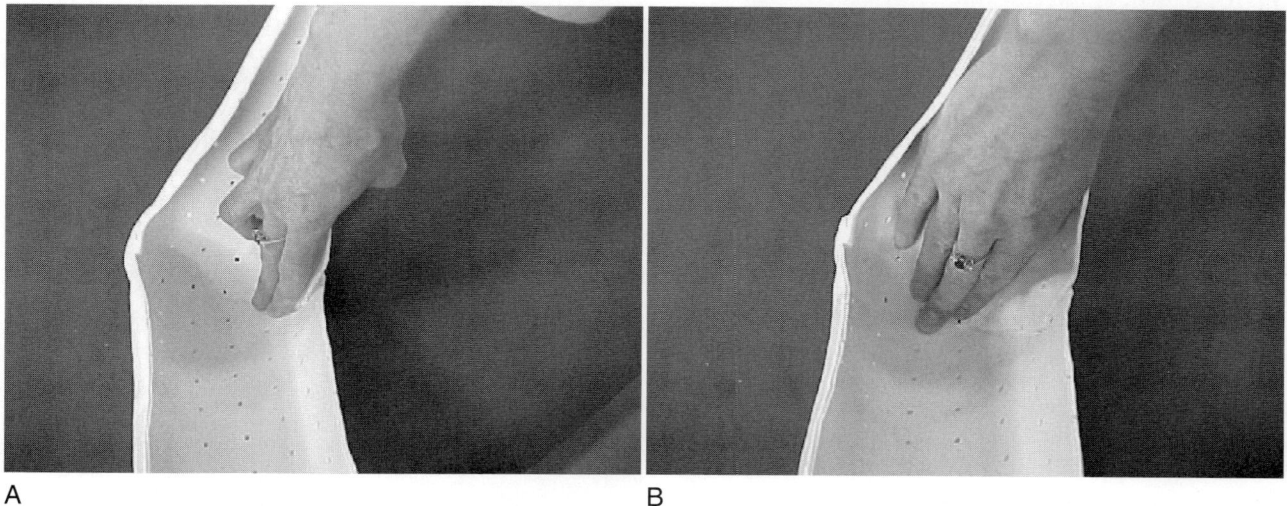

Figure 10-19 (A and B) Elbow seams are smoothed and a space for pressure relief over the olecranon is created. [Courtesy of Carol Page, PT, CHT.]

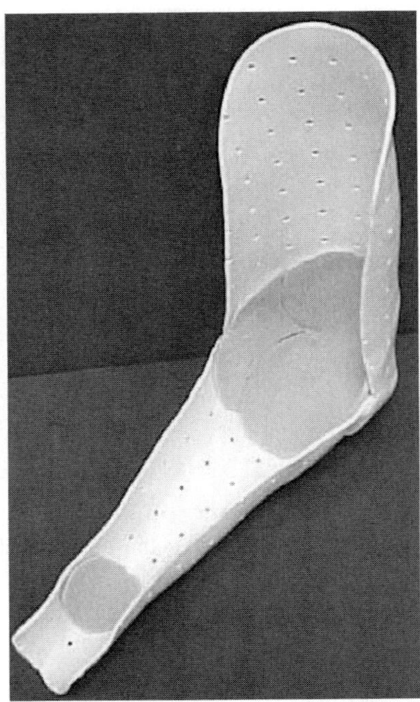

Figure 10-20 Padding is inserted into the splint. [Courtesy of Carol Page, PT, CHT.]

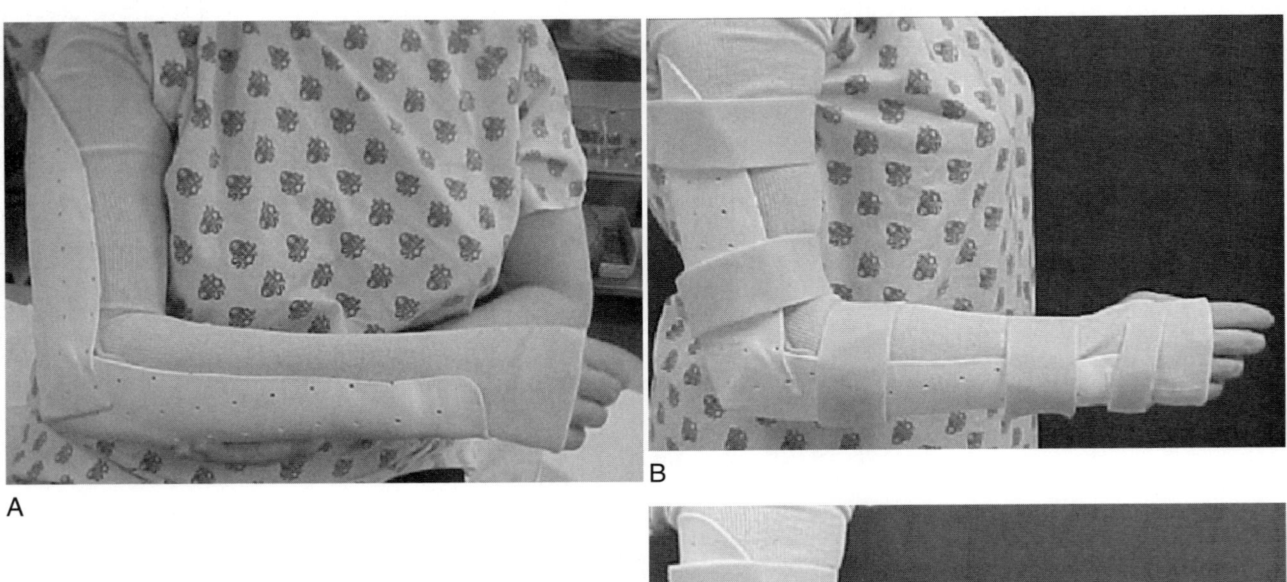

A

B

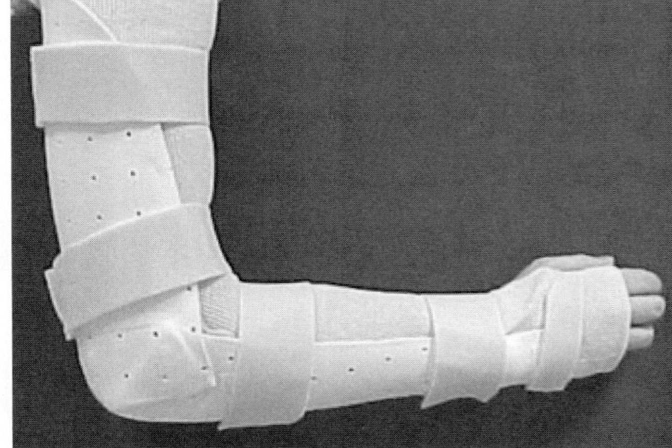

C

Figure 10-21 (A) Fit is checked. (B) Velcro straps are applied. (C) Splint is applied and fit rechecked. [Courtesy of Carol Page, PT, CHT.]

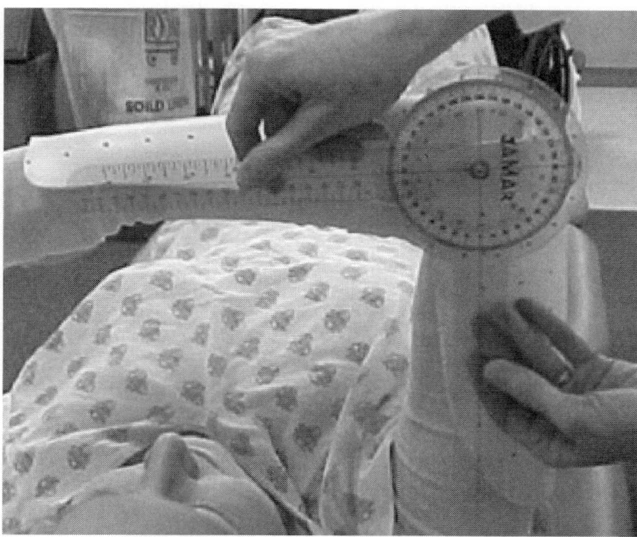

Figure 10-22 A goniometer is used to check the angle at the elbow before the material cools. [Courtesy of Carol Page, PT, CHT.]

- Always determine that the client has full finger and thumb range of motion when wearing the splint by having him or her flex the digits and oppose the thumb.
- Make sure the elbow, wrist, and forearm are at the correct angle. A frequent fabrication mistake when molding in the supine position is for the elbow to push into more extension during the molding process. To avoid this, continue to check the position of the elbow until the splint material is completely cool. Use a goniometer to check the position before the material cools (Figure 10-22).
- Make sure the wrist is in neutral extension and deviation. It is common for the wrist to posture in flexion and ulnar deviation in the supine position. This mistake can occur because of a lack of careful monitoring of the person's wrist position as the thermoplastic material is cooling. The therapist should closely monitor the wrist position in any splint that positions the wrist in neutral, because it is easy for the wrist to move in slight flexion. A quick spot check before the thermoplastic material is completely cool can address this problem.
- The forearm position should be carefully monitored so that the forearm does not posture in either pronation or supination.
- Make sure the splint extends as high as possible up the axilla, particularly on the lateral side. This will provide adequate support and leverage to properly immobilize the elbow.
- Make sure the medial side of the proximal portion clears the axilla to prevent irritation.

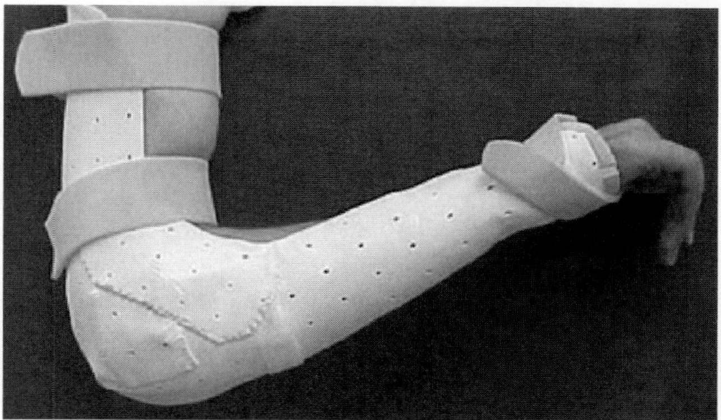

Figure 10-23 A thermoplastic strut provides lateral support at the elbow. [Courtesy of Carol Page, PT, CHT.]

- Be careful not to wrap the Ace wrap tightly around the warm thermoplastic. This will leave marks and distort the material. It can also compress the proximal and forearm portion, making it too narrow. This will dig into the arm and forearm. To avoid this problem, lightly Ace wrap the material and while the material is still pliable pull the edges lightly away from the arm.
- If a mistake occurs, it is better to remold the entire splint rather than spot one area.
- Make sure there is enough material to support the elbow laterally and medially (two-third the circumference of the elbow). Often in larger individuals a thermoplastic strut must be added to provide adequate support (Figure 10-23).
- In large-frame individuals a figure-of-eight strap may be required to properly secure the elbow in the splint.

- If you have access to assistance, an extra pair of hands is helpful in molding these large splints.

Precautions for Elbow Immobilization Splints

- Pad all bony prominences.
- Smooth all edges and line with moleskin or padding for clients with sensitive skin, particularly under the axilla and at the distal palmar crease and thumb web space.
- Edema in the elbow is common after injury or surgery to the joint. Make sure the client is scheduled for a follow-up visit within several days to modify and adjust the splint to accommodate for changes in edema.
- Open, draining, or infected wounds may require an alternative posterior elbow shell to protect and immobilize the joint while avoiding pressure over the wound (Figure 10-24).

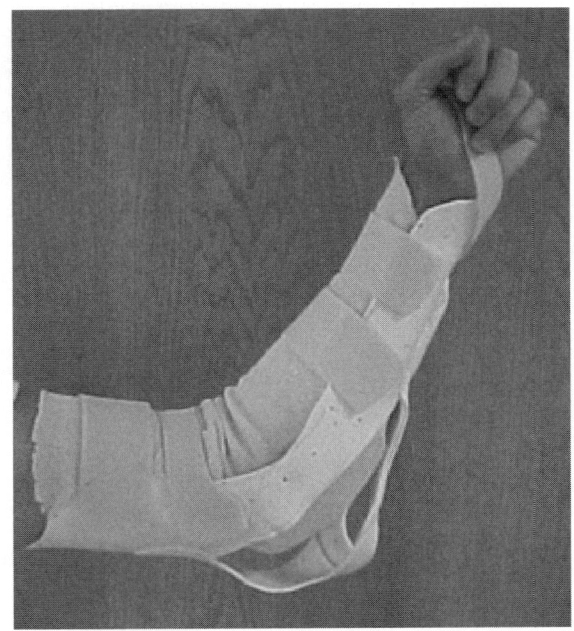

Figure 10-24 Alternative design: posterior immobilization splint to avoid posterior pressure.

SELF-QUIZ 10-1*

Circle either true (T) or false (F).

1. T F Elbow immobilization splints can be posterior or anterior.
2. T F It is better that the wrist be left free in elbow splints to allow for more functional motion.
3. T F Perforated material is not preferable for elbow splints because the holes lessen the strength of the material.
4. T F Following a total elbow replacement, the elbow can be immobilized in either a brace or posterior elbow splint.
5. T F Posterior splints are preferred for cubital tunnel syndrome.
6. T F The angle of elbow immobilization is dictated by the client's comfort.
7. T F Ace wrapping the material helps position and mold the material while the therapist continues to support the arm in the correct position.
8. T F An anterior elbow splint is appropriate for preventing or correcting elbow flexion contractures and for blocking elbow flexion.
9. T F The best splint for an extension contracture of the elbow of greater than 45 degrees is a serial static elbow extension splint.
10. T F Generally, biceps tendon repairs are immobilized with the elbow in complete extension.

*See Appendix A for the answer key.

Laboratory Exercise 10-1 Making an Elbow Shell Pattern

1. Practice making a posterior elbow shell pattern on another person. Use the detailed instructions provided to take measurements and draw the pattern.
2. Cut out your pattern and check for proper fit.

Laboratory Exercise 10-2 Fabricating an Elbow Splint

Practice fabricating an elbow immobilization splint on a partner. Before starting, determine the correct position for your partner's elbow. Measure the angle of elbow flexion/extension with a goniometer to ensure a correct position. After fitting your splint and making all adjustments, use Form 10-1 as a self-evaluation of the elbow immobilization splint, and use Grading Sheet 10-1 as a classroom grading sheet.

FORM 10-1* Elbow immobilization splint

Name: ______________________________

Date: ______________________________

Type of elbow immobilization splint:

Posterior ❍ Anterior ❍

Elbow position: ______________________________

After the person wears the splint for 30 minutes, answer the following questions. (Mark *NA* for nonapplicable situations.)

Evaluation Areas				**Comments**
Design				
1. The elbow position is at the correct angle.	Yes ❍	No ❍	NA ❍	
2. The elbow has adequate medial and lateral support (two-thirds the circumference of the elbow).	Yes ❍	No ❍	NA ❍	
3. The splint supplies sufficient proximal/lateral support (1 inch proximal to axillary crease).	Yes ❍	No ❍	NA ❍	
4. The splint is two-thirds the circumference of the upper arm.	Yes ❍	No ❍	NA ❍	
5. Distally the splint extends to the distal palmar crease.	Yes ❍	No ❍	NA ❍	
6. The splint is two-thirds the circumference of the forearm.	Yes ❍	No ❍	NA ❍	
Function				
1. The splint allows full thumb and digit motion.	Yes ❍	No ❍	NA ❍	
2. The splint allows full shoulder motion.	Yes ❍	No ❍	NA ❍	
3. The splint provides adequate elbow support to properly secure the elbow in the splint and prevent elbow motion.	Yes ❍	No ❍	NA ❍	
Straps				
1. The straps are secure and rounded.	Yes ❍	No ❍	NA ❍	
Comfort				
1. The splint edges are smooth with rounded corners.	Yes ❍	No ❍	NA ❍	
2. The proximal end is flared.	Yes ❍	No ❍	NA ❍	
3. The splint does not cause impingements or pressure sores.	Yes ❍	No ❍	NA ❍	
4. The splint does not irritate bony prominences.	Yes ❍	No ❍	NA ❍	
Cosmetic Appearance				
1. The splint is free of fingerprints, dirt, and pencil and pen marks.	Yes ❍	No ❍	NA ❍	
2. The splinting material is not buckled.	Yes ❍	No ❍	NA ❍	
Therapeutic Regimen				
1. The person has been instructed in a wearing schedule.	Yes ❍	No ❍	NA ❍	
2. The person has been provided splint precautions.	Yes ❍	No ❍	NA ❍	
3. The person demonstrates understanding of the education.	Yes ❍	No ❍	NA ❍	
4. Client/caregiver knows how to clean the splint.	Yes ❍	No ❍	NA ❍	

Continued

FORM 10-1* Elbow immobilization splint—cont'd

Discuss possible splint adjustments or changes you should make based on the self-evaluation. (What would you do differently next time?)

*See Appendix B for a perforated copy of this form.

GRADING SHEET 10-1* Elbow immobilization splint

Name: ____________________

Date: ____________________

Type of elbow immobilization splint:

Posterior ❍ Anterior ❍

Elbow position: ____________________

Grade:

1 = beyond improvement, not acceptable
2 = requires maximal improvement
3 = requires moderate improvement
4 = requires minimal improvement
5 = requires no improvement

Evaluation Areas						**Comments**
Design						
1. The elbow position is at the correct angle.	1	2	3	4	5	
2. The elbow has adequate medial and lateral support (two-thirds the circumference of the elbow).	1	2	3	4	5	
3. The splint supplies sufficient proximal/lateral support (1 inch proximal to axillary crease).	1	2	3	4	5	
4. The splint is two-thirds the circumference of the upper arm.	1	2	3	4	5	
5. Distally the splint extends to the distal palmar crease.	1	2	3	4	5	
6. The splint is two-thirds the circumference of the forearm.	1	2	3	4	5	
Function						
1. The splint allows full thumb and digit motion.	1	2	3	4	5	
2. The splint allows full shoulder motion.	1	2	3	4	5	
3. The splint provides adequate elbow support to properly secure the elbow in the splint and prevent elbow motion.	1	2	3	4	5	
Straps						
1. The straps are secure and rounded.	1	2	3	4	5	
Comfort						
1. The splint edges are smooth with rounded corners.	1	2	3	4	5	
2. The proximal end is flared.	1	2	3	4	5	
3. The splint does not cause impingements or pressure sores.	1	2	3	4	5	
4. The splint does not irritate bony prominences.	1	2	3	4	5	
Cosmetic Appearance						
1. The splint is free of fingerprints, dirt, and pencil and pen marks.	1	2	3	4	5	
2. The splinting material is not buckled.	1	2	3	4	5	

*See Appendix C for a perforated copy of this sheet.

CASE STUDY 10-1*

Read the following scenario and use your clinical reasoning skills to answer the questions based on information in this chapter.

Laura is a 47-year-old attorney who slipped on the ice and fractured and dislocated her left elbow. She was first treated at the local emergency room, where she was casted. One week later, she was operated on by an orthopedist—who reduced the fracture with internal fixation (ORIF) to the radial head and repaired the ruptured lateral ligament of the elbow. Two days post-surgery she is referred for therapy (prior to discharge from the hospital) for a posterior elbow splint in 110 to 120 degrees of flexion. She lives alone and has two active dogs she cares for.

1. Describe the appropriate splint for this client. List all joints you would include in this splint.

____

____

____

____

2. What position will the client assume for fabrication of this splint?

____

____

____

____

3. Which bony prominences require extra protection in the splint? How is this accomplished?

____

____

____

____

4. What wearing schedule will you provide to this client?

____

____

____

____

*See Appendix A for the answer key.

CASE STUDY 10-2*

Read the following scenario and use your clinical reasoning skills to answer the questions based on information from this chapter.

John is a right-hand-dominant 34-year-old sporting goods executive who ruptured the distal portion of his right biceps tendon when attempting to catch a falling box. The tendon was repaired surgically 2 weeks post-injury. He was discharged from the hospital with a bulky dressing and half cast immobilizing his elbow in 90 degrees. At his first postoperative visit, the cast and dressing are removed. The client is sent to therapy in a sling with a prescription for a splint in 90 degrees of flexion and instructions to progress into extension beginning 2 weeks postoperatively.

1. What splint or brace is most appropriate for this client?

____

____

____

____

2. What wearing schedule and instructions will you provide to this client?

____

____

____

____

*See Appendix A for the answer key.

REVIEW QUESTIONS

1. What are three main indications for use of an elbow immobilization splint?
2. What are the precautions for splinting the elbow?
3. When might a therapist consider serial splinting with an elbow immobilization splint?
4. What are the purposes of immobilization splinting of the elbow?
5. What are the advantages of a custom splint over a commercial splint?
6. What are the advantages of a commercial splint over a custom splint?
7. What are indications for anterior elbow splinting?
8. What are the positions for molding an elbow splint?

References

Barenholtz A, Wolff A (2001). Elbow fractures and rehabilitation. Orthopedic Physical Therapy Clinics of North America 10(4):525-539.

Blackmore S (2000). Therapist's management of ulnar nerve compression at the elbow. In EJ Mackin, AD Callahan, TM Skirven, et al. (eds.), *Rehabilitation of the Hand and Upper Extremity, Fifth Edition*. St Louis: Mosby.

Cabanela MF, Morrey BF (2000). Fractures of the olecranon. In BF Morrey (ed.), *The Elbow and Its Disorders, Third Edition*. Philadelphia: Saunders, pp. 365-379.

Cooney W (2000). Elbow arthroplasty: Historical perspective and current concepts. In BF Morrey (ed.), *The Elbow and Its Disorders, Third Edition*. Philadelphia: Saunders, pp. 583-601.

Fess E, Gettle K, Philips C, Janson J (2005). Splinting for work, sports and the performing arts. In E Fess, K Gettle, C Philips, J Janson (eds.), *Hand and Upper Extremity Splinting: Principles and Methods, Third Edition*. St Louis: Mosby, pp. 470-471.

Flowers KR, LaStayo P (1994). Effect of total end range time on improving passive range of motion. Journal of Hand Therapy 7(3):150-157.

Gelinas JJ, Faber KJ, Patterson SD, et al. (2000) The effectiveness for turnbuckle splinting for elbow contractures. Journal of Bone and Joint Surgery (Br) 82(1):74-78.

Griffith A (2002). Therapist's management of the stiff elbow. In EJ Mackin, AD Callahan, TM Skirven, et al. (eds.), *Rehabilitation of the Hand and Upper Extremity, Fifth Edition*. St Louis: Mosby, pp. 1245-1262.

Hotchkiss R (1996). Fractures and dislocations of the elbow. In DP Green (ed.), *Rockwood and Green's Fractures in Adults, Fourth Edition*. Philadelphia: Lippincott-Raven.

Jupiter JB, Morrey BF (2000). Fractures of the distal humerus in adults. In BF Morrey (ed.), *The Elbow and Its Disorders, Third Edition*. Philadelphia: Saunders, pp. 293-330.

Kannus P, Natri A (1997). Etiology and pathophysiology of tendon ruptures in sports. Scandinavian Journal of Science and Sports 7(2):107-112.

Morrey BF (2000a). Anatomy of the elbow joint. In BF Morrey (ed.), *The Elbow and Its Disorders, Third Edition*. Philadelphia: Saunders, pp. 13-42.

Morrey BF (2000b). Complications of elbow replacement surgery. In BF Morrey (ed.), *The Elbow and Its Disorders, Third Edition*. Philadelphia: Saunders, pp. 667-677.

Morrey BF (2000c). Radial head fractures. In BF Morrey (ed.), *The Elbow and Its Disorders, Third Edition*. Philadelphia: Saunders, pp. 341-364.

Morrey BF, Adams RA, Bryan RS (1991). Total replacement for post traumatic arthritis of the elbow. Journal of Bone and Joint Surgery 73(4):607-612.

O'Driscoll S (2000). Elbow dislocations. In BF Morrey (ed.), *The Elbow and Its Disorders, Third Edition*. Philadelphia: Saunders, pp. 409-420.

Rayan G (1992). Ulnar nerve compression. Hand Clinics 8:325.

Regan W, Morrey BF (2000). Coronoid process and monteggia fractures. In BF Morrey (ed.), *The Elbow and Its Disorders, Third Edition*. Philadelphia: Saunders, pp. 396-408.

Wolff A (2000). Postoperative management after total elbow replacement. Techniques in Hand and Upper Extremity Surgery 4(3): 213-220.

Wolff A, Altman E (2006). Contracture release of the elbow. In J Mosca, JB Cahill, et al. (eds.), *Hopsital for Special Surgery: Cioppa-Postsurgical Rehabilitation Guidelines for the Orthopedic Clinician*. Philadelphia: Mosby.

CHAPTER 11

Mobilization Splints: Dynamic, Serial-Static, and Static Progressive Splinting

Jean Wilwerding-Peck, OTR/L, CHT

Key Terms

Mobilization splint
Torque
Mechanical advantage
End feel
Outrigger
Finger loop
Static progressive tension

Chapter Objectives

1. Understand the biomechanics of dynamic splinting.
2. Identify effects of force on soft tissue.
3. Understand the way to apply appropriate tension.
4. Identify common uses of dynamic splinting.
5. List the goals of dynamic splinting.
6. List the materials necessary for fabrication of a dynamic splint.
7. Explain the risks of applying dynamic force.
8. Identify contraindications for application of a dynamic splint.
9. Understand the fabrication steps of three dynamic splints.
10. Identify instances in which dynamic splinting is appropriate.
11. Explain sources of force in dynamic splinting.

Mobilization splints or dynamic splints have movable parts and are designed to apply force across joints [Brand 2002]. Mobilization splints use constant or adjustable tension, or both, to achieve one of the following goals [Fess 2002]:

- Substitute for loss of muscle function
- Correct deformities caused by muscle-tendon tightness or joint contractures
- Maintain active or passive range of motion
- Provide controlled motion after tendon repair or joint arthroplasty
- Aid in fracture alignment and wound healing

This chapter provides basic information on the principles of dynamic splinting. Specifically, this chapter reviews the construction process of dynamic splints for a flexor tendon repair, radial nerve injury, and proximal interphalangeal (PIP) flexion contracture. Even though early attempts at dynamic splint construction may seem challenging, the process becomes easier with practice and experience.

Implications of Mobilization Splints

There are many implications for the use of dynamic splinting that become more familiar to the therapist with increased exposure to various hand injuries. Some specific indications for the use of dynamic splints are presented in this chapter.

However, it is important to note that the therapist must first understand the person's injury, surgical procedures, and physician's protocol for treatment. If any of these conditions are in question, the therapist should seek clarification prior to splinting.

Substitution for Loss of Motor Function

Whether the person has a peripheral nerve injury, spinal cord injury, or other debilitating disease, a splint can increase the functional use of a hand. The goals of splinting for loss of muscle function are to substitute for loss of motor use, prevent overstretching of nonfunctioning muscles, and prevent joint deformity. Both dynamic and static splints can accomplish these goals [Fess et al. 2005].

A common peripheral nerve injury is high radial nerve palsy. A hand with radial nerve damage has limited functional use due to the inability to extend the wrist and metacarpophalangeal (MCP) joints, and because of the lack of palmar abduction and radial abduction of the thumb. A splint that provides passive assistance to the wrist and MCP joints in extension while allowing active composite flexion of the fingers will greatly increase the functional use of the hand (see also Chapter 13, Figure 13-8).

Another example of substitution for loss of motor function involves persons with spinal cord injuries. A person who has a C7 lesion may also benefit from dynamic splinting. The person's active wrist extension will become the force to transmit motion for finger flexion in a tenodesis splint (Figure 11-1).

Finally, persons who have debilitating diseases such as amyotrophic lateral sclerosis, Guillain-Barré syndrome, or other neurologic disorders may benefit from specialized dynamic splints. However, the presence of spasticity might preclude candidates for dynamic splinting (see Chapter 14).

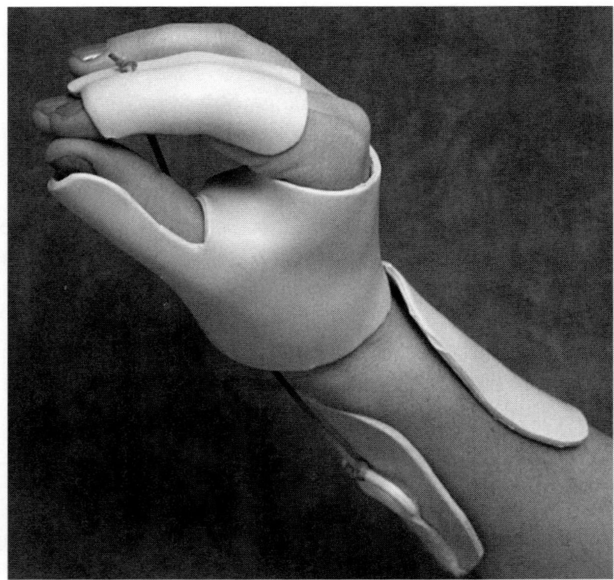

Figure 11-1 A tenodesis splint uses active wrist extension to aid passive finger flexion.

Correction of a Joint Deformity

Limited passive joint range of motion might be a result of multiple factors, including prolonged immobilization, trauma, or significant scar formation. A person who exhibits limited passive joint motion may be a candidate for a dynamic splint. However, if a large discrepancy exists between active and passive joint motion the goal of treatment should focus on active range of motion and strengthening prior to splinting. If active range of motion and passive range of motion are similar, greater active motion can be gained through mobilization splinting [Colditz 2002a].

The best results from dynamic splinting are attained when the therapist initiates treatment soon after edema and pain are under control. As mentioned previously in this text, the best way to lengthen tissue is to provide a tolerable force over a long period of time. Research indicates a direct correlation between the length of time a stiff joint is held at its end range and the resulting gain achieved with passive joint motion [Flowers and LaStayo 1994]. The focus of dynamic splinting should be on increasing the length of time the splint is worn rather than increasing the force. However, certain conditions (such as dense ligaments or scar tissue) generally always require a greater amount of force to achieve tissue remodeling.

Application of external force necessitates careful attention to the distribution of pressures over the skin surface because the skin is always the weak link in the system. A general goal for a mobilization splint is to increase passive joint range of motion by 10 degrees per week [Brand 2002]. Should passive range of motion not improve following two weeks of splinting, the splinting and treatment program should be reevaluated [Fess and McCollum 1998].

Provision of Controlled Motion

Therapists use dynamic splinting to control motion after the completion of joint implant arthroplasty and flexor tendon repairs. Because of the altered joint mechanics of a person who has arthritis and undergoes joint replacement surgery, the dynamic splint has multiple functions. First, dynamic splints provide controlled motion and precise alignment of the repaired soft tissue while minimizing soft-tissue deformity. For example, after joint replacement the splint may provide forces on one finger in both extension and radial deviation. Second, the splint maintains alignment of the joints for the healing structures while allowing guarded movement of the joint [Fess et al. 2005].

After flexor tendon repairs, the therapist uses a dynamic splint to provide controlled motion to the healing structures. The reasons for controlled motion are threefold. First, moving the tendons increases the flow of nutrient-rich synovial fluid to enhance healing. Second, tendons allowed early mobilization have demonstrated increased tensile strength compared to immobile tendons. Third, by allowing 3 to 5 mm of tendon excursion adhesion formation between tendons and surrounding structures is minimized [Stewart and van Strien 2002].

Aid in Fracture Alignment and Wound Healing

Dynamic traction should be used for the treatment of selected intra-articular fractures of the finger [Hardy 2004]. A dynamic traction splint involves the use of static tension while allowing joint movement. Traction provides tension to the ligaments, which incorporates the use of ligamentotaxis to bring boney fragments back into anatomic alignment. With constant traction applied throughout the range of motion, the splint allows the fracture to heal while maintaining adequate glide of surrounding soft tissues. Mobilization splints may also be used following a severe burn to assist in wound healing. The use of such splinting during wound healing will facilitate proper collagen alignment and scar formation.

Biomechanics of Dynamic Splinting

Anatomic Considerations

To fabricate a dynamic splint accurately, a therapist must understand the principles of hand biomechanics and must know in what ways the application of external force affects normal hand function [Fess 2002]. Knowledge of complex mathematical calculations is not required for a therapist to have a basic understanding of the biomechanics of dynamic splinting.

The goal of a mobilization splint is to restore a joint's normal range of motion, and to minimize the effects of inflammation and scar tissue. Application of an external force to healing joint structures raises the following questions. During what stage in the healing process should a splint be used to apply force? How much force should the splint apply? Where should the force be applied? The therapist should exercise caution when applying force to an injured joint until the inflammation and pain are under control. Mild inflammation is acceptable, but edema should not fluctuate significantly. A mobilization splint applied too early after injury might result in increased inflammation and decreased motion.

Soft-tissue structures respond to prolonged stress by changing or reforming. This activity is called *creep* and results from the application of prolonged force [Brand and Hollister 1993b]. Soft tissue responds to excessive force with increased pain and a reintroduction of the inflammatory process [Fess and McCollum 1998]. By applying controlled stress to the tissue over a prolonged period of time, the therapist can create tension gentle enough to allow creep without tissue injury. Provided it remains within elastic limits, the stress from a mobilization splint can positively affect the gradual realignment of collagen fibers (resulting in increased tensile strength of the tissue) without causing microscopic tearing of the tissue. The ability to alter collagen formation is greatest during the proliferative stage of wound healing but continues to a lesser degree for several months during scar maturation [Colditz 2002].

Torque and Mechanical Advantage

To provide the greatest benefit from a mobilizing splint, the therapist must understand relevant theories of physics. *Mechanical advantage* involves the consideration of various forces applied by the splint base and the dynamic portion of the splint. As seen in Figure 11-2, *Fa* refers to the applied force and *Fr* refers to the resistance force. *Fm* is determined by the sum of the opposing forces (Fa + Fr) [Fess 1995]. Mechanical advantage is defined as [Brand 2002]:

- Length of the lever arm of the applied force (*la*)
- Length of the lever arm of the applied resistance (*lr*)

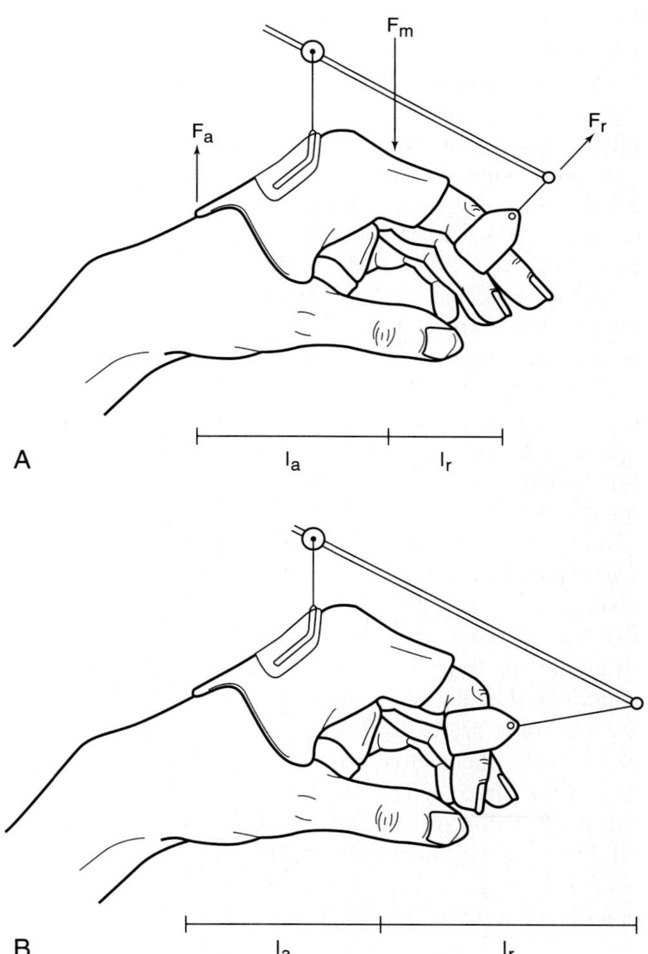

Figure 11-2 Mechanical advantage is determined by the ratio of the lever arm length (*la*) of the applied force (*Fa*) to the lever arm (*lr*) of the applied resistance (*Fr*). Splint A has a better mechanical advantage than splint B.

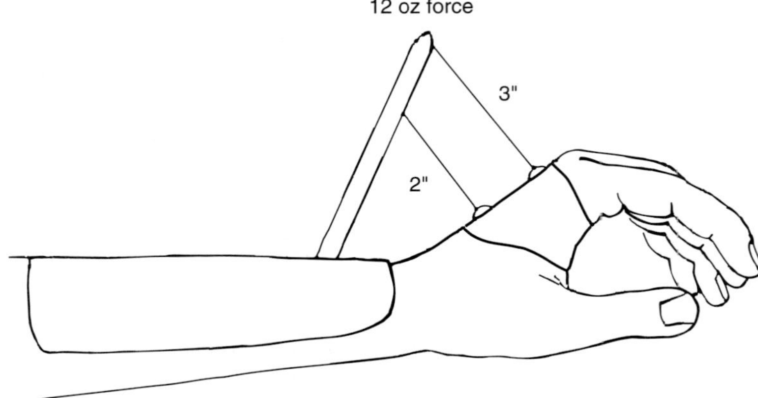

Figure 11-3 The 2-inch moment arm produces 24 inch ounces of torque. The 3-inch moment arm produces 36 inch ounces of torque.

By adjusting the length of the splint base or the length of the outrigger, the mechanical advantage can be altered (Figure 11-2) [Smith et al. 1996]. The goal of a splint is to maintain a mechanical advantage of between 2/1 and 5/1, meaning that the lever arm of the applied force is at least twice as long as the lever arm of the applied resistance [Brand 2002]. A splint with a greater mechanical advantage will be more comfortable and durable [Fess 1995]. A mobilizing MCP flexion splint that is forearm and hand based rather than just hand based will disperse pressures in addition to providing a greater mechanical advantage due to the longer lever areas of the applied force.

Torque is defined as the effect of force on the rotational movement of a point [Fess et al. 2005]. The amount of torque is calculated by multiplying the applied force by the length of the moment arm (Figure 11-3). A correlation exists between the distance from a pivot point and the amount of force required. To achieve the same results, a force applied close to the pivot point (i.e., short moment arm) must be greater than the force applied on a longer moment arm. This force is called *torque* because it acts on the rotational movement of a joint.

In practical terms, the therapist should place the force as far as possible from the mobilized joint without affecting other joints [Brand and Hollister 1993b]. A forearm-based dynamic wrist extension splint should be constructed so that its mobilizing force is on the most distal aspect of the palm, while not affecting MCP movement. An exception to placing the force as far from the mobilized joint as possible occurs when rheumatoid arthritis is involved. If the joint is unstable, a force applied too far from the joint will result in tilt rather than a gliding motion of the joint (Figure 11-4) [Hollister and Giurintano 1993]. Therefore, when splinting a hand with rheumatoid arthritis the force should be applied as close to the mobilizing joint as possible.

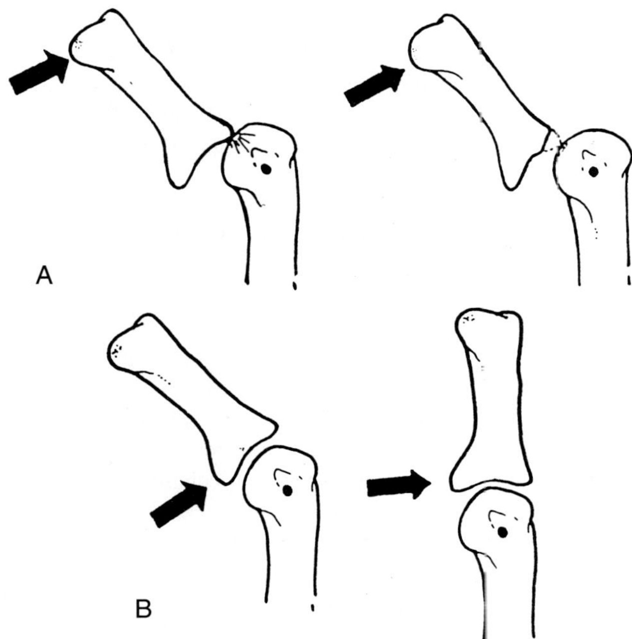

Figure 11-4 A force applied too far from an unstable joint will result in "tilt" (A) rather than glide (B). (From Hunter JM, Mackin EJ, Callahan AD (eds.) (1995). Rehabilitation of the Hand, Fourth Edition. St. Louis: Mosby p. 1586.)

Application of Force

In dynamic splinting, the therapist applies force to a joint or finger through the application of nail hooks, finger loops, or a palmar bar. When applying force to increase passive joint range of motion, the therapist must keep the direction of pull at a 90-degree angle to the axis of the joint and perpendicular to the axes of rotation [Cannon et al. 1985]. As range of motion increases, the therapist must adjust the outrigger to maintain the 90-degree angle (Figure 11-5) [Fess et al. 2005]. The outrigger should not pull the finger or hand toward ulnar or radial deviation.

When excessive force is applied to the skin for a prolonged period, tissue damage can result. The amount of pressure the skin can tolerate dictates the maximum tolerable force. As a general rule, the amount of acceptable pressure or force per unit area is 50 g/cm^2 [Brand and Hollister 1993a]. As the

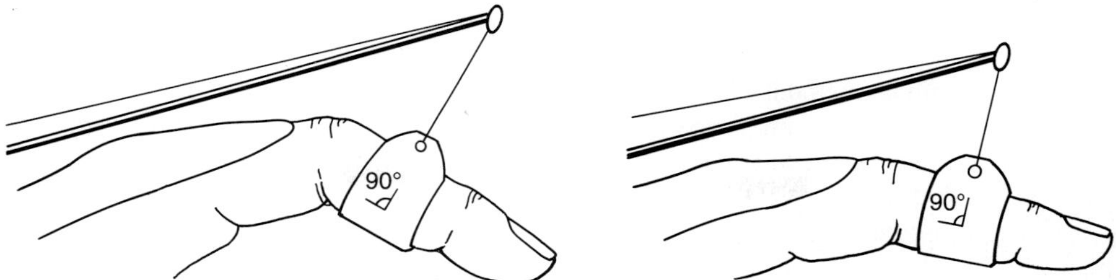

Figure 11-5 The line of tension must be maintained at 90 degrees from the long axis of the bone.

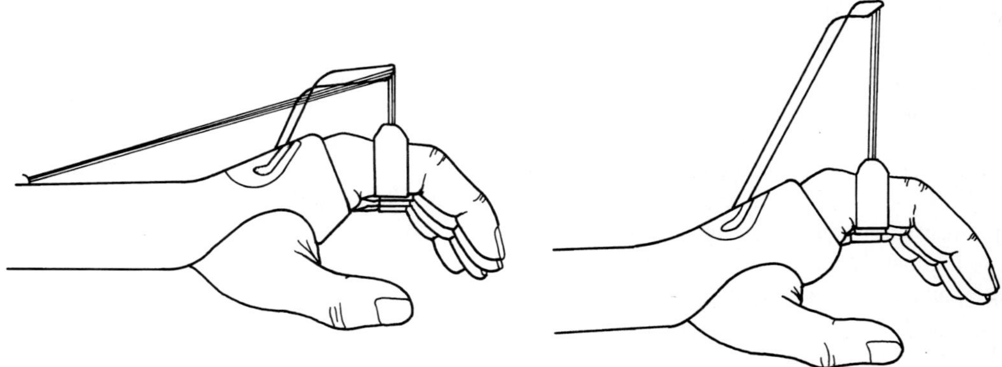

Figure 11-6 A low-profile outrigger (left) versus a high-profile outrigger (right).

area over which force is applied becomes larger, the pressure per unit area becomes less. A leather sling with a skin contact area on a finger of approximately 4 cm^2 should provide a maximum pressure of 200 g [Fess at al. 2005]. A smaller sling with less skin contact area concentrates the pressure and is less tolerable.

Skin grafts, immature scar tissue, and fragile skin of older persons have less tolerance for sling pressure. The person's tolerance ultimately determines the amount of force. The person should report the sensation of a *gentle* stretch, not pain [Fess 2002]. To avoid harm, the therapist should monitor the splint for the first 20 to 30 minutes of wear and at every treatment session thereafter. The person must also be educated on the importance of monitoring the splint for signs of pressure areas and skin breakdown, as well as how to don and doff the splint properly.

Features of a Mobilization Splint

Two features unique to mobilization splinting are the use of an outrigger and the application of force. The outrigger is a projection from the splint base the therapist uses to position a mobilizing force. The outrigger material depends on the amount and position of the desired force. If the outrigger and attachment to the base are not secure, the direction of the mobilizing force may change—reducing the effectiveness of the splint [Colditz 1983].

An outrigger can be a high or low profile (Figure 11-6). Each type has advantages and disadvantages. With a significant change in range of motion, the high-profile outrigger will result in slightly less deviation from the 90-degree angle of pull than the low-profile outrigger. Clients should be seen in the clinic frequently enough that increases in range of motion can be accommodated by regular adjustments to the outrigger, thus maintaining the 90-degree angle of pull [Austin et al. 2004]. It should be noted that a high-profile outrigger, on the other hand, is bulky and may decrease the person's compliance with wearing the splint. A low-profile outrigger requires adjustments more frequently but is more aesthetically pleasing and less cumbersome.

Various materials might be used for outriggers. The therapist may roll a thermoplastic material that has a high level of self-adherence to form a thick, tubular outrigger. This material offers easy adjustment by reshaping the plastic. However, a thermoplastic material outrigger may make the splint more cumbersome and thus reduce the person's compliance with the wearing schedule. There are also commercially available low-temperature tubes that are easily formed and less cumbersome.

A therapist can form an outrigger from ⅛-inch wire rod. This diameter is thick enough to provide stability yet pliable enough to manipulate with pliers. Construction of an outrigger using a wire rod requires precise shaping, a skill that necessitates practice. Commercial adjustable wire outrigger kits are also available. Although the use of a commercial kit may increase the material cost of the splint, the application of the adjustable components is easier and may thus reduce splintmaking time. The therapist should bear in mind that charges for fabrication time are the most costly part of the splint.

The therapist can use various methods for applying dynamic force to a joint. Finger loops from strong pliable material are usually best because of the increased conformability to the shape of the finger [Fess et al. 2005]. The therapist can supply force by using rubber bands, springs, or elastic thread. Although rubber bands are more readily available and easy to adjust, springs offer more consistent tension throughout the range. A long rubber band stretched over the maximum length of the splint provides more constant tension than a short rubber band [Brand and Hollister 1993a]. Elastic thread is the easiest to apply and adjust. A nonstretchable string or outrigger line is necessary to connect the finger loop to the source of the force (Figure 11-7). The choice is usually based on clinical experience and preference.

Another method of applying force is through static progressive tension. Rather than providing the variable tension of a dynamic splint, a static tension splint uses nonelastic tension to provide a constant force. An advantage of properly applied static tension is that tissue is not stretched beyond the elastic limit [Schultz-Johnson 2002]. In place of the rubber band or spring (as used on a dynamic tension splint) the therapist may use a Velcro tab, turnbuckle, or commercially available static progressive components to apply the force (Figure 11-8). Tension is increased by gradually moving the Velcro tab more proximally on the splint base or adjusting the turnbuckle. The force is static rather than dynamic but is readily adjustable by the person throughout the wearing time (Figure 11-9). Because the person has control over the amount of applied tension, the static progressive splint is more tolerable to wear than a dynamic tension splint [Schultz-Johnson 2002].

In determining whether to apply dynamic or static tension, the therapist must identify the "end feel" of a joint. End feel is assessed by passively moving a joint to its maximal end range. A joint with a soft or springy end feel indicates immature scar tissue. A joint with a hard end feel indicates a more mature scar tissue or long-standing contracture. A splint with static or dynamic tension is appropriate for a joint with a soft end feel, whereas a joint with a hard end feel will respond only to static tension. Regardless of the end feel, static tension will increase passive range of motion faster than dynamic tension for any joint [Schultz-Johnson 1996].

Another determinant in selecting the type of tension to be used with mobilization splinting is the stage of tissue healing. As seen in Figure 11-10, different types of splints are more appropriate at various stages of healing. The acute stage is primarily characterized as the initial inflammatory stage. The proliferative stage occurs after the initial inflammation subsides and tissues are in the early stages of reorganization. The chronic stage is attained when the cells have realigned and the joint response to stress is a hard end feel [Colditz 1995].

Technical Tips for Dynamic Splinting

When applying an outrigger to the base, the therapist must ensure that both surfaces to be bonded are clean. If a plastic has a glossy finish, the two surfaces might require light scratching or a bonding agent to increase self-adherence. After placing the outrigger on the base appropriately, the therapist should hold the surfaces firmly together and smooth the edges until the plastic cools. To speed hardening, a vapocoolant spray may be used.

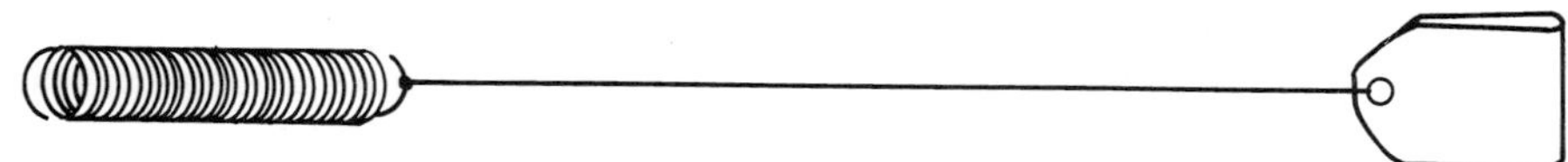

Figure 11-7 The therapist uses nonstretchable nylon string to attach finger loops to the source of tension.

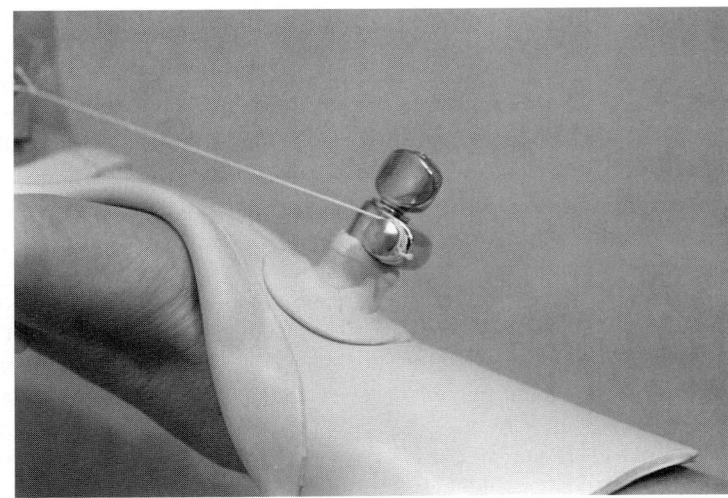

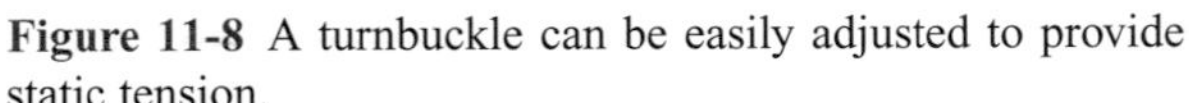

Figure 11-8 A turnbuckle can be easily adjusted to provide static tension.

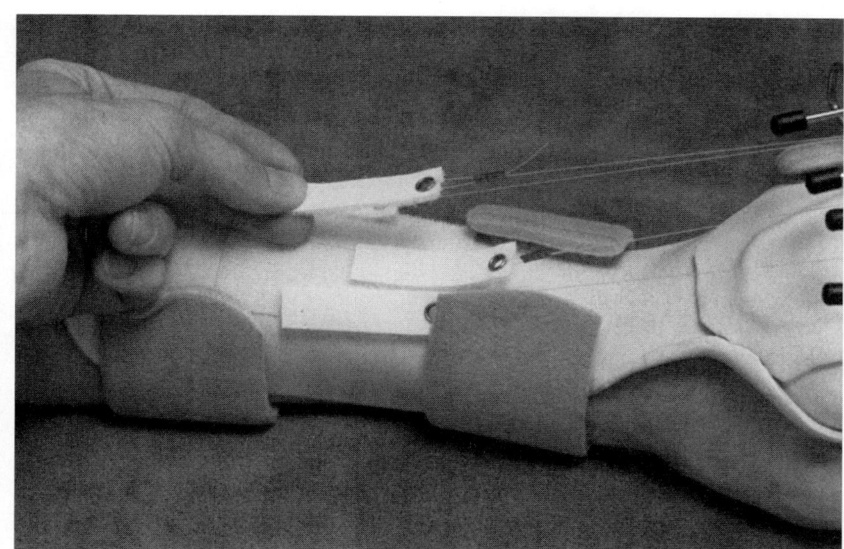

Figure 11-9 The person may adjust Velcro tabs used for static progressive tension.

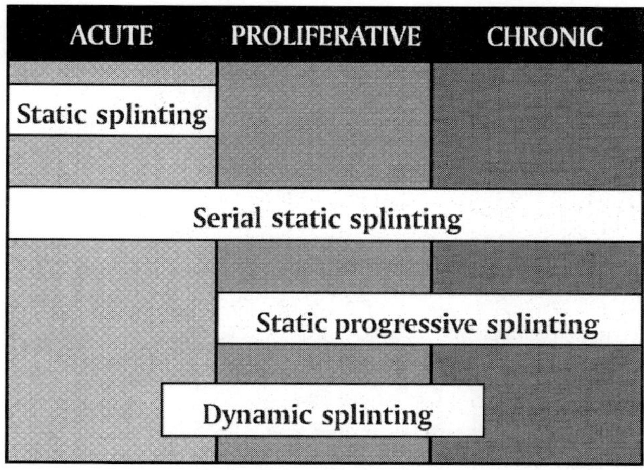

Figure 11-10 The stage of healing helps to determine the most appropriate type of splint. (From Hunter JM, Mackin EJ, Callahan AD (eds.) (1995). Rehabilitation of the Hand, Fourth Edition. St. Louis: Mosby 1155.)

The therapist should use caution when spot heating near an outrigger wire. Wire conducts heat more greatly than plastic, and thus the wire may push through the thermoplastic material. When splinting over bandages or a dressing, the therapist may place a damp paper towel or stockinette over the area to prevent the thermoplastic material from adhering to the dressing. The therapist should check the line of pull so that a 90-degree angle is present on the finger loops when axial and lateral views are observed. Finally, all joints should be checked from various angles to ensure that joints are not being pulled into hyperextension, ulnar deviation, or radial deviation.

Materials and Equipment for a Dynamic Splint

In addition to the equipment necessary to fabricate a static splint, a variety of items are required to fabricate a dynamic splint. The following is a list of materials and equipment

SELF-QUIZ 11-1*

Circle either true (T) or false (F).

1. T F A therapist should apply a dynamic splint to an extremity only when pain and inflammation are well controlled.
2. T F Creep occurs when soft tissue adapts through application of a prolonged force.
3. T F Persons who have new tissue or skin grafts have a high tolerance for pressure over those areas.
4. T F The focus of mobilization splinting should be on increasing the tension rather than increasing the amount of time the splint is worn.
5. T F A general goal for a dynamic splint is to increase passive range of motion by 10 degrees per week.
6. T F Joint end feel must be taken into consideration when determining whether to use static or dynamic tension.

*See Appendix A for the answer key.

therapists use for dynamic splinting, although all items are not necessary for every splint.

- Thermoplastic material with a high level of self-adhesion
- Finger loops
- Nail hooks, an emery board, and super-glue
- Solvent
- Nonstretchable nylon string (outrigger line)
- An outrigger kit
- A wire rod (⅛ inch) with tools to bend
- Rubber bands, springs, elastic string, Velcro tabs, turnbuckles, or commercially available static progressive components
- Safety pins or other material to make a hook
- Pliers, wire bender

Mobilization splinting can be both fun and challenging. Three common mobilization splints include the flexor tendon splint, the mobilization PIP extension splint, and the radial palsy splint. These are described in the sections that follow.

Fabrication of a Flexor Tendon Splint

One common use of a dynamic splint is for a person who has an injury to one or more finger flexor tendons. The goals of postoperative *flexor* tendon repair are to [Loth and Wadsworth 1998]:

- Prevent re-rupture of the healing tendon
- Increase tensile strength of the repaired tendon
- Limit scar formation that will reduce tendon excursion

The splint assists in attaining these goals by maintaining the hand in a protected position while allowing controlled motion of the fingers [May et al. 1992]. This type of dynamic splint is one of the least complicated to fabricate because an outrigger is not required. However, it is a very demanding splint because initially it must be worn 24 hours per day (with removal only for therapy). Therefore, the fit must be very good to ensure comfort and to prevent migration of the splint. The therapist should also check the physician's preference in regard to the type of splint and wearing schedule because various protocols exist for tendon repairs. Although no protocol is universally accepted, two of the most common are the Kleinert [1983] and the Duran and Houser [1975] [Stewart and van Strien 2002]. The following splint is a modification of both protocols:

1. Apply the nail hooks to the person's fingernails so that the super-glue thoroughly dries before application of the force. Explain to the person the reason for the application of the hooks, and assure the person that removal of the hooks is possible. To increase the adherence of the hook, roughen the fingernail with an emery board and then clean the fingernail with an alcohol wipe. The hook may require an adjustment with two pairs of pliers to fit the contour of the nail (Figure 11-11A). Position the hooks so that they face the person. Hooks should be applied to the proximal nail bed to prevent avulsion of the fingernail (Figure 11-11B). When applying the hook, do not use on an excessive amount of glue. Glue that comes in a gel form may be easier to manage. Give the person extra hooks and application instructions because hooks may occasionally break off. Alternatives to the nail hooks are adhesive Velcro loop applied to the nail and sutures placed through physician-created holes in the nail during surgery.
2. Construct the pattern for a dorsal hand and forearm splint, similar to that shown in Figure 11-12. Select thermoplastic material with a property of drapability.

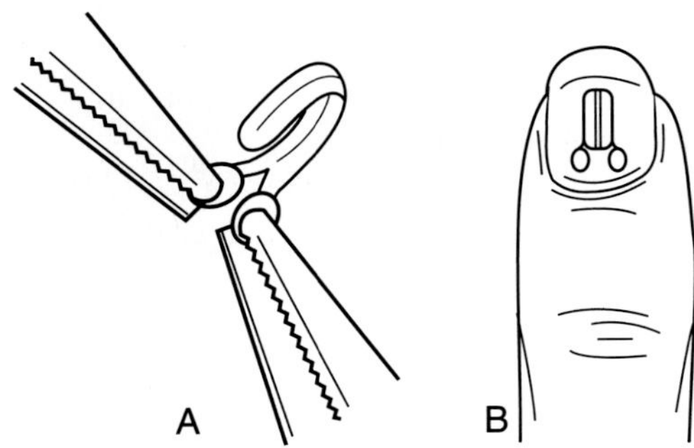

Figure 11-11 (A) Pliers may be used to adjust the hook to fit the contour of the fingernail. (B) The nail hook is applied to the proximal nail bed.

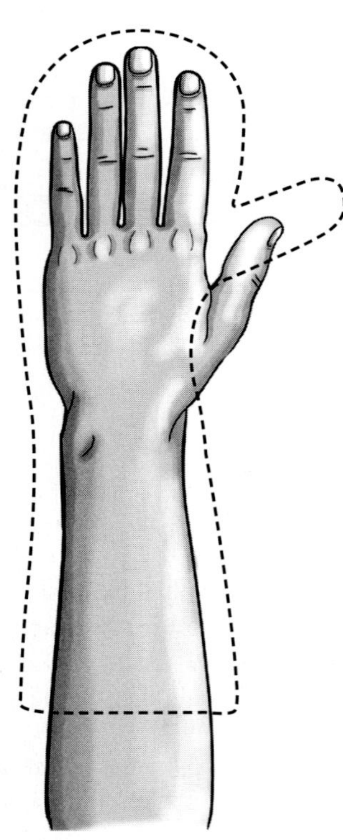

Figure 11-12 Pattern for a dorsal block splint that is used after flexor tendon repair.

Remember to design the pattern to cover two-thirds the length of the forearm and half the circumference of the forearm. The distal end of the splint should extend about 1 inch beyond the tips of the fingers. Form the splint base over the dorsal surface of the forearm, wrist, and hand while molding the palmar bar. The ideal hand position is 30 to 45 degrees of wrist flexion, 50 to 70 degrees of MCP flexion, and the interphalangeals (IPs) in full extension [May et al. 1992] (Figure 11-13). If the hand has just been removed from the postoperative bulky dressing, the person may not tolerate the ideal position. If this occurs, splint as close as possible to the ideal position and adjust the splint when tolerable. Plastics with memory are helpful in reforming the splint's positions.

3. Use a heat gun to create a bubble over the radial styloid and distal ulna to avoid pressure, or pad the bony prominence.
4. Apply straps with hook-and-loop Velcro at the following locations: across the palmar bar, at the wrist, 3 inches proximal to the wrist, and across the forearm (Figure 11-14).

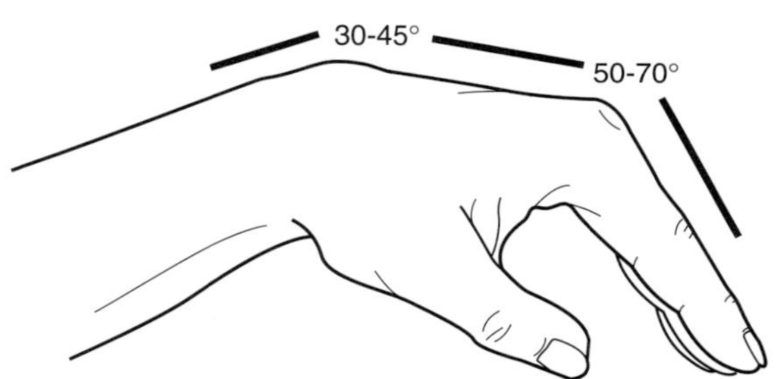

Figure 11-13 The ideal position after flexor tendon repair is 30 to 45 degrees of wrist flexion, 50 to 70 degrees of metacarpal phalangeal flexion, and full interphalangeal extension.

5. Attach a safety pin to the strap that crosses the wrist approximately 3 inches proximal to the wrist crease (see Figure 11-14).
6. Apply traction using elastic thread attached to the nail hooks at the distal end and to the safety pin at the proximal end. Use elastic thread due to its ability to stretch while maintaining a fairly constant tension. Apply the force to hold the fingers in flexion, but allow the person to achieve full active extension of the IP joints against the force of the elastic (Figure 11-15). It may take a few days before full IP extension is attained if the client had been immobilized previously with the fingers flexed. As IP extension improves, adjust the splint elastic tension to maintain passive finger flexion while allowing full active extension.

Achieving full PIP and distal IP extension is important because flexion contractures are a common complication following flexor tendon repair [Jebson and Kasdan 1998]. If the person is unable to attain full PIP extension, a wedge may be placed behind the involved finger(s). The purpose of the wedge is to increase MCP flexion, thus decreasing flexor tension and increasing PIP extension (Figure 11-16).

Zone II Flexor Tendon Repairs

Due to the confined arrangement of tendons within the pulley system, flexor tendon injuries in zone II are highly susceptible to adhesions (Figure 11-17) [Duran et al. 1990]. A palmar pulley might provide greater excursion of tendons from these lesions. This pulley can be created by firmly securing an additional piece of thermoplastic with eyelets for each finger (Figure 11-18). The palmar bar also serves to maintain the palmar arch and prevents splint migration. The elastic thread runs through the palmar pulley as the person actively performs approximately 10 repetitions of active finger extension every hour. The treatment rationale is to

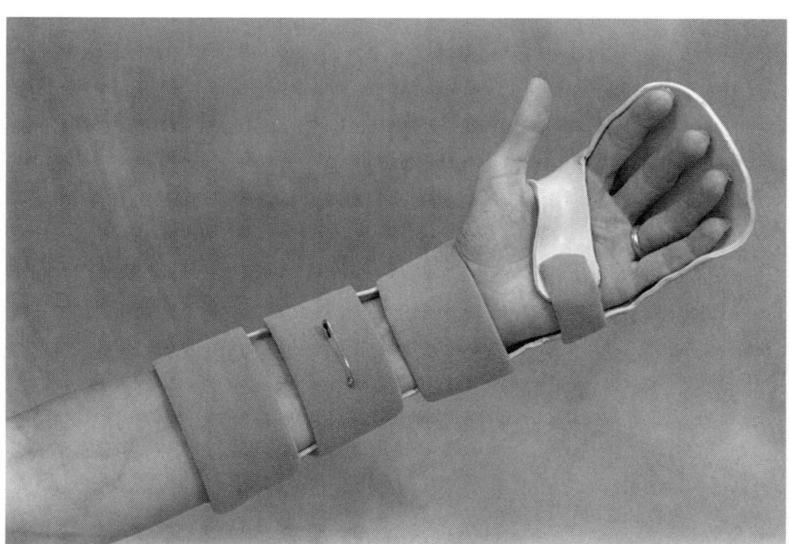

Figure 11-14 Straps are applied across the palmar bar, at the wrist, 3 inches proximal to the wrist, and at the forearm. The safety pin is fixed to the strap 3 inches proximal to the wrist crease.

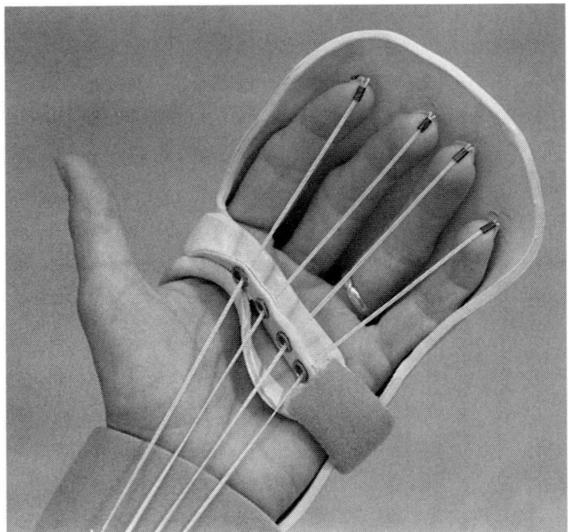

Figure 11-15 The person must be able to attain full IP active extension against the force of the tension.

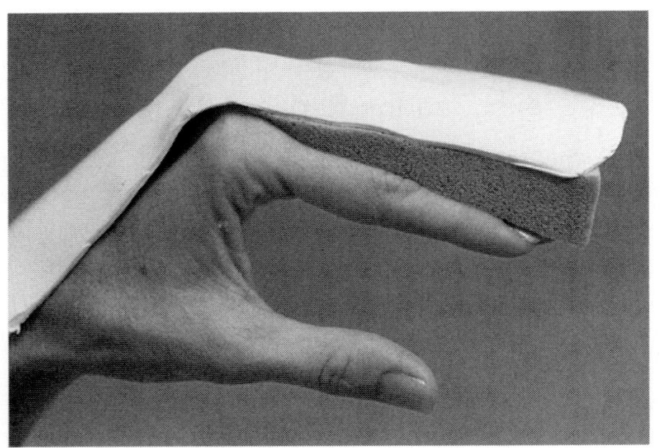

Figure 11-16 To attain full PIP extension, a wedge may be inserted.

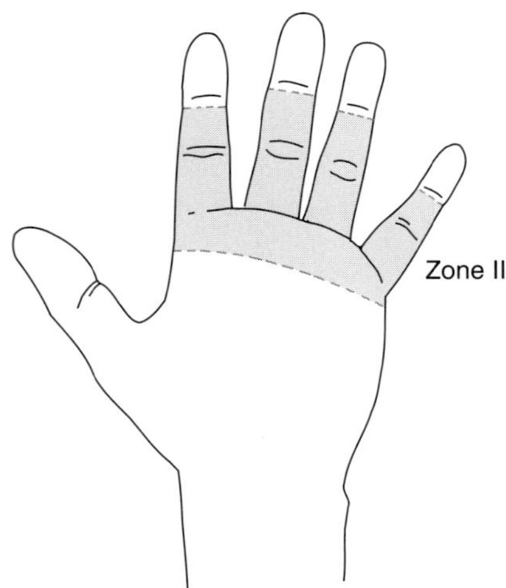

Figure 11-17 A palmar pulley may be best for tendon injuries in zone II.

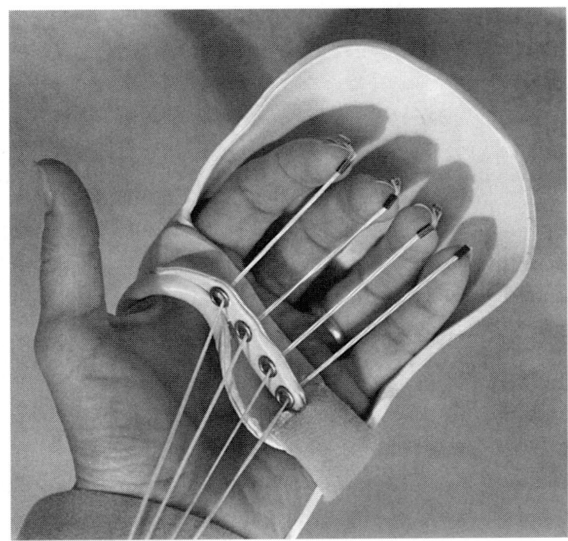

Figure 11-18 An attachment may be added to the palmar bar to increase tendon excursion in zone II injuries.

increase excursion of the tendon, limit scar formation, and increase tensile strength of the repair [May et al. 1992].

The therapist may apply a strap to the distal aspect of the fingers in order to maintain full IP extension (Figure 11-19). This application may also reduce the loss of extension at the IP joints [May et al. 1992]. Generally, the strap is intended only for night wear—traction being maintained throughout the day. If, however, the person has developed or is developing an IP flexion contracture the person may alternate between flexion traction and the extension strap during the day. The therapist should issue the person a written home program consisting of a splint-wearing schedule, instructions regarding splint care, and therapeutic exercises.

Fabrication of a Mobilizing PIP Extension Splint

The PIP joint is the most important joint of the finger with regard to functional hand use. A PIP joint that cannot fully extend limits the ability of the hand to grasp large objects, inhibits the person's ability to place a hand in a pocket, and hinders other functional activities [Prosser 1996]. A mobilizing PIP extension splint is designed to help regain limited passive extension of the PIP joint. A loss of PIP extension may occur following soft-tissue damage at the PIP joint; crush injury, burn, or fracture around the PIP joint; or flexor tendon repair. There are many splint options to regain PIP motion, including both custom-fit and prefabricated splints.

For a custom-fit splint, an outrigger kit with extender rods is practical to use due to the ease of adjustment as the person's range of motion increases. The commercial outrigger usually contains a wire outrigger, extender rod, Allen wrench, rubber cap for the rod, and adjustment wheel to

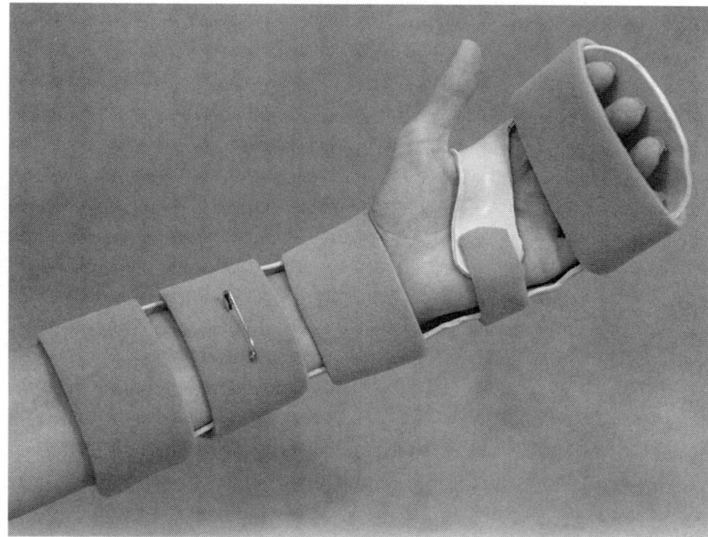

Figure 11-19 The person may use a strap to secure fingers in extension for night wear.

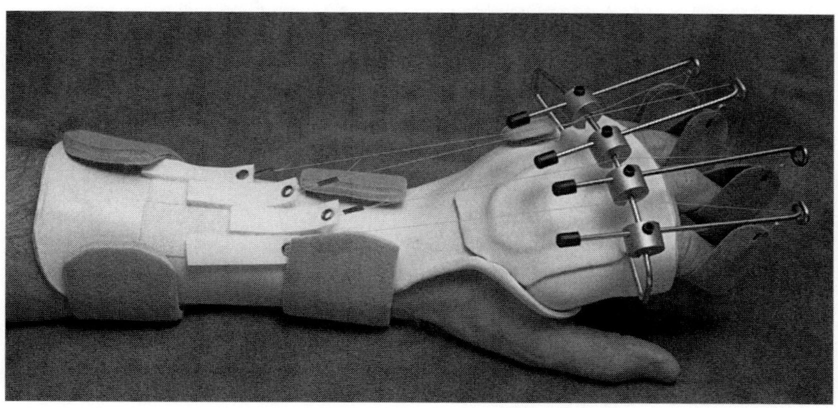

Figure 11-20 A splint to increase PIP extension at the index through small fingers.

secure the rods to the outrigger. This PIP extension splint is hand based in order to prevent immobilization of the non-involved wrist joint. Instead of springs or Velcro tabs, the therapist uses a rubber band to provide a dynamic progressive force. Multiple-finger outrigger kits are also available for this type of splint (Figure 11-20). The following are instructions for creating a hand-based splint.

1. Fabricate a pattern for a hand-based splint. The splint is primarily dorsally based, with the MCP joint of the involved finger immobilized (Figure 11-21A). A thermoplastic material that has high drapability is the most appropriate for this splint. As the splint is conformed to the person's hand, maintain a 45-degree angle of MCP flexion while molding the splint around the proximal phalanx and the first web space. If necessary, the ulnar bar may be reheated later and conformed to the ulnar aspect and palm of the hand. The following is a checklist for the splint base (letters in parentheses correspond to those in Figure 11-21B).
    - The distal aspect of the splint must be proximal to the PIP joint in order to allow unrestricted motion (A).
    - At the first web space, the splint should not limit thumb opposition (B). This edge of the splint may be rolled if necessary.
    - MCP extension of non-involved fingers should not be limited (C).
    - Wrist motion should not be limited by the proximal aspect of the splint (D).
2. Remove the splint from the person. Using a leather punch, make a small hole in the dorsal ulnar aspect of the splint (Figure 11-21B). Using the heat gun, warm the area around the hole. With an Allen wrench, lift the area (Figure 11-21C) to form a site for later attachment of the rubber band. The rubber band may also be attached using and adhesive strap with a D-ring.
3. Reapply the splint to the person. Attach the outrigger as follows:
    a. With the adjustment wheel and extender rod loosely attached to the outrigger, position the outrigger on the splint so that the rod is parallel to and centered on the proximal phalanx.
    b. With the outrigger in place, mark the splint where the ends of the wire are to be attached to the base (Figure 11-21D).

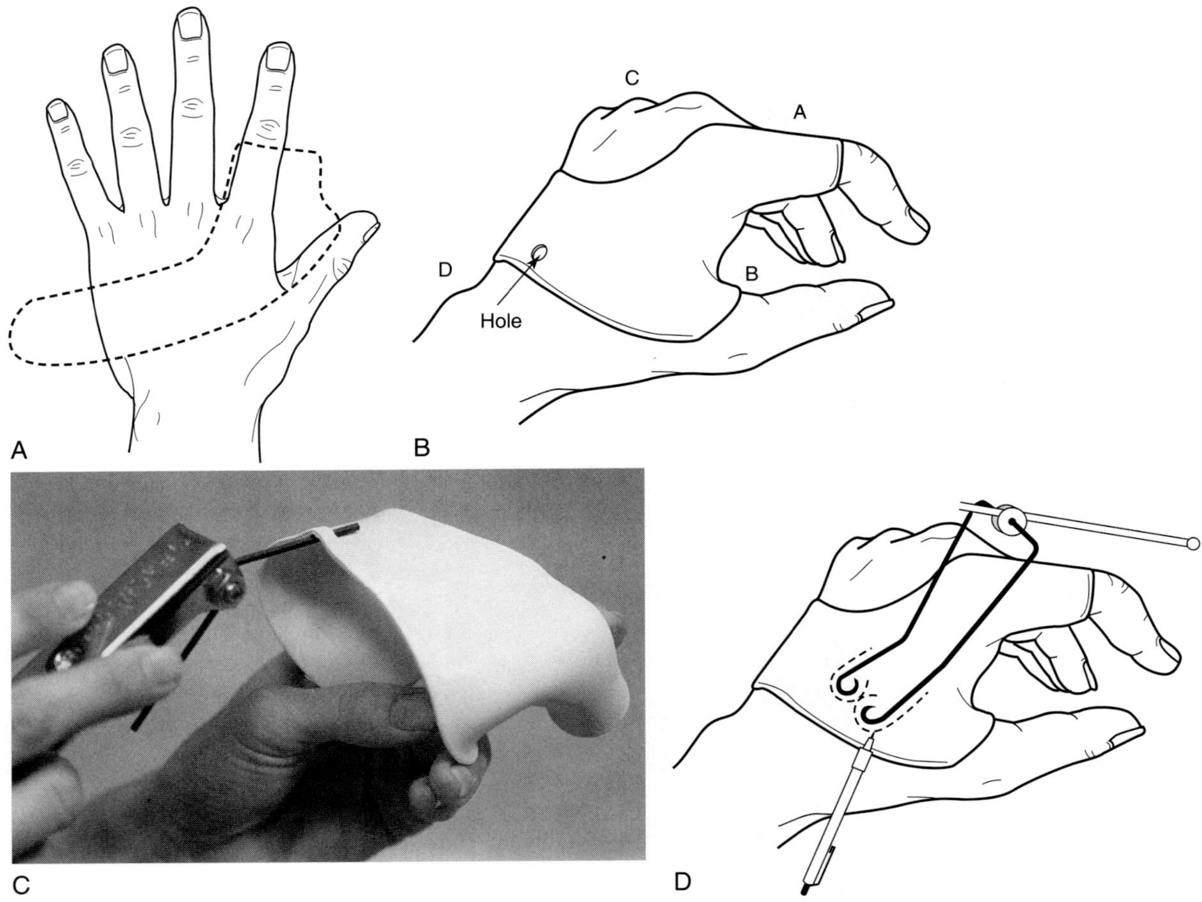

Figure 11-21 (A) Splint pattern for a hand-based PIP extension splint. (B) Splint base checklist. (C) An Allen wrench or other small tool may be used to raise the edge of the splint to form a site for attachment of the elastic tension. (D) With the extender rod appropriately positioned above the finger, the therapist draws an outline of the outrigger on the splint base.

4. Remove the splint from the person. If the extender rod is in the way, remove it before attaching the outrigger to the base.
5. Cut a piece of thermoplastic material large enough to extend beyond the outrigger base by at least ½ inch on each side.
6. Heat the outrigger wire over a heat gun, and slightly embed the wire into the splint base.
7. Lightly scratch the surface or apply solvent to the warm piece of thermoplastic material to increase the bonding.
8. Place the warm thermoplastic material over the outrigger base, and secure the material to the splint base by pressing the material securely around the outrigger wire.
9. Loosely reattach the extender rod to the outrigger.
10. Apply the splint to the person's hand.
11. If a prefabricated finger loop is not available, one can be made using soft leather or polyethylene. A sling that is 4 inches long and 1 inch wide will be appropriate for most adult fingers. Holes are punched at the two ends of the sling for the line attachment. The long edges may need slight trimming so that the sling does not interfere with movement of non-involved joints. With the loop in place on the middle phalanx and nylon string placed through the rod, position the extender rod to obtain a 90-degree angle of pull (Figure 11-22A). Gently tighten the rods in place using the Allen wrench.
12. Secure the appropriate rubber band to the nylon string so that the tension pulls the joint to a well-tolerated end range (Figure 11-22B).
13. Remove the splint from the person and finish securing the extender rod. If the rods extend more than ½ inch proximal to the adjustment wheels, the rod may be cut using heavy-duty wire cutters. For safety reasons, snip the excess extender rod when the person is not wearing the splint.
14. Place a protective rubber cap on the end of the rod.

Fabrication of a Composite Finger Flexion Splint with Static Progressive Tension

Following trauma to the wrist or hand, a person may often experience joint pain or stiffness that limits the ability to attain composite finger flexion. Whereas therapy will focus

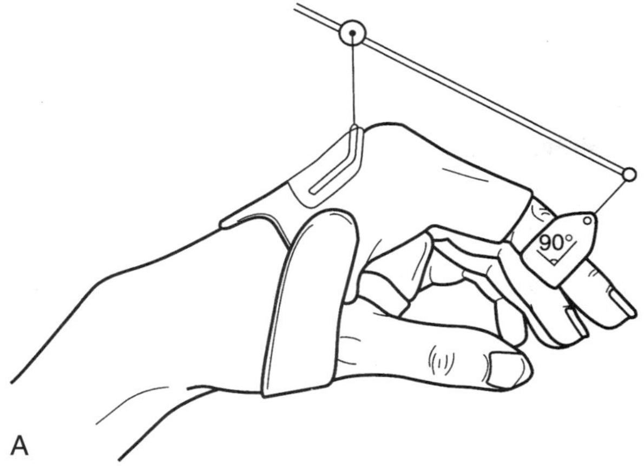

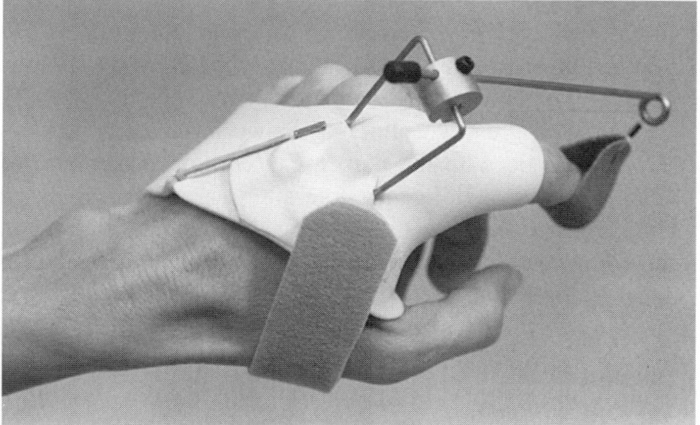

Figure 11-22 (A) The extender rod is adjusted to provide a 90-degree angle of pull on the middle phalanx. (B) A rubber band or elastic thread is attached to nylon string and adjusted to provide appropriate tension.

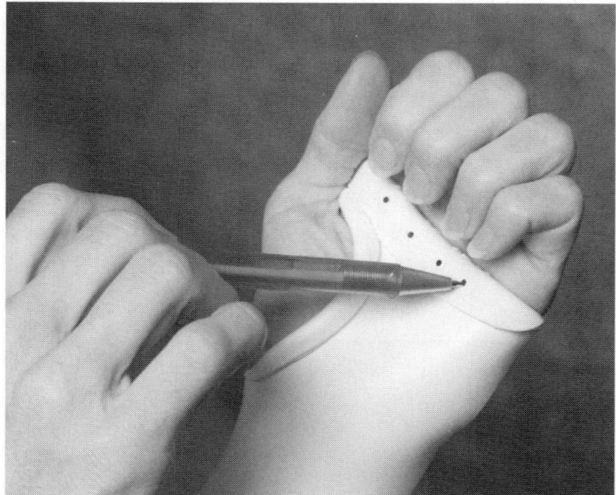

Figure 11-23 A mark is applied to the palmar bar at the point where each finger achieves composite flexion.

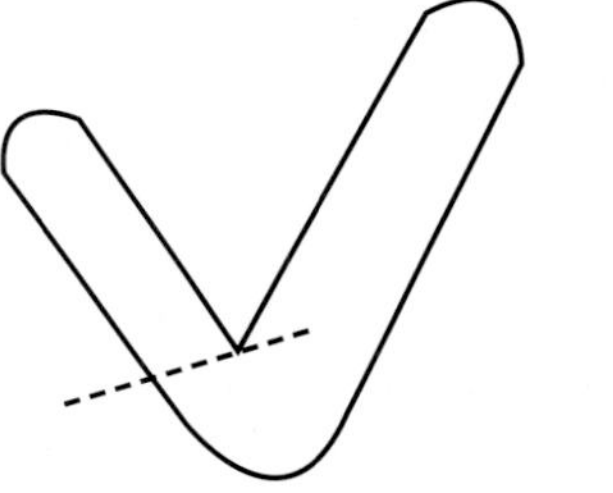

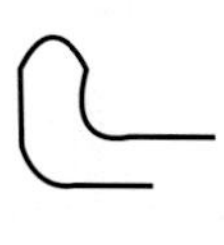

Figure 11-24 Using pliers, bend the wire at a half-way mark to form a 90-degree angle.

on restoring joint range of motion of the individual joints in addition to composite finger flexion, a splint that focuses on providing a low-load prolonged stress to all of the joints will maximize the return of function. This splint uses static progressive tension to allow the person to control the amount of force required to maintain the tissue at a maximum tolerable stretch [Schultz-Johnson 2002]. Although a custom-made component will be utilized for this splint, a commercially available "Bio-dynamic" component for finger sleeves is available through Smith-Nephew, Roylan.

1. Fabricate a volar-based wrist immobilization splint with straps as directed in Chapter 7. Ensure that the distal aspect of the splint does not limit MCP flexion of the index through small fingers.
2. With the splint applied to the person, mark on the distal palmar bar where the fingers would touch with full composite finger flexion (Figure 11-23a). Remove the splint from the person.
3. A line guide for the monofilament will be created using a metal non rubber-coated paper clip. Using wire cutters, snip a section of the paper clip to form a ?-inch loop. With pliers, bend at the midsection to form a 90-degree angle (Figure 11-24).

4. Grasping the bent paper clip with a pair of pliers, hold over a heat gun for approximately 10 seconds. *Carefully* insert the metal clip into the rolled aspect of the palmar bar where previously marked (Figure 11-25).
5. For each finger to be included in the splint, two finger sleeves will be required: one for the proximal phalanx and one for the distal phalanx. Cut two ¾-inch by 3-inch pieces of Velfoam or other similar hook-and-loop material for each finger.
6. On the proximal sleeve, punch four (4) small holes at the midpoint and on the distal sleeve punch two small holes at the midpoint. As in Figure 11-26, the monofilament thread or other suitable material is threaded through the proximal sleeve to the distal sleeve and returning to the proximal sleeve.
7. Following reapplication of the thermoplastic splint, the finger sleeves are secured on the proximal and distal phalanges with a piece of Velcro hook. The monofilament pulley line will be located at the midpoint on the volar aspect of the finger. Note that the finger sleeve may need to be trimmed for a secure fit.
8. The long ends of the monofilament are threaded through the metal line guide.
9. While applying light tension to the finger sleeves, secure a Velcro hook tab to the end of the monofilament thread. Be sure to secure the tab on the distal end of the Velcro loop strip so as to allow improvements in range of motion without having to make further adjustments.
10. The person is then asked to secure the Velcro tab at a place that provides a gentle stretch to the finger(s). After 5 to 10 minutes of wearing the splint, the person may be able to increase the amount of tension. A mark may be placed on the Velcro loop where the tab is located in order for the person to note improvements as progress is made in range of motion and the tab is moved more proximally (Figure 11-27).

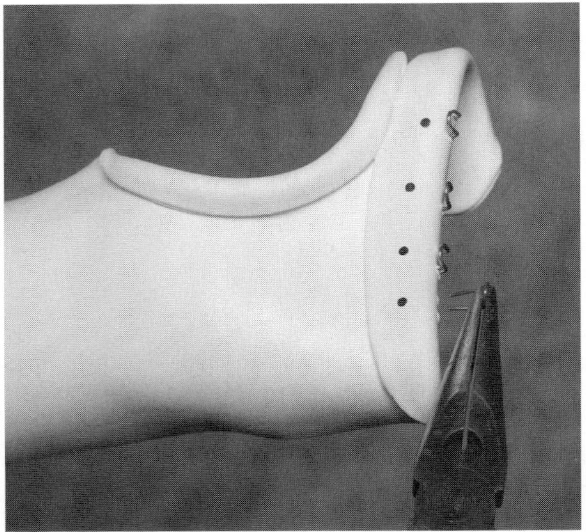

Figure 11-25 Using pliers, the open end of the heated wire is pushed through the distal aspect of the palmar bar where previously marked.

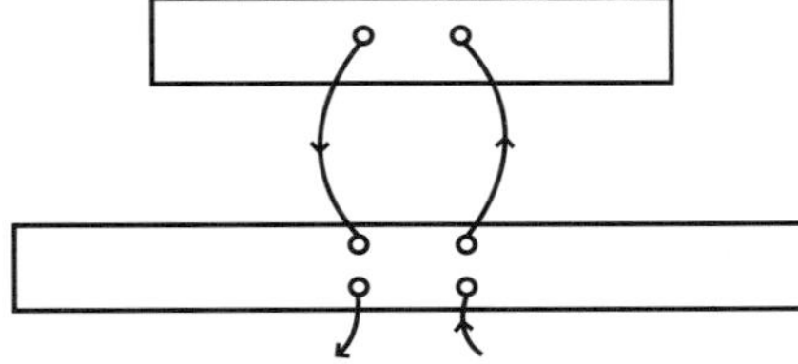

Figure 11-26 The monofilament is threaded through the finger sleeves in this manner.

Finger Flexion Splint Wearing Schedule

Initially the person is instructed to wear the splint for 30 minutes three to four times per day. If there are no complications, the splint wear time can be increased significantly. The static progressive splint may be worn for extended periods of time because the person can control the amount of tension. Some people may tolerate wearing the splint at night, thus eliminating the need for daytime splinting when the splint may interfere with functional activities [Schultz-Johnson 2002].

Fabrication of a Radial Palsy Splint

The radial nerve palsy splint does not involve the application of force to "mobilize" a joint, a process that typically defines dynamic splinting. Instead of a dynamic force, the splint uses a static line to support the fingers [Colditz 2002b]. The splint does, however, use an outrigger—which makes the construction similar to that of a dynamic splint. The splint described by the following instructions was initially designed by Crochetiere and was modified by Hollis and Colditz [Colditz 2002b].

A lesion to the radial nerve above the elbow results in loss of active wrist, thumb, and finger MCP extension.

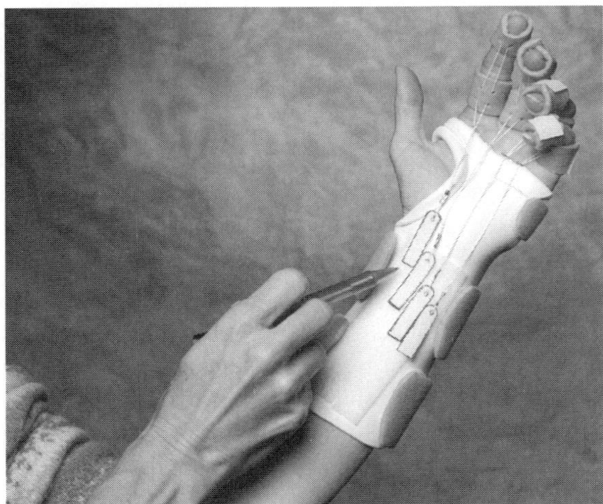

Figure 11-27 A pen mark is placed at the proximal border of the tab to identify improvements.

The inability to actively extend and stabilize the wrist and fingers limits the functional use of the hand. For many people with a high radial nerve injury, a static wrist support that maintains wrist extension will greatly enhance the function of the hand. However, for tasks that require full finger extension (such as keyboarding, grasping large objects, and repetitive factory work) a splint that provides thumb and MCP support is necessary. The goal of this splint is to create a limited tenodesis action to allow functional grip [Colditz 1987]. The splint includes a dorsal base with a low-profile outrigger that spans from the wrist to the proximal phalanx of each finger.

1. Draw a pattern that is the circumference and two-thirds the length of the forearm (Figure 11-28). Fabricate the dorsal forearm base of the radial nerve splint from a thermoplastic material that has self-adherence and drapability properties. Position the splint on the dorsal aspect of the forearm. Construct the splint so that it extends from the proximal aspect of the forearm to just proximal to the distal ulna. The base must be at least half the circumference of the forearm to prevent distal migration of the splint.
2. Apply straps to stabilize the splint base during formation of the outrigger.
3. Make the outrigger from ⅛-inch wire rod. The outrigger must be wider than the hand at the level of the MCPs by approximately ½ inch (Figure 11-29).
4. To form the outrigger properly, draw an outline of the hand and mark the MCP and PIP joints. Draw a curved line halfway between the joints and extend it ½ inch beyond the hand on each side. Form the distal aspect of the outrigger along this curved line (Figure 11-29).
5. Conform the proximal end of the outrigger wire to the splint base. The wire will have a slight dorsal angle at the level of the wrist (Figure 11-29). Excessive outrigger wire may be snipped. After forming the outrigger, secure it to the base with a piece of thermoplastic material prepared with solvent.
6. Drape an additional piece of thermoplastic material over the distal aspect of the outrigger (over the phalanges). Punch holes directly above each finger.
7. To decrease wear on the cord, metal eyelet reinforcements may be placed in each hole.
8. Form a hook from a paper clip and place it in the middle of the dorsal forearm splint (Figure 11-30). Apply the hook to the base with a small piece of thermoplastic material prepared with solvent.
9. Place the splint on the person to secure the finger loops and cord. The length of the cord should allow full finger extension when the wrist drops to neutral (Figure 11-31). During active finger flexion, the wrist should extend slightly. If the finger loops impinge on the MCP or PIP joints, the loops can be trimmed on the volar surface.

Radial Palsy Splint Wearing Schedule

This splint should be worn throughout the day as tolerated to assist the person with functional activities. When not completing specific activities, and during the night, the radial nerve splint is replaced with a static wrist support splint for greater comfort.

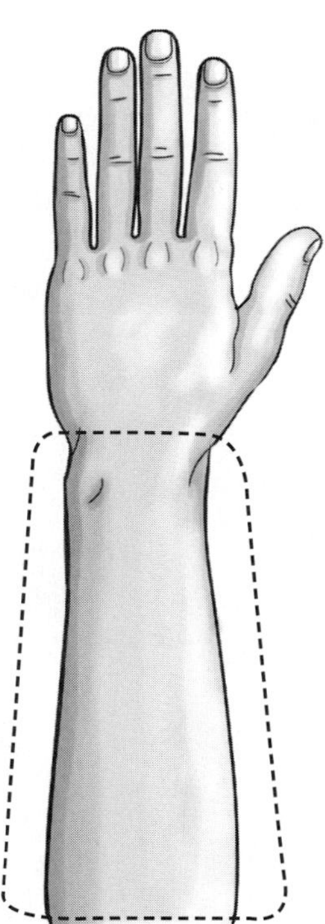

Figure 11-28 Pattern for radial nerve palsy splint.

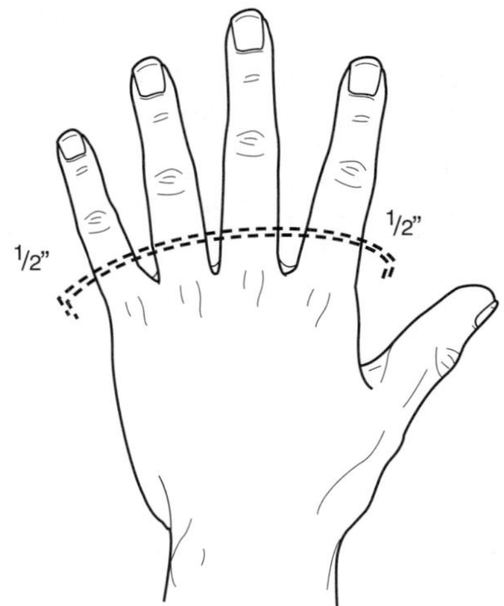

Figure 11-29 The curved outrigger must extend ½ inch beyond the hand at the level of the MCPs.

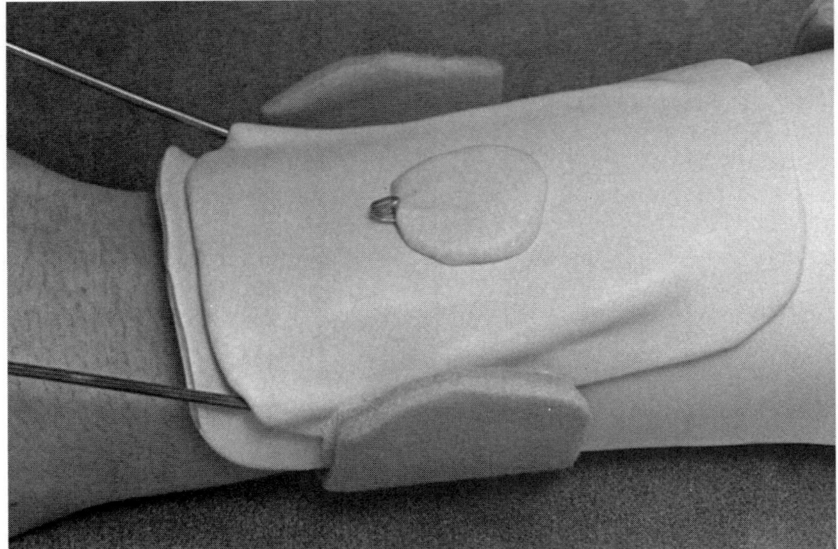

Figure 11-30 An anchor hook formed from a paper clip.

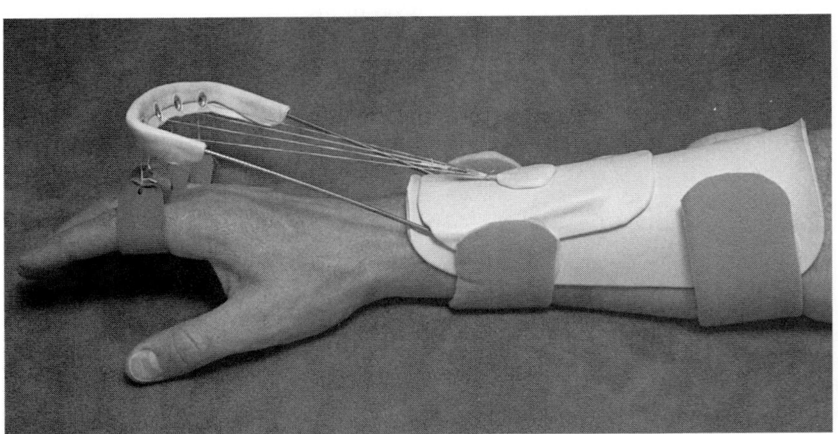

A

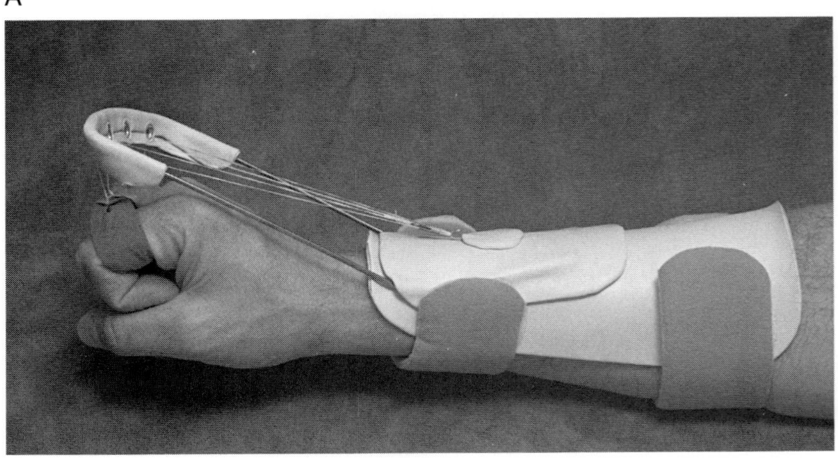

B

Figure 11-31 Neither the outrigger (A) nor the line (B) must impede composite flexion.

Laboratory Exercise 11-1 Fabricating a Radial Nerve Splint

Practice fabricating a radial nerve splint on a partner. After fitting the splint and making all adjustments, use Form 11-1. This check-off sheet is a self-evaluation of the radial nerve splint. Use Grading Sheet 11-1 as a classroom grading sheet.

Precautions for Dynamic Splinting

Therapists should consider specific precautions during application of dynamic splints. The first rule of dynamic splinting, and of all treatment, is to do no harm. Therapists should follow this rule by adhering to the following guidelines [Fess 2002].

- The person must be responsible enough to care for the splint and to follow a guided wearing schedule. A mobilization splint is not appropriate for a child or adult who cannot follow instructions.
- Keep in mind normal functional anatomy and biomechanics of the extremity.
- Apply minimal force. The amount of force should provide a low-grade stretch that is tolerable over a long period of time [Colditz 1990]. Signs indicating too much force include reddened pressure areas, cyanosis of the fingertips, and complaints of pain or numbness. A person will most likely not wear a splint that causes discomfort.
- Keep in mind the risks of wearing an ill-fitted splint (e.g., pressure points, skin breakdown, prolonged immobilization of noninvolved structures).
- Remember aesthetics. A person is more likely to wear a splint that has a finished, professional appearance. A low-profile splint may be more aesthetically pleasing.
- Monitor and adjust the splint frequently for accurate fit.
- Listen to the person. The splint must fit well, have a tolerable amount of tension, and cause minimal interference with daily activities. Complaints by the person require reevaluation of the splint's fit.
- Use extreme caution when applying an external force to a hand that has decreased sensation. An increased risk of skin breakdown exists if a splint creates an excessive amount of force in the absence of sensory feedback.
- The altered joint mechanics of a person who has rheumatoid arthritis make static splinting more appropriate than dynamic splinting. A therapist may use dynamic splinting on a person who has rheumatoid arthritis, but only if specific indications are met. A dynamic splint may be used with rheumatoid arthritis with only very gentle tension applied as close to the joint as possible. The goal of splinting is to gently stretch involved soft tissue or to provide gentle resistance to strengthen weakened muscles [Cailliet 1994]. The therapist must be careful to avoid adverse reactions.

FORM 11-1* Radial nerve splint

Name: ______________________

Date: ______________________

Answer the following questions after the person wears the splint for 30 minutes. (Mark *NA* for nonapplicable situations.)

Evaluation Areas				Comments
Design				
1. The forearm trough is the proper length and width.	Yes ❍	No ❍	NA ❍	
2. The outrigger wire is at the appropriate angles and ½ inch wider than the MCPs at the level of the hand.	Yes ❍	No ❍	NA ❍	
3. The thermoplastic material on the MCP aspect of the outrigger is secure.	Yes ❍	No ❍	NA ❍	
4. The line to the outrigger is at a 90-degree angle from the long axis of the bone when the hand is at rest.	Yes ❍	No ❍	NA ❍	
5. The anchor hook is secure.	Yes ❍	No ❍	NA ❍	
6. The thermoplastic material patch adequately secures the outrigger.	Yes ❍	No ❍	NA ❍	
Function				
1. The wrist is maintained in neutral when the fingers are in extension.	Yes ❍	No ❍	NA ❍	
2. The outrigger or lines do not impede composite flexion of the fingers.	Yes ❍	No ❍	NA ❍	
3. The fit of the trough and straps prevents distal migration of the splint.	Yes ❍	No ❍	NA ❍	
4. The slings do not migrate distally with finger flexion and extension.	Yes ❍	No ❍	NA ❍	
Comfort				
1. Excessive pressure is not present on the radial or ulnar styloids.	Yes ❍	No ❍	NA ❍	
2. The edges are smooth with rounded corners.	Yes ❍	No ❍	NA ❍	
3. The proximal and distal ends are flared.	Yes ❍	No ❍	NA ❍	
4. Impingements or pressure areas are not present.	Yes ❍	No ❍	NA ❍	
5. Slings are durable enough to allow hand function over a long period of time.	Yes ❍	No ❍	NA ❍	
Therapeutic Regimen				
1. The person has been instructed in a wearing schedule.	Yes ❍	No ❍	NA ❍	
2. The person has been provided splint precautions.	Yes ❍	No ❍	NA ❍	
3. The person demonstrates understanding of the education.	Yes ❍	No ❍	NA ❍	
4. Client/caregiver knows how to clean the splint.	Yes ❍	No ❍	NA ❍	

*See Appendix B for a perforated copy of this form.

GRADING SHEET 11-1*

Radial Nerve Splint

Name: ____________________

Date: ____________________

Wrist position at rest:

Grade: ___________

1 = beyond improvement, not acceptable
2 = requires maximal improvment
3 = requires moderate improvement
4 = requires minimal improvement
5 = requires no improvement

Evaluation Areas						Comments
Design						
1. The forearm trough is the proper length and width.	1	2	3	4	5	
2. The outrigger wire is at the appropriate angles and ½ inch wider than the MCPs at the level of the hand.	1	2	3	4	5	
3. The thermoplastic material on the MCP aspect of the outrigger is secure.	1	2	3	4	5	
4. The line to the outrigger is at a 90-degree angle from the long axis of the bone when the hand is at rest.	1	2	3	4	5	
5. The anchor hook is secure.	1	2	3	4	5	
6. The thermoplastic material patch adequately secures the outrigger.	1	2	3	4	5	
Function						
1. The wrist is maintained in neutral when the fingers are in extension.	1	2	3	4	5	
2. The outrigger or lines do not impede composite flexion of the fingers.	1	2	3	4	5	
3. The fit of the trough and straps prevents distal migration of the splint.	1	2	3	4	5	
4. The slings do not migrate distally with finger flexion and extension.	1	2	3	4	5	
Cosmesis						
1. Excessive pressure is not present on the radial or ulnar styloids.	1	2	3	4	5	
2. The edges are smooth with rounded corners.	1	2	3	4	5	
3. The proximal and distal ends are flared.	1	2	3	4	5	
4. Impingements or pressure areas are not present.	1	2	3	4	5	

GRADING SHEET 11-1*—cont'd

Radial Nerve Splint

Comments:

____

____

____

____

____

____

____

____

____

____

*See Appendix C for a perforated copy of this grading sheet.

CASE STUDY 11-1*

Read the following scenario and answer the questions based on information in this chapter.

Michael is a 12-year-old right-handed boy who is out of school for the summer. After a rough landing from his bike ramp, he was unable to move his right elbow without significant pain. At the hospital the physician determined that Michael had a comminuted fracture of the right humerus. In addition, Michael was unable to actively extend his thumb, wrist, and MCPs, and he was unable to abduct his thumb. An electromyogram revealed damage to the radial nerve. The physician has ordered occupational therapy for fabrication of a splint.

1. Which clinical evaluation is required before fabrication of the splint?
   a. Evaluate ability to actively extend wrist, MCPs, and thumb
   b. Evaluate sensory deficits
   c. Evaluate functional use of injured hand
   d. All of the above
2. What is the primary goal for this splint?
   a. Prevent further injury
   b. Protect damaged nerve by immobilizing wrist
   c. Increase functional use of hand
   d. Limit composite flexion of fingers
3. Which outrigger is most appropriate for this splint?
   a. High-profile
   b. Low-profile
   c. No outrigger
4. What is the most desirable source of finger and wrist support for this splint?
   a. Static tension
   b. Rubber band tension
   c. Spring tension
   d. Elastic string tension
5. What is the position of the wrist during composite flexion of the fingers?
   a. Flexion of 30 degrees
   b. Neutral
   c. Extension up to 45 degrees

*See Appendix A for the answer key.

REVIEW QUESTIONS

1. What are four possible goals of mobilizing splinting?
2. What are the complications associated with application of too much force?
3. What is the angle of pull between the long axis of the bone and the outrigger line the therapist must maintain?
4. What is the acceptable force per unit area for sling pressure?
5. What patient information should the therapist gather before considering a person for a mobilizing splint?
6. What is the difference between a high-profile and a low-profile outrigger? What are the advantages and disadvantages of each?
7. What are three methods for the application of force?
8. What criteria are used to determine whether to use static tension or elastic/dynamic tension?
9. What are the steps for attaching an outrigger wire to a splint base?
10. What are three precautions with mobilizing splinting?

References

Austin G, Slamett M, Cameron D, Austin N (2004). A comparison of high-profile and low-profile dynamic mobilization splint designs. Journal of Hand Therapy 17:335-343.

Brand PW, Hollister A (1993b). External stress: Effects at the surface. In *Clinical Mechanics of the Hand*. St. Louis: Mosby.

Brand PW, Hollister A (1993a.). Terminology, how joints move, mechanical resistance, and external stress: Effect at the surface. In *Clinical Mechanics of the Hand*. St. Louis: Mosby.

Brand PW (2002). The forces of dynamic splinting. Ten questions before applying a dynamic splint to the hand. In *Rehabilitation of the Hand, Fifth Edition*. St. Louis: Mosby.

Cailliet, R (1993). Functional anatomy and joints: Injuries and disease. In *Hand Pain and Impairment, Fourth Edition*. Philadelphia: F. A. Davis 243-245.

Cannon N, Foltz R, Koepfer J, Lauck M, Simpson D, Bromley R (1985). Mechanical principles. In *Manual of Hand Splinting*. New York: Churchill Livingstone p. 6-7.

Colditz J (1983). Low profile dynamic splinting of the injured hand. American Journal of Occupational Therapy 37:182-188.

Colditz JC (1987). Splinting for radial nerve palsy. Journal of Hand Therapy 1:18-23.

Colditz JC (2002a). Dynamic splinting of the stiff hand. In JM Hunter, EJ Mackin, AD Callahan (eds.), *Rehabilitation of the Hand, Fifth Edition*. St. Louis: Mosby.

Colditz JC (2002b). Splinting the hand with a peripheral nerve injury. In JM Hunter, EJ Mackin, AD Callahan (eds.), *Rehabilitation of the Hand, Fifth Edition*. St. Louis: Mosby.

Colditz, JC (1995). Therapist's management of the stiff hand. In *Rehabilitation of the Hand*. St. Louis: Mosby.

Duran RJ, Coleman CR, Nappi JF, Klerekoper LA (1990). In JM Hunter, LH Schneider, EJ Mackin, AD Callahan (eds.), *Rehabilitation of the Hand*. St. Louis: Mosby.

Fess EE (1990). Principles and methods of splinting for mobilization of joints. In JM Hunter, LH Schneider, EJ Mackin, AD Callahan (eds.), *Rehabilitation of the Hand, Third Edition*. St. Louis: Mosby.

Fess EE (1995). Splints: Mechanics versus convention. J Hand Therapy 8:124-130.

Fess EE, McCollum M (1998). The influence of splinting on healing tissues. J Hand Therapy 11:125-130.

Fess EE, Gettle K, Philips C, Janson J (2005). *Hand and Upper Extremity Splinting: Principles and Methods, Third Edition*. St. Louis: Mosby.

Flowers K, LaStayo P (1994). Effect of total end range time on improving passive range of motion. J Hand Ther 7:150-157.

Hardy M (2004). Principles of metacarpal and phalangeal fracture management: A review of rehabilitation concepts. Journal of Orthopaedic and Sports Physical Therapy 34:781-799.

Hollister A, Giurintano D (1993). *How Joints Move: Clinical Mechanics of the Hand*. St. Louis: Mosby.

Jebson PL, Kasdan ML (1998). *Hand Secrets*. Philadelphia: Hanley & Belfus.

Loth TS, Wadsworth CT (1998). *Orthopedic Review for Physical Therapists*. St. Louis: Mosby.

May E, Silfverskiold K, Sollerman C (1992). Controlled mobilization after flexor tendon repair in zone Il: A prospective comparison of three methods. J Hand Surg 17A:942-952.

May E, Silfverskiald K, Sollerman C (1992). The correlation between controlled range of motion with dynamic traction and results after flexor tendon repair in zone II. J Hand Surg 17:1133-1139.

Prosser R (1996). Splinting in the management of proximal interphalangeal joint flexion contracture. Journal of Hand Therapy 9: 378-386.

Schultz-Johnson K (1996). Splinting the wrist: Mobilization and protection. Journal of Hand Therapy 9:165-176.

Schultz-Johnson K (2002). Static progressive splinting. Journal of Hand Therapy 15:163-178.

Smith LK, Weiss EL, Lehmkuhl LD (1996). *Brunnstrom's Clinical Kinesiology, Fifth Edition*. Philadelphia: F. A. Davis.

Stewart KM, van Strien G (2002). Postoperative management of flexor tendon injuries. In JM Hunter, LH Schneider, EJ Mackin, AD Callahan (eds.), *Rehabilitation of the Hand, Fifth Edition*. St. Louis: Mosby.

CHAPTER 12

Splinting for the Fingers

Cynthia Cooper, MFA, MA, OTR/L, CHT
Lisa Deshaies, OTR/L, CHT

Key Terms

Boutonniere deformities
Buddy straps
Central extensor tendon
Collateral ligaments
Extensor lag
Finger sprain
Flexion contracture
Fusiform swelling
Lateral bands
Mallet finger
Oblique retinacular ligament
Swan-neck deformities
Terminal extensor tendon
Transverse retinacular ligament
Volar plate

Chapter Objectives

1. Explain the functional and anatomic considerations for splinting the fingers.
2. Identify diagnostic indications for splinting the fingers.
3. Describe a mallet finger.
4. Describe a boutonniere deformity.
5. Describe a swan-neck deformity.
6. Name three structures that provide support to the stability of the proximal interphalangeal (PIP) joint.
7. Explain what buddy straps are.
8. Apply clinical reasoning to evaluate finger splints in terms of materials used, strapping type and placement, and fit.
9. Discuss the process of making a mallet splint, a gutter splint, and a PIP hyperextension block splint.

Depending on the diagnosis, finger problems may require splints that cross the hand and wrist—or they may be treated with splints that are smaller. This chapter describes the smaller splints that are finger based, crossing the PIP and/or distal interphalangeal (DIP) joint—leaving the metacarpophalangeal (MCP) joint free.

Functional and Anatomic Considerations for Splinting the Fingers

The PIP and DIP joints are hinge joints. These joints have collateral ligaments on each side that provide joint stability and restraint against deviation forces. The radial collateral ligament protects against ulnar deviation forces, and the ulnar collateral ligament protects against radial deviation forces. On the palmar (or volar) surface is the volar plate, which is a fibrocartilaginous structure that prevents hyperextension. The central extensor tendon crosses the PIP joint dorsally and is part of the PIP joint dorsal capsule. It is implicated in boutonniere deformities. The lateral bands, which are contributions from the intrinsic muscles, and the transverse retinacular ligament are additional structures that contribute to the delicate balance of the extensor mechanism at the PIP joint. They are implicated in boutonniere deformities and swan-neck deformities. The terminal extensor tendon attaches to the distal phalanx and is implicated in mallet finger injuries (Figure 12-1) [Campbell and Wilson 2002].

For any finger problem, it is always important to prioritize edema control. Treatment for edema can often be incorporated into the splinting process. Examples of this would be the use of self-adherent compressive wrap under the splint or to secure the splint on the finger. For diagnoses that require splint use 24 hours per day but permit washing of the

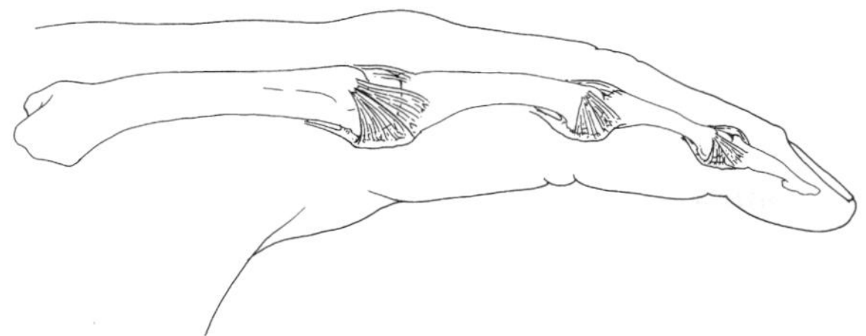

Figure 12-1 Structures that provide PIP joint stability include the accessory collateral ligament, the proper collateral ligament, the dorsal capsule with the central extensor tendon, and the volar plate. [From Mackin EJ, Callahan AD, Skirven TM, Schneider LH, Osterman AL. Hunter (2002). *Mackin & Callahan's Rehabilitation of the Hand and Upper Extremity, Fifth Edition.* St. Louis: Mosby.]

digit, it may be appropriate to fabricate one splint for shower use and another for use during the rest of the day. In general, thinner LTT is typically used on digits because it is less bulky yet strong enough to support or protect these relatively small body parts. On a stronger person or a person with larger hands, 3/32-inch material may be better to use than 1/16-inch thickness. Selecting perforated versus nonperforated splinting material is partly a matter of personal choice, but use caution with perforated materials because the edges may be rougher and there can be the possibility of increased skin problems or irregular pressure—particularly if there is edema. Smaller perforations seen in microperforated materials minimize the risk.

Because finger splints are so small, there is an increased possibility of them being pulled off in the covers during sleep or during activity. It is often necessary to tape them into place in addition to using Velcro straps. Be careful not to apply the tape circumferentially so as not to cause a tourniquet effect. An alternative solution is to use a long Velcro strap to anchor the splint around the hand or wrist.

Diagnostic Indications

Commonly seen diagnoses that require finger splints are mallet fingers, boutonniere deformities, swan-neck deformities, and finger sprains. These diagnoses are discussed separately in the sections that follow in terms of splinting indications, including consideration of wearing schedule and fabrication tips. Prefabricated splinting options are also addressed.

Mallet Finger

A mallet finger presents as a digit with a droop of the DIP joint (Figure 12-2). This posture often occurs as a result of axial loading with the DIP extended or flexion force to the fingertip. The terminal tendon is avulsed, causing a droop of the DIP. A laceration to the terminal tendon may also cause this problem [Hofmeister et al. 2003].

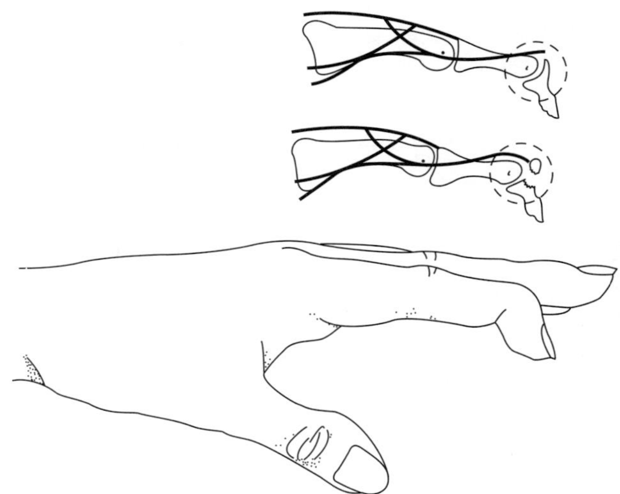

Figure 12-2 Mallet finger deformity. [From American Society for Surgery of the Hand (1983). *The Hand: Examination and Diagnosis, Second Edition.* Edinburgh: Churchill Livingstone.]

With a mallet injury, the DIP joint can usually be passively extended to neutral—but the client is not able to actively extend it himself. This is called a DIP extensor lag. If the DIP joint cannot be passively extended, this is called a DIP flexion contracture. It is unlikely the DIP joint will develop a flexion contracture early on, but this can be seen in more long-standing cases.

Splinting for Mallet Finger

The goal of splinting for mallet finger is to prevent DIP flexion. Some physicians prefer the DIP joint to be splinted in slight hyperextension, whereas others prefer a neutral DIP position. It is good to clarify this with the doctor. If hyperextension is desired, care must be taken not to excessively hyperextend because this may compromise blood flow to the area. Either way, it is very important that the splint does not impede PIP flexion unless there are specific associated issues such as a secondary swan-neck deformity that would justify limiting the PIP joint's mobility.

The DIP joint should be splinted for about 6 weeks to allow the terminal tendon to heal. This terminal tendon is a very delicate structure, and for this reason the joint should not be left unsupported or be allowed to flex for even a moment during this 6-week interval. It can be challenging to achieve this continuous DIP support because there is also the need for skin care and air flow. Practice with the client so that there is good understanding of techniques to support the DIP joint while performing skin hygiene and when applying and removing the splint [Cooper 2007].

After about 6 weeks of continual splinting and with medical clearance, the client is weaned off the splint. It is usually still worn at night for several weeks. At this time, it is very important to watch for the development of a DIP

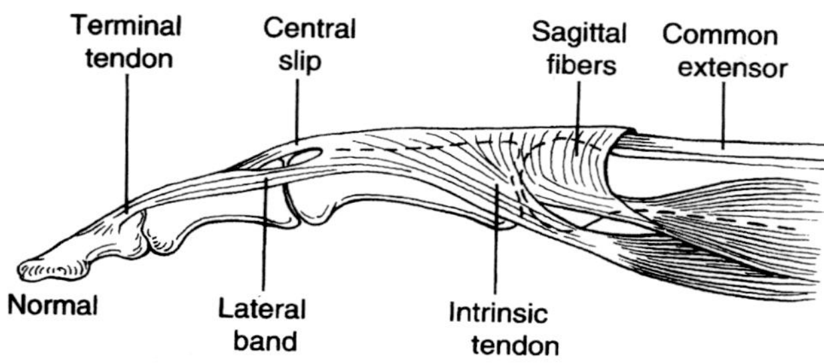

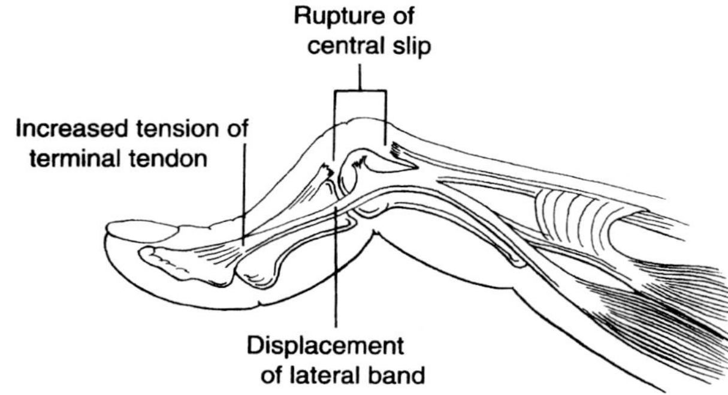

Figure 12-3 Normal anatomy and anatomy of boutonniere deformity. [From Burke SL, Higgins J, McClinton MA, Saunders R, Valdata L (2006). *Hand and Upper Extremity Rehabilitation: A Practical Guide, Third Edition.* St. Louis: Churchill Livingstone.]

extensor lag. If this is noticed, resume use of the splint and consult the physician.

Boutonniere Deformity

A boutonniere deformity is a finger that postures with PIP flexion and DIP hyperextension (Figure 12-3). This deformity can result from axial loading, tendon laceration, burns, or arthritis. The central extensor tendon (also called the central slip) is disrupted, which leads to the imbalance of the extensor mechanism as the lateral bands displace volarly. If not treated in a timely manner, the PIP joint extensor lag may become a flexion contracture. In addition, the DIP joint may lose flexion motion due to tightness of the oblique retinacular ligament (ORL), also called the ligament of Landsmeer.

Splinting for Boutonniere Deformity

The goal of splinting for boutonniere deformity is to maintain PIP joint extension while keeping the MCP and DIP joints free for about 6 to 8 weeks. If there is a PIP flexion contracture, a prefabricated dynamic three-point extension splint might be used—or a static splint can be adjusted serially with the goal of achieving full passive PIP extension. There are various types of splints for boutonniere deformity, including simple volar gutter splints. Figure 12-4 depicts some common options for splinting the PIP joint in extension while keeping the DIP joint free. In some cases, including the DIP joint in the splint may be preferable because this will increase the mechanical advantage. It is usually acceptable to do this if the ORL is not tight.

Serial casting is also an option with this diagnosis (Figure 12-5). This technique requires training and practice before being used on clients [Bell-Krotoski 2002, 2005]. After 6 to 8 weeks of splinting and with medical clearance, the client is weaned off the splint. At this time, it is important to watch for loss of PIP extension. If this is noted, adjust splint usage accordingly.

Swan-neck Deformity

A swan-neck deformity is seen when the finger postures with PIP hyperextension and DIP flexion (Figure 12-6). Positionally, the swan-neck deformity at the PIP and DIP is

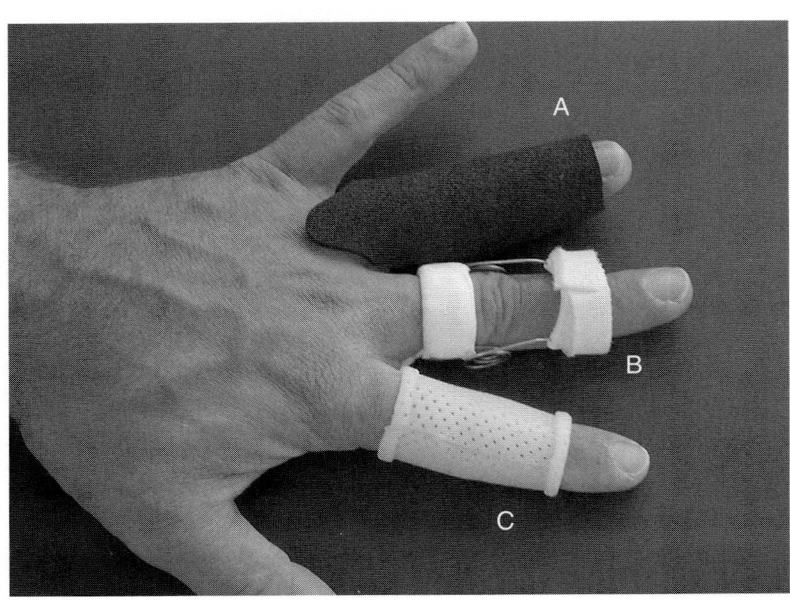

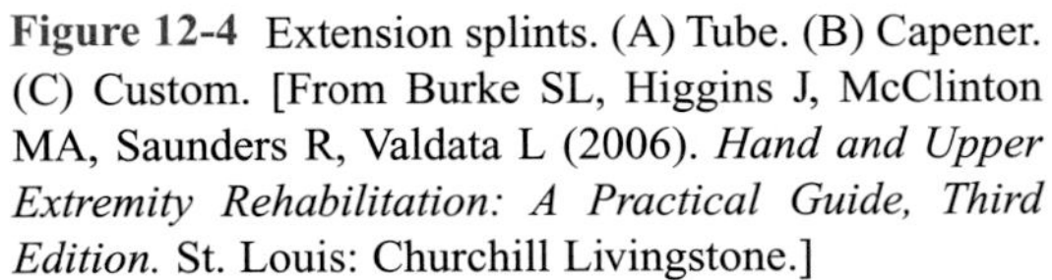

Figure 12-4 Extension splints. (A) Tube. (B) Capener. (C) Custom. [From Burke SL, Higgins J, McClinton MA, Saunders R, Valdata L (2006). *Hand and Upper Extremity Rehabilitation: A Practical Guide, Third Edition.* St. Louis: Churchill Livingstone.]

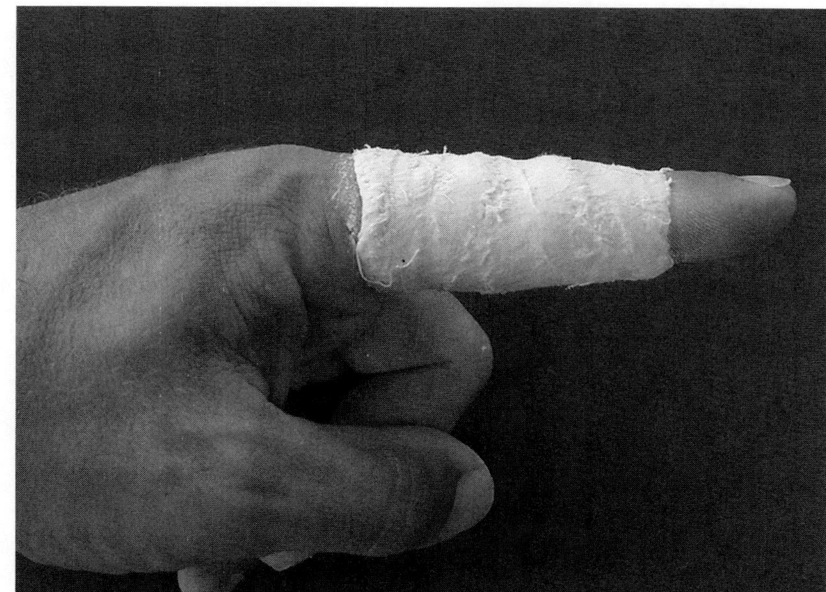

Figure 12-5 Serial cast. [From Burke SL, Higgins J, McClinton MA, Saunders R, Valdata L (2006). *Hand and Upper Extremity Rehabilitation: A Practical Guide, Third Edition.* St. Louis: Churchill Livingstone.]

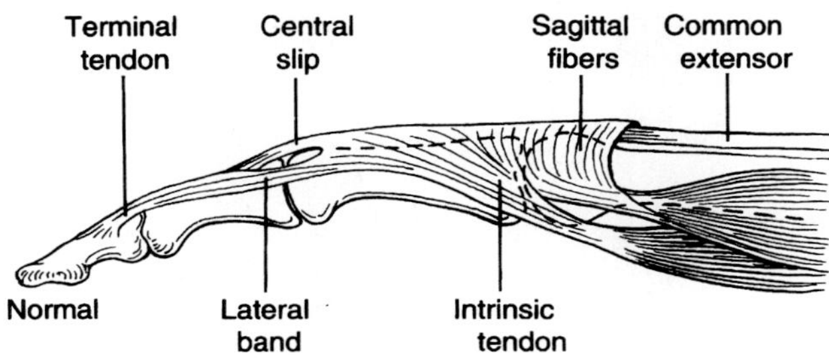

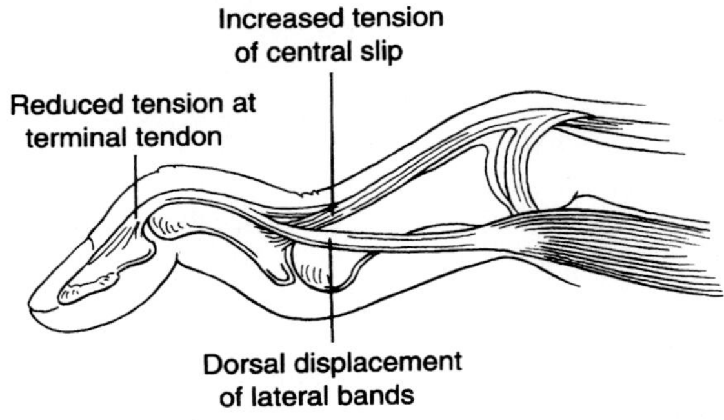

Figure 12-6 Normal finger anatomy and anatomy of swan neck deformity. [From Burke SL, Higgins J, McClinton MA, Saunders R, Valdata L (2006). *Hand and Upper Extremity Rehabilitation: A Practical Guide, Third Edition.* St. Louis: Churchill Livingstone.]

the opposite of the boutonniere deformity. It may be possible to correct the PIP and DIP joints passively—or they may be fixed in their deformity positions. There are multiple possible causes of this deformity that may occur at the level of the MCP, the PIP, or the DIP joints. As with boutonniere deformity, the result is an imbalance of the extensor mechanism—but with a swan-neck deformity the lateral bands displace dorsally. In addition to other traumatic causes, it is not uncommon for people with rheumatoid arthritis to demonstrate swan-neck deformities [Alter et al. 2002, Deshaies 2006].

Splinting for Swan-neck Deformity

The goal of splinting for swan-neck deformity is to prevent PIP hyperextension and to promote DIP extension while not restricting PIP flexion. A dorsal gutter with the PIP joint in slight flexion (about 20 degrees) can be made. If the DIP demonstrates an extensor lag, the splint can cross the DIP and a strap can be added to support the DIP in neutral. Less restrictive styles of splints are shown in Figure 12-7. These are three-point splints that prevent PIP hyperextension but allow PIP flexion. They can be either custom formed or prefabricated.

Finger PIP Sprains

Finger sprains may be ignored by clients as trivial injuries, but they can be very painful and functionally debilitating—with the potential for chronic swelling and stiffness and surprisingly long recovery time. Uninjured digits are at risk of losing motion and function, which further complicates the picture. Prompt treatment can favorably affect the client's outcome and expedite return to occupations impacted by the injury.

PIP sprains are graded in terms of severity, from grade I to grade III. Box 12-1 describes these grades and identifies proper treatment. PIP joint dislocations are also described in terms of the direction of joint dislocation (i.e., dorsal, lateral, or volar). PIP joint sprains are associated with fusiform swelling, which is fullness at the PIP joint and

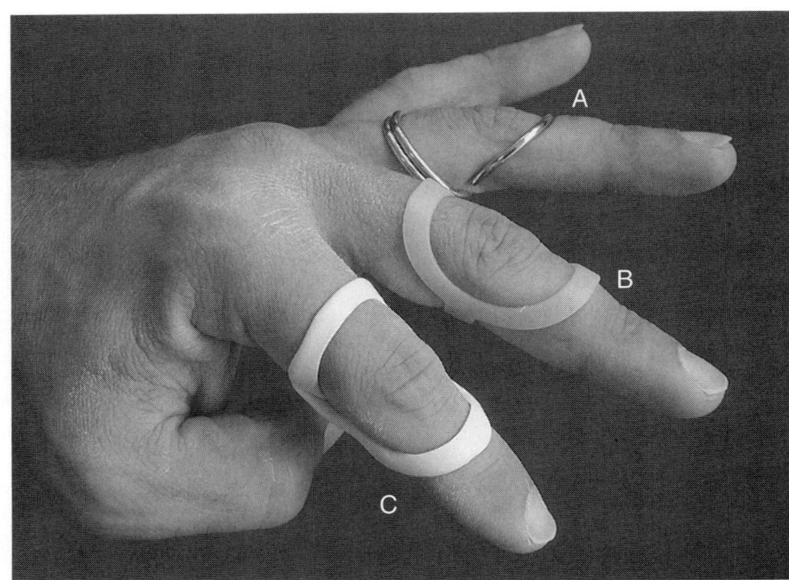

Figure 12-7 PIP hyperextension block (swan-neck) splints. (A) Custom-ordered silver ring splint. (B) Prefabricated polypropylene Oval 8 splint. (C) Custom low-temperature thermoplastic splint. [From Burke SL, Higgins J, McClinton MA, Saunders R, Valdata L (2006). *Hand and Upper Extremity Rehabilitation: A Practical Guide, Third Edition.* St. Louis: Churchill Livingstone.]

Box 12-1 Grades of Ligament Sprain Injuries

Mild Grade I Sprain

No instability with active or passive ROM; macroscopic continuity with microscopic tears. The ligament is intact but individual fibers are damaged.

- Treatment: Immobilize the joint in full extension if comfortable and available. Otherwise, immobilize in a small amount of flexion.
- When pain has subsided, begin AROM and protect with buddy taping or buddy strapping.

Grade II Sprain

Abnormal laxity with stress; the collateral ligament is disrupted. AROM is stable but passive testing reveals instability.

- Treatment: Immobilize the joint in full extension for 2 to 4 weeks. The MD may recommend early ROM, but avoid any lateral stress.

Grade III Sprain

Complete tear of the collateral ligament along with injury to the dorsal capsule or the volar plate. The finger has usually dislocated with injury.

- Treatment: Early surgical intervention is often recommended.

proximal and distal tapering. Edema control is critical with this diagnosis.

Splinting for Finger PIP Sprains

The goal of splinting finger PIP sprains is to support the PIP joint and promote healing and stability. Splinting options for the injured PIP joint with extension limitations are similar to those used for boutonniere deformities. If there is a PIP flexion contracture, dynamic or serial static PIP extension splinting is used—or serial casting may be considered. If there has been a volar plate injury, a dorsal gutter is fabricated to block about 20 to 30 degrees of PIP extension while allowing PIP flexion (Figure 12-8).

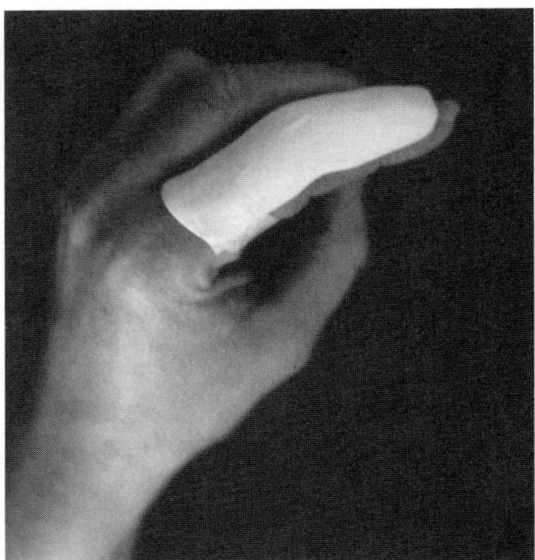

Figure 12-8 Dorsal gutter splint blocking about 20 to 30 degrees of PIP extension. [From Fess EE, Gettle KS, Philips CA, Janson RJ (2005). *Hand and Upper Extremity Splinting: Principles and Methods, Third Edition.* St. Louis: Mosby.]

Buddy straps (Figure 12-9) are used to promote motion and support the injured digit. There are many different styles to choose from [Campbell and Wilson 2002]. An offset buddy strap may be needed, especially for small finger injuries due to the length discrepancy between the small and ring fingers.

The physician will indicate what arc of motion is safe, according to the injury and joint stability. It is important not

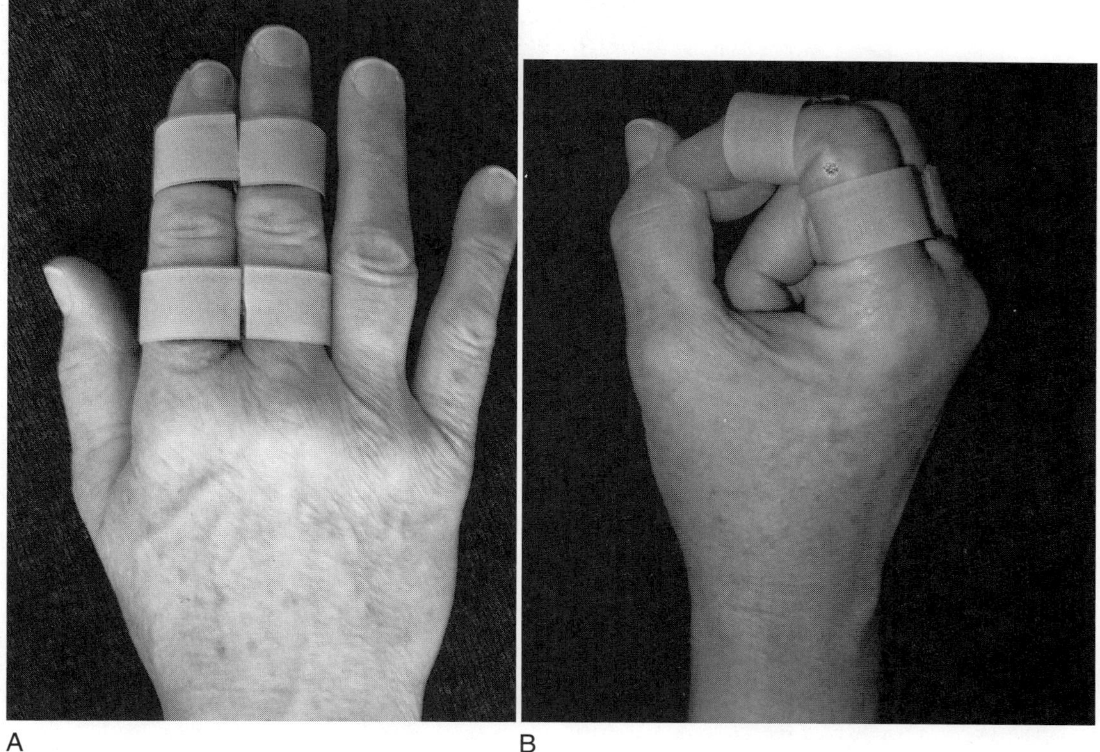

Figure 12-9 Examples of buddy straps for proximal interphalangeal collateral ligament injuries. [From Burke SL, Higgins J, McClinton MA, Saunders R, Valdata L (2006). *Hand and Upper Extremity Rehabilitation: A Practical Guide, Third Edition.* St. Louis: Churchill Livingstone.]

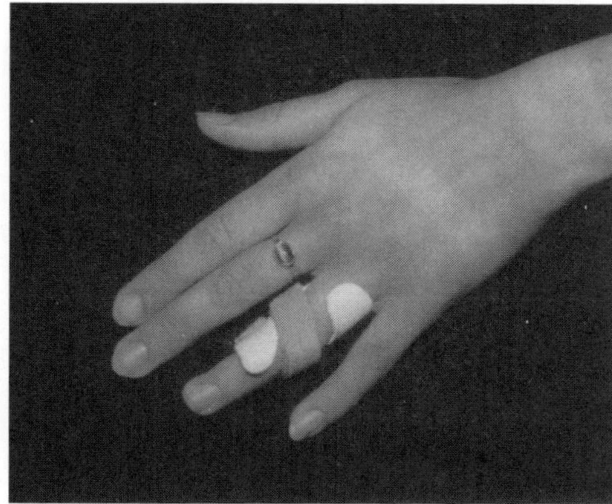

Figure 12-10 PIP extension splint with lateral support. [From Fess EE, Gettle KS, Philips CA, Janson RJ (2005). *Hand and Upper Extremity Splinting: Principles and Methods, Third Edition.* St. Louis: Mosby.]

to apply lateral stress to the injured tissues. For example, if the index finger has an injury to the radial collateral ligament do not put ulnar stress on it. Lateral pinch would also be problematic in this instance. Sometimes it is necessary to custom fabricate a PIP gutter that corrects lateral position as well. Figure 12-10 shows a digital splint that provides lateral support.

Generally, PIP finger sprains are at risk for stiffness and are prone to developing flexion contractures. For this reason, a night PIP extension splint is often appropriate to use. However, this type of injury may also present problems achieving PIP/DIP flexion as well. In this instance, splinting can be provided along with exercises to gain flexion passive range of motion. Examples of flexion splints are shown in Figure 12-11. Such choices must be applied very gently, and tissue tolerances should be monitored carefully.

Precautions for Finger Splints

- Monitor skin for signs of maceration and/or pressure both on the splinted finger and adjacent fingers that come into contact with the splint.
- Check splint edges and straps for signs of tightness.
- Provide written instructions, and practice with clients so that they are correctly following guidelines for splint care and use.

Occupation-Based Splinting

Some finger splints may help with hand function by decreasing pain and providing stability. However, many finger splints can certainly interfere with daily hand use. Understandably, clients may be tempted to remove their splints in order to participate in activities they enjoy. To help prevent this from happening, therapists should incorporate an occupation-based approach.

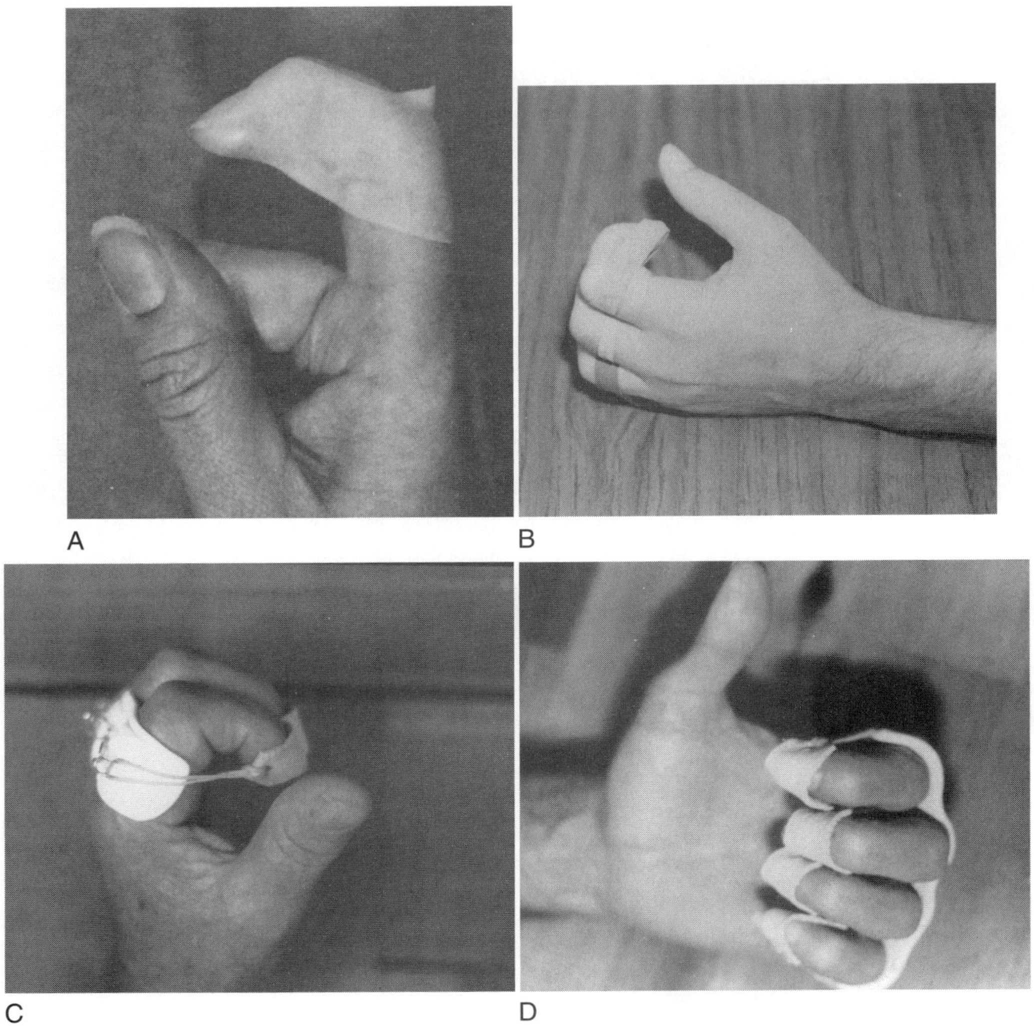

Figure 12-11 Examples of PIP/DIP flexion splints. [From Fess EE, Gettle KS, Philips CA, Janson RJ (2005). *Hand and Upper Extremity Splinting: Principles and Methods, Third Edition.* St. Louis: Mosby.]

SELF-QUIZ 12-1*

Circle either true (T) or false (F).

1. T F PIP joints are hinge joints.
2. T F A mallet finger is represented by loss of extension at the PIP joint.
3. T F An extensor lag is when there is loss of passive extension at the joint.
4. T F Finger sprains of the PIP joints are always trivial injuries.
5. T F Buddy straps promote motion and support an injured digit.

*See Appendix A for the answer key.

Examples of Occupation-Based Finger Splinting

An elderly retired male enjoyed woodworking but was unable to use his woodworking tools comfortably due to arthritis-related pain and instability of the index finger PIP joint. He expressed interest in a PIP joint protective gutter splint to help him use his tools. To determine the best position of the PIP joint splint, he brought his tools to therapy and demonstrated the finger position he needed. A splint was made that provided support during this task.

A client with a mallet injury came to a clinic with maceration under the splint. He stated that he was wearing his splint in the shower and keeping the wet splint on his

Laboratory Exercise 12-1*

1. The following picture shows a mallet finger gutter splint. What is wrong with this splint?

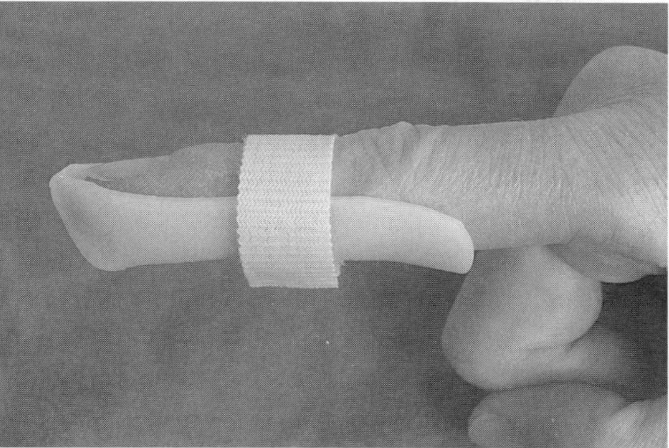

____

____

2. The following picture shows a PIP gutter splint. What is wrong with this splint?

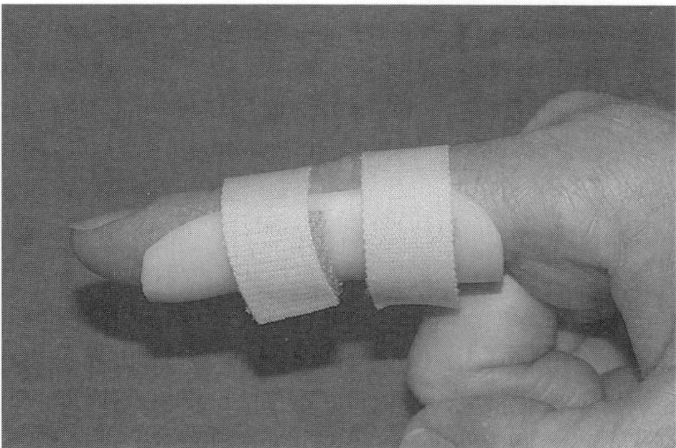

____

____

3. The following picture shows a PIP hyperextension block splint. What is wrong with this splint?

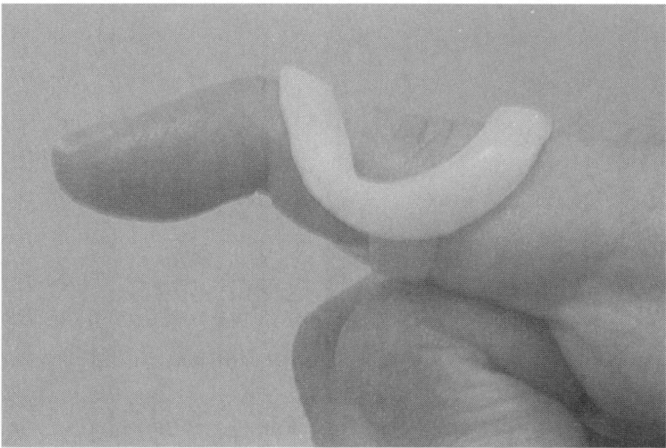

____

____

*See Appendix A for the answer key.

Laboratory Exercise 12-2

Practice fabricating a dorsal-volar mallet splint on a partner with the DIP joint in neutral. Check to be sure the PIP crease is not blocked and that full PIP AROM is available. Use Form 12-1 as a check-off sheet for a self-evaluation of the dorsal-volar mallet splint. Use Grading Sheet 12-1 as a classroom grading sheet.

FORM 12-1* Finger splint

Name: ______________________

Date: ______________________

After the person wears the splint for 30 minutes, answer the following questions. (Mark *NA* for nonapplicable situations.)

Evaluation Areas				**Comments**
Design				
1. The PIP position is at the correct angle.	Yes ❍	No ❍	NA ❍	
2. The DIP position is at the correct angle.	Yes ❍	No ❍	NA ❍	
3. The splint provides adequate support and is not constrictive.	Yes ❍	No ❍	NA ❍	
4. The splint length is appropriate.	Yes ❍	No ❍	NA ❍	
5. The splint width is appropriate.	Yes ❍	No ❍	NA ❍	
6. The splint is snug enough to stay in place yet loose enough to apply and remove.	Yes ❍	No ❍	NA ❍	
Function				
1. The splint allows full MCP motion.	Yes ❍	No ❍	NA ❍	
2. The splint allows full PIP motion.	Yes ❍	No ❍	NA ❍	
3. The splint allows full DIP motion.	Yes ❍	No ❍	NA ❍	
4. The splint enables as much hand function as possible.	Yes ❍	No ❍	NA ❍	
Straps				
1. The straps are secure and the terminal edges are rounded.	Yes ❍	No ❍	NA ❍	
Comfort				
1. The splint edges are smooth, rounded, contoured, and flared.	Yes ❍	No ❍	NA ❍	
2. The splint does not cause pain or pressure areas.	Yes ❍	No ❍	NA ❍	
Cosmetic Appearance				
1. The splint is free of fingerprints, dirt, and pencil/pen marks.	Yes ❍	No ❍	NA ❍	
2. The splinting material is not buckled.	Yes ❍	No ❍	NA ❍	
Therapeutic Regimen				
1. The client or caregiver has been instructed in a wearing schedule.	Yes ❍	No ❍	NA ❍	
2. The client or caregiver has been provided splint precautions.	Yes ❍	No ❍	NA ❍	
3. The client or caregiver demonstrates understanding of the splint program.	Yes ❍	No ❍	NA ❍	
4. The client or caregiver demonstrates proper donning and doffing of splint.	Yes ❍	No ❍	NA ❍	
5. The client or caregiver knows how to clean the splint and straps.	Yes ❍	No ❍	NA ❍	

Discuss possible splint adjustments or changes you should make based on the self-evaluation (What would you do differently next time?):

____

____

____

____

____

____

____

*See Appendix B for a perforated copy of this form.

GRADING SHEET 12-1*

Name: ______________________________

Date: ______________________________

Type of finger splint:

Mallet finger ❍ PIP gutter ❍ PIP hyperextension block ❍ Other __________

Grade: ___________

1 = beyond improvement, not acceptable
2 = requires maximal improvement
3 = requires moderate improvement
4 = requires minimal improvement
5 = requires no improvement

Evaluation Areas						**Comments**
Design						
1. The PIP position is at the correct angle.	1	2	3	4	5	
2. The DIP position is at the correct angle.	1	2	3	4	5	
3. The splint provides adequate support and is not constrictive.	1	2	3	4	5	
4. The splint length is appropriate.	1	2	3	4	5	
5. The splint width is appropriate.	1	2	3	4	5	
6. The splint is snug enough to stay in place yet loose enough to apply and remove.	1	2	3	4	5	
Function						
1. The splint allows full MCP motion.	1	2	3	4	5	
2. The splint allows full PIP motion.	1	2	3	4	5	
3. The splint allows full DIP motion.	1	2	3	4	5	
4. The splint enables as much hand function as possible.	1	2	3	4	5	
Straps						
1. The straps are secure and the terminal edges are rounded.	1	2	3	4	5	
Comfort						
1. The splint edges are smooth, rounded, contoured, and flared.	1	2	3	4	5	
2. The splint does not cause pain or pressure areas.	1	2	3	4	5	
Cosmetic Appearance						
1. The splint is free of fingerprints, dirt, and pencil/pen marks.	1	2	3	4	5	
2. The splinting material is not buckled.	1	2	3	4	5	

*See Appendix C for a perforated copy of this sheet.

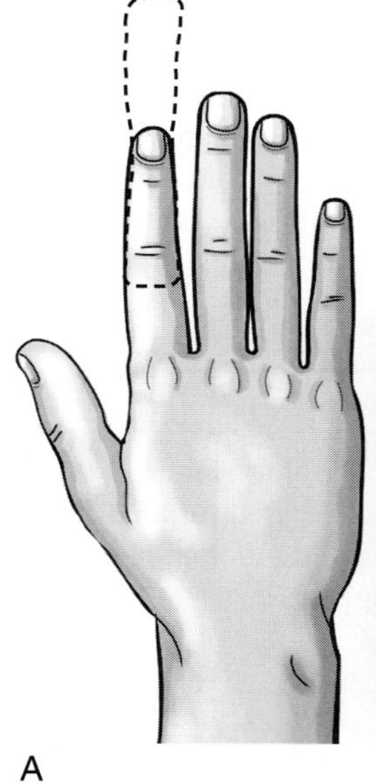

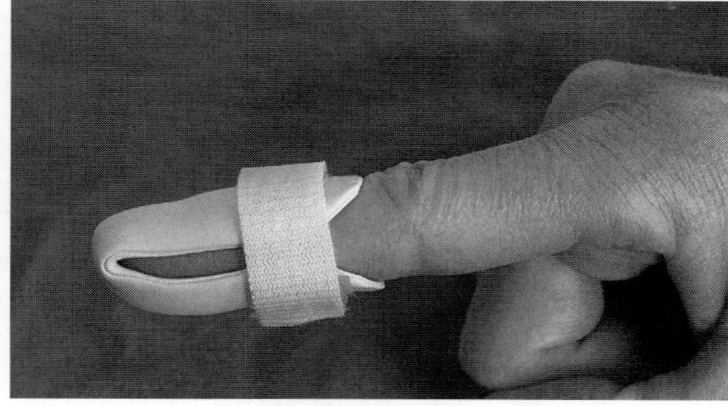

A B

Figure 12-12 (A) Dorsal-volar mallet splint pattern. (B) Completed dorsal-volar mallet splint.

finger all day. In addition to reviewing skin care guidelines and practicing safe protected donning and doffing of the splint, an additional splint was made to use while showering. This allowed him to apply a dry splint after his shower. With this solution, he was able to avoid further skin maceration.

Fabrication of a Dorsal-Volar Mallet Splint

This splint is indicated for a mallet injury. Figure 12-12A represents a detailed pattern that can be used for any finger. Figure 12-12B shows a completed splint. This splint has some adjustability for fluctuations in edema, which can be advantageous (3⁄32-inch nonperforated material works well for this splint). An alternative splint design is a DIP gutter splint. Figure 12-13 represents a detailed pattern for this alternative.

1. Mark the length of the finger from the PIP joint to the tip.
2. Mark the width of the finger.
3. Cut out the pattern and round the four edges.
4. Trace the pattern on a sheet of thermoplastic material.
5. Warm the material slightly to make it easier to cut the pattern out of the thermoplastic material.
6. Heat the thermoplastic material.
7. Apply the material to the client's finger, clearing the volar PIP crease. Be gentle with the amount of hand pressure over the dorsal DIP because this is usually quite tender.
8. Maintain the DIP in extension or slight hyperextension, depending on the physician's order.
9. Allow the material to cool completely before removing the splint.

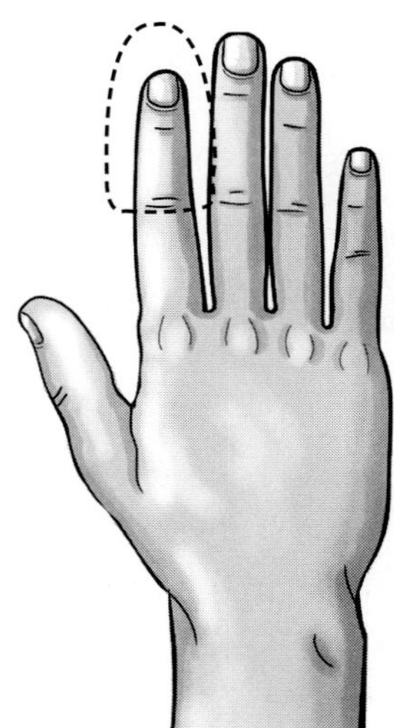

Figure 12-13 DIP gutter splint pattern.

10. Ensure proper fit of the splint. It should stay in place securely with a thin 1⁄2-inch Velcro strap.
11. Trim edges as needed.
12. Smooth all edges completely.

Technical Tips for Proper Fit of Mallet Splints

- Finger splints may seem easy to make because they are small. However, it may actually take extra time to fabricate them precisely. Do not be surprised if you wind up needing extra time to make and fine-tune these small splints.
- Ordinary Velcro loop straps may feel bulky on small finger splints. Thinner strap material that is ½ inch in

width and less bulky can be very effective with finger splints.

Prefabricated Mallet Splints

Figure 12-14 shows various styles of mallet splints. If there has been surgery and the client has a percutaneous pin, the splint must accommodate this. The DIP splint can be a volar gutter splint, a volar-dorsal splint, or a stack splint. A prefabricated Alumifoam splint is sometimes used, but there may be inconveniences as well as skin issues associated with the adhesive tape used to secure it. Prefabricated or custom fabricated stack splints need to be monitored for clearance at the dorsal distal edge because this is an area prone to tenderness and edema related to the injury itself.

Mallet Finger Impact on Occupation

Mallet injuries can result in awkward hand use and can also limit the freedom of flexion of uninvolved digits. It is very important to teach clients to maintain active PIP motion of the involved digit and to use compensatory skills such as relying on uninjured fingertips for sensory input.

Fabrication of a PIP Gutter Splint

This splint is indicated for a PIP sprain injury. Figure 12-15A represents a detailed pattern that can be used for any finger. Figure 12-15b shows a completed splint (3/32-inch nonperforated material works well for this splint).

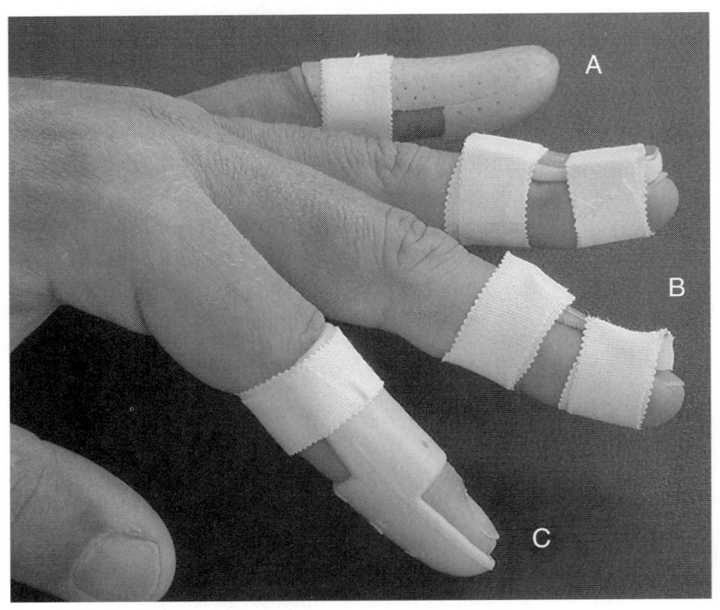

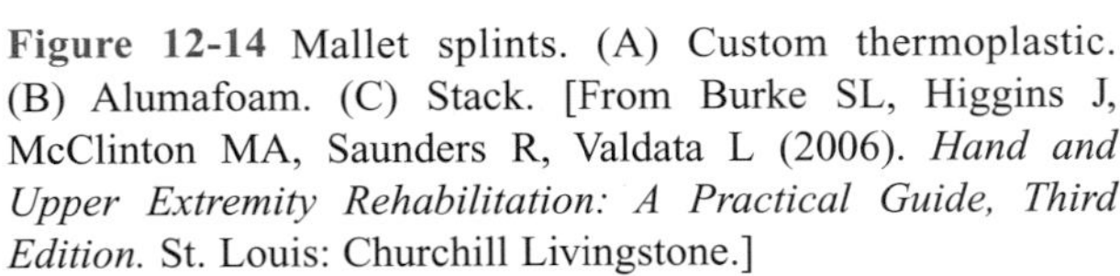

Figure 12-14 Mallet splints. (A) Custom thermoplastic. (B) Alumafoam. (C) Stack. [From Burke SL, Higgins J, McClinton MA, Saunders R, Valdata L (2006). *Hand and Upper Extremity Rehabilitation: A Practical Guide, Third Edition.* St. Louis: Churchill Livingstone.]

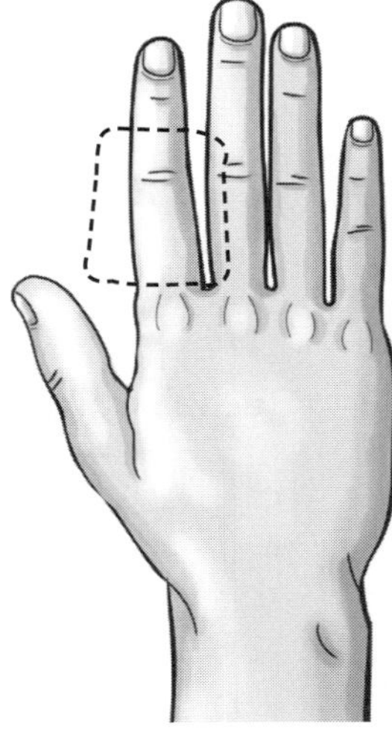

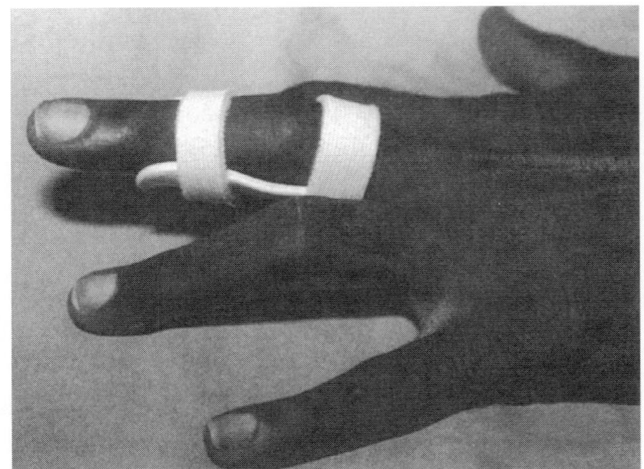

Figure 12-15 (A) PIP gutter splint pattern. (B) Completed PIP gutter splint. [From Clark GL, Shaw Wilgis EF, Aiello B, Eckhaus D, Eddington LV (1998). *Hand Rehabilitation: A Practical Guide, Second Edition.* New York: Churchill Livingstone.]

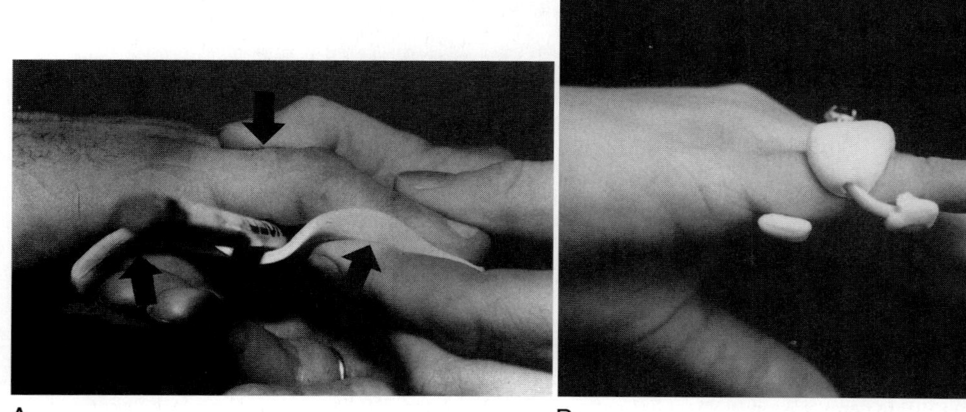

Figure 12-16 (A) Prefabricated PIP extension splint that crosses the DIP. (B) Prefabricated PIP extension splint with DIP free. [From Fess EE, Gettle KS, Philips CA, Janson RJ (2005). *Hand and Upper Extremity Splinting: Principles and Methods, Third Edition.* St. Louis: Mosby.]

1. Mark the length of the finger from the web space to the DIP joint.
2. Mark the width of the finger, adding approximately ¼ to ½ inch on each side—depending on the size of the digit.
3. Cut out the pattern and round the four edges.
4. Trace the pattern on a sheet of thermoplastic material.
5. Warm the material slightly to make it easier to cut the pattern out of the thermoplastic material.
6. Heat the thermoplastic material.
7. Position the client's hand with the palm up so that the material can drape nicely.
8. Apply the material to the client's finger, clearing the MP and DIP creases and positioning the PIP joint in the desired position (this is typically the available passive extension). Be gentle with the amount of hand pressure used over the PIP joint and over the sides of the joint.
9. Roll the edges of the splint as needed for comfort and clearance of MP and DIP joint motions.
10. Allow the material to cool completely before removing the splint.
11. Ensure proper fit of the splint.
12. Trim edges as needed.
13. Smooth all edges completely.

Technical Tips for Proper Fit of PIP Gutter Splints

- Straps should not be too tight because this can cause edema. However, they must fit closely enough to provide a secure fit.
- Modify the height of finger splint edges so that straps can have contact with the skin. If the edges are too high, the straps will not be effective.
- If you are trying to achieve full PIP extension, consider placing a strap directly over the PIP joint. However, be careful to closely monitor skin tolerance.

Prefabricated PIP Splints

Figure 12-16 shows examples of prefabricated PIP extension splints. Remember that prefabricated splints do not always fit well or accommodate edema. In addition, there can be problems associated with distribution of pressure and skin tolerance and with excessive joint forces.

Impact of PIP Injuries on Occupations

PIP joint injuries can limit the flexibility and function of the entire hand. Reaching into the pocket or grasping a tool may be impeded. Pain can interfere with comfort doing a simple but socially significant thing such as a handshake. Rings may no longer fit over the injured joint. Early appropriate therapy can help restore these functions to our clients.

Fabrication of a PIP Hyperextension Block (Swan-Neck Splint)

This splint is indicated for a finger with a flexible swan-neck deformity. Figure 12-17A represents a detailed pattern that can be used for any finger. Figure 12-17B shows a completed splint. An alternative splint design involves wrapping a thin strip or tube of thermoplastic material in a spiral fashion (Figure 12-18). A properly fitting splint will effectively block the PIP in slight flexion when the finger is actively extended and allow unrestricted active PIP flexion. A thin (1/16 inch) nonperforated thermoplastic material (such as Orfit or Aquaplast) works well for this splint. It is especially important to minimize bulk if multiple fingers need to be

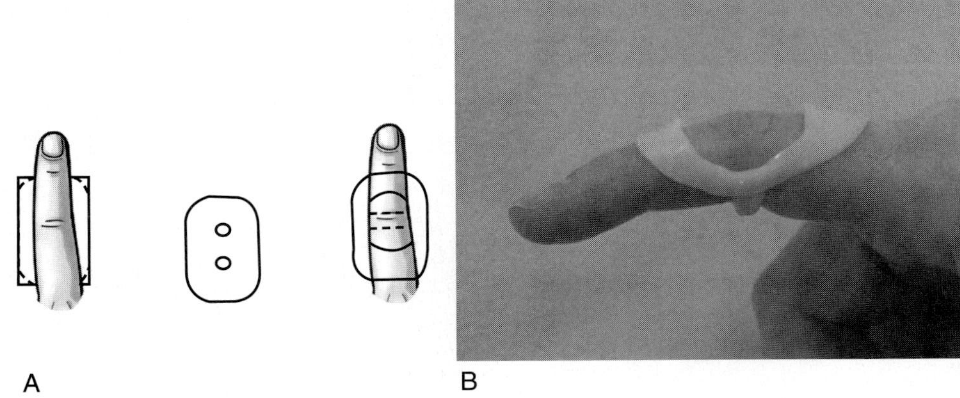

Figure 12-17 (A) PIP hyperextension block splint pattern. (B) Completed PIP hyperextension block splint.

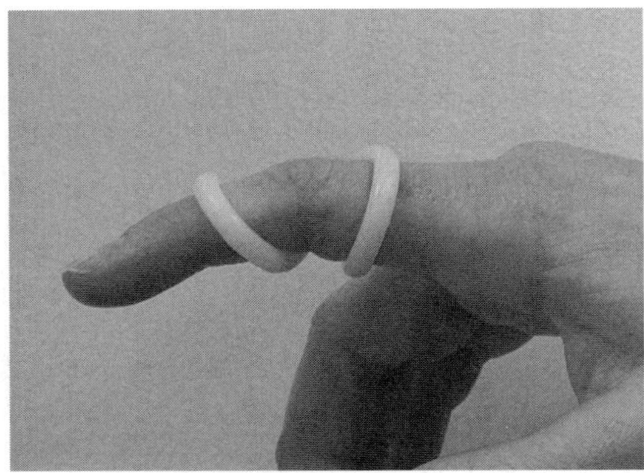

Figure 12-18 Spiral design PIP hyperextension block splint.

splinted on the same hand—so that splints do not get caught on each other.

1. Mark the length of the finger from the web space to the DIP joint.
2. Mark the width of the finger, adding approximately ¼ inch on each side.
3. Cut out the pattern and round the four edges.
4. Trace the pattern on a sheet of thermoplastic material.
5. Cut the pattern out of the thermoplastic material. Cutting thin material does not require heating of the plastic first.
6. Mark location for holes, leaving an approximately ¼- to ½-inch bar of material in the center of the splint.
7. Punch holes.
8. Apply a light amount of lotion to the finger to enable material to slide over the finger easily.
9. Heat the thermoplastic material.
10. Slightly stretch the holes so that they are just large enough to slide the finger through. Be careful not to overstretch because the splint will be too loose.
11. Slide the material over the finger, weaving the finger up through the proximal hole and down through the distal hole.
12. Center the volar thermoplastic bar directly under the PIP joint, and the dorsal distal and proximal ends of the splint over the middle and proximal phalanges.
13. Keep the PIP in slight flexion (approximately 20 to 25 degrees) as you form the splint on the finger.
14. Roll the edges of the volar thermoplastic bar as needed to allow unrestricted PIP flexion.
15. Fold the lateral sides of the splint volarly and contour the material to the finger.
16. Allow the material to cool completely before removing the splint.
17. Ensure proper fit of the splint. The splint should be loose enough to slide over the PIP joint yet snug enough to not migrate or twist on the finger. It should allow full PIP flexion and effectively prevent the PIP from going into hyperextension.
18. Trim edges as needed.
19. Smooth all edges completely.

Technical Tips for Proper Fit of Hyperextension Block (Swan-neck Splint)

- A common mistake is to allow the PIP joint to go into extension while fabricating the splint. Closely monitor PIP position to make sure it remains in slight flexion during the splinting process.
- If the PIP joint is enlarged or swollen, it may be very difficult to slide the splint off the finger once the splint is made. This can be avoided by gently sliding the splint back and forth over the PIP joint a few times before the thermoplastic material is fully cooled.
- Because this splint is meant to enable function, make sure to minimize splint bulk by flattening the volar

PIP bar and lateral edges as much as possible so they do not impede the grasping of objects.

Prefabricated Hyperextension Block Splints

Swan-neck splints are commercially available, and offer some advantages over custom-fabricated thermoplastic splints. They are more durable, less bulky, and often more cosmetically pleasing to clients. Therapists use ring sizers to determine the splint size needed for each finger. Custom-ordered ring splints made of silver or gold (Figure 12-19) are attractive, unobtrusive, and flexible enough to be adjusted for fluctuations in joint swelling. However, they are more costly. Prefabricated splints made of polypropylene (Figure 12-20) are a less expensive alternative that offer durability and a streamlined fit. Their fit can be slightly modified by a therapist using a heat gun, but they cannot be adjusted by clients in response to variations in joint swelling.

Impact of Swan-neck Deformities on Occupations

Swan-neck deformities often cause difficulty with hand closure. PIP tendons and ligaments can catch during motion, and the long finger flexors have less mechanical advantage to initiate flexion when the PIP starts from a hyperextended position. A PIP hyperextension block should improve the client's hand function by allowing the PIP to flex more quickly and easily, enabling the ability to grasp objects.

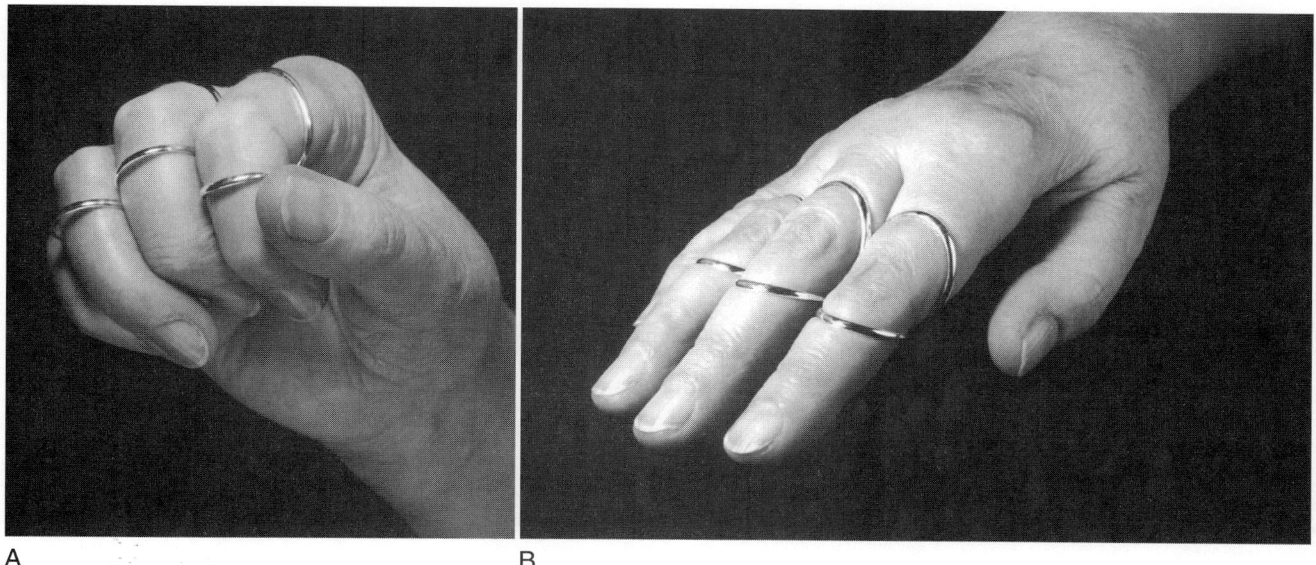

Figure 12-19 Custom-ordered PIP hyperextension block splints. [Courtesy the Silver Ring Splint Company, Charlottesville, Virginia.]

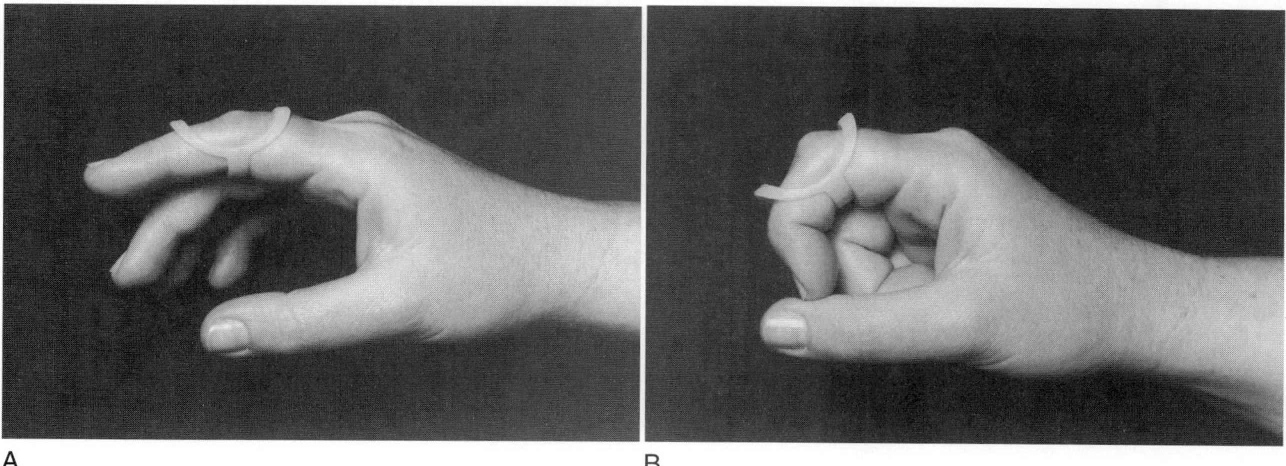

Figure 12-20 Prefabricated PIP hyperextension block splints. [Courtesy 3-Point Products, Stevensville, Maryland.]

Table 12-1 Efficacy Study of Silver Ring Splints

AUTHOR'S CITATION	DESIGN	NO. OF PARTICIPANTS	DESCRIPTION	RESULTS	LIMITATIONS
Zijlstra TR, Heijnsdijk L, Rasker JJ (2004). Silver ring splints improve dexterity in clients with rheumatoid arthritis. Arthritis Rheum, 51: 947–951.	Prospective study	17 clients	Clients with stable disease and finger deformities were seen by two therapists, who decided by consensus which deformities a silver ring splint (SRS) might be appropriate for. SRS size was measured and temporary thermoplastic splints were made. Seventeen clients received a total of 72 SRSs (64 PIP, 5 DIP, 3 thumb IP). Measurements were taken on dexterity, self-reported hand function, pain, grip and pinch strength, and client satisfaction at time of SRS delivery and at 1 month, 3 months, and 12 months.	There was a statistically significant improvement in observed dexterity ($P = 0.005$ at 3 months; $P = 0.026$ at 12 months). There was no statistically significant change in self-reported hand function, pain, or strength. After 1 year 48 SRSs were still regularly used by clients. Twenty-four SRSs (21 PIP, 2 DIP, 1 thumb IP) were discontinued, with main reasons cited as paresthesias and pressure on bony edges or rheumatoid nodules. Eleven of 15 clients completing a survey said they would continue to wear their SRSs.	Small sample size. Non-blinded observers. Authors cite some outcome measures used may have lacked sensitivity to change. Decisions to treat clients with SRSs were made by therapists without input from clients' point of view.

Conclusions, Evidence-Based Practice Information Chart

Table 12-1 presents one study published on PIP hyperextension block splints. Considering how frequently finger splints are used, there is a surprising lack of evidence to support their efficacy. This explains why only one study was located.

Despite the lack of evidence for their use, finger splints are a mainstay of care for many common finger problems. Finger biomechanics are very complicated. Added to this, there are multiple custom and prefabricated splints to select from. These challenges can understandably obfuscate decision making, particularly for newer therapists. We hope this chapter helps you use sound clinical reasoning to work collaboratively with clients. This will ensure that the best splint is selected based on each client's clinical needs and occupational demands.

CASE STUDY 12-1*

Read the following scenario and use your clinical reasoning skills to answer the questions based on information in this chapter.

RC is a 23-year-old right dominant male who jammed his right long finger while playing softball. He developed pain and swelling of the distal finger, along with a droop of the DIP joint. His doctor diagnosed a mallet injury and sent him to occupational therapy for splint fabrication.

1. What joint(s) should his finger splint cross?

____

____

2. What is the recommended wearing schedule of the splint?

____

____

3. Name two different types of splints RC could use.

____

____

4. How long is RC likely to need to wear his splint?

____

____

*See Appendix A for the answer key.

CASE STUDY 12-2*

Read the following scenario and use your clinical reasoning skills to answer the questions based on information in this chapter.

DS is a 62-year-old left dominant female who fell and developed pain and swelling of her left long finger PIP joint. She was diagnosed with a PIP joint injury to the radial collateral ligament and volar plate.

1. Should DS have a dorsal or volar finger splint?

____

____

2. What joint(s) should the splint cross and what position should they be in?

____

____

3. Which fingers would be good to buddy tape or buddy strap together, and why?

____

____

4. DS loved to play tennis. When she was medically cleared to play again, she experienced recurrence of swelling at the long finger PIP joint. What might help her manage her pain and swelling so that she could play tennis again?

____

____

*See Appendix A for the answer key.

CASE STUDY 12-3*

Read the following scenario and use your clinical reasoning skills to answer the questions based on information in this chapter.

AW is a 41-year-old right dominant law firm receptionist who has a three-year history of rheumatoid arthritis. She was referred to occupational therapy for evaluation of splinting needs. She presents with recent development of swan-neck deformities of all fingers of both hands. She is able to actively flex her PIPs, but it is awkward and effortful to do so. She reports having difficulty with home and work tasks that involve grasping objects.

1. Do you think AW would benefit from PIP hyperextension block splints, and why?

2. How could you and AW determine if splinting will improve her hand function?

3. What key client factors and splint options would you consider in selecting the best splints for AW?

4. When should AW wear her splints?

*See Appendix A for the answer key.

REVIEW QUESTIONS

1. What is a mallet finger?
2. What is the posture of a finger with a boutonniere deformity?
3. What is the posture of a finger with a swan-neck deformity?
4. What is fusiform swelling?
5. What structures provide joint stability and restraint against PIP deviation forces?
6. What is the difference between an extensor lag and a flexion contracture?
7. What type of finger splint is typically used for a swan-neck deformity?
8. What position is the DIP splinted in when treating a mallet finger?
9. What position is the PIP splinted in when treating a boutonniere deformity?
10. What position is the PIP splinted in when treating a swan-neck deformity?

References

Alter S, Feldon P, Terrono AL (2002). Pathomechanics of deformities in the arthritic hand and wrist. In EJ Mackin, AD Callahan, TM Skirven, LH Schneider, AL Osterman (eds.), *Rehabilitation of the Hand and Upper Extremity, Fifth Edition*. St. Louis: Mosby pp. 1545-1554.

Bell-Krotoski J (2002). Plaster cylinder casting for contractures of the interphalangeal joints. In EJ Mackin, AD Callahan, TM Skirven, LH Schneider, AL Osterman (eds.), *Rehabilitation of the Hand and Upper Extremity, Fifth Edition*. St. Louis: Mosby pp. 1839-1845.

Bell-Krotoski J (2005). Plaster serial casting for the remodeling of soft tissue, mobilization of joints, and increased tendon excursion. In EE Fess, KS Gettle, CA Philips, JR Janson (eds.), *Hand and Upper Extremity Splinting: Principles and Methods, Third Edition*. St. Louis: Mosby pp. 599-606.

Campbell PJ, Wilson RL (2002). Management of joint injuries and intraarticular fractures. In EJ Mackin, AD Callahan, TM Skirven, LH Schneider, AL Osterman (eds.), *Rehabilitation of the Hand and Upper Extremity, Fifth Edition*. St. Louis: Mosby pp. 396-411.

Cooper C (2007). Common finger sprains and deformities. In C Cooper (ed.), *Fundamentals of Hand Therapy: Clinical Reasoning and Treatment Guidelines for Common Diagnoses of the Upper Extremity*. St. Louis: Mosby pp. 301-319.

Deshaies L. Arthritis (2006). In HM Pendleton, W Schultz-Krohn (eds.), *Pedretti's Occupational Therapy: Practice Skills for Physical Dysfunction, Sixth Edition*.St. Louis: Mosby pp. 950-982.

Hofmeister EP, Mazurek MT, Shin AY, Bishop AT (2003). Extension block pinning for large mallet fractures. Journal of Hand Surgery pp. 28A:453-459.

CHAPTER 13

Splinting for Nerve Injuries

Helene Lohman, MA, OTD, OTR/L
Brenda M. Coppard, PhD, OTR/L

Key Terms

Axonotmesis
Cubital tunnel syndrome
Cumulative trauma disorders
Double crush
Median nerve
Neurapraxia
Neurotmesis
Posterior interosseous nerve syndrome
Pronator tunnel syndrome
Radial nerve
Radial tunnel syndrome
Ulnar nerve
Wallerian degeneration
Wartenberg's neuropathy

Chapter Objectives

1. Identify the components of a peripheral nerve.
2. Describe a peripheral nerve's response to injury and repair.
3. List the operative procedures used for nerve repair.
4. List the three purposes for splinting nerve palsies.
5. Describe the nerve injury classification.
6. Identify the locations for low and high peripheral nerve lesions.
7. Explain causes of radial, ulnar, and median nerve lesions.
8. Review the sensory and motor distributions of the radial, median, and ulnar nerves.
9. Explain the functional effects of radial, ulnar, and median nerve lesions.
10. Identify the splinting approaches and rationale for radial, ulnar, and median nerve injuries.
11. Use clinical judgment to evaluate a problematic splint for a nerve lesion.
12. Use clinical judgment to evaluate a fabricated hand-based ulnar nerve splint.
13. Apply documentation skills to a case study.
14. Understand the importance of evidence-based practice with provision of splints for nerve conditions.

Splint interventions for nerve lesions require that therapists have a thorough knowledge of static (immobilization) and dynamic (mobilization) splinting principles and sound critical-thinking skills. Comprehension of kinesiology, physiology, and anatomy is paramount to understanding the motor, sensory, and vasomotor implications of a nerve injury. Competence in manual muscle-testing skills is also necessary to evaluate the muscles as nerves recover from injuries [Colditz 2002]. This chapter includes information on peripheral nerve anatomy; nerve injury classifications; nerve repair; and types, effects, and treatments for radial, ulnar, and median nerve injuries.

Peripheral Nerve Anatomy

As shown in Figure 13-1, a peripheral nerve consists of the epineurium, perineurium, endoneurium, fascicles, axons, and blood vessels [Jebson and Gaul 1998]. The epineurium is made of loose collagenous connective tissue. There are external and internal types of epineurium. The external epineurium contains blood vessels. The internal epineurium protects the fascicles from pressure and allows gliding of fascicles. The amount of epineurium varies among persons, nerve types, and along each individual nerve. The perineurium surrounds fascicles, and the endoneurium surrounds the axons. A fascicle consists of a group of axons that are surrounded by endoneurium and are covered by

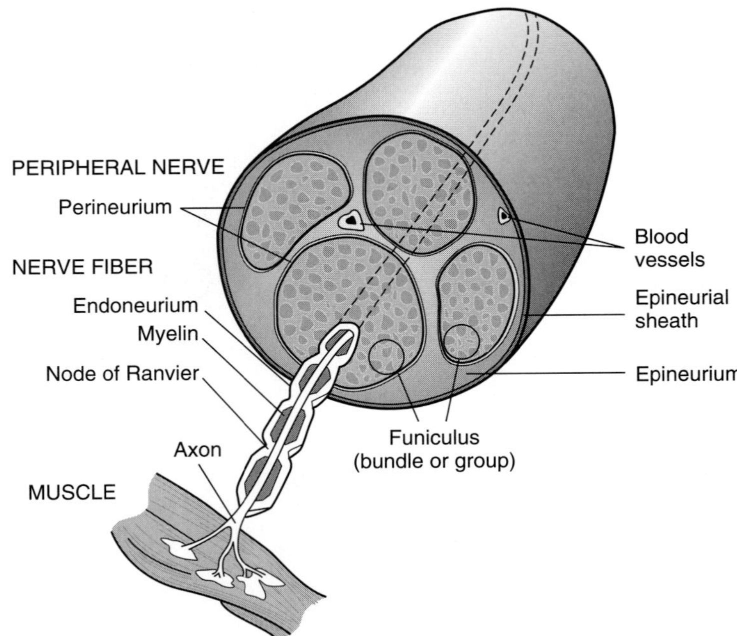

Figure 13-1 Components of a peripheral nerve.

a sheath of perineurium. An individual fascicle contains a mix of myelinated and unmyelinated fibers. The myelin sheath encapsulates the axon. Myelin is a lipoprotein, which allows for conduction of fast impulses. Each nerve contains a varied number and size of fascicles.

Nerves are at risk for injury when laceration, avulsion, stretch, crush, compression, or contusion occurs [Callahan 1984]. In addition, peripheral nerves can be attacked by viruses, bacteria, or the body's immune system [Greene and Roberts 2005]. Often bone, tendon, ligament, vessel, and soft-tissue injuries accompany nerve injuries.

Nerve Injury Classification

Nerve injuries are categorized by the extent of damage to the axon and sheath [Skirven 1992]. Nerve compression lesions often contribute to peripheral neuropathies. When a specific portion of a peripheral nerve is compressed, the peripheral axons within the nerve sustain the greatest injury. Initial changes occur in the blood/nerve barrier followed by subperineural edema. This results in a thickening of the internal and external perineurium [Novak and Mackinnon 1998]. As the compression worsens, the motor, proprioceptive, light touch, and vibratory sensory axons become more vulnerable [Spinner 1990]. All the fibers may be paralyzed after enduring severe and prolonged compression. Seddon [1943] originally described three levels of nerve injury: (1) neurapraxia, (2) axonotmesis, and (3) neurotmesis (Figure 13-2). Later in 1968, Sunderland extended the classification to five levels, which are termed as first- through fifth-degree injuries.

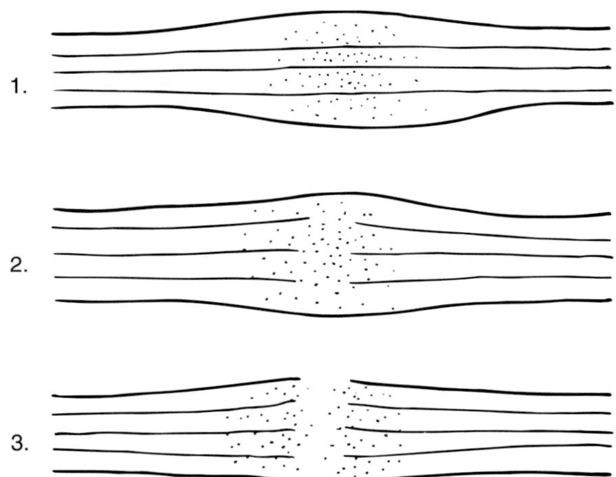

Figure 13-2 The three classifications of nerve injuries are (1) neurapraxia, (2) axonotmesis, and (3) neurotmesis.

First-degree Injury

A first-degree injury involves the demylination of the nerve, which temporarily blocks conduction [Boscheinen-Morrin et al. 1987, Novak and Mackinnon, 2005]. The prognosis for persons with neurapraxia is extremely good; recovery is usually spontaneous within three months [Spinner 1990].

Second-degree Injury

When a second-degree injury occurs, the axon is severed and the sheath remains intact. Wallerian degeneration occurs when a nerve is completely severed or the axon and myelin sheath are damaged, and the endoneurial tube remains intact. The segment of axon and the motor and sensory end receptors distal to the lesion suffer ischemia and begin to degenerate 3 to 5 days after the injury [Jebson and Gaul 1998]. The intact endoneurial tube allows for potential regrowth for the proximal part of the nerve to reattach to the distal portion of the nerve. With the ideal scenario the rate of regeneration is approximately 1 inch per month. Complete recovery usually occurs if regeneration happens in a timely manner before muscle degeneration [Novak and Mackinnon 2005].

Third-degree Injury

A third-degree injury is a more severe form of a second-degree injury with the addition of the "continuity of the endoneurial tube destroyed from a disorganization of the internal structures of the nerve bundles" [Sunderland 1968, p.132]. Recovery is more complicated with possible delayed or incomplete axonal growth [Sunderland 1968]. Because fibers are often mismatched, clients benefit from motor and sensory reeducation [Novak and Mackinnon 2005].

Fourth-degree Injury

At this level of injury "the involved segment is ultimately converted into a tangled strand of connective tissue, Schwann cells, and regenerating axons which can be enlarged to form a neuroma" [Sunderland 1968, p. 135]. The effects are more severe than a third-degree injury with increased neuronal degeneration, misdirected axons, and less axon survival [Sunderland 1968]. Surgical intervention is necessary to remove the neuroma (a tumor of nerve fibers and cells).

Fifth-degree Injury

A fifth-degree injury results in partial or complete severance of the axon and the sheath with loss of motor, sensory, and sympathetic function [Sunderland 1968]. Without the directional guidance from an intact endoneurial tube, misdirected axon growth may lead to a complicated recovery. Microsurgery is required to reestablish axon direction. Occasionally, grafting is necessary if the gap is too large for approximation of the two nerve ends [Spinner 1990].

Nerve Repair

Peripheral nerve lesions often occur to the median, radial, and ulnar nerves. The location of the lesion determines the impairment of sudomotor, vasomotor, muscular, sensory, and functional involvement [Boscheinen-Morrin et al. 1987]. Sometimes nerves can be compressed at more than one site, which is called *double crush injury* [Upton and McComas 1973, Rehak 2001]. Therefore, it is important to be aware of key diagnostic procedures to determine the extent of compression.

Operative Procedures for Nerve Repair

There are four procedures used to surgically repair nerves: (1) decompression, (2) repair, (3) neurolysis, and (4) grafting [Saidoff and McDonough 1997]. Nerve decompression is the most common operation performed on nerves. An example of surgical decompression is the transection of the transverse carpal ligament to decompress the median nerve (this is also known as a carpal tunnel release).

Surgical nerve repairs involve microsurgical sutures to repair the epineurium. Surgical nerve repairs are classified as primary, delayed primary, or secondary [Jebson and Gaul 1998]. A primary repair occurs within hours of the injury. A delayed primary repair occurs within 5 to 7 days after the injury. Any surgical repair performed beyond seven days is a secondary repair.

Neurolysis is a procedure performed on a nerve that has become encapsulated in dense scar tissue, which compresses the nerve to surrounding soft tissues and prevents it from gliding. When the client attempts to move in a way that would normally glide the nerve, it instead stretches, affecting circulation and chemical balance. Scars may physically interfere with the axon regeneration.

Nerve grafting is necessary when there is a large gap in a nerve and end-to-end nerve repair is not possible. An autograft donated by a cutaneous nerve, such as the sural nerve, can fill the gap. Although the outcome from a nerve graft is somewhat unreliable, occasionally it is the only option for repair.

Purposes for Splinting Nerve Injuries

The three purposes for splinting an extremity that has a nerve injury are protection, prevention, and assistance with function [Arsham 1984]. If a nerve has undergone surgical repair, the physician may initially order application of a cast or splint to place the hand, wrist, or elbow in a protective position, thus reducing the amount of tension on the repaired nerve. Avoiding tension on a repaired nerve is extremely important because results of nerve repairs are directly related to the amount of tension across the repair site [Skirven and Callahan 2002].

Prevention of contractures is important because nerve lesions result in various degrees of muscle denervation. For example, a short opponens splint prevents a contracture of the thumb web space after a median nerve injury [Fess et al. 2005]. Sometimes a client does not seek immediate medical attention after the occurrence of a nerve injury, and a resulting contracture develops and requires splint intervention. For example, if a person presents with a clawhand deformity as a result of an ulnar nerve injury the therapist may choose to fabricate a mobilizing ulnar gutter splint to remodel the soft tissues to increase passive extension of the ring and little fingers' proximal interphalangeal (PIP) joints [Callahan 1984].

Once metacarpophalangeal (MCP) and PIP stiffness have occurred treatment should focus on regaining maximum passive range of motion (PROM). After normal PROM is reestablished, splinting interventions for the muscle imbalance become an option [Fess 1986].

Often, function after a nerve injury can be enhanced by splint intervention. For example, a client may be better able to grasp and release objects after a radial nerve injury if he or she is wearing an elastic tension MCP and wrist extension splint. This splint assists the MCP joints to extend to open the hand for grasp release. Without the splint, the wrist and MCP joints are unable to extend, and difficulty with grasp and grasp release activities results.

Upper Extremity Compression Neuropathies

Cumulative trauma disorder (CTD) is not a medical diagnosis but an etiologic label for a range of disorders [Melhorn 1998]. The cause of CTD is not solely work activities. Social activities, activities of daily living (ADL), and leisure pursuits may also enhance the development and exacerbation of CTD [Melhorn 1998]. The first step in controlling the CTD is to understand the compressive neuropathies of the upper extremity [Vender et al. 1998]. Table 13-1 outlines the nature and treatment of compressive neuropathies that can occur at the wrist, elbow, and forearm. The compressive neuropathies are discussed in more detail later in this chapter.

Table 13-1 Upper Extremity Compression Neuropathies

	PRESENTATION	SPLINTING INTERVENTION
Wrist		
Carpal tunnel syndrome	Complaints of numbness, tingling, and paresthesias in the median nerve distribution. Persons may complain of dropping objects or cramping and aching, especially during sleep and driving. In severe cases, thenar atrophy or loss of strength of palmar abduction of the thumb will be present. Positive Phalen's and Tinel's signs and night pain are present.	Splinting involves prefabricated or custom-made wrist splint with the wrist in neutral. Splint regimens vary, but most include nighttime wear.
Ulnar nerve entrapment at the wrist (ulnar tunnel syndrome)	Entrapment of the ulnar nerve usually occurs in the Guyon's canal. Sensory changes involve the fifth digit and ulnar side of the fourth digit. True ulnar nerve entrapment is not common.	Splinting involves a dorsal hand-based splint with fourth and fifth digit in 30 to 45 degrees of flexion at the metacarpophalangeal (MCP) joint to block MCP hyperextension. Splint can be dynamic or static. Splint is worn until the nerve has regenerated.
Elbow and Forearm		
Pronator syndrome	Compression of the median nerve as it crosses the elbow at the origin of the pronator teres. It is associated with pain in the proximal forearm and is aggravated by resisted forearm pronation when the elbow is flexed.	Initial splinting may include splinting the forearm in neutral between supination and pronation, wrist in neutral to slight flexion, and with or without the elbow in flexion. If the elbow is included, position in 90 degrees of flexion. If conservative treatment fails and there are signs of muscle atrophy, surgical decompression may be considered.
Anterior interosseous syndrome	Compression of the anterior interosseous branch of the median nerve is associated with pain in the proximal volar forearm followed by loss of ability to flex the interphalangeal (IP) joint of the thumb and the distal interphalanged (DIP) joint of the second and third digits. There are usually no sensory complaints.	Physicians may recommend 8 to 12 weeks of observation, during which extreme forearm pronation/supination is avoided and extension of the elbow is limited. Splinting may include immobilizing the elbow in 90 degrees of flexion with the forearm in neutral. Another option is to fabricate small splints to block index DIP and thumb IP extension or hyperextension (see Figure 13-17).
Radial tunnel syndrome	True radial tunnel syndrome is rare and is often misdiagnosed as lateral epicondylitis. Radial tunnel syndrome presents with pain and discomfort in the extensor-supinator muscle mass in the proximal forearm. Radial tunnel syndrome has pain as the presenting symptom, not motor dysfunction.	Conservative treatment involves splinting the elbow in 90 degrees flexion with the forearm in supination and the wrist in 20 to 30 degrees of extension. If no improvement is noted within about 4 weeks, surgical decompression may be considered. Another option is fabricating a thumb immobilization splint.

Table 13-1 Upper Extremity Compression Neuropathies—cont'd

	PRESENTATION	SPLINTING INTERVENTION
Posterior interosseous nerve syndrome	Presentation is similar to radial tunnel syndrome. However, posterior interosseous syndrome includes weakness or paralysis of any muscles innervated by the posterior interosseous nerve and does not involve sensory loss. The ability to extend the wrist in radial deviation is present, but extension of the wrist is impaired in neutral or ulnar deviation. Loss of thumb extension and abduction and active extension of the MCP joints are also present.	Conservative treatment involves splinting the elbow in flexion with the forearm in neutral or slightly supinated and the wrist in 20 to 30 degrees of extension. If no improvement is noted within about 12 weeks, surgical decompression may be considered. Another option is fabricating a tenodesis splint.
Cubital tunnel syndrome	Presents with localized pain to the medial side of the proximal forearm and elbow. There is numbness and tingling of the fifth digit and the medial side of the fourth digit. Advanced compression will present with hypothenar eminence atrophy. A positive Froment's sign may accompany this syndrome.	Conservative treatment includes avoidance of direct pressure on the medial aspect of the elbow and on the flexor carpi ulnaris. An elbow pad may help to distribute pressure over the nerve. Splinting for nighttime includes positioning the elbow in 30 to 45 degrees of flexion. If the wrist is included, it is positioned in 20 degrees of extension. During the daytime, prolonged elbow flexion should be avoided and with continuous symptoms the splint should be worn all the time.
Radial sensory entrapment (Wartenberg's neuropathy)	Compression of the superficial radial nerve usually includes numbness, tingling, and pain of the dorsoradial aspect of the forearm, wrist, and hand. Symptoms occur during ulnar deviation of the wrist, thumb composite flexion, and forceful pronation and supination of the forearm.	Conservative treatment includes avoidance of motions at the wrist and forearm. A wrist immobilization splint with the wrist in 20 to 30 degrees of extension may be effective. If pain occurs with thumb motion, the thumb should also be incorporated into the splint.

Locations of Nerve Lesions

The location of a nerve lesion determines the sensory and motor result. Lesions are referred to as low or high. Low lesions occur distal to the elbow, and high lesions occur proximal to the elbow [Barr and Swan 1988]. High lesions affect more muscles and may affect a larger sensory distribution than low lesions. Therefore, knowledge of relevant anatomy is important.

Substitutions

When a nerve lesion occurs, "there is no opposing balancing force to the intact active muscle group" [Colditz 2002, p. 622]. If a nerve lesion remains unsplinted, the intact musculature overpowers the denervated muscles. Intact musculature takes over and produces movement normally generated by the dennervated muscles [Clarkson and Gilewich 1989]. The person learns to adapt to the imbalance [Posner 2000, Colditz 2002]. An example of a substitution or trick movement is the pinch that develops after a low-level median nerve injury. With the help of the adductor pollicis, the flexor pollicis longus pinches objects against the radial side of the index finger. A therapist may mistakenly think that motor return has occurred for the abductor pollicis brevis, flexor pollicis brevis, opponens pollicis, and first and second lumbricals. However, the pinch movement observed is actually a substitution.

Prognosis

Many factors affect the prognosis of recovery from a nerve injury. These factors include the extent of the injury, the cleanliness of the wound, the method of repair, and the client's age [Skirven 1992, Skirven and Callahan 2002]. Other factors that alter nerve repair include the amount of tension on the repair, the person's general health, and whether the person smokes. Correct alignment of axons and avoidance of tension on the damaged nerve improve the prognosis. A clean wound has a better prognosis than a dirty wound [Boscheinen-Morrin et al. 1987]. Sharply severed nerves recover better than frayed nerve damage resulting from a crush or gunshot wound [Frykman 1993]. Nerve microsurgery "timed appropriately according to the nature

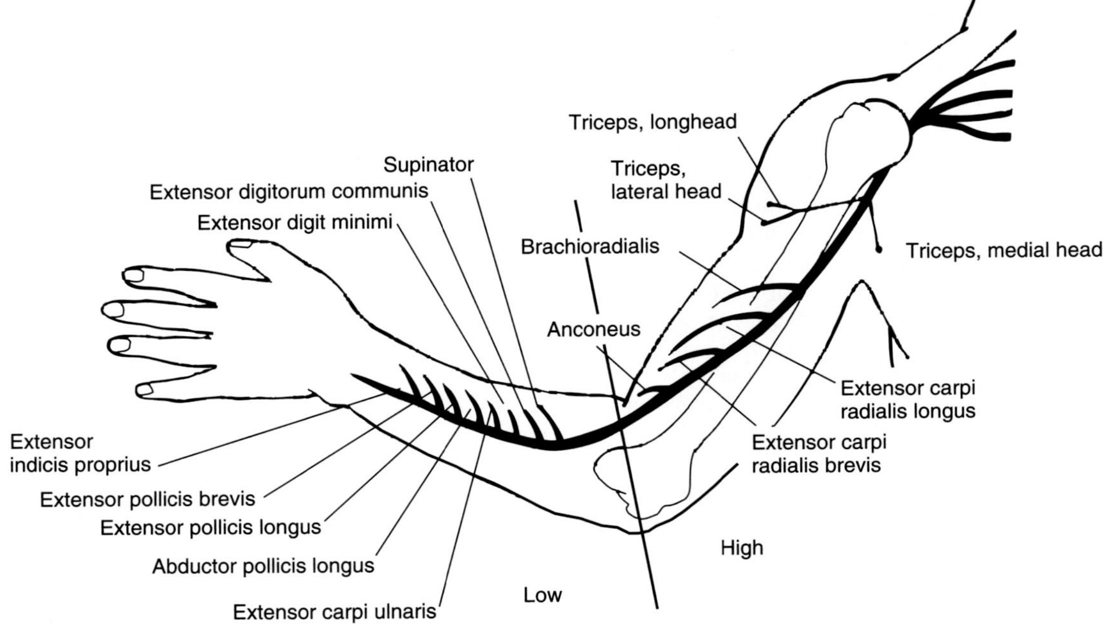

Figure 13-3 Radial nerve motor innervation.

and extent of the injury is essential for a favorable outcome" [Skirven 1992, p. 324]. Age is also a factor in the speed of recovery. A child's potential for regeneration is greater than an adult's [Skirven 1992]. Full sensory and motor return occurs often in a child but rarely in an adult.

The rate of axonal regeneration in human beings is 1 to 3 mm per day. Because nerve regeneration is slow, the therapist conducts periodic monitoring (and splinting is often part of the treatment protocol). In addition, the therapist documents results of the evaluation and any changes to the splinting or exercise program.

Radial Nerve Injuries

Radial nerve palsies are very common and typically occur from midhumeral fractures or compressions [Arsham 1984, Colditz 1987]. Other causes of superficial radial nerve palsies at the wrist include pressure, edema, and trauma on the nerve from crush injuries; de Quervain's tendonitis; handcuffs; and a tight or heavy wristwatch [Eaton and Lister 1992]. The location of the radial nerve injury determines which muscles are affected (Figure 13-3).

Three lesions are possible when the radial nerve is injured [Colditz 2002]. The first type of lesion involves a high injury at the level of the humerus that results in wrist drop and lack of finger MCP extension (Figure 13-4). With this type of lesion, the triceps are rarely affected unless the injury is extremely high.

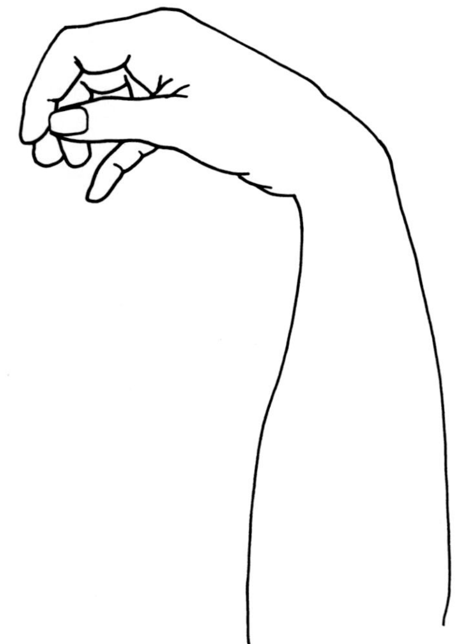

Figure 13-4 Wrist drop deformity from a radial nerve injury.

The second type of lesion involves the posterior interosseous nerve. After spiraling around the humerus and crossing the elbow, the radial nerve divides into a motor and a sensory branch [Eaton and Lister 1992]. The motor branch is the posterior interosseous nerve, and the sensory branch is the superficial branch of the radial nerve. Compression usually causes this palsy, but lacerations or stab wounds can also be sources of lesions to the posterior interosseous nerve. Radial tunnel syndrome and posterior interosseous nerve compression are two distinct types of compression syndromes that can occur in the same tunnel and with the same nerve. As Gelberman et al. [1993, p. 1870] state, "It is difficult for the conscientious diagnostician to accept the reality that the same nerve compressed in the same anatomical site can result in two entirely different symptom complexes." Compression of the radial nerve just distal to the elbow between the radial head and the supinator muscle is typically called *radial tunnel syndrome* [Izzi et al. 2001, Skirvern and Callahan 2002] and is linked to repetitive forearm rotation [Cohen and Garfin 1997]. With radial tunnel syndrome, complaints of pain are usually in the radial nerve distribution of the distal forearm [Hornbach and Culp 2002] and will involve sensory problems without muscle weakness [Eaton and Lister 1992, Gelberman et al. 1993].

Posterior interosseous nerve compression results in rapid motor loss [Gelberman et al. 1993], with no sensory loss [Eaton and Lister 1992, Gelberman et al. 1993, Kleinert and Mehta 1996]. It is characterized by aching on the lateral side of the elbow, difficulty with MCP finger and thumb extension, and difficulty with thumb abduction. Wrist extension is intact, but the wrist tends to radially deviate due to muscle imbalance [Kleinert and Mehta 1996].

The third type of lesion is damage to the sensory branch of the radial nerve. This type of lesion does not result in a functional loss. However, compression symptoms include numbness, tingling, burn, and pain over the dorsoradial surface of the hand [Skirven and Osterman 2002]. Compression of this superficial branch is called Wartenberg's syndrome [Nuber et al. 1998].

Functional Involvement from Radial Nerve Lesions

Table 13-2 outlines the muscles and motions that are affected and the lesion locations in radial nerve lesions. After crossing the elbow and dropping below the supinator, the radial nerve divides and forms the posterior interosseous nerve [Colditz 2002]. Lesions and compressions of the posterior interosseous nerve at the forearm level can affect the following muscles:

- Extensor digitorum communis
- Extensor carpi ulnaris
- Abductor pollicis longus
- Extensor pollicis longus
- Extensor pollicis brevis
- Extensor indicis proprius
- Extensor digiti minimi

Loss of these muscles results in a loss of MCP extension of all the digits, loss of thumb radial abduction, and loss of thumb extension. With attempts at wrist extension, strong wrist radial deviation is present. With attempts at finger extension, the MCPs flex and the PIPs extend because the extensor digitorum muscle is affected. In addition to the muscles just indicated, a radial nerve injury at the elbow level can affect the following muscles:

- Extensor carpi radialis longus
- Extensor carpi radialis brevis
- Supinator

Table 13-2 Radial Nerve Lesions

AFFECTED MUSCLES	WEAK OR LOST MOTIONS
Forearm Level (Posterior Interosseous Nerve)	
Extensor digitorum communis	Metacarpophalangeal (MCP) extension of digits 2 through 5
Extensor carpi ulnaris	Wrist extension and wrist ulnar deviation
Extensor indicis proprius	Extension of the MCP, proximal interphalangeal (PIP), distal interphalangeal (DIP) of the second digit
Extensor digiti minimi	Extension of the MCP, proximal interphalangeal (PIP), distal interphalangeal (DIP) of the fifth digit
Abductor pollicis longus	Thumb abduction
Extensor pollicis longus	Thumb extension
Extensor pollicis brevis	MCP extension and assist CMC extension
Elbow Level	
Extensor carpi radialis longus	Radial wrist extension
Extensor carpi radialis brevis	Radial wrist extension
Supinator	Supination
Extensor digitorum communis	MCP extension of digits 2 through 5
Extensor carpi ulnaris	Wrist extension and ulnar deviation
Extensor indicis proprius	Extension of the MCP, PIP, DIP of the second digit
Extensor digiti minimi	Extension of the MCP, PIP, DIP of the fifth digit
Abductor pollicis longus	Thumb abduction
Extensor pollicis longus	Thumb extension
Extensor pollicis brevis	MCP extension and assist CMC extension
Axilla Level	
Brachioradialis	Elbow flexion
Triceps	Elbow extension
Extensor carpi radialis longus	Radial wrist extension
Extensor carpi radialis brevis	Radial wrist extension
Supinator	Supination
Extensor digitorum communis	MCP extension of digits 2 through 5
Extensor carpi ulnaris	Wrist extension and ulnar deviation
Extensor indicis proprius	Extension of the MCP, PIP, DIP of the second digit
Extensor digiti minimi	Extension of the MCP, PIP, DIP of the fifth digit
Abductor pollicis longus	Thumb abduction
Extensor pollicis longus	Thumb extension
Extensor pollicis brevis	MCP extension and assist CMC extension

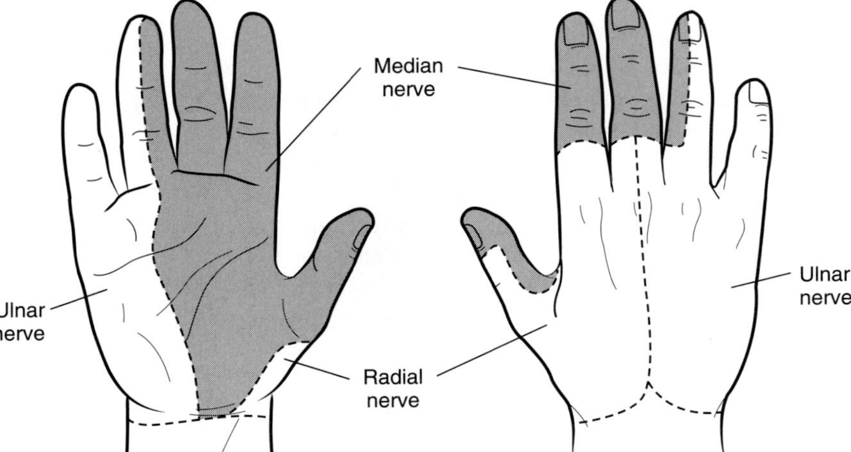

Figure 13-5 Radial, median, and ulnar nerve sensory distribution.

In addition to the motions lost at the forearm level, an injury at the elbow level involves a loss of radial wrist extension, MCP joint extension, thumb extension, thumb radial abduction, and weakened forearm supination.

When a high-level lesion or compression occurs in the upper arm (i.e., axilla level), the injury can affect the triceps and brachioradialis muscles. Loss of these muscles results in lost elbow extension, weak supination, absent wrist and finger extensors, and lost thumb extension and abduction.

The functional results of an axilla-level lesion are a loss of wrist stabilization in an extended position, loss of finger and thumb extension, and loss of thumb abduction. A client with a high radial nerve lesion has poor grip and coordination because of the lack of wrist extensor opposition to the flexors [Fess 1986, Bosheinen-Morrin et al. 1987]. The resulting deformity is called *wrist drop.*

Significant loss of sensation is not present with radial nerve injuries. The superficial sensory branch of the radial nerve supplies sensation to the dorsum of the index and middle fingers and half of the ring finger to the PIP joint level. Figure 13-5 shows a representation of hand sensory distribution from the radial nerve. Laceration or contusion to the sensory branch of the radial nerve can be annoying. This often occurs in conjunction with de Quervain's release. Sensory compromise over the dorsum of the thumb may result in hypersensitivity. Sometimes a splint or padded device can protect the area while a desensitization program is implemented [personal communication, K. Schultz-Johnson, October 1999].

Radial Nerve Injury Splint Intervention

The client benefits from a splint intervention in addition to a therapeutic program. There are several splint options for radial nerve injuries. Splints specific for diagnoses are discussed first, followed by various design options of splints.

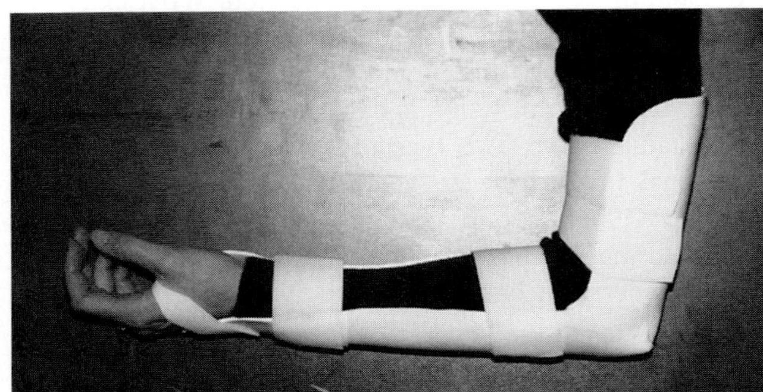

Figure 13-6 Long-arm elbow and wrist splint for radial tunnel syndrome. [From Alba CD (2002). Therapist's management of radial tunnel syndrome. In EJ Mackin, AD Callahan, TM Shirven, LH Schneider, AL Osterman (eds.), *Rehabilitation of the Hand and Upper Extremity, Fifth Edition.* St. Louis: Mosby, pp. 696-700.]

Splinting for Radial Tunnel Syndrome

For this condition, the elbow is positioned in approximately 90 degrees flexion, forearm in full supination, and the wrist in slight wrist extension (20 to 30 degrees) [Gelberman et al. 1993, Alba 2002]. Positioning the forearm in supination decompresses pressure on the radial nerve. The splint (Figure 13-6) is worn all the time, with removal for hygiene [Alba 2002]. Kleinert and Mehta [1996] suggest the splinting approach of fabricating a thermoplastic thumb immobilization splint (see Chapter 8).

Splinting for Posterior Interosseous Nerve Syndrome

A couple of splinting options are suggested for posterior interosseous nerve syndrome. One option is to fabricate a long-arm elbow and wrist splint with the elbow in flexion,

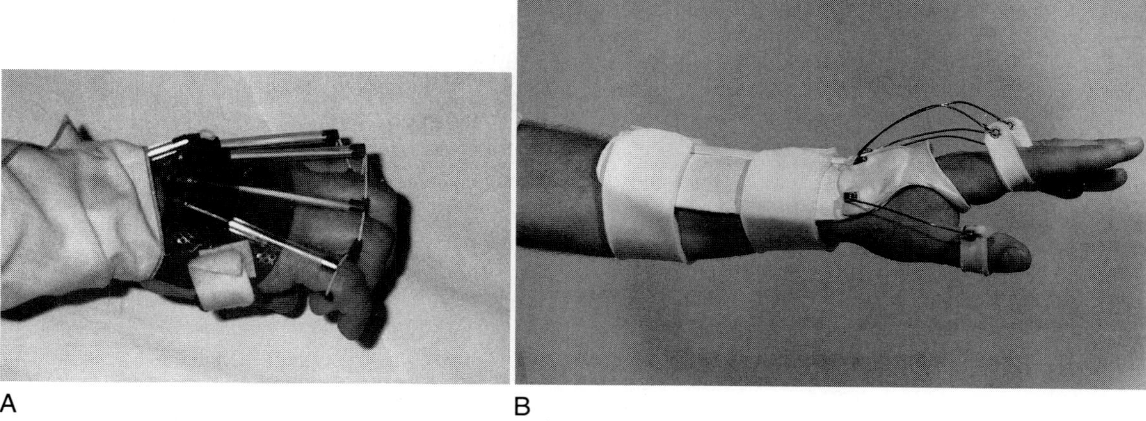

A B

Figure 13-7 Low-profile designs with pre-purchased outrigger parts. [From Fess EE, Gettle KS, Philips CA, Janson JR (2005). *Hand and Upper Extremity Splinting: Principles and Methods, Third Edition*. St. Louis: Elsevier/Mosby.]

forearm in neutral or slightly supinated, and the wrist in 20 to 30 degrees of extension. Another option is to fabricate a tenodesis splint because it encourages wrist and finger function [Eaton and Lister 1992]. The tenodesis splint is discussed later in this chapter.

Splinting for Wartenberg's Neuropathy

For Wartenberg's neuropathy, a wrist immobilization splint is fabricated with the wrist in 20 to 30 degrees of extension. If pain occurs with thumb motion, the thumb is also incorporated into the splint. Refer to Chapter 8 on how to fabricate a thumb splint.

Wrist Immobilization Splint

The therapist can use a wrist immobilization splint to place the wrist in a functional position of 30 degrees of extension [Cannon et al. 1985]. A client can usually extend the fingers to release an object by using the intrinsic hand muscles [Boscheinen-Morrin et al. 1987]. The therapist keeps in mind the advantages, disadvantages, and patterns of volar and dorsal wrist splints (see Chapter 7). A wrist immobilizer splint may be appropriate to wear on occasions when the client desires a more inconspicuous design than a mobilization splint. A wrist immobilization splint may also be more appropriate for nighttime wear than a mobilization splint.

Wearing a mobilization splint at night may result in damage to the outrigger and injury to the client. Some persons who have heavy demands on their hands prefer the simple wrist immobilization splints to the more fragile outrigger-mobilization designs. A therapist may offer both a wrist immobilization splint and a wrist mobilization splint to the person. Alternating the splints may maximize function.

Mobilization Extension Splints

Mobilization splinting for a radial nerve injury promotes functional hand use [Borucki and Schmidt 1992]. The therapist fabricates a dorsal wrist immobilizer splint as the base for a mobilization extension splint (using elastic for the source of tension) [Arsham 1984]. The dynamic component for this splint positions the MCPs in extension. Several low-profile options exist that can be made with purchased outrigger parts (Figure 13-7). However, Colditz [2002, p. 633] remarks that "one should be cautioned against designs for dynamic wrist and finger extension, because the powerful unopposed flexors often overcome the force of the dynamic splint during finger flexion."

A mobilization MCP extension splint for radial nerve injury substitutes for the absent muscle power by assisting the MCP extensors. This splint is worn throughout the day until the impaired musculature reaches a manual muscle test (MMT) grade of fair (3) [Callahan 1984]. A client who does not show clinical improvement in three months should return to a physician for consideration of surgical intervention [Eaton and Lister 1992]. Because wrist control usually returns first, the therapist modifies the splint design and uses a hand-based mobilization splint after the forearm-based mobilization splint has been worn [Arsham 1984, Ziegler 1984]. If only one finger is lagging in extension, the therapist dynamically incorporates that finger into the splint [Ziegler 1984].

Another type of mobilization splint a therapist uses for radial nerve injuries is a mobilization splint that reestablishes the tendonesis pattern of the hand [Crochetiere et al. 1975; Colditz 1987, 2002]. The tenodesis splint includes a dorsal base splint with a low-profile outrigger that spans from the wrist to each proximal phalanx. This splint is sometimes called a dynamic tenodesis suspension splint [Hannah and Hudak 2001]. Finger loops are worn on each proximal phalanx, and a nylon cord attached from the finger loops is stretched to a point on the dorsal base. A tenodesis pattern occurs when the client flexes the wrist and the fingers extend and when the client extends the wrist and the fingers flex (Figure 13-8).

The splint design using the tenodesis pattern has many advantages. First, the design allows the palmar surface of the hand to be relatively free for sensory input and normal grasp [Colditz 2002]. The wrist is not immobilized. It only moves with the natural tenodesis effect and the thumb can move independently [Colditz 1987, 2002]. In addition, the hand arches are maintained [Colditz 2002]. As wrist extension returns, the client can continue to wear the splint because it does not immobilize the wrist and it enhances the strength of the wrist extensors for functional tasks [Colditz 2002]. Therefore a hand-based splint is not required. The low-profile design also enhances the performance of functional tasks. However, the tenodesis splint design is usually not sturdy enough for people with high load demands on their hands [personal communication, K. Schultz-Johnson, October 1999].

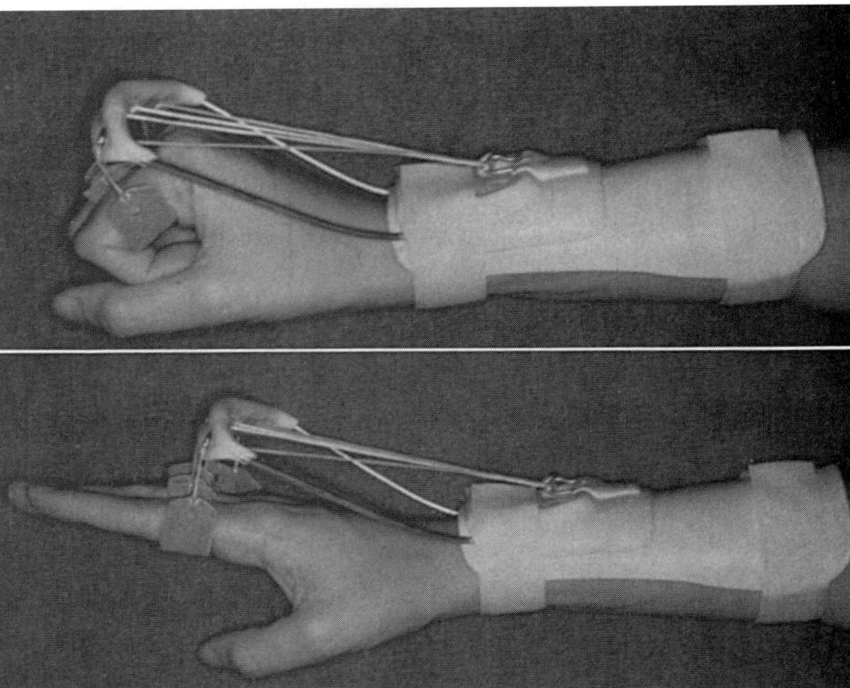

Figure 13-8 A splint for radial nerve injury. [From Colditz JC (2002). Splinting the hand with a peripheral nerve injury. In EJ Mackin, AD Callahan, TM Shirven, LH Schneider, AL Osterman (eds.), *Rehabilitation of the Hand and Upper Extremity, Fifth Edition*. St. Louis: Mosby, pp. 622-634.]

*Laboratory Exercise 13-1

Read the following scenario and answer the questions based on information from the chapter.

Ricardo is a 36-year-old right-handed man who presents with pronator syndrome. The physician referred Ricardo to a therapist for splint fabrication and a home program. The therapist wrote the following SOAP note.

S: "I really want to get better fast."

O: Pt. presented with a left forearm-level radial nerve injury. MMT scores for the extensor digitorum communis, extensor digiti minimi, extensor indicis, abductor pollicis longus, and extensor carpi ulnaris were all 0 (zero). Pt. reports no pain in the LUE. A left dorsal hand-based dynamic MCP extension splint was fabricated and fitted. Pt. was instructed how to don and doff the splint and how to grasp and release objects. *Pt. was also instructed verbally and given written information on the wearing schedule, splint care, and precautions. Pt. was given a home program to be completed 5×/day.*

A: Pt. was receptive to splint and home program. Pt. was able to independently grasp objects while wearing the splint. Anticipate compliance with wearing schedule and home program.

P: Will monitor needs for modifications of the splint and home program.

Several appointments later, the client regained muscle strength with an MMT score of fair (3). The therapist fabricated a left dynamic MCP extension hand-based splint.The therapist encouraged the patient to continue with ADL and the home program. The therapist initiated gentle strengthening activities. The therapist also modified the splint-wearing schedule and home program and told the client to complete the program 5×/day. The client had no complaints and was able to independently grasp light objects while wearing the splint. Write the next progress note.

____

____

____

____

____

____

____

*See Appendix A for the answer key

Ulnar Nerve Injuries

Ulnar compression syndromes are the second most common compression neuropathies in the upper extremity [Posner 2000]. An ulnar nerve lesion can occur in conjunction with a median nerve lesion [Enna 1988]. Lesions to the ulnar nerve commonly happen as a result of a fracture of the medial epicondyle of the humerus, a fracture of the olecranon process of the ulna, or a laceration or ganglia at the wrist. Most commonly, compression of the ulnar nerve at the elbow takes place at the epicondylar groove, or where the ulnar nerve courses between the two heads of the flexor carpi ulnaris muscle [Posner 2000]. Ulnar nerve compressions at the wrist level within the Guyon's canal are less common [Posner 2000]. Wrist-level injuries usually result from compression because of the superficial nature of ulnar nerve within the Guyon's canal [Posner 2000] (see Table 13-1).

McGowan [1950] developed a grading system for ulnar nerve conditions, with grade I manifesting with paresthesias and clumsiness, grade II exhibiting interosseous weakness and some muscle wasting, and grade III involving paralysis of the ulnar intrinsic muscles. Ulnar nerve injuries at the elbow are classified as acute, subacute, or chronic [Possner 2000]. Acute injuries result from trauma. Subacute develop over time and involve continual elbow compression, such as a factory worker who continuously positions his elbow on a table while doing work. Both acute and subacute injuries respond to conservative interventions, such as reducing elbow flexion during tasks and/or splinting.

Chronic conditions require surgery, especially if daily living tasks are severely impacted [Posner 2000]. Clinically, a person with an ulnar nerve compression at the elbow (cubital tunnel syndrome) will complain of discomfort on the medial side of the arm and numbness and tingling in digits 4 and 5 [Hong et al. 1996]. Prolonged flexion and force from occupations or sports such as baseball and tennis are common causation factors [Fess et al. 2005].

Regardless of the cause or location of an ulnar lesion, if a deformity results it is called a *clawhand*. Anatomically, this deformity occurs because the MCP joints of the ring and little fingers are positioned in hyperextension. The fourth and fifth digits are incapable of fully extending the PIP and distal interphalangeal (DIP) joints because of the unopposed action of the extensor digitorum communis and the extensor digiti minimi (Figure 13-9). In addition, the lumbricals and the intrinsic muscles responsible for interphalangeal (IP) extension are paralyzed [Boscheinen-Morrin et al. 1987].

Functional Implications of Ulnar Nerve Injuries

In the early stages of an ulnar nerve injury, a person may have difficulties performing ADL and may experience hand fatigue. Muscle weakness is not usually evident until the condition has progressed [Possner 2000]. Table 13-3 identifies the muscles the ulnar nerve innervates in a low-level or wrist lesion and a high-level lesion that occurs at or above the elbow.

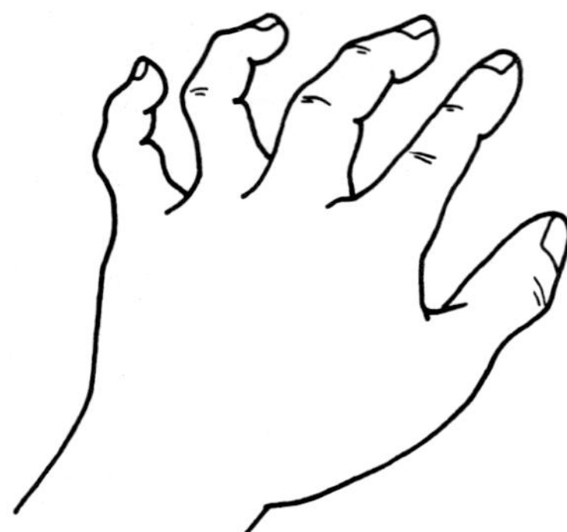

Figure 13-9 A clawhand deformity caused by an ulnar nerve injury.

If an ulnar nerve lesion occurs just distal to the elbow, the extrinsic muscles of the hand are lost because they are innervated distal to the elbow. At the wrist level, compression of the ulnar nerve in the distal part of the ulnar tunnel results in different functional effects based on the zone location of the nerve [Gross and Gelberman 1985, Possner 2000].

Generally, the functional result from a high- or low-level ulnar nerve lesion is loss of pinch and power grip strength [Fess 1986, Skirven 1992]. The client is not able to grasp an object fully because of the denervation of the finger abductors, atrophy of the hypothenar eminence, inability to oppose the little finger to the thumb, and ineffective pinch of the thumb [Boscheinen-Morrin et al. 1987, Salter 1987]. The loss of the first dorsal interosseous muscle and the abductor pollicis leads to unstable pinching of the thumb and index finger [Boscheinen-Morrin et al. 1987]. Loss of lateral finger movements and diminished sensory feedback can affect functional occupational activities such as typing on a computer [Salter 1987].

With a high lesion the loss of the flexor digitorum profundus of the ring and small fingers further compromises hand grasp [Skirven 1992]. In addition, the client presents with weakened wrist ulnar deviation.

Another characteristic of ulnar nerve injuries is a posture called *Froment's sign*, which functionally results in flexion of the thumb IP joint during pinching activities [Cailliet 1994]. Froment's sign is apparent because the adductor pollicis brevis, the deep head of the flexor pollicis brevis, and first dorsal interosseous muscle are not working. Because of these losses, performance of the fine dexterity tasks of daily living is remarkably affected.

The sensory distribution of the ulnar nerve typically innervates the little finger and the ulnar half of the ring finger on the volar and dorsal surfaces of the hand (see Figure 13-5). Clients who have ulnar nerve compression can experience numbness, tingling, and paresthesia in this nerve distribution and equal sensory loss in high and low lesions. When splinting for ulnar nerve lesions, the therapist monitors the areas of decreased sensation for pressure sores. Figure 13-10 illustrates the muscles an ulnar nerve lesion affects.

Table 13-3 Ulnar Nerve Lesions

AFFECTED MUSCLES	WEAK AND LOST MOTIONS
Low Level (Wrist Level)	
Abductor digiti minimi	Metacarpophalangeal (MCP) abduction of the fifth digit
Flexor digiti minimi	MCP flexion of the fifth digit and opposition
Opponens digiti minimi	Opposition of the fifth digit
Lumbricals to the fourth and fifth digits	MCP finger flexion and interphalangeal (IP) extension to the forth and fifth digits
Dorsal interossei	MCP abduction of the digits
Palmar interossei	MCP adduction of the digits
Flexor pollicis brevis (deep head)	MCP and CMC flexion of the thumb and opposition
Adductor pollicis	Adduction of the CMC joint and MCP flexion
High Level (At or Above the Elbow Level)	
Flexor carpi ulnaris	Wrist flexion and adduction
Flexor digitorum profundus of the fourth and fifth digits	Flexion of the distal interphalangeal (DIP) joint of the fourth and fifth digits
Abductor digiti minimi	MCP abduction of the fifth digit
Flexor digiti minimi	MCP flexion of the fifth digit and opposition
Opponens digiti minimi	Opposition of the fifth digit
Lumbricals to the fourth and fifth digits	MCP flexion and IP extension to the fourth and fifth digits
Dorsal interossei	MCP abduction of the digits
Palmar interossei	MCP adduction of the digits
Flexor pollicis brevis (deep head)	MCP and CMC flexion of the thumb and opposition
Adductor pollicis	Adduction of the CMC joint and MCP flexion

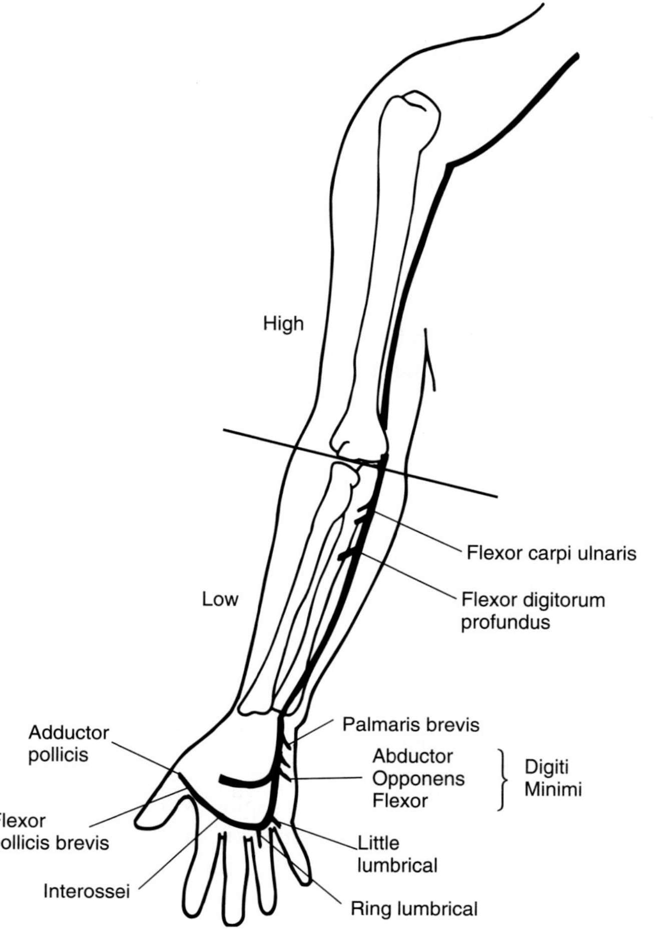

Figure 13-10 Ulnar nerve motor innervation.

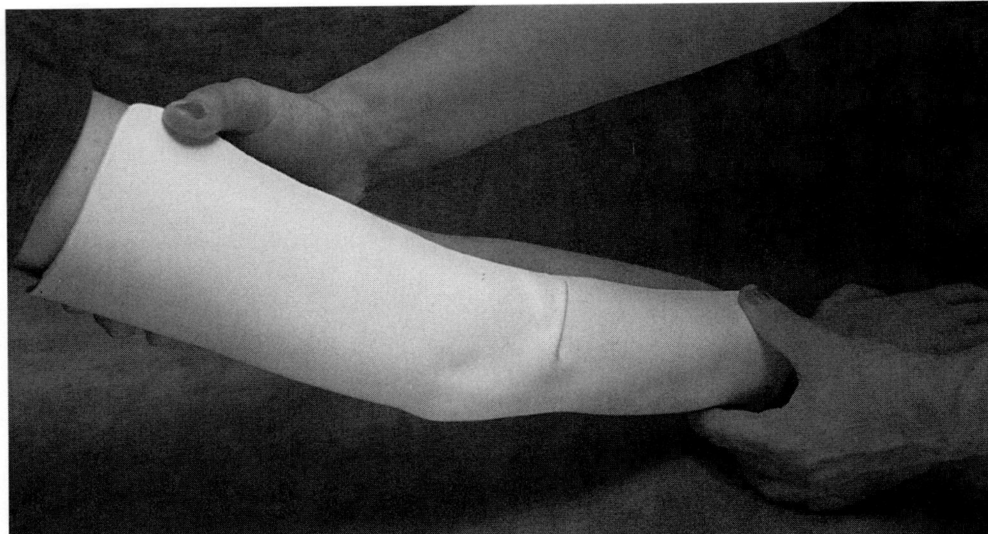

Figure 13-11 The arm and elbow position during molding of an elbow splint.

Ulnar Nerve Injury Splint Interventions

Treatments for ulnar nerve compression or injury at the elbow and wrist levels require that the client be trained to modify activities that contribute to the development of the problem.

Splinting for Ulnar Nerve Compression at the Elbow

A commonly discussed treatment for compression at the cubital tunnel is an elbow splint with the elbow flexed 30 to 45 degrees [Harper 1990, Aiello 1993]. If included, the wrist is positioned in neutral to 20 degrees of extension. Including the wrist decreases the effects from flexor carpi ulnaris contraction [Posner 2000].

The elbow splint helps to prevent repetitive or prolonged elbow flexion, especially beyond 60 to 90 degrees. Prolonged elbow flexion can stress the ulnar nerve via traction [Harper 1990, Seror 1993] and can increase pressure in the cubital tunnel [MacNicol 1980]. This position commonly occurs during sleep or with computer usage [Seror 1993, Cailliet 1994]. For sporadic or mild symptoms, the elbow splint may be worn during the night for approximately 3 weeks [Blackmore 2002]. If demonstrating dysthesia, decreased sensibility, and continuous symptoms, the client may wear the elbow splint all the time [Cannon 1991, Posner 2000, Blackmore 2002].

Many therapists recommend a soft splinting approach. Several soft elbow splints allow some movement but limit flexion to less than 45 degrees. When fabricating a rigid elbow splint, the therapist chooses a thermoplastic material with the following properties: (1) rigidity so that the thermoplastic material is strong enough to support the weight of the elbow, (2) self-bonding to help with formulation of the crease at the elbow, and (3) conformability and drapability to mold the material over the bony olecranon process (see Chapter 3). When fabricating the splint, the therapist should have an assistant help stabilize the arm or use an elastic wrap bandage. A tuck in the splinting material should be close to the elbow joint, as shown in Figure 13-11. Care must be taken that strapping the thermoplastic material does not provide pressure over the medial elbow area, where the nerve crosses [Posner 2000].

According to one study [Hong et al. 1996] (n = 10), splinting for ulnar nerve compression at the elbow was more effective than steroid injections to the site. Over 6 months, subjects experienced relief from wearing the splint during the night and during activities that were irritating the compression condition.

Hand-based Ulnar Nerve Splint Intervention

As shown in Figure 13-12, the splint for an ulnar nerve lesion involves positioning the ring and little fingers in 30 to 45 degrees of MCP flexion [Callahan 1984, Cannon et al. 1985]. This position prevents attenuation of the denervated intrinsic muscles and the MCP volar plates of the ring and little fingers [Colditz 2002]. In addition, this position corrects the clawhand posture of MCP hyperextension and PIP flexion. With the MCPs blocked in flexion, the power of the extensor digitorum communis is transferred to the IP joints and allows them to extend in the absence of the intrinsic muscles. Ultimately, this splint will help facilitate the functional grasp of the client [Skirven 1992].

The therapist splints the hand in this position with a mobilizing (dynamic) or immobilizing (static) splint. A client usually

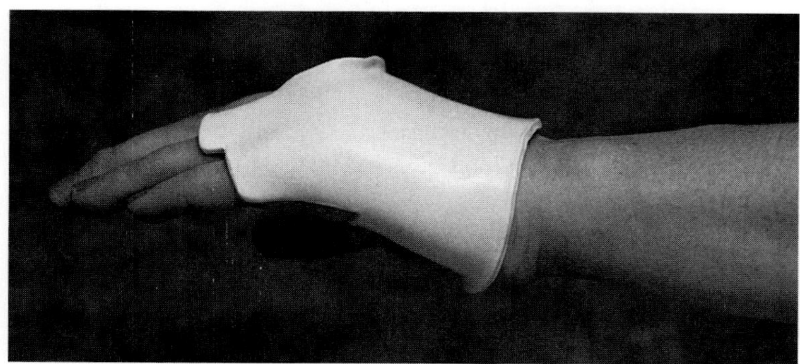

Figure 13-12 The hand position for splinting an ulnar nerve injury.

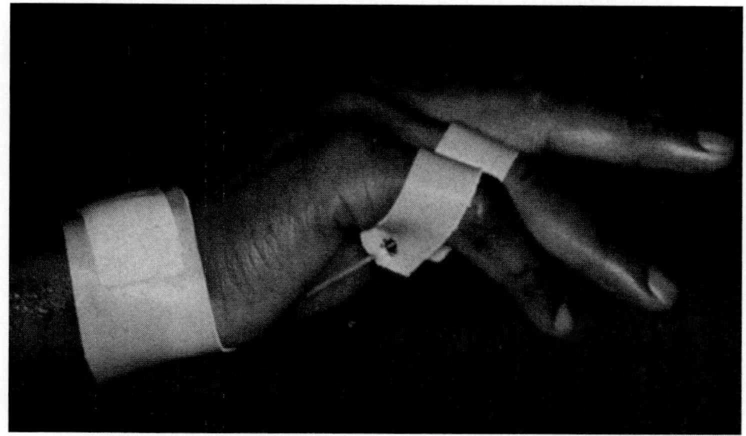

Figure 13-13 A dynamic extension splint for an ulnar nerve injury. [From Colditz JC (2002). Splinting the hand with a peripheral nerve injury. In EJ Mackin, AD Callahan, TM Shirven, LH Schneider, AL Osterman (eds.), *Rehabilitation of the Hand and Upper Extremity, Fifth Edition*. St. Louis: Mosby, pp. 622-634.]

wears an immobilization splint continuously, with removal only for hygiene and exercise. Colditz [2002] suggests the fabrication of a less bulky splint to keep from impeding the palmar sensation and function of the hand. One such splint is the figure-of-eight splint design Kiyoshi Yasaki developed at the Hand Rehabilitation Center in Philadelphia, Pennsylvania [Callahan 1984].

Mobilization Splints for Ulnar Nerve Injuries

The therapist can use a mobilization splint design that includes finger loops attached to the ring and little fingers' proximal phalanges (Figure 13-13). The rubber band traction pulls the two fingers into MCP flexion and is connected to a soft wrist cuff. The client wears the splint throughout the day, with removal for hygiene and exercise. Physicians usually prescribe this type of splint when there is a need for a strong force to prevent hyperextension contractures at the MCP joints. To supplement this type of splint, a positioning (immobilization) nighttime splint may be necessary. An immobilization hand-based pattern for an ulnar nerve injury (Figure 13-14) is useful for providing a strong counterforce to prevent a clawhand deformity [Callahan 1984].

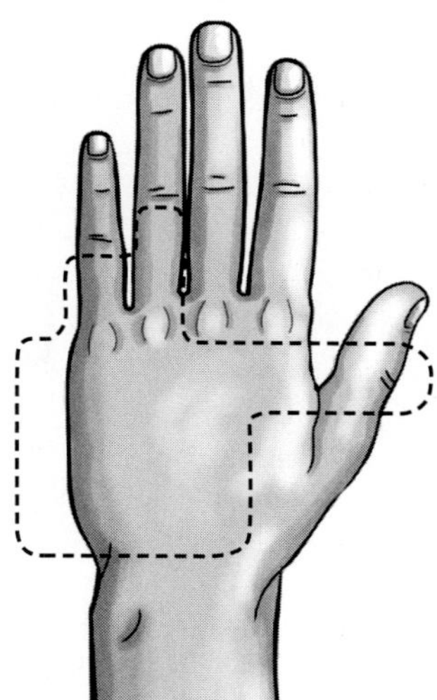

Figure 13-14 A hand-based pattern for an ulnar nerve splint.

Another option for splinting the ulnar nerve lesion is a spring-wire-and-foam splint, which is available commercially or can be custom made. Persons appreciate the low-profile design of the spring-wire-and-foam splint, and compliance tends to be high [personal communication, K. Schultz-Johnson, October 1999].

Laboratory Exercise 13-2

On a partner, practice fabricating a hand-based splint in the anticlaw position for a client who has an ulnar nerve lesion. Before starting, determine the position in which to place the person's hand. Remember to position the MCP joints of the ring and little fingers in approximately 30 to 45 degrees of flexion.

After fitting the splint and making all adjustments, use Form 13-1. This check-off sheet is a self-evaluation of the splint. Use Grading Sheet 13-1 as a classroom grading sheet.

Median Nerve Lesions

Traumatic median nerve lesions can result from humeral fractures, elbow dislocations, distal radius fractures, dislocations of the lunate into the carpal canal, and lacerations of the volar wrist [Skirven 1992]. The classic deformity is called an *ape* (or *simian*) *hand* because with denervation of the thenar eminence it appears flattened. A loss of thumb opposition occurs (Figure 13-15). The thumb is positioned in extension and adduction next to the index finger because of the unopposed action of the extensor pollicis longus and the adductor pollicis [Boscheinen-Morrin et al. 1987]. The thumb web space may contract, and the fingers may show trophic changes. In addition, a slight claw deformity of the index and middle fingers may occur because of the loss of the lumbrical innervation [Salter 1987].

Functional Involvement from a Median Nerve Injury

The median nerve in a low-level or wrist lesion and a high-level lesion involving the elbow or neck area innervates the muscles depicted in Figure 13-16 (Table 13-4). The impact on function from a median nerve lesion results in clumsiness with pinch and a decrease in power grip [Boscheinen-Morrin et al. 1987]. Whether a low or high injury, the sensory loss of a median nerve injury is the same. With lack of sensation in the fingers, skilled functions are difficult to perform with the hand. Power grip is affected because the thumb is no longer a stabilizing force as a result of loss of the abductor pollicis brevis, flexor pollicis brevis, and the opponens pollicis. Weakness in the lumbricals of the index and middle fingers further affects skilled movements of the hand [Borucki and Schmidt 1992]. The sensory areas innervated by the median nerve are used for identifying objects, temperature, and texture [Arsham 1984].

Higher lesions can weaken or impair forearm pronation, wrist flexion, thumb IP flexion, and flexion of the proximal and distal IP joints of the index and middle fingers. Compression syndromes that can occur from higher median nerve injuries are pronator syndrome and anterior interosseous syndrome. Pronator syndrome often results from strong and repetitive pronation and supination motions, with the most common compression site between the two heads of the pronator teres [Nuber et al. 1998]. Anterior interosseous syndrome is rare and is distinguished by a vague discomfort in the proximal forearm. It usually involves compression of the deep head of the pronator teres. Clinically, the person presents with an inability to make an O with the thumb and index finger [Nuber et al. 1998].

Thoracic outlet syndrome is sometimes considered an ulnar nerve injury initially or a high-level median nerve injury because it can initially resemble a median nerve compression [Messer and Bankers 1995]. Because median nerve injuries can occur throughout the extremity, it is possible that a person can be mistakenly thought to have one type of median nerve injury when he or she actually has another. Therefore, the astute therapist carefully considers the symptoms presented by the person. For example, a person may have pronator syndrome instead of carpal tunnel syndrome

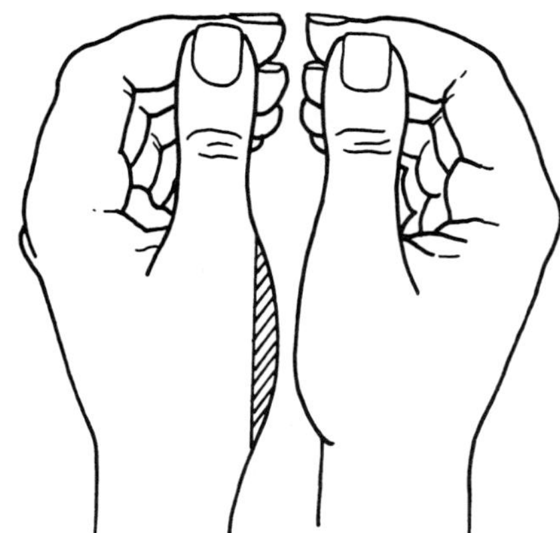

Figure 13-15 The classic median nerve deformity called an ape (or simian) hand. Note the thenar muscle atrophy of the left hand.

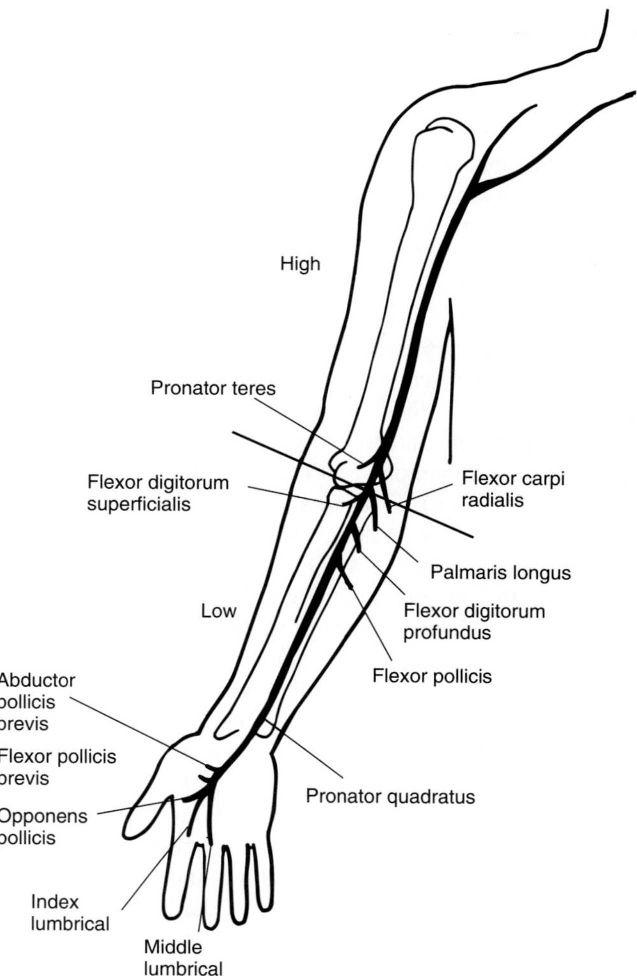

Figure 13-16 Median nerve motor innervation.

Table 13-4 Median Nerve Lesions

AFFECTED MUSCLES	WEAK AND LOST MOTIONS
Low Level (Wrist Level)	
Abductor pollicis brevis	Abduction of the CMC and metacarpophalangeal (MCP) joints of the thumb, weak extension of the interphalangeal (IP) joint, and opposition
Flexor pollicis brevis (superficial head)	Flexion of the MCP and CMC joints and opposition
Opponens pollicis	Thumb opposition
First and second lumbricals	IP extension and MCP flexion of the second and third digits
High Level (Elbow or Neck Level)	
Flexor pollicis longus	IP thumb flexion and weakness with flexion of the MCP and CMC joints
Lateral half of the flexor digitorum profundus to the second and third digits	Distal interphalangeal (DIP) flexion of the second and third digits
Pronator quadratus	Forearm pronation and elbow flexion
Pronator teres	Forearm pronation and elbow flexion
Flexor carpi radialis	Flexion and abduction of the wrist
Palmaris longus	Wrist flexion
Flexor digitorum superficialis	Flexion of the proximal interphalangeal (PIP) joints second through fifth digits and weak flexion of the MCP joints and wrist flexion
Abductor pollicis brevis	Abduction of the CMC and MCP joints of the thumb, weak extension of the IP joint, and opposition
Flexor pollicis brevis (superficial head)	Flexion of the MCP and CMC joints and opposition
Opponens pollicis	Thumb opposition
First and second lumbricals	IP extension and MCP flexion of the second and third digits

(CTS) if (1) pain is experienced with resisted pronation and passive supination activities, (2) a positive Tinel's sign at the proximal forearm is present, (3) tenderness of the pronator muscle is evident, (4) "numbness in the thenar eminence in the distribution of the palmar cutaneous branch of the median nerve" is present [Rehak 2001, p. 535], (5) nocturnal symptoms are absent, (6) muscle fatigue is present, (7) thenar atrophy is absent, or (8) Phalen's test is negative [Saidoff and McDonough 1997, Nuber et al. 1998, Rehak 2001]. CTS is a likely diagnosis for persons who have complaints of night pain, symptoms with repetitive wrist movements (especially flexion), weakness in thumb opposition and abduction, a positive Phalen's test, and a positive Tinel's sign at the wrist [Saidoff and McDonough 1997]. If a person is referred with a diagnosis of CTS and actually has symptoms of pronator syndrome, the therapist calls the referring physician and discusses examination findings.

Frequently, in persons with these syndromes surgical procedures are required to decompress the nerve [Borucki and Schmidt 1992]. On occasion, a physician may request a splint for conservative management of mild cases. For example, for a mild case of pronator tunnel syndrome the physician may prescribe an elbow splint to position the forearm in neutral between pronation and supination and the elbow in flexion (Table 13-5) [Cailliet 1994]. This elbow position takes tension off the nerve, and the forearm position prevents compression via pronator contraction or stretch.

The median nerve's classic course and sensory distribution include the volar surface of the thumb, index, middle, and radial half of the ring fingers and the dorsal surface of the distal phalanxes of the thumb, index, middle, and radial half of the ring finger (see Figure 13-5). Clients who have median nerve compression can experience numbness, tingling, and paresthesia in this nerve distribution. Because the area of sensory distribution is large, the therapist monitors and educates clients or caregivers about the associated risks and prevention of skin injury or breakdown.

Splinting Interventions for Median Nerve Injuries

Understanding the functional effects of the muscular loss resulting from a median nerve injury or compression syndrome is important because it influences the therapist's splint provision. Usually, with a median nerve lesion if the therapist is able to maintain good passive mobility of the joints, extensive splinting may not be necessary and occasional night splinting may be sufficient [Fess 1986].

Splinting for Pronator Syndrome

Clients with pronator syndrome should avoid resisted pronation and passive supination [Saidoff and McDonough 1997]. Other than changing activities that contribute to pronator syndrome, the person may benefit from splinting.

Table 13-5 Splint Interventions for Peripheral Nerve Lesions

SPLINT	POSITION
Radial	
Wrist immobilization splint	Wrist in 30 degrees of extension
Mobilization dorsal-based MCP extension splint	Wrist in 30 degrees of extension; MCPs in dynamic extension
Tenodesis splint (described by Colditz)	Dorsal base using the tenodesis effect with MCPs in dynamic extension
Ulnar	
Elbow splint	Elbow in 30 to 45 degrees of flexion
Hand-based immobilization anticlaw splint	MCPs of forth and fifth digits in 30 to 45 degrees of MCP flexion
Median	
Dorsal- or volar-based wrist splint	Wrist in neutral
Ulnar gutter wrist splint	Wrist in neutral
Thumb web spacer splint or C bar splint	Thumb in 40 to 45 degrees of palmar abduction

One splint option is to place the elbow in 90 degrees flexion, forearm neutral, and the wrist in neutral to slight flexion [Nuber et al. 1998].

Splinting for Anterior Interosseous Nerve Compression

Other than the suggestion of avoidance of elbow extension and extreme forearm pronation and supination, a couple of splinting options are recommended. One option is to immobilize the elbow in 90 degrees flexion and the forearm in neutral. As discussed, absence of this nerve results in difficulty making an O with the thumb and index finger flexed. To compensate for this deficit, the therapist fabricates a small thermoplastic splint to block thumb IP and index distal interphalangeal (DIP) extension [Colditz 2002] (Figure 13-17).

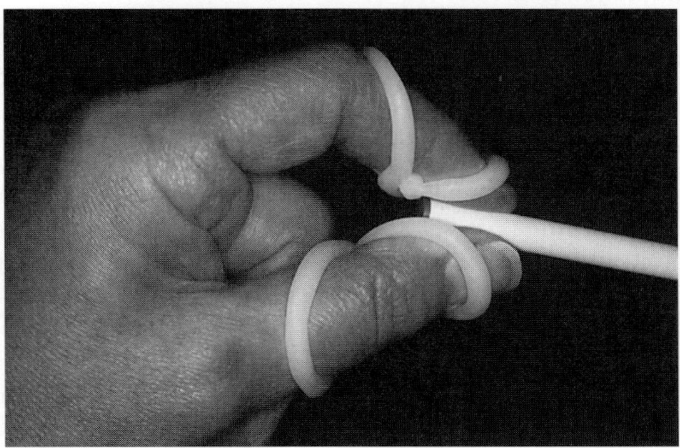

Figure 13-17 To encourage finger tip to thumb prehension, these small splints help someone with anterior interosseus nerve palsy. [From Colditz JC (2002). Splinting the hand with a peripheral nerve injury. In EJ Mackin, AD Callahan, TM Shirven, LH Schneider, AL Osterman (eds.), *Rehabilitation of the Hand and Upper Extremity, Fifth Edition*. St. Louis: Mosby, pp. 622-634.]

Splinting for Carpal Tunnel Syndrome

The most common type of median nerve compression is CTS, which compresses the median nerve at the wrist. Compression at the wrist occurs because of a discrepancy in volume of the rigid carpal canal and its content, consisting of the median nerve and flexor tendons. Some conditions (such as diabetes, pregnancy, Dupuytren's disease, and CMC arthritis) can be associated with CTS. Home, leisure, and occupational activities involving repetitive or sustained wrist flexion, extension, and ulnar deviation; forearm supination; forceful gripping; and pinching contribute to the development and exacerbation of CTS. Vibration, cold temperatures, and constriction over the wrist can also be contributing factors [Feldman et al. 1987, Wieslander et al. 1989, Barnhart et al. 1991, Schottland et al. 1991, Ostorio et al. 1994]. When manifestations are primarily sensory and occur from overuse or occupational causes, splinting of the wrist often helps reduce pain and symptoms [Borucki and Schmidt 1992].

Often, other therapeutic interventions need to accompany the splinting program. These include ergonomic adaptations for home, leisure, and work environments; education on prevention; activity modifications; a range-of-motion program with emphasis on tendon and nerve gliding exercises; and edema-control techniques [Sailer 1996]. See Chapter 7 for an overview of efficacy studies on carpal tunnel intervention.

Usually, any splint for CTS positions the wrist as close to neutral as possible. This helps maximize available carpal tunnel space, minimize median nerve compression, and provide pain relief [Kruger et al. 1991, Messer and Bankers 1995]. A wrist immobilization splint is commonly worn at night, and sometimes during home, leisure, or work activities that involve repetitive stressful wrist movements. As discussed in Chapter 7, the wearing schedule can vary but it is usually important at minimum to require nighttime wear to prevent extreme wrist postures that can occur during sleep [Sailer 1996]. The wearing schedule should be carefully monitored to prevent weakening of the muscles as a result of inactivity [Messer and Bankers 1995]. In addition, the splint may exacerbate symptoms if the person wearing it fights against it [personal communication, K. Schultz-Johnson, October 1999].

Volar Wrist Immobilization Splint

Some clients and therapists prefer volar wrist splints, which provide adequate support to the wrist. A volar wrist splint with a gel sheet or elastomer putty insert may be beneficial to control scar formation after carpal tunnel release surgery. A disadvantage of the volar wrist splint design for CTS is that the splint may interfere with palmar sensation [Borucki and Schmidt 1992]. Positioning the wrist in the splint is important. A poorly designed wrist splint may compress the carpal tunnel area of the wrist.

Dorsal or Ulnar Gutter Wrist Immobilization Splint

Other splinting approaches for CTS include fabrication of dorsal, ulnar gutter, or circumferential wrist splints. An advantage of the dorsal wrist splint is that there is no thermoplastic material directly over the carpal tunnel, thus avoiding compression. However, a disadvantage of the dorsal wrist splint is that it may not provide as much support and distribute pressure as well as the volar wrist splint. However, some therapists fabricate the splint with a larger palmar area for more support. An ulnar gutter wrist splint may also position the wrist in neutral and is less likely to compress the carpal tunnel. A circumferential wrist splint results in a high degree of immobilization of the wrist (see Chapter 7).

Some clients may be more comfortable with soft prefabricated wrist splints. The therapist checks the splint on the person to ensure a correct fit for function [Arsham 1984].

Splinting Median Nerve Injuries with Thumb Involvement

For a client who has a median nerve injury involving the thumb, as in the later stages of CTS, the therapist addresses loss of thumb opposition for functional grasp and pinch. The therapist positions and splints the thumb in opposition and palmar abduction, which assists the thumb for tip prehension. A C bar between the thumb and the index finger helps maintain the thumb web space. The thumb web space is a common site for muscular shortening of the adductor pollicis after median nerve damage. The splint design is usually static. A static splint for a median nerve injury with thumb involvement may benefit from a hand-based thumb spica splint (see Chapter 8).

For a low-level median nerve injury, the therapist may choose to fabricate a thumb web spacer splint (Figure 13-18).

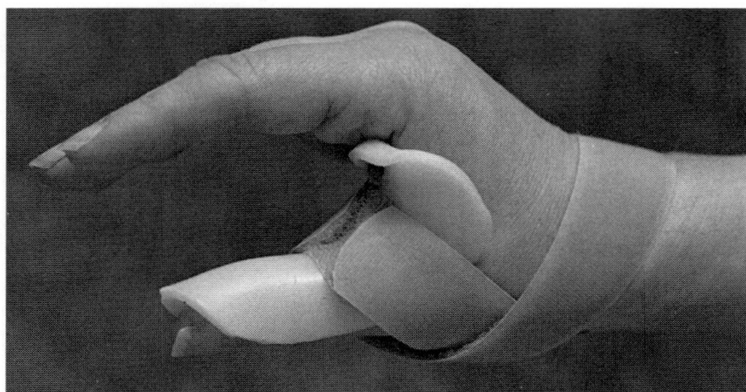

Figure 13-18 A thumb web spacer splint for a median nerve injury.

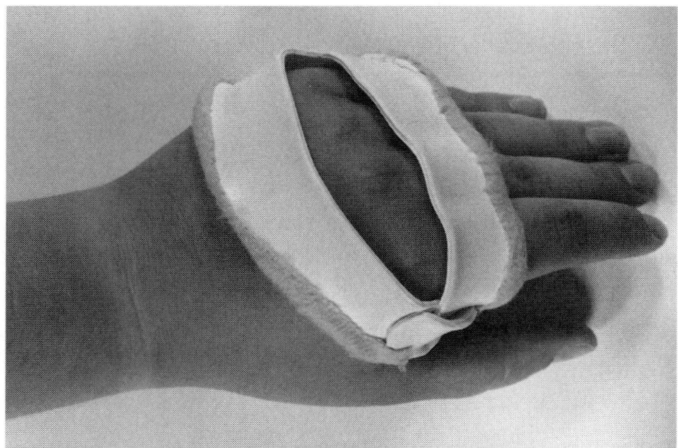

Figure 13-19 This splint inhibits MP extension with a combined median and ulnar nerve. [From Fess EE, Gettle KS, Philips CA, Janson JR (2005). *Hand and Upper Extremity Splinting: Principles and Methods, Third Edition*. St. Louis: Elsevier Mosby.]

The web spacer splint allows free wrist mobility [Borucki and Schmidt 1992]. If the therapist fabricates a mobilization thumb splint, a static thumb spica splint may be incorporated into the splint-wearing program for nighttime wear.

Splinting for Combined Median Ulnar Nerve Injuries

Sometimes with extensive injuries both median and ulnar nerves are involved. In that case, splinting to prevent further deformities involves splint designs that look similar to a singular nerve injury but with all digits included. The thumb may be included if it is affected (Figure 13-19).

Summary

Splinting for nerve injuries involves a comprehensive knowledge of the muscular, sensory, and functional implications. There are various splinting interventions for nerve injuries (Table 13-6). However, the therapist must note that these are general guidelines and that physicians and experienced therapists may have other specific protocols for positioning and splinting.

Table 13-6 Splinting for Radial and Ulnar Nerve Deficits

AUTHOR'S CITATION	DESIGN	# OF PARTICIPANTS	DESCRIPTION	RESULTS	LIMITATIONS
Hannah SD, Hudak PL (2001). Splinting and radial nerve palsy: A single-subject experiment. *Journal of Hand Therapy* 14:195-201.	Single-subject experimental design	Single-subject (1 study participant)	The aim of this study was to compare the client's response to four treatment interventions: no splint (baseline), static volar wrist cock-up splint, dynamic tenodesis suspension splint and dorsal wrist cock-up with dynamic finger extension splint. The participant wore each splint for 3 weeks, documenting time worn and activities performed.	Following the three 3-week trials, the study participant was allowed to choose whichever splint she felt was most beneficial for another 3-week trial. She chose both the static volar wrist cock-up splint and the dynamic finger extension splint. Using the DASH, the TEMPA, and the COPM, the dynamic finger extension splint showed the most improvement in perceived disability, functional abilities and satisfaction with performance. Despite lack of improvement with the volar cock-up splint, the participant chose it because she found it supportive, easy to put on and less conspicuous than the others.	Researchers were not blind to the interventions (types of splints). No re-administration of the TEMPA was completed at the end of each 3-week interval. The two dynamic splints had an added thumb component to assist in grasp and release of objects, which may have exaggerated findings of the functional differences among splints. Alternative research methods are needed to further understand the affects of splinting for radial nerve palsy and other nerve conditions. Another limitation is that both the tenodesis suspension splint and dorsal wrist dynamic finger extension splint had components that encouraged thumb abduction for grasp and release. This may have magnified the functional differences between the dynamic splints and the volar wrist cock-up splint.

Continued

Table 13-6 Splinting for Radial and Ulnar Nerve Deficits—cont'd

AUTHOR'S CITATION	DESIGN	# OF PARTICIPANTS	DESCRIPTION	RESULTS	LIMITATIONS
Hong CZ, Long HA, Kanakamedala V, Chang YM, Yates L (1996). Splinting and local steroid injection for the treatment of ulnar neuropathy at the elbow: Clinical and electrophysiological evaluation. *Archives of Physical Medicine Rehabilitation* 77:573-576.	Randomized control trial	10 participants (12 nerves)	The aim of this study was to compare the effects of splinting at the elbow to the effects of splinting combined with steroid treatment for ulnar neuropathy. The study participants were randomized with Group A receiving a steroid injection and a splint and Group B, the splint alone. Splint wearing was monitored and participants were disqualified if they did not meet the required time. Motor nerve conduction was measured by patient report and also myoelectrically to detect returns in ulnar nerve function. Participants were tested at 1 month and 6 months.	The study demonstrated that splint application offered a significant decrease in symptoms and increase in conduction velocity for both groups at 1 and 6 months. The addition of a steroid injection did not appear to create a significant difference in reducing symptoms of study participants. Based on this study, it seems as though splinting is an adequate treatment for ulnar neuropathy at the elbow as the addition of steroid injection did not appear to offer additional benefits.	One limitation of this study was the lack of population diversity. The participants in this study were gathered from a local VA facility and were all males with an average age of 59.1 years. Authors of the study cite this as a possible reason for poor response to local steroid injection.

SELF-QUIZ 13-1*

In regard to the following questions, circle either true (T) or false (F).

1. T F With neurapraxia the prognosis is extremely good because recovery is usually spontaneous.
2. T F Functionally, a client suffering from a radial nerve injury has a poor grip.
3. T F The main purpose of splinting a nerve injury is to immobilize the extremity.
4. T F The clawhand deformity occurs only with a low-level ulnar nerve injury.
5. T F The therapist should position an elbow splint in 90 degrees of flexion for a client who has an ulnar nerve compression at the elbow level.
6. T F For an ulnar nerve splint the therapist should position the ring and little fingers in approximately 30 to 45 degrees of MCP flexion.
7. T F The proper splint for a radial nerve injury is a wrist immobilization or dynamic wrist and MCP extension splint.
8. T F The therapist should immobilize radial, ulnar, and median nerve injuries only in static splints.
9. T F Froment's sign is an identifying posture of a median nerve injury.
10. T F Functionally, a client suffering from an ulnar nerve injury has loss of pinch strength and power grip.
11. T F The therapist may use a thumb web spacer splint for a median nerve injury.
12. T F Low-level nerve injuries occur only distal to the wrist.

*See Appendix A for the answer key.

FORM 13-1* Anticlaw splint

Name: ____________________

Date: ____________________

Answer the following questions after the splint has been worn for 30 minutes. (Mark NA for nonapplicable situations.)

Evaluation Areas				Comments
Design				
1. The splint prevents hyperextension of the MCP joints of the ring and little fingers.	Yes ❍	No ❍	NA ❍	
Function				
1. The splint allows full wrist motions.	Yes ❍	No ❍	NA ❍	
2. The splint allows full function of the middle and index fingers.	Yes ❍	No ❍	NA ❍	
Straps				
1. The straps avoid bony prominences.	Yes ❍	No ❍	NA ❍	
2. The straps are secure and rounded.	Yes ❍	No ❍	NA ❍	
Comfort				
1. The edges are smooth with rounded corners.	Yes ❍	No ❍	NA ❍	
2. The proximal end is flared.	Yes ❍	No ❍	NA ❍	
3. Impingements or pressure areas are not present.	Yes ❍	No ❍	NA ❍	
4. Splint pressure is well distributed over the proximal phalanx of the ring and little fingers.	Yes ❍	No ❍	NA ❍	
Cosmetic Appearance				
1. The splint is free of fingerprints, dirt, and pencil or pen marks.	Yes ❍	No ❍	NA ❍	
2. The splinting material is smooth and free of buckles.	Yes ❍	No ❍	NA ❍	
Therapeutic Regimen				
1. The person has been instructed in a wearing schedule.	Yes ❍	No ❍	NA ❍	
2. The person has been provided with splint precautions.	Yes ❍	No ❍	NA ❍	
3. The person demonstrates understanding of the education.	Yes ❍	No ❍	NA ❍	
4. Client/caregiver knows how to clean the splint.	Yes ❍	No ❍	NA ❍	

Discuss possible adjustments or changes you would make based on the self-evaluation.

____

____

____

____

____

____

*See Appendix B for a perforated copy of this form.

GRADING SHEET 13-1* Anticlaw splint

Name: ______________________

Date: ______________________

Grade: ______________

1 = beyond improvement, not acceptable
2 = requires maximal improvement
3 = requires moderate improvement
4 = requires minimal improvement
5 = requires no improvement

Evaluation Areas						Comments
Design						
1. The splint prevents hyperextension of the MCP joints of the ring and little fingers.	1	2	3	4	5	
Function						
1. The splint allows full wrist motions.	1	2	3	4	5	
2. The splint allows full function of the middle and index fingers.	1	2	3	4	5	
Straps						
1. The straps avoid bony prominences.	1	2	3	4	5	
2. The straps are secure and rounded.	1	2	3	4	5	
Comfort						
1. The edges are smooth with rounded corners.	1	2	3	4	5	
2. The proximal end is flared.	1	2	3	4	5	
3. Impingements or pressure areas are not present.	1	2	3	4	5	
4. Splint pressure is well distributed over the proximal phalanx of the ring and little fingers.	1	2	3	4	5	
Cosmetic Appearance						
1. The splint is free of fingerprints, dirt, and pencil or pen marks.	1	2	3	4	5	
2. The splinting material is not buckled.	1	2	3	4	5	

Comments:

____

____

____

____

____

*See Appendix C for a perforated copy of this grading sheet.

CASE STUDY 13-1*

Read the following scenario and answer the questions based on information in this chapter. Indicate all answers that are correct.

Mark is a 51-year-old man employed as a truck driver. While driving his truck he tends to position his left upper extremity resting on the window frame. Over time he develops compression of the ulnar nerve at the elbow, which is manifested by interosseous weakness. Mark complains of discomfort on the medial side of the arm and continuous numbness and tingling in digits 4 and 5.

1. Functionally, what might Mark have difficulty doing?
2. What is the correct splint for his condition?
3. What are the correct positions for his joints in this splint?
4. After being fitted with a custom thermoplastic splint, Mark complains that he does not like the hard feel of the material. What will you do?
5. What would be your suggested wearing schedule?
6. What other lifestyle adjustments would be suggested?

*See Appendix A for the answer key.

CASE STUDY 13-2*

Read the following scenario and answer the questions based on information in this chapter.

Kevin is employed part-time in the local symphony orchestra as a violinist. During one very busy season he develops the following symptoms: pain on the lateral aspect of the elbow, motor weakness with extension of the MCP joints of the fingers and thumb, and difficulty abducting the thumb. Although he can extend the wrist, it tends to deviate radially. He does not have sensory loss.

1. What condition does he have?
   a. Posterior interosseous nerve syndrome
   b. Radial tunnel syndrome
   c. Wartenberg syndrome
   d. Cubital tunnel syndrome

2. What does this condition have in common with posterior interosseous nerve syndrome?
   a. Both occur in the same tunnel and involve the same nerve but have different symptoms
   b. Both are components of a double crush syndrome
   c. Both result from repetitive wrist extension
   d. Both result from compression of the ulnar nerve

3. Why does Kevin's wrist deviate radially?
   a. Because the extensor carpi ulnaris in still intact
   b. Because the extensor carpi radialis is still intact

4. What type of splint should the therapist provide?
   a. Volar wrist splint
   b. Dynamic tenodesis suspension splint
   c. Thumb immobilization splint
   d. Elbow extension splint

5. What is the functional advantage of this splint?
   a. The design allows the dorsal surface of the hand to be relatively free
   b. The wrist and thumb can move
   c. The fingers are not immobilized
   d. The hand is completely free to move

6. What would be your suggested wearing schedule?
   a. Only during painful activities
   b. All the time, with removal for hygiene

*See Appendix A for the answer key.

REVIEW QUESTIONS

1. Which factors are important in the prognosis of a peripheral nerve lesion?
2. What are the deformities resulting from radial, ulnar, and median nerve lesions?
3. What are the functional results of radial, ulnar, and median nerve lesions?
4. What are the splinting options for radial nerve injuries? In which position should the therapist splint the hand?
5. What is the proper type, position, and thermoplastic material needed for fabrication of a splint for ulnar nerve compression at the elbow?
6. What is the proper splinting position for a clawhand deformity? Why is this a good position?
7. What are the advantages and disadvantages of the different approaches to wrist splinting for carpal tunnel syndrome?
8. What is the appropriate position in which to splint a hand with a median nerve lesion that includes thumb symptoms?

References

Aiello B (1993). Ulnar nerve compression in cubital tunnel. In GL Clark, EF Shaw, WB Aiello, D Eckhaus, LV Eddington (eds.), *Hand Rehabilitation: A Practical Guide*. New York: Churchill Livingstone.

Alba CD (2002). Therapist's management of radial tunnel syndrome. In EJ Mackin, AD Callahan, TM Shirven, LH Schneider (eds.), *Rehabilitation of the Hand, Fifth Edition*. St. Louis: Mosby, pp. 696-700.

Arsham NZ (1984). Nerve injury. In EM Ziegler (ed.), *Current Concepts in Orthotics: A Diagnosis-related Approach to Splinting*. Germantown, WI: Rolyan Medical Products.

Barnhart S, Demers PA, Miller M, Longstreth WT, Rosenstock L (1991). Carpal tunnel syndrome among ski manufacturing workers. Scandinavian Journal of Work Environmental Health 17:46-52.

Barr NR, Swan D (1988). *The Hand: Principles and Techniques of Splintmaking*. Boston: Butterworth Publishers.

Blackmore SM (2002). Therapist's management of ulnar nerve neuropathy at the elbow. In EJ Mackin, AD Callahan, TM Shirven, LH Schneider (eds.), *Rehabilitation of the Hand, Fifth Edition*. St. Louis: Mosby, pp. 679-689.

Borucki S, Schmidt J (1992). Peripheral neuropathies. In ML Aisen (ed.), *Orthotics in Neurologic Rehabilitation*. New York: Demos Publications.

Boscheinen-Morrin J, Davey V, Conolly WB (1987). Peripheral nerve injuries (including tendon transfers). In J Boscheinen-Morrin, V Davey, WB Conolly (eds.), *The Hand: Fundamentals of Therapy*. Boston: Butterworth Publishers.

Cailliet R (1994). *Hand Pain and Impairment, Fourth Edition*. Philadelphia: F. A. Davis.

Callahan A (1984). Nerve injuries. In MH Malick, MC Kasch (eds.), *Manual on Management of Specific Hand Problems*. Pittsburgh: American Rehabilitation Educational Network.

Cannon NM (ed.), (1991). *Diagnosis and Treatment Manual for Physicians and Therapists, Third Edition*. Indianapolis: The Hand Rehabilitation Center of Indiana.

Cannon NM, Foltz RW, Koepfer JM, Lauck MF, Simpson DM, Bromley RS (1985). *Manual of Hand Splinting*. New York: Churchill Livingstone.

Chan RKY (2002). Splinting for peripheral nerve injury in the upper limb. Hand Surgery 7(2):251-259.

Clarkson HM, Gilewich GB (1989). *Musculoskeletal Assessment: Joint Range of Motion and Manual Muscle Strength*. Baltimore: Williams & Wilkins.

Cohen MS, Garfin SR (1997). Nerve compression syndromes: Finding the cause of upper-extremity symptoms. Consultant 37:241-254.

Colditz JC (1987). Splinting for radial nerve palsy. J Hand Ther 1:18-23.

Colditz JC (2002). Splinting the hand with a peripheral nerve injury. In EJ Mackin, AD Callahan, TM Shirven, LH Schneider (eds.), *Rehabilitation of the Hand, Fifth Edition*. St. Louis: Mosby, pp. 622-634.

Crochetiere WJ, Goldstein SA, Granger GV, Ireland J (1975). The Granger Orthosis for Radial Nerve Palsy. Orthotics and Prosthetics 29(4):27-31.

Eaton CJ, Lister GD (1992). Radial nerve compression. Hand Clinics 8(2):345-357.

Enna CD (1988). *Peripheral Denervation of the Hand*. New York: Alan R. Liss.

Feldman RG, Travers PH, Chirico-Post J, Keyserling WM (1987). Risk assessment in electronic assembly workers: Carpal tunnel syndrome. Journal of Hand Surgery (Am) 12(5):849-855.

Fess EE (1986). Rehabilitation of the patient with peripheral nerve injury. Hand Clinics 2(1):207-215.

Fess EE, Gettle KS, Philips CA, Janson JR (2005). *Hand Splinting Principles and Methods, Third Edition*. St. Louis: Elsevier Mosby.

Frykman GK (1993). The quest for better recovery from peripheral nerve injury: Current status of nerve regeneration research. Journal of Hand Therapy 6(2):83-88.

Gelberman RH, Eaton R, Urbanisk JR (1993). Peripheral nerve compression. Journal of Bone and Joint Surgery 75A:1854-1878.

Greene DP, Roberts SL (1999). *Kinesiology Movement in the Context of Activity*. St. Louis: Mosby.

Gross MS, Gelberman RH (1985). The anatomy of the distal ulnar tunnel. Clinical Orthopedics and Related Research 196:238-247.

Hannah SD, Hudak PL (2001). Splinting and radial nerve palsy: A single-subject experiment. Journal of Hand Therapy 14:195-201.

Harper BD (1990). The drop-out splint: An alternative to the conservative management of ulnar nerve entrapment at the elbow. Journal of Hand Therapy 3:199-210.

Hong CZ, Long HA, Kanakamedala V, Chang YM (1996). Splinting and local steroid injection for the treatment of ulnar neuropathy at the elbow: Clinical and electrophysiological evaluation. Archives of Physical Medicine and Rehabilitation 77:573-576.

Hornbach & Culp. (2002). Radial tunnel syndrome. In EJ Mackin, AD Callahan, TM Shirven, LH Schneider (ed.), *Rehabilitation of the Hand, Fifth Edition*. St. Louis: Mosby.

Izzi J, Dennison D, Noerdlinger M, Dasilva M, Akelman E (2001). Nerve injuries of the elbow, wrist, and hand in athletes. Clinics in Sports Medicine 20(1):203-217.

Jebson PJL, Gaul JS (1998). Peripheral nerve injury. In PJL Jebson, ML Kasdan (eds.), *Hand Secrets*. Philadelphia: Hanley & Belfus.

Kleinert MJ, Mehta S (1996). Radial nerve entrapment. Orthopedic Clinics of North America 27:30.

Kruger VL, Kraft GH, Deitz JC, Ameis A, Polissar L (1991). Carpal tunnel syndrome: Objective measures and splint use. Archives of Physical Medicine and Rehabilitation 72(7):517-520.

MacNicol MF (1980). Mechanics of the ulnar nerve at the elbow. Journal of Bone and Joint Surgery (Br) 62B:53, 518.

McGowan AJ (1950). The results of transposition of the ulnar nerve for traumatic ulnar neuritis. Journal of Bone and Joint Surgery (Br) 23B:293-301.

Melhorn JM (1998). Cumulative trauma disorders and repetitive strain injuries: The future. Clinical Orthopaedics and Related Research 351:107-126.

Messer RS, Bankers RM (1995). Evaluating and treating common upper extremity nerve compression and tendonitis syndromes... without becoming cumulatively traumatized. Nurse Practitioner Forum 6(3):152-166.

Novak CB, Mackinnon SE (1998). Nerve injury in repetitive motion disorders. Clinical Orthopaedics and Related Research 351:10-20.

Novak CB, Mackinnon SE (2005). Evaluation of nerve injury and nerve compression in the upper quadrant. Journal of Hand Therapy 18:230-240.

Nuber GW, Assenmacher J, Bowen MK (1998). Neurovascular problems in the forearm, wrist, and hand. Clinics in Sports Medicine 17(3):585-610.

Omer G (1990). Nerve response to injury and repair. In JM Hunter, LH Schneider, EJ Mackin, AD Callahan (eds.), *Rehabilitation of the Hand, Third Edition*. St. Louis: Mosby.

Ostorio AM, Ames RG, Jones J, Castorina J, Rempel D, Estrin W, Thompson D (1994). Carpal tunnel syndrome among grocery store workers. American Journal of Internal Medicine 25:229-245.

Posner MA (2000). Compressive neuropathies of the ulnar nerve at the elbow and wrist. AAOS Instructional Course Lectures 49:305-317.

Rehak DC (2001). Pronator syndrome. Clinics in Sports Medicine 20(30):531-540.

Saidoff DC, McDonough AL (1997). *Critical Pathways in Therapeutic Intervention: Upper Extremities*. St. Louis: Mosby.

Sailer SM (1996). The role of splinting and rehabilitation. Hand Clinics 12(2):223-240.

Salter MI (1987). *Hand Injuries: A Therapeutic Approach*. Edinburgh, London: Churchill Livingstone.

Schottland JR, Kirschberg GJ, Fillingim R, Davis VP, Hogg F (1991). Median nerve latencies in poultry processing workers: An approach to resolving the role of industrial "cumulative trauma" in the development of carpal tunnel syndrome. Journal of Occupational Medicine 33:627-631.

Seddon HJ (1943). Three types of nerve injury Brain: A journal of neurology, 66:237-288.

Seror P (1993). Treatment of ulnar nerve palsy at the elbow with a night splint. Journal of Bone and Joint Surgery (Br) 75(2):322-327.

Skirven T (1992). Nerve injuries. In BG Stanley, SM Tribuzi (eds.), *Concepts in Hand Rehabilitation*. Philadelphia: F. A. Davis, pp. 322-338.

Skirven TM, Callahan AD (2002). Therapist's management of peripheral-nerve injuries. In EJ Mackin, AD Callahan, TM Shirven, LH Schneider (eds.), *Rehabilitation of the Hand, Fifth Edition*. St. Louis: Mosby, pp. 599-621.

Skirven T, Osterman AL (2002). Clinical examination of the wrist. In EJ Mackin, AD Callahan, TM Shirven, LH Schneider (eds.), *Rehabilitation of the Hand, Fifth Edition*. St. Louis: Mosby, pp. 1099-1116.

Spinner M (1990). Nerve lesions in continuity. In JM Hunter, LH Schneider, EJ Mackin, AD Callahan (eds.), *Rehabilitation of the Hand, Third Edition*. St. Louis: Mosby, pp. 523-529.

Sunderland S (1968). The peripheral nerve trunk in relation to injury: A classification of nerve injury. In S Sunderland (ed.), *Nerves and Nerve Injuries*. Baltimore: Williams & Wilkins, pp. 127-137.

Upton AR, McComas AJ (1973). The double crush in nerve entrapment syndromes. Lancet 2:359-362.

Vender MI, Truppa KL, Ruder JR, Pomerance J (1998). Upper extremity compressive neuropathies. Physical Medicine and Rehabilitation: State of the Art Reviews 12(2):243-262.

Wieslander G, Norback D, Gothe C, Juhlin L (1989). Carpal tunnel syndrome (CTS) and exposure to vibration, repetitive wrist movements and heavy manual work: A case-referent study. British Journal of Industrial Medicine 46:43-47.

Ziegler EM (1984). *Current Concepts in Orthotics: A Diagnosis-related Approach to Splinting*. Germantown, WI: Rolyan Medical Products.

CHAPTER 14

Antispasticity Splinting

Michael Lohman, MEd, OTR/L, CO
Omar Aragón, OTD, OTR/L

Key Terms

Cylindrical foam
Fiberglass bandage
Hard cone
Inflatable splint
Maximum range
Neoprene
Orthokinetics
Orthosis
Plaster bandage
Spasticity
Submaximum range
Trough

Chapter Objectives

1. Identify and describe the two historic trends in upper extremity tone-reduction splinting (orthotics). (Note: The authors use the terms *splint* and *orthosis* interchangeably in this chapter.)
2. Compare the strengths and weaknesses of dorsal and volar forearm platforms (troughs). (Note: The authors use the terms *platform* and *trough* interchangeably in this chapter.)
3. Discuss the neurophysiologic rationale supporting the use of the finger spreader and hard cone.
4. Discriminate between the passive and dynamic components of spasticity.
5. Describe the difference between submaximum and maximum ranges as they relate to tone-reduction splints.
6. Identify and describe the two major components of orthokinetic splints.
7. Describe one unique characteristic for each of the following materials: plaster bandage, fiberglass bandage, inflatable splints, cylindrical foam, neoprene.
8. Successfully fabricate and clinically evaluate the proper fit of a thermoplastic hard cone.
9. Use clinical judgment to correctly analyze two case studies.

The status of tone-reduction wrist/hand orthotics is like an amorphous quicksand waiting to engulf the unwary therapist. Rehabilitation literature reflects the universal lack of consensus, which Fess et al. [2005, p. 518] summarize with the following statement: "Some physicians and therapists feel strongly that the hypertonic extremity should not be splinted, whereas others are equally adamant that splinting has beneficial results. Even among proponents of splinting, numerous disagreements exist concerning splint design, surface of splint application, wearing times and schedules, joints to be splinted, and specific construction materials for splints and splint components."

Current professional standards of practice dictate that significant cumulative data and consistent scientific analysis provide the foundation for objective evaluations and treatment protocols. Literature in tone-reduction splinting does not reflect the development of this core body of knowledge. Lannin and Herbert [2003, p. 807] conducted a systematic review of published literature on the use of hand splints following stroke and concluded that there is "insufficient evidence to either support or refute the effectiveness of hand splinting for adults following stroke who are not receiving prolonged stretches to their upper limb." The paucity of data on the effectiveness of tone-reduction splinting has fostered confusion and contradiction. In the absence of a well-established practice protocol, this chapter is restricted to a discussion of current theoretical and experimental rationales and splint designs. Each practitioner is ultimately responsible for justifying the effectiveness of these techniques in client treatment.

Basmajian et al. [1982, p. 1382] define *spasticity* as "a state of increased muscular tone with exaggeration of the tendon reflexes." Clients who have upper motor neuron (UMN) lesions such as cerebrovascular accidents (CVAs), closed-head injuries, spinal cord injuries, and cerebral palsy often exhibit spasticity [Bishop 1977]. Spasticity can cause deformity [Bloch and Evans 1977] and limit functional movement [Doubilet and Polkow 1977]. Hand splinting is one treatment technique used to prevent joint deformity and influence muscle tone [Mills 1984].

Historically, experts have documented two major trends in hemiplegic hand splinting. Until the 1950s, the direct application of mechanical force to correct or prevent joint contractures (i.e., biomechanical approach) was the preferred practice in dealing with the effects of spasticity. During the 1950s, emphasis shifted to the underlying causes of spasticity. This viewpoint focuses on the effects of sensory feedback provided by splints in altering muscle tone and promoting normal movement patterns (i.e., neurophysiologic approach) [Neuhaus et al. 1981]. As differing neurophysiologic theories emerged in the 1950s, therapists advocated divergent treatment and splint management principles. At present, several prevalent neurophysiologic rationales recommend a variety of designs composed of a variety of elements related to design position and material options, including the following: (1) platform design, (2) finger and thumb position, (3) static and dynamic prolonged stretch, and (4) material properties.

Some authors have limited their splint designs to one elemental concern, whereas other authors have combined several design elements to support specific treatment rationales. Several commercially available antispasticity hand splints incorporate a variety of design elements. Although this chapter reviews each design element separately, therapists must remember that neurophysiologic splint-design concepts are interrelated and that many splints encompass combinations of design elements.

Forearm Platform Position

A forearm platform is a design element that provides a base of support to control wrist position. Many frequently used tone-reduction splint designs do not affect wrist control but attempt only to influence the digits [Dayhoff 1975, Bloch and Evans 1977, Jamison and Dayhoff 1980, Langlois et al. 1991]. Other designs attempt to influence wrist position but do not address digit position [MacKinnon et al. 1975, Switzer 1980].

Lannin and Herbert [2003, p. 807] stated that "there is insufficient evidence to either support or refute the effectiveness of dorsal or volar hand splinting in the treatment of adults following stroke who are not receiving an upper limb stretching programme." Isolated joint control constitutes a fundamental design flaw that can produce a predictable outcome because the tendons of the extrinsic flexors cross the wrist, fingers, and thumb. If the digits are positioned in extension, the unsplinted wrist assumes a greater attitude of flexion [Fess et al. 2005]. This compensatory sequence can lead to decreased passive motion and contracture development.

Rehabilitation science literature contains adherents for volar-based forearm platforms [Brennan 1959, Zislis 1964, Peterson 1980] and dorsal-based forearm platforms [Kaplan 1962, Charait 1968, Snook 1979, Carmick 1997]. Other authors report that the two positions are equally effective in tone reduction [McPherson et al. 1982, Rose and Shah 1987].

National distributors market ulnar-based platform splints designed to reduce spasticity [Sammons Preston Roylan 2005], although the literature does not appear to mention ulnar-based forearm platforms (Figure 14-1). A therapist can secure all orthotic forearm platforms to the forearm by using straps, resulting in skin contact with volar and dorsal surfaces simultaneously [Rose and Shah 1987, Langlois et al. 1989]. The corresponding cutaneous stimulation provided to flexors or extensors by the forearm platform and straps may be facilitatory or inhibitory. The literature has not yet described research that examines the exact relationship between these variables [Langlois et al. 1991]. These variables are, however, discussed later in this chapter.

Research does not indicate which, if any, of these forearm-platform designs provide the best results to reduce spasticity. However, each forearm-platform design has individual qualities that may be relevant in a clinical decision regarding forearm-platform design. A volar forearm platform that extends into the hand provides greater support for the transverse metacarpal arch. Volar designs do not extend thermoplastic material over the ulnar styloid, thus avoiding the possibility of pressure over this key bony prominence.

A dorsal forearm platform frees the palmar area and enhances sensory feedback. This style is easier to apply and remove if wrist flexion tightness is present. Pressure is also more evenly distributed over the larger thermoplastic surface of the dorsal forearm platform as opposed to the smaller strap surface the volar style provides. An ulnar forearm platform provides a more even distribution of pressure for a client who exhibits a strong component of wrist ulnar deviation with wrist flexion spasticity (Figure 14-1).

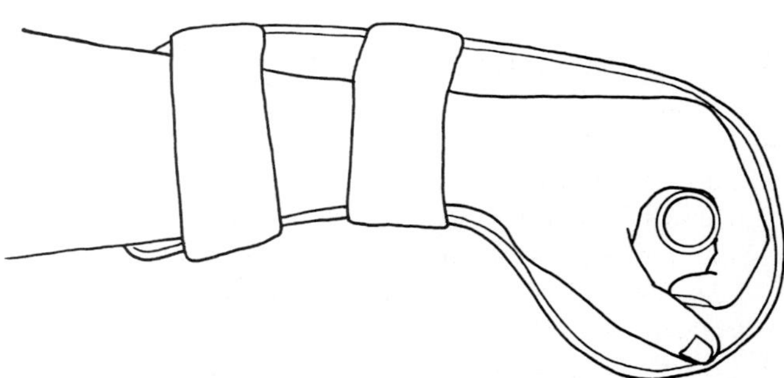

Figure 14-1 A hard cone attached to an ulnar platform: spasticity cone splint [Sammons Preston 1995].

Finger and Thumb Position

The finger spreader and hard cone are examples of splint designs based on divergent neurophysiologic treatment theories. Both positioning devices are designed to be adjuncts to specific treatment techniques that promote voluntary hand motion [Bobath 1978, Farber 1982, Davies 1985].

The neurodevelopmental treatment (NDT) theory advocates the use of reflex-inhibiting patterns (RIP) to inhibit abnormal spasticity. Finger and thumb abduction is a key point of control that facilitates extensor muscle tone and inhibits flexor muscle tone [Bobath 1978, Davies 1985]. The finger-spreader design assists in maintaining the reflex-inhibiting pattern.

Therapists have constructed recent adaptations of the finger-spreader design from rigid thermoplastic material [Doubilet and Polkow 1977, Langlois et al. 1991]. Bobath's [1970] original soft foam material has dynamic qualities that are sacrificed when the therapist substitutes rigid, more durable, and cosmetically appealing materials [Langlois et al. 1989] (Figure 14-2). Doubilet and Polkow [1977] state that positioning the thumb in palmar abduction with the metacarpophalangeal (MCP) and proximal interphalangeal (PIP) joints extended is preferable to radial abduction of the thumb because palmar abduction provides greater fitting security, positions the thumb more comfortably, and produces similar results in spasticity reduction.

In addition to deciding the thumb position, the therapist considers wrist and interphalangeal joint control. Although some researchers have not extended their RIP designs to include the wrist or interphalangeal joints [Doubilet and Polkow 1977, Langlois et al. 1991], other experts have included extension of the interphalangeal joints of the fingers, thumb, and wrist [Snook 1979, McPherson et al. 1985, Scherling and Johnson 1989]. The resulting design provides a continuous chain of stabilizing forces throughout the wrist and digits. This chain is necessary to prevent compensatory patterns that transfer the forces of spasticity to the unsplinted joint.

Cones

Rood [1954] first advocated the inhibition of flexor spasticity by using a firm cone to provide constant pressure over the palmar surface. The device should provide skin contact over the entire palmar surface for maximal effect but should not apply stretch to the wrist and finger flexor muscles. Farber and Huss [1974] observed that the hard cone has an inhibitory effect on flexor muscles because this device places deep tendon pressure on the wrist and finger-flexor insertions at the base of the palm. Farber [1982] also observed that the total contact from the hard cone provides maintained pressure over the flexor surface of the palm, thus assisting in the desensitization of hypersensitive skin.

Hard cones are typically constructed of cardboard or thermoplastic material (Figure 14-3). This hollow structure is positioned with the smaller end placed radially and the larger end placed ulnarly to provide maximum palmar contact.

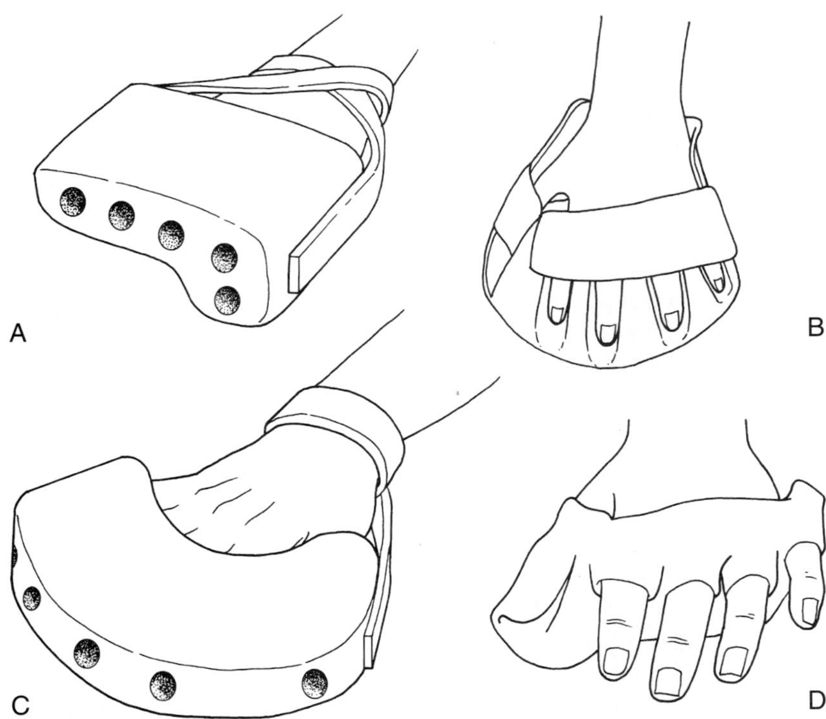

Figure 14-2 Finger spreader designs: (A) palmar abduction [Sammons-Preston 2005], (B) radial abduction [Smith & Nephew Rolyan 1998], (C) radial abduction [Sammons-Preston 2005], and (D) palmar abduction [Doubiet and Polkow 1977].

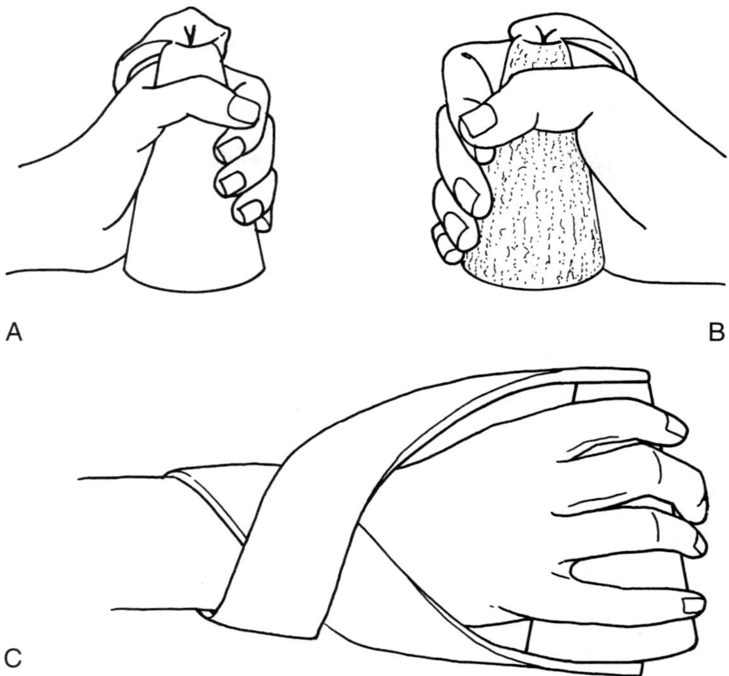

Figure 14-3 Hard-cone designs: (A) hand plastic [Sammons Preston 2005], (B) terry cloth covering [Sammons Preston 2005], and (C) crossover strap system [Contour Fabricator 1983].

Kiel [1974, 1982] recommends the provision of a thenar groove to relieve web-space pressure.

Design criteria for hard cones as cited in the literature does not include the use of forearm platforms to control wrist position. Although Kiel [1974] uses a volar platform with a hard cone in the orthokinetic wrist splint (Figure 14-4), the movable wrist joint allows free motion to occur in wrist flexion and extension. Hard cones attached to ulnar platforms (Figure 14-1) are commercially available [Sammons Preston Rolyan 2005], but the literature does not appear to discuss the combination of forearm platforms and hard-cone elements designed to control wrist and finger position.

When using a firm cone without a forearm platform, the therapist secures the cone to the hand by using a wide [e.g., 2.5-cm (1-inch)] elastic or nonelastic strap over the dorsum of the hand (Figure 14-4) [Dayhoff 1975, Jamison and Dayhoff 1980]. Dayhoff [1975] reports that contact with soft material on the palmar surface appears to increase flexor tone. This soft stimulus may activate the primitive grasp response [Farber 1982]. Brunnstrom [1970] describes this response as

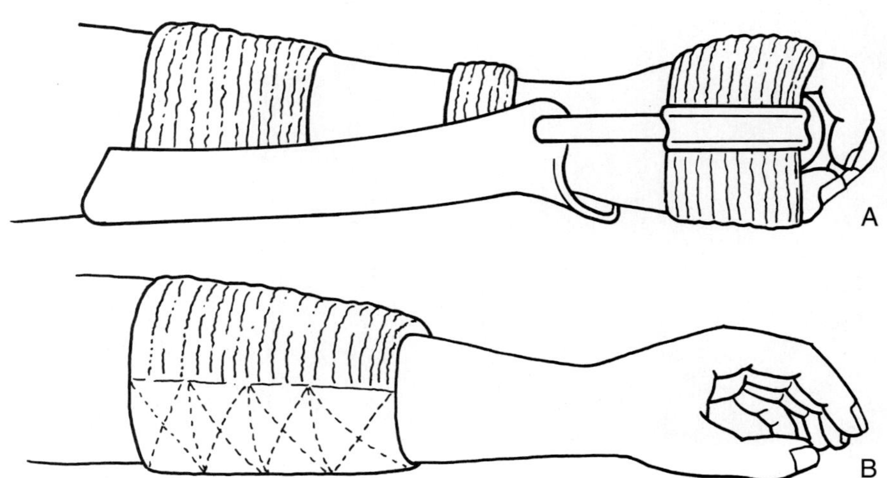

Figure 14-4 Orthokinetic material placement: (A) orthokinetic wrist splint [Kiel 1974] and (B) forearm cuff [Farber and Huss 1974].

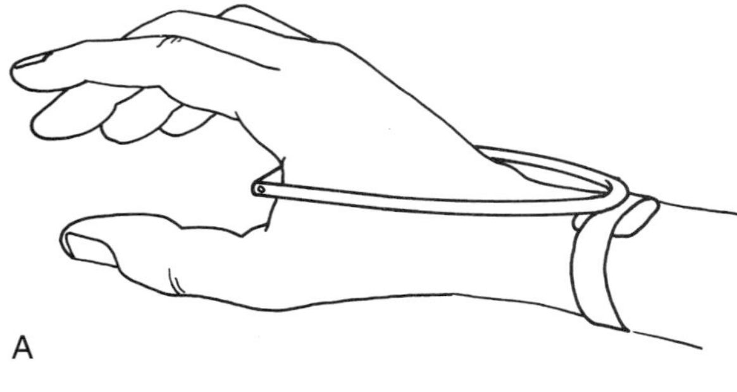

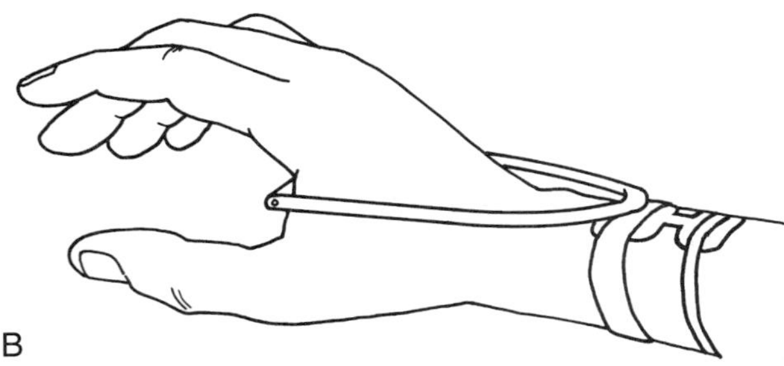

Figure 14-5 Adapted hard-cone designs: (A) MacKinnon [1975] and (B) Exner and Bunder [1983].

the instinctive grasp reaction. Commercially available soft-palm protectors [Sammons Preston Rolyan 2005] may be contraindicated for clients who exhibit the primitive grasp reaction.

MacKinnon et al. [1975] adapted the standard hard cone to increase sensory awareness and improve hand function. They altered the design from a 4- to 5-cm diameter hollow cone shape to a 0.3- to 1.3-cm diameter cylindrical shape by using a solid wood dowel. Placement of the dowel is critical to design rationale. Pressure over the palmar aspect of the metacarpal heads may be a key to activating hand intrinsics. In response to increased intrinsic activity, muscle tone is reduced in finger flexors and the thumb adductor. Placement of the dowel more distally shifts the maximum contact area from the palm to the metacarpal heads and exposes a larger palmar surface to sensory feedback, thus enhancing awareness and use of the hand.

The original MacKinnon splint incorporates a dorsal forearm platform consisting of a small rectangle of thermoplastic material attached to the dorsum of the wrist with a volar Velcro strap [MacKinnon et al. 1975]. This platform serves as the base for plastic tubing secured to the palmar dowel. The intention of this platform is not to position the wrist forcefully in extension but to position the dowel to apply maximal pressure to the metacarpal heads. Exner and Bonder [1983] enlarged this dorsal forearm platform because it was insufficient to control the forces of marked wrist flexion spasticity. The design alteration relieves skin pressure, provides increased wrist control, and ensures greater comfort (Figure 14-5).

Hard-Cone Splint Construction for the Wrist and Hand

1. Determine the correct cone size by positioning an acrylic cone in the client's palm. (Use a small Sammons Preston BK-1500 or a large BK-1502 acrylic cone, as shown in Figure 14-6A.) The therapist must

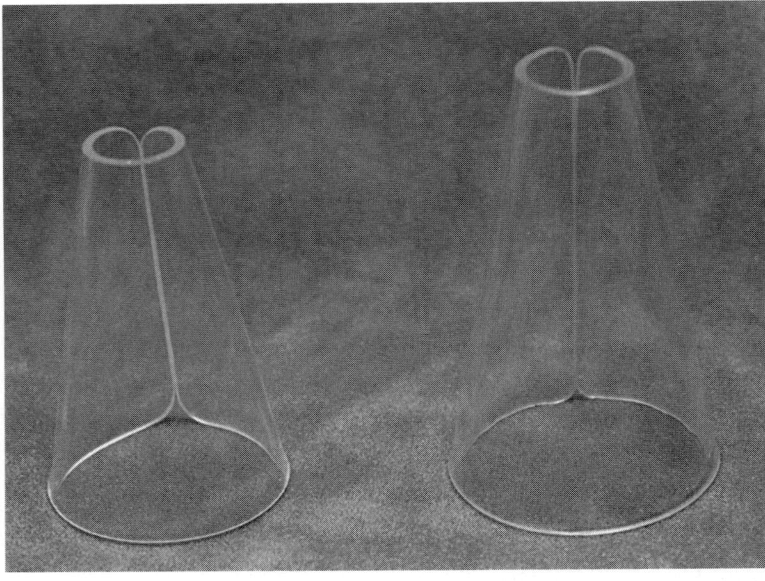

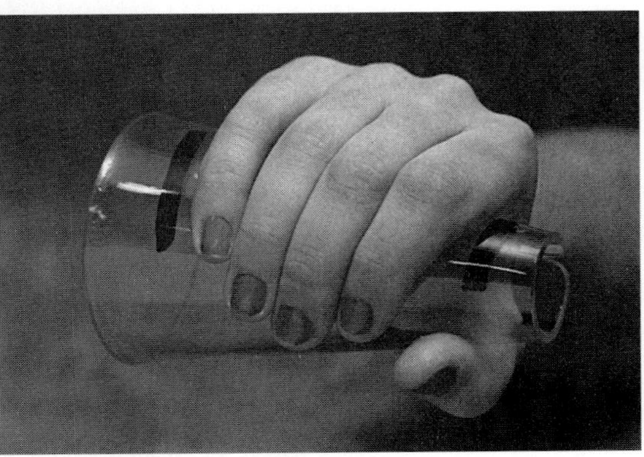

Figure 14-6 (A) Small and large acrylic hand cones. (B) A hand cone correctly positioned on a client with medial and lateral borders marked.

establish the correct amount of palm pressure the client can tolerate without application of stretch to the fingers and thumb. Slide the cone onto the client's hand to determine the correct position (Figure 14-6B).

2. Establish the wrist position by using a goniometer to measure the submaximum or maximum amount of wrist extension the client can tolerate. This measurement must take place while the client wears the acrylic cone (Figure 14-7). Mark on the material the medial and lateral borders of the hand while the cone is positioned in the palm (Figure 14-6B).
3. Using the template provided (Figure 14-8), trace and cut out the pattern from thermoplastic material (Figure 14-9).
4. Apply dishwashing liquid to the acrylic cone as a parting agent.
5. Wrap heated thermoplastic material around the cone (Figure 14-10).
6. Using a sharp pair of scissors, cut the place where the material meets to create a smooth seam edge (Figure 14-11).
7. Slide the thermoplastic cone off the acrylic cone before the material cools to prevent removal difficulty (Figure 14-12).
8. Fit the thermoplastic cone to the client's hand (Figure 14-13), and mark the following on the cone.
   a. Medial border
   b. Lateral border

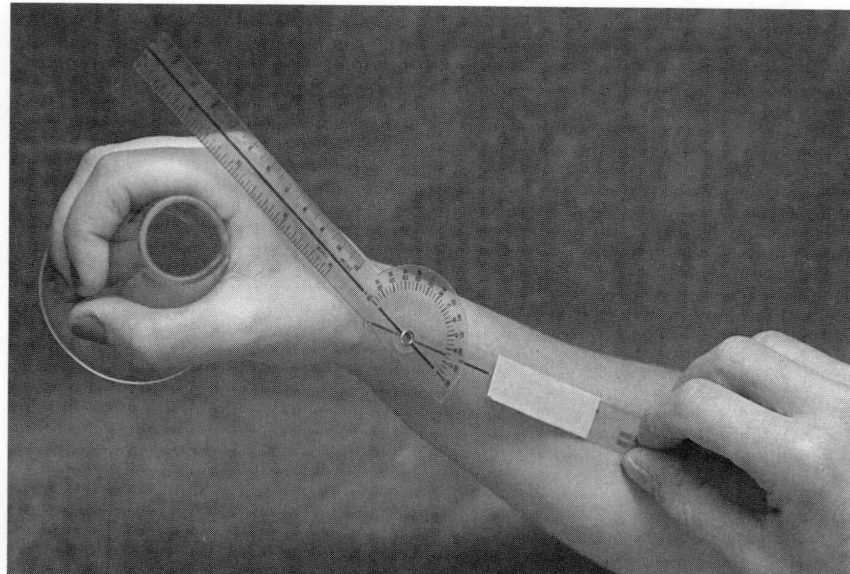

Figure 14-7 Use a goniometer to measure the wrist position.

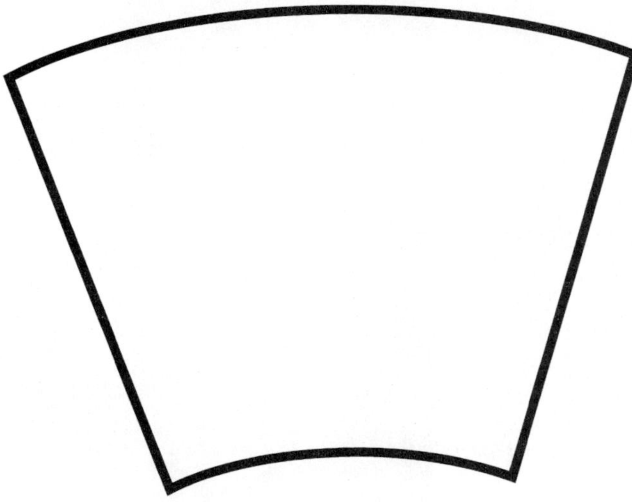

Figure 14-8 A template.

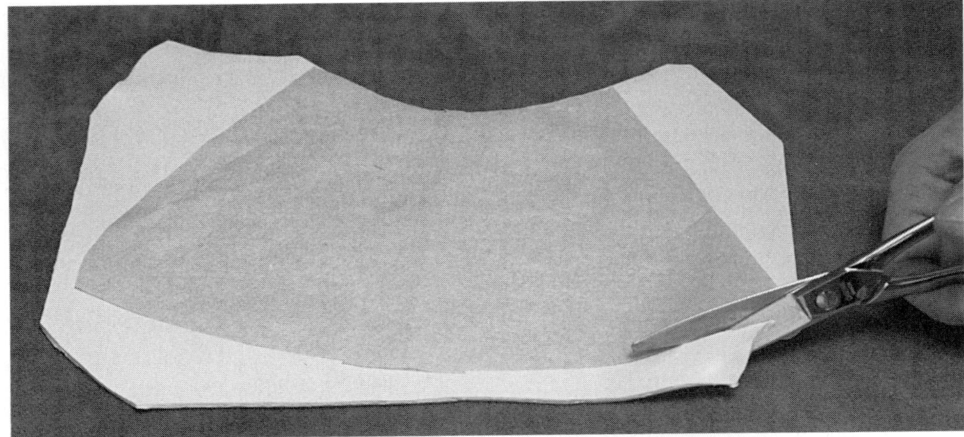

Figure 14-9 Use a template to trace and cut out the pattern.

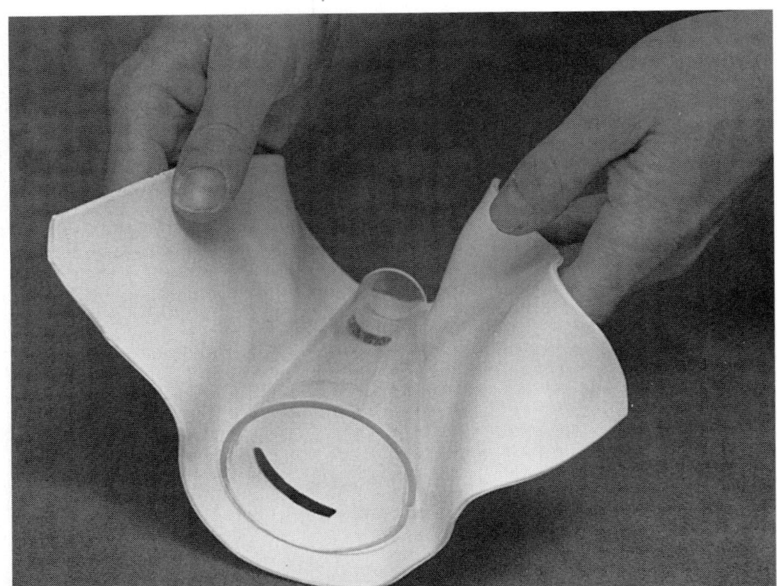

Figure 14-10 Wrap the heated material around the cone.

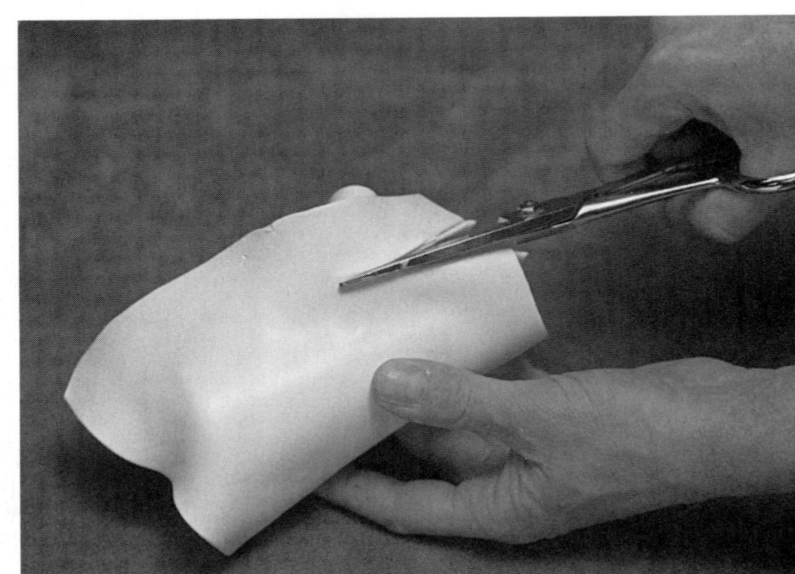

Figure 14-11 Use sharp scissors to create a smooth seam.

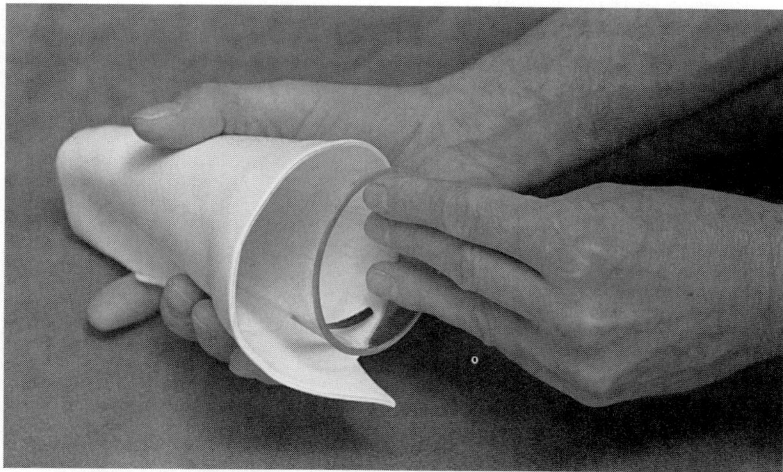

Figure 14-12 Slide the thermoplastic cone off the acrylic cone before the material cools.

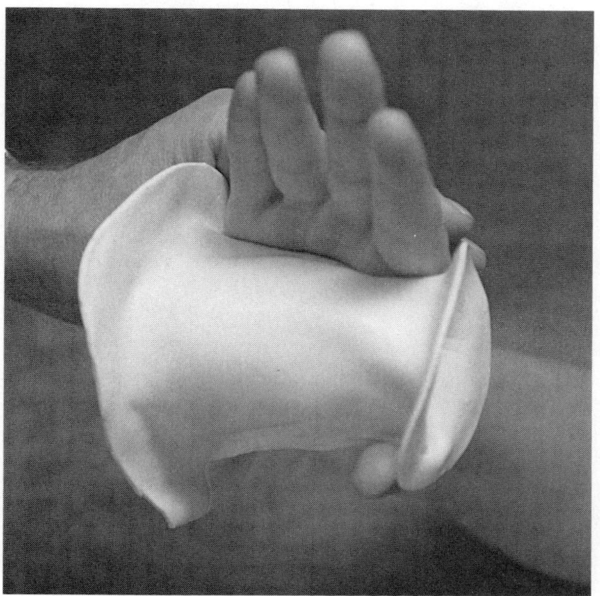

Figure 14-13 Fit the cone to the client's hand.

c. Thumb position
d. Metacarpal arch support

9. Spot heat each of the following areas separately and mold them to the client (Figure 14-14).
   a. Radial support
   b. Ulnar support
   c. Thumb groove
   d. Metacarpal arch support
10. Using a paper pattern, fabricate a dorsal forearm platform (Figure 14-15) that is one-half the width of the forearm and two-thirds the length of the forearm.
11. Warm two pieces of thermoplastic material that are 2 inches wide and 8 inches long. After doing this, fold and seam the pieces lengthwise to create radial and ulnar supports that connect the forearm platform to the cone (Figure 14-16).
12. Position the completed cone and forearm platform on the client (Figure 14-17), maintaining the wrist in proper alignment.

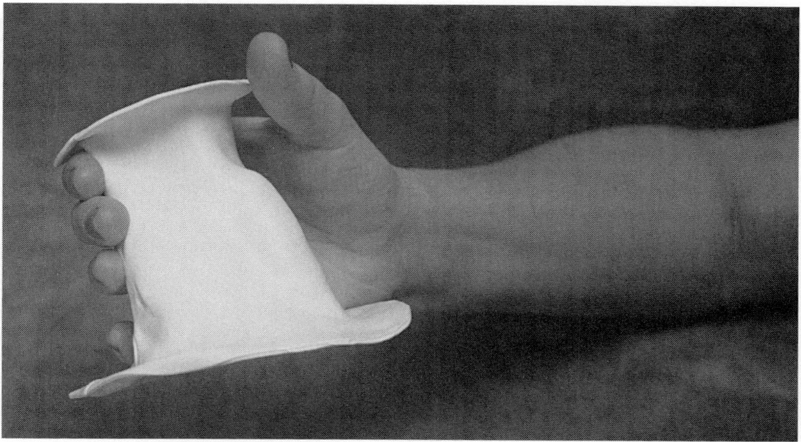

Figure 14-14 Spot heat the mold areas *A* through *D* separately.

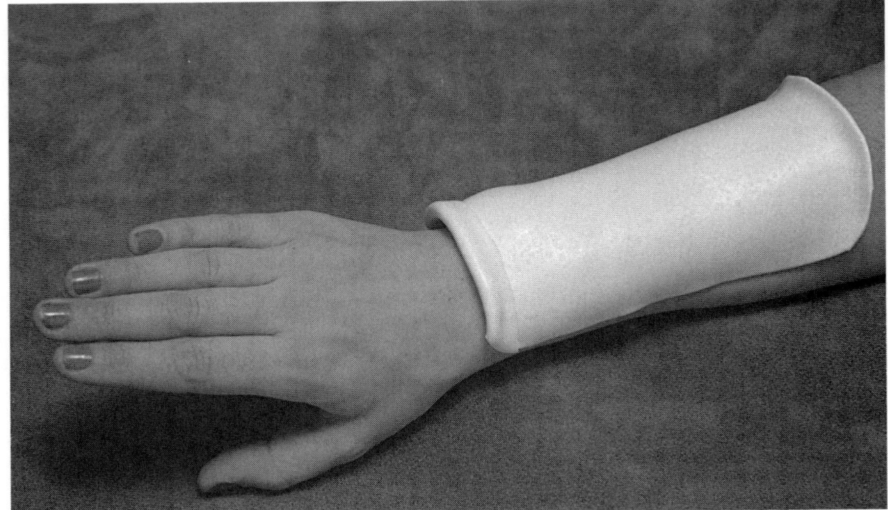

Figure 14-15 Fabricate a dorsal platform.

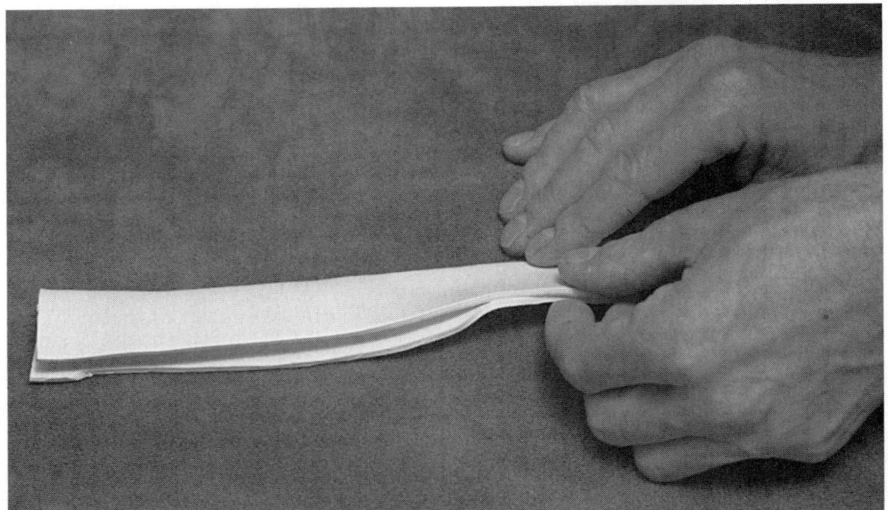

Figure 14-16 Fold and seam the material lengthwise.

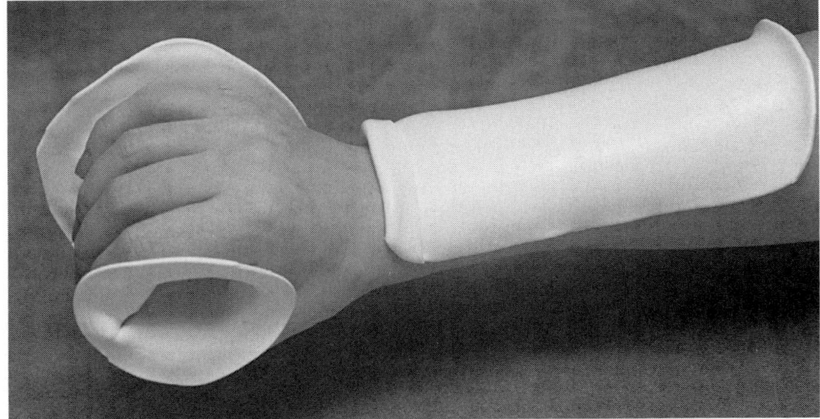

Figure 14-17 Position the completed cone and forearm platform on the client.

13. Apply the radial and ulnar supports (Figure 14-18).
14. After the supports have finished cooling, apply two forearm straps and one strap across the dorsum of the hand to complete the splint (Figure 14-19).
15. Use a goniometer to measure the client's wrist position while the client is secured in the completed orthosis to ensure proper wrist position.

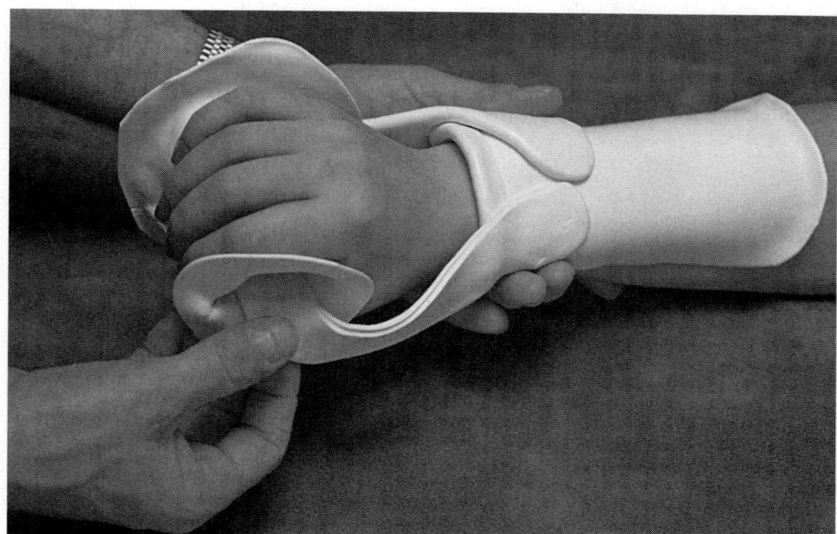

Figure 14-18 Apply the radial and ulnar supports.

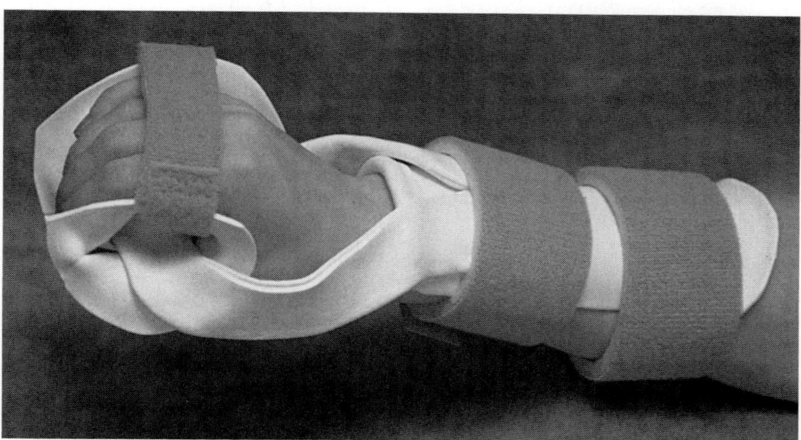

Figure 14-19 Apply the straps.

Laboratory Exercise 14-1

1. Practice fabricating a hard-cone wrist and hand splint on a partner. Use a goniometer and an acrylic cone to position the hand and wrist correctly.
2. After fitting the cone, use Form 14-1. This is a check-off sheet for self-evaluation of the hard-cone wrist and hand splint. Use Grading Sheet 14-1 as a classroom grading sheet.

Static and Dynamic Prolonged Stretch

Spasticity is a positive symptom of upper motor neuron lesion damage because it is an exaggeration of normal muscle tone [Tona and Schneck 1993]. Therapists commonly evaluate muscle tone by measuring the amount of resistance a muscle offers to quick-passive stretch or elongation [Trombly and Scott 1989]. Abnormal resistance to passive movement (i.e., stretch reflex) may be a static (i.e., passive) response to the muscle's maintained state of stretch or a dynamic response to the force and velocity of movement during stretching of the muscle.

The static component (i.e., the nonreflexive, elastic properties of the muscle) and the dynamic component (i.e., the reflexive or active tension of the muscle during stretch) contribute to exaggerated stretch reflex or spasticity [Jansen 1962, McPherson 1981]. The stretch reflex can be triggered at any point of the range-of-motion arc, thus limiting free range of motion. This reflex may also be a significant force to pull the wrist or finger muscles into an abnormal, shortened resting state. This activity creates *hypertonus*, which is defined as a force of spasticity sufficient to move the limb toward an abnormal resting state [McPherson et al. 1985].

Researchers concur that positioning the wrist and finger flexors in gentle, continuous stretch reduces the passive component of spasticity [McPherson 1981, McPherson et al. 1985, Rose and Shah 1987, Scherling and Johnson 1989]. Some authors recommend a static thermoplastic splint that positions the spastic flexor muscle in less than maximum available passive range of motion (i.e., submaximum range) but beyond the point the stretch reflex is triggered [Peterson 1980, Rose and Shah 1987, Tona and Schneck 1993]. Other authors advocate a static thermoplastic splint that positions the spastic flexor muscle in a fully elongated state (i.e., maximum range) [Farber and Huss 1974, Snook 1979]. Ushiba et al. [2004] reports using a wrist splint to provide prolonged wrist extension. Results of the study indicate inhibitory effects on flexor tone in 82% of the 17 subjects who had spasticity.

A dynamic thermoplastic design is also advocated because it provides a more sustained, consistent stretch to the spastic muscle. The use of an elastic or spring-metal force (Figure 14-20) may ensure slow stretch that does not trigger stretch-reflex receptors [McPherson et al. 1985, Scherling and Johnson 1989].

Material Properties

Orthokinetic Materials

Dr. Julius Fuchs, an orthopedic surgeon, developed orthokinetic (righting-of-motion) principles in 1927. Some experts have described, refined, and adapted these principles

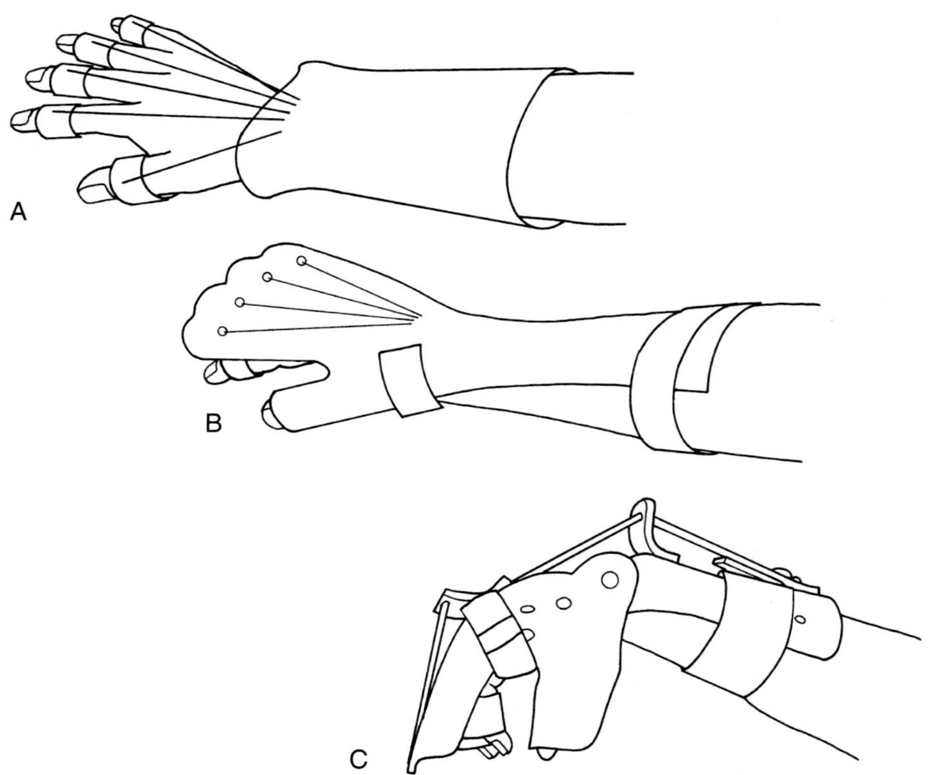

Figure 14-20 Elastic and spring-metal dynamic designs: (A) spring wire [McPherson and Becker 1985], (B) elastic [Scherling and Johnson 1988], and (C) elastic [Rolyan 1993].

[Blashy and Fuchs 1959; Neeman 1971, 1973; Farber and Huss 1974; Kiel 1974, 1982; Farber 1982; Neeman and Neeman 1984]. The term *field* refers to material qualities in orthokinetic terminology.

Dr. Fuch's hand-splint design consists of an orthokinetic tube or cuff (Figure 14-4) that uses dynamic forces to increase range of motion rather than a static device that often contributes to pain and immobilization [Farber and Huss 1974]. The cuff is constructed of an active or facilitatory field the therapist places over the agonist muscle belly. The therapist places the passive or inhibitory field over the antagonist muscle belly. The elastic bandage-material construction of the active field provides minute pinching motions to the dermatome of the agonist muscle (i.e., exteroproprioceptive stimulation) as the muscle contracts and relaxes [Farber 1982]. The inactive field is constructed of layers of elastic bandage sewn or stitched together and provides continuous nonchanging input to the antagonist dermatome.

Because the facilitatory effects of the orthokinetic cuff are activated during the contraction and relaxation of the muscle, this device is most effective when active range of motion is present [Farber 1982]. Other authors recommend alternative materials for construction of inactive fields. Kiel [1974, 1982] uses the unchanging thermoplastic surface of the volar forearm platform in her design of the orthokinetic wrist splint (Figure 14-4). Exner and Bonder [1983] substitute Velfoam as the nonelastic material (Figure 14-5). Kiel [1974, 1982] also suggests that foam lining over a thermoplastic surface transforms that surface from a passive field to an active field as the foam material changes shape to provide facilitatory stimulation.

Serial and Inhibition Casting

Circumferential casting techniques involve specialized fabrication skills and use orthopedic casting materials. Solid serial casting is designed to increase range of motion and decrease contractures caused by spasticity through a series of periodic cast changes. Typically, the affected joint is cast in submaximal range (5 to 10 degrees below maximum passive range). Cast change schedules range from every day for recent contractures to every 10 days for chronic contractures. Blood circulation, edema, skin condition, sensation, and range of motion should be closely monitored during the casting process. The casting program is discontinued when range-of-motion gains are not noted between several cast changes.

Final casts are usually bivalved and applied daily to maintain range-of-motion gains [Feldman 1990]. Therapists routinely use casts to decrease joint contractures. Frequent, periodic cast changes (serial casting) provide prolonged continuous pressure to gradually lengthen muscles and soft tissue. Plaster is a cost-effective choice if the practitioner desires to gradually increase passive range of motion by using a series of static splints. Fiberglass materials are more costly and should not be used without specialized training. King [1982] describes a plaster, serial, dropout cast designed to maintain elbow flexion and stretch and to encourage increased elbow extension (Figure 14-21).

Orthopedic casting materials include plaster or fiberglass bandages that are water activated. Both materials require six to eight layers of thickness for adequate strength, and they harden in 3 to 8 minutes (depending on water temperature). The materials emit heat as a byproduct in the curing process. Plaster splints are not water resistant, do not clean easily, may cause allergic reactions, and pose limitations because of their weight. A plaster bandage is relatively inexpensive, is easy to handle, and conforms/drapes easily to body parts. Fiberglass splints are water resistant, cleanable, lightweight, and not prone to allergic reactions. In addition, fiberglass materials are significantly more expensive and more difficult to handle than plaster. The therapist typically applies several layers of cotton cast padding to the extremity before the application of layers of plaster or fiberglass for skin protection. Specialized casting tools include the following:

- Electric cast saw
- Hand cast spreader
- Bandage scissors

Casting program materials include the following:

- Plaster or fiberglass casting tape (2-inch, 3-inch, 4-inch, 5-inch)
- Nylon or cotton stockinette (2-inch, 3-inch, 4-inch, 5-inch)
- Rubber gloves (specialized casting gloves for fiberglass)
- Plastic water bucket
- Drop sheet to protect client
- Cast padding

Plaster Casting Procedures [Feldman 1990]

1. Measure and record joint range of motion.
2. The client should be sitting or lying comfortably and should be draped with sheets or towels to protect clothing and skin. Explain the procedure to the client clearly and reassure as needed. Some clients with brain injuries may be agitated during the casting procedure.

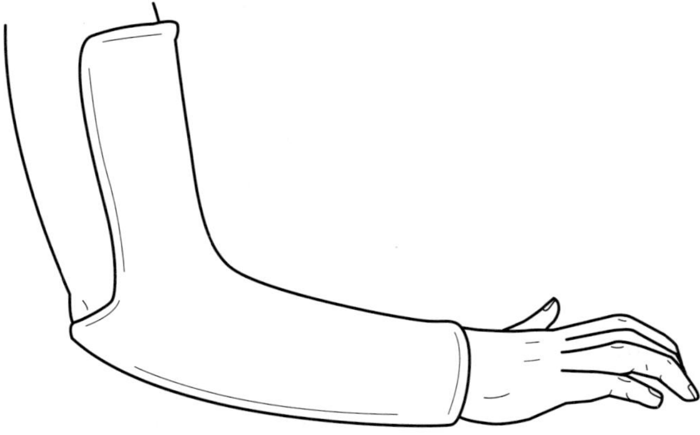

Figure 14-21 Elbow dropout cast.

Premedicating such clients with a sedative can be considered.

3. Tubular stockinette is placed over the extremity to be casted, extending at either end 4 to 6 inches beyond where the cast will end.
4. Determine the targeted position of the extremity. Direct another person (therapist or aid) how and where to hold the extremity.
5. Strips of stick-on foam can be placed on either side of an area that may be susceptible to skin breakdown.
6. Apply cast padding in a taut fashion around the extremity, ending after three or four layers have been applied. Extra padding or felt may be added if needed over bony prominences. Padding is applied 1 to 2 inches above the end of the stockinette.
7. Dip the plaster roll five to six times in warm water. Squeeze excess moisture from the roll.
8. Apply plaster to the extremity in a spiral fashion, moving proximally to distally.
9. Direct the person assisting to stretch the joint minimally as the plaster is being applied. The casting assistant should not apply direct pressure to the plaster as it is setting (breakdown or ischemia inside the cast can occur from this loading point effect). Rather, the assistant should stretch the joint above and below the cast or apply pressure with the entire surface of the hand to evenly distribute pressure.
10. Four to five layers of plaster should be applied. The plaster should be smoothed with the surface using the hand surface in a circular fashion as the plaster sets. Special attention must be paid to smoothing proximal and distal edges to prevent skin breakdown.
11. Before applying the last layer, turn back the ends of stockinette onto the cast. This gives a smooth finished surface to cast edges. Apply the last layer of plaster just below this edge.
12. Instruct the casting assistant to maintain stretch on the joint until the plaster has set (3 to 8 minutes).
13. The plaster will be completely dry in 24 hours. Weight bearing on the casted extremity should be avoided until then.
14. Clean any dripped plaster from the client's skin, elevate the extremity comfortably, and check either end of the cast for tightness. Check the client's circulation regularly. Some authors [Copley et al. 1996] recommend a post-casting management program of bivalve splinting in order to maintain increased range of motion and tone reduction.

Fiberglass Casting Procedures [Feldman 1990]

1. Plastic gloves should be worn by anyone touching the fiberglass material during fabrication. Initially and throughout the procedure, the plastic gloves should be coated with petroleum jelly or lotion. Fiberglass adheres to the skin or unlubricated gloves and is difficult to remove. Prepare the limb with padding and stockinette. Practice with the casting assistant to position the joint in the manner desired.
2. Submerge the fiberglass roll in cool water and gently squeeze six to eight times. Remove the roll from the water and apply it dripping wet to the extremity to facilitate handling of the material.
3. Fiberglass roll packages should be opened one at a time and applied within minutes. Fiberglass hardens and does not bond to itself when left exposed to air.
4. Fiberglass must overlap itself by half a tape width.
5. FirBLy blot the exterior of the cast with an open palm in a circular fashion after all layers have been applied. This is to facilitate maximum bonding of all layers. Rubbing in a longitudinal fashion disrupts the fiberglass bond.
6. If one layer of the cast is allowed to cure (harden), subsequent layers do not bond well. All three to four layers should be applied in efficient succession.
7. During the first 2 minutes after immersion, the fiberglass can be molded while the extremity is maintained in the desired position. The extremity should be held stationary during the last few minutes of the 5- to 7-minute setting time.
8. The cast will be completely set in 7 to 10 minutes. It can be removed after that with a cast saw. Cast saws should be operated only by those individuals with training and experience.

The fiberglass cast can be made into a working bivalve in the following manner [Feldman 1990].

1. Using the cast saw, cut the cast into anterior and posterior sections. Remove the cast with the cast spreader.
2. Remove the padding and stockinette from the extremity with the cast scissors and discard them.
3. Inspect both fiberglass shells for protrusions and rough edges. Trim the edges of each shell and file smooth.
4. When the cast padding has been soiled, use cotton padding to reline the shells, taking care to rip padding edges off to provide a smooth inner surface with no ripples. Reline with the same amount of padding used to fabricate the original cast. Extend the padding over all edges and sides of shells.
5. Fold the padding over the edges of the shells and secure with adhesive tape.
6. Cut a length of the stockinette approximately 4 to 6 inches longer than the length of the shell. Line each shell with stockinette. Secure both ends with adhesive tape.
7. Fashion straps using wide webbing and buckles. These can be taped or sewn onto stockinette covering the shell. Bivalves can also be secured with Ace wraps.
8. Carefully wean the client into the bivalve, modifying and adjusting as needed.

Summary: Serial and Inhibition Casting

Therapists also use plaster and fiberglass materials for inhibition or tone-reducing casting. The exact mechanism for

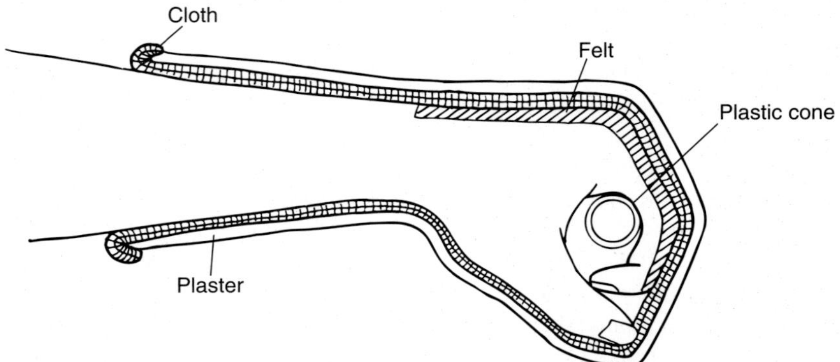

Figure 14-22 An inhibitive cast with a hard plastic cone.

the inhibitory effect of these materials is not known [Tona and Schneck 1993]. Gentle, passive stretching and the neutral warmth of the underlying cotton padding may serve as primary relaxing agents [King 1982]. Some authors believe that inhibitive casting materials are more effective than thermoplastic materials at providing deep pressure, prolonged demobilization, neutral warmth, and consistent tactile stimulation [Tona and Schneck 1993]. These authors advocate the use of a separate thermoplastic inhibitive splint (hard cone) incorporated into an inhibitive cast to enhance the tone-reducing effects of both materials (Figure 14-22).

Lower extremity tone-reduction orthotic literature includes the use of a separate footboard as an inhibitive element in the plaster-negative model-casting procedure. The end product of this process is a continuous one-piece thermoplastic orthosis [Hylton 1990]. Current lower extremity tone-reduction orthotic literature focuses on the incorporation of various inhibitive and facilitatory design elements into one total-surface-contact thermoplastic splint [Lohman and Goldstein 1993].

Other Materials

Authors have reported the spasticity-reduction effectiveness of other materials that provide neutral warm and passive stretch. Pneumatic-pressure arm splints that are orally inflatable (Figure 14-23) are especially effective as adjuncts to upper extremity weight bearing [Bloch and Evans 1977; Johnstone 1981; Poole et al. 1990, 1992; Lofy et al. 1992]. These tubular devices are open at the distal end, allowing the therapist to place the client's wrist and hand into the desired position of extension. Wallen and O'Flaherty [1991] have devised a cylindrical foam splint (Figure 14-24) that reduces the muscle tone of the upper extremity. The foam material reacts dynamically and automatically adjusts to greater degrees of extension. Mackay and Wallen [1996] report a significant increase in passive elbow extension after use of soft foam splint.

Elastic tubular bandages have been successful in providing relaxation of upper extremity hypertonicity through the application of neutral warmth and deep pressure [Johnson and Vernon 1992]. Takami et al. [1992] describe the use of a titanium metal alloy that gradually changes shape in

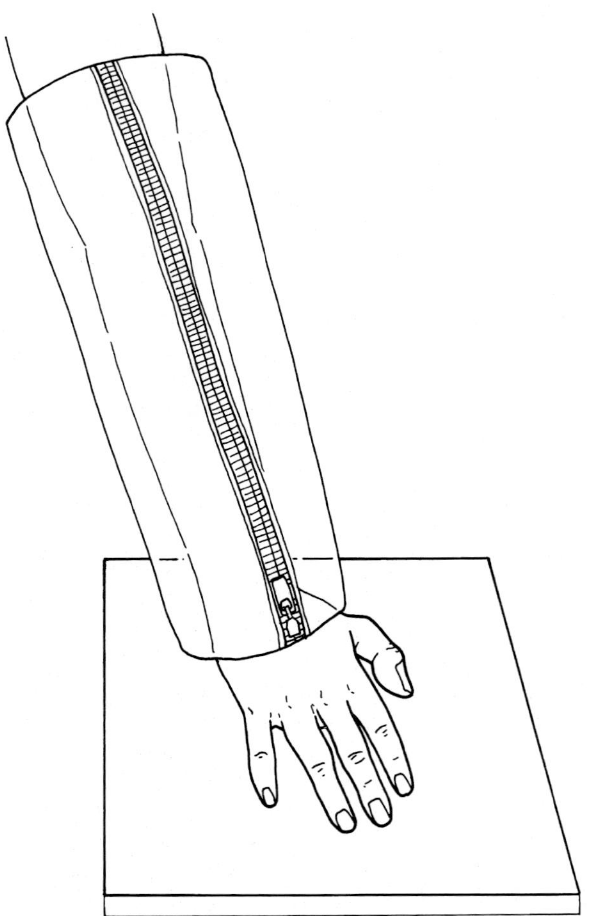

Figure 14-23 An orally inflatable pneumatic-pressure arm splint.

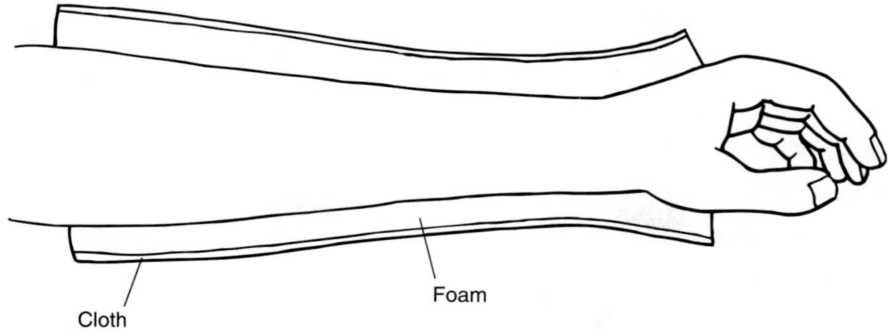

Figure 14-24 A cylinder foam splint.

response to room temperature and provides gentle passive stretch to spastic wrist flexors. In addition, neoprene material provides a dynamic force that produces gentle stretch. The neoprene thumb abduction supination splint (TASS) (Figure 14-25) facilitates key-point positioning of the upper extremity, thus reducing spasticity [Casey and Kratz 1988]. Gracies et al. [2000] report success in reducing wrist and finger flexor spasticity using a Lycra sleeve and glove. Lycra is thinner than neoprene but provides a similar dynamic force, thus promoting gentle stretch.

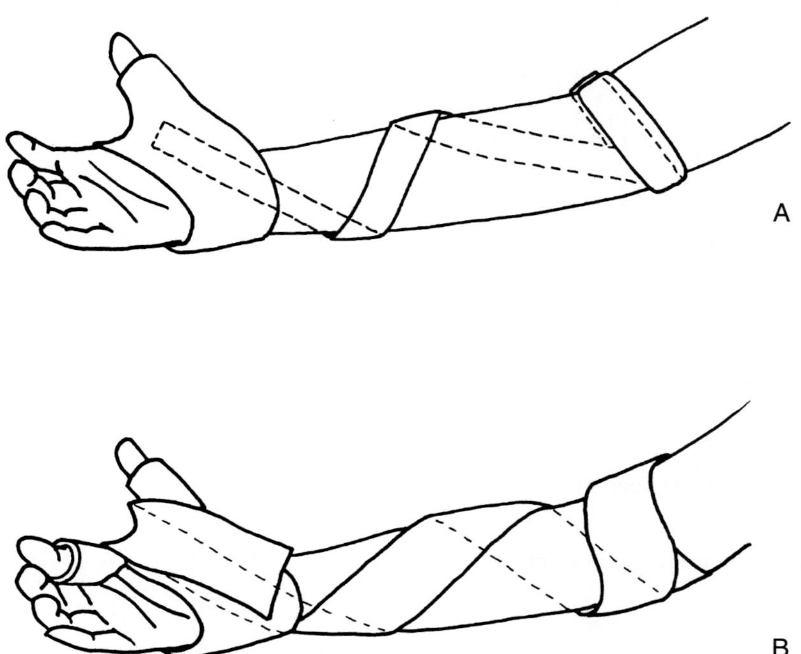

Figure 14-25 Neoprene splint designs: (A) TASS [Casey and Kratz 1988], (B) tap [Smith & Nephew Rolyan 1998].

FORM 14-1* Hard-cone wrist and hand splint

Name: ______________________________

Date: ______________________________

Type of cone wrist and hand splint:

Volar platform ❍ Dorsal platform ❍

Answer the following questions after the splint has been worn for 30 minutes. (Mark *NA* for nonapplicable situations.)

Evaluation Areas				Comments
Design				
1. The wrist position is at the correct angle.	Yes ❍	No ❍	NA ❍	
2. The correct cone-diameter size reflects the palm width and web-space size.	Yes ❍	No ❍	NA ❍	
3. The small end of the cone is placed radially and the large end is placed ulnarly.	Yes ❍	No ❍	NA ❍	
4. The thumb is positioned in palmar abduction with the web space preserved.	Yes ❍	No ❍	NA ❍	
5. The splint is two-thirds the length of the forearm.	Yes ❍	No ❍	NA ❍	
6. The splint is half the width of the forearm.	Yes ❍	No ❍	NA ❍	
Function				
1. The wrist is positioned in submaximal or maximal range.	Yes ❍	No ❍	NA ❍	
2. The fingers are positioned to provide firm pressure but not stretch the flexors.	Yes ❍	No ❍	NA ❍	
Straps				
1. The straps avoid bony prominences.	Yes ❍	No ❍	NA ❍	
2. The straps are secure and rounded.	Yes ❍	No ❍	NA ❍	
3. The active field materials are used over the extensor muscle bellies.	Yes ❍	No ❍	NA ❍	
4. The passive field materials are used over the flexor muscle bellies.	Yes ❍	No ❍	NA ❍	
Comfort				
1. The edges are smooth with rounded corners.	Yes ❍	No ❍	NA ❍	
2. The proximal end is flared.	Yes ❍	No ❍	NA ❍	
3. Impingements or pressure areas are not present. (The ulnar styloid is relieved.)	Yes ❍	No ❍	NA ❍	
Cosmetic Appearance				
1. The splint is free of fingerprints, dirt, and pencil or pen marks.	Yes ❍	No ❍	NA ❍	
2. The splinting material is not buckled.	Yes ❍	No ❍	NA ❍	
Therapeutic Regimen				
1. The person/caregiver has been instructed in a wearing schedule.	Yes ❍	No ❍	NA ❍	
2. The person/caregiver has been provided with splint precautions.	Yes ❍	No ❍	NA ❍	

FORM 14-1* Hard-cone wrist and hand splint—cont'd

3. The person/caregiver demonstrates understanding of the education. Yes ❍ No ❍ NA ❍
4. Person/caregiver knows how to clean the splint. Yes ❍ No ❍ NA ❍

Discuss adjustments or changes you would make based on the self-evaluation.

*See Appendix B for a perforated copy of this form.

GRADING SHEET 14-1* Hard-cone wrist and hand splint

Name: ______________________

Date: ______________________

Type of cone wrist and hand splint:

Volar platform ❍ Dorsal platform ❍

Grade: ____________

1 = beyond improvement, not acceptable
2 = requires maximal improvement
3 = requires moderate improvement
4 = requires minimal improvement
5 = requires no improvement

Evaluation Areas						Comments
Design						
1. The wrist position is at the correct angle.	1	2	3	4	5	
2. The correct cone-diameter size reflects the palm width and web-space size.	1	2	3	4	5	
3. The small end of the cone is placed radially and the large end is placed ulnarly.	1	2	3	4	5	
4. The thumb is positioned in palmar abduction with the web space preserved.	1	2	3	4	5	
5. The splint is two-thirds the length of the forearm.	1	2	3	4	5	
6. The splint is half the width of the forearm.	1	2	3	4	5	
Function						
1. The wrist is positioned in submaximal or maximal range.	1	2	3	4	5	
2. The fingers are positioned to provide firm pressure but not stretch the flexors.	1	2	3	4	5	
Straps						
1. The straps avoid bony prominences.	1	2	3	4	5	
2. The straps are secure and rounded.	1	2	3	4	5	
3. The active field materials are used over the extensor muscle bellies.	1	2	3	4	5	
4. The passive field materials are used over the flexor muscle bellies.	1	2	3	4	5	
Comfort						
1. The edges are smooth with rounded corners.	1	2	3	4	5	
2. The proximal end is flared.	1	2	3	4	5	
3. Impingements or pressure areas are not present. (The ulnar styloid is relieved.)	1	2	3	4	5	
Cosmetic Appearance						
1. The splint is free of fingerprints, dirt, and pencil or pen marks.	1	2	3	4	5	
2. The splinting material is not buckled.	1	2	3	4	5	

*See Appendix C for a perforated copy of this grading sheet.

CASE STUDY 14-1

Read the following scenario and answer the questions based on information in this chapter.

BL experienced a CVA 2 months ago and is presently residing in a skilled nursing facility. Over a 4-week period of flaccidity, upper extremity wrist and finger-flexion spasticity has gradually increased. Pain-free range of motion is limited to 5 degrees of wrist extension. No active wrist and finger motion is present. A strong stretch reflex is elicited at 10 degrees of wrist flexion. The nursing staff is concerned that BL will develop palm maceration because his fingers rest in a tightly clenched position. A rolled washcloth was positioned in his palm to reduce the likelihood of skin breakdown, but nursing notes indicate that use of this device has increased finger-flexion tightness. The thumb is tightly flexed across the palm, thus causing skin irritation to the thumb-web space.

1. Which of the following orthotic designs is most appropriate for BL? Explain your answer.
   a. A dorsal-based forearm platform and finger spreader that positions the wrist and fingers statically in maximum extension
   b. A volar-based forearm platform and hard cone that positions the wrist and fingers dynamically in submaximum extension
   c. An orthokinetic cuff positioned on the forearm that leaves the wrist and fingers unsplinted
   d. An inhibitive cast that places the wrist in maximum extension and the fingers in a current resting position
   e. A neoprene thumb-abduction splint that leaves the wrist and fingers unsplinted

2. The nursing staff is resistant to discontinuing BL's present soft hand-positioning device. How would you approach the staff members to convince them to change the splint management of this client?

Three weeks have passed. BL has been wearing the new tone-reduction splint consistently for several hours daily. Nursing reports indicate that tight fist clenching has reduced significantly. Passive range of motion has increased to 30 degrees of wrist extension. Minimum stretch reflex can be felt at 20 degrees of wrist extension. Weak wrist and finger extension is present when the extremity is positioned with gravity eliminated. The thumb, however, remains tightly flexed into the palm.

3. Which of the following orthotic designs is the most appropriate for BL at this time? Explain your answer.
   a. A finger spreader that positions the thumb in radial abduction and leaves the wrist unsplinted
   b. A hard cone that positions the thumb in opposition and leaves the wrist unsplinted
   c. An orthokinetic cuff on the forearm that leaves the fingers and thumb unsplinted
   d. An orally inflatable splint that leaves the wrist, fingers, and thumb in extension
   e. A neoprene thumb-abduction and extension orthosis that leaves the wrist and fingers unsplinted

4. What specific suggestions would you offer the nursing staff to encourage increased functional hand skills while BL is wearing tone-reduction orthosis?

*See Appendix A for the answer key.

REVIEW QUESTIONS

1. How do the biochemical and neurophysiological approaches to hand splinting differ?
2. What are the strengths and weaknesses of dorsal versus volar forearm platform?
3. What are the three rationales supporting the use of the finger spreader and the hand cone?
4. Why are passive and dynamic components of spasticity critical in splint design?
5. What are the two major components of other kinetic splinting?
6. What are two major characteristics for each of the below materials?
   - Plaster Bandage
   - Fiberglass Bandage
   - Inflatable splints
   - Cylindrical foam
   - Neoprene

References

Basmajian J, Burke M, Burnett G, Campbell C, Cohn W, Corliss C, et al. (1982). *Illustrated Stedman's Medical Dictionary, Twenty-fourth Edition*. London: Williams & Wilkins.

Bishop B (1977). Spasticity: Its physiology and management. Part III. Identifying and assessing the mechanisms underlying spasticity. Physical Therapy 57:385-395.

Blashy MRM, Fuchs (Neeman) RI (1959). Orthokinetics: A new receptor facilitation method. American Journal of Occupational Therapy 13:226-234.

Bloch R, Evans M (1977). An inflatable splint for the spastic hand. Archives of Physical Medicine and Rehabilitation 58:179-180.

Bobath B (1970). *Adult Hemiplegia: Evaluation and Treatment*. London: William Heinemann, Medical Books.

Bobath B (1987). *Adult Hemiplegia: Evaluation and Treatment*. London: William Heinemann, Medical Books.

Brennan J (1959). Response to stretch of hypertonic muscle groups in hemiplegia. British Medical Journal 1:1504-1507.

Brunnstrom S (1970). *Movement Therapy in Hemiplegia*. New York, Evanston, and London: Harper & Row, Publishers.

Carmick J (1997). Case report: Use of neuromuscular electrical stimulation and a dorsal wrist splint to improve the hand function of a child with spastic hemiparesis. Physical Therapy 77(6):661-671.

Casey CA, Kratz EJ (1988). Soft splinting with neoprene: The thumb abduction supinator splint. American Journal of Occupational Therapy 42(6):395-398.

Charait S (1968). A comparison of volar and dorsal splinting of the hemiplegic hand. American Journal of Occupational Therapy 22:319-321.

Copley J, Watson-Will A, Dent K (1996). Upper limb casting for clients with cerebral palsy: A clinical report. Australian Occupational Therapy Journal 43:39-50.

Davies P (1985). *Steps to Follow: A Guide to the Treatment of Hemiplegia*. New York: Springer-Verlag.

Dayhoff N (1975). Re-thinking stroke soft or hard devices to position hands. American Journal of Nursing 75(7):1142-1144.

Doubilet L, Polkow L (1977). Theory and design of a finger abduction splint for the spastic hand. American Journal of Occupational Therapy 32:320-322.

Exner C, Bonder B (1983). Comparative effects of three hand splints on bilateral hand use, grasp, and arm-hand posture in hemiplegic children: A pilot study. Occupational Therapy Journal Research 3:75-92.

Farber SD (1982). Neurorehabilitation: A multidisciplinary approach. Toronto: WB Saunders.

Farber SD, Huss AJ (1974). *Sensorimotor Evaluation and Treatment Procedures for Allied Health Personnel*. Indianapolis: Indiana University Foundation.

Feldman PA (1990). Upper extremity casting and splinting. In MD Glenn, J Whyte (eds.), *The Practical Management of Spasticity in Children and Adults*. Malvern, PA: Lea & Febiger.

Fess EE, Gettle KS, Philips CA, Janson JR (2005). *Hand and Upper Extremity Splinting: Principles and Methods*. St. Louis: Elsevier/Mosby.

Fuchs J (1927). *Technische Operationen in der Orthopaedie Orthokinetik*. Berlin: Verlag Julius Springer.

Gracies J-M, Marosszeky JE, Renton R, Sandanam J, Gandevia SC. Burke D (2000). Short-term effects of dynamic lycra splints on upper limb in hemiplegic patients. Archives Physical Medical Rehabilitation 81:1547-1555.

Hylton NM (1990). Postural and functional impact of dynamic AFOs and FOs in a pediatric population. Journal of Prosthetic Orthotics 2(1):40-53.

Jamison S, Dayhoff N (1980). A hard hand-positioning device to decrease wrist and finger hypertonicity: A sensorimotor approach for the client with non-progressive brain damage. Nursing Research, 29:285-289.

Jansen JKS (1962). Spasticity: Functional aspects. Acta Neurologica Scandinavica 38(3):41-51.

Johnson J, Vernon DC (1992). Elastic tubular bandages: An adjunctive treatment approach to abnormal muscle tone. Gerontology Special Interest Selection Newsletter 15(2):3-4.

Johnstone M (1981). Control of muscle tone in the stroke client. Physiology 67:198.

Kaplan N (1962). Effect of splinting on reflex inhibition and sensorimotor stimulation in treatment of spasticity. Archives of Physical Medicine and Rehabilitation 43:565-569.

Kiel J (1974). *Dynamic Orthokinetic Wrist Splint: Sensorimotor Evaluation and Treatment Procedures*. Indianapolis: Indiana-Purdue University.

Kiel J (1982). *Orthokinetic Wrist Splint for Flexor Spasticity: Neurorehabilitation*. Toronto: W. B. Saunders.

King T (1982). Plaster splinting as a means of reducing elbow flexor spasticity: A case study. American Journal of Occupational Therapy 36:671-674.

Langlois S, MacKinnon JR, Pederson L (1989). Hand splints and cerebral spasticity: A review of the literature. Canadian Journal of Occupational Therapy 56(3):113-119.

Langlois S, Pederson L, MacKinnon JR (1991). The effects of splinting on the spastic hemiplegic hand: Report of a feasibility study. Canadian Journal of Occupational Therapy 58(1):17-25.

Lannin NA, Herbert RD (2003). Is hand splinting effective for adults following stroke? A systematic review and methodological critique of published research. Clinical Rehabilitation 17:807-816.

Lofy S, Pereida L, Spores M (1992). Air splints: Technique propels stroke rehab. Occupational Therapy Week 6(18):18-19.

Lohman M, Goldstein H (1993). Alternative strategies in tone-reducing AFO design. Journal of Prosthetic Orthotics 5(1):21-24.

Mackay S, Wallen M (1996). Re-examining the effects of the soft splint on acute hypertonicity at the elbow. Australian Occupational Therapy Journal 43:51-59.

MacKinnon J, Sanderson E, Buchanan D (1975). The MacKinnon splint: A functional hand splint. Canadian Journal of Occupational Therapy 42:157-158.

McPherson J (1981). Objective evaluation of a splint designed to reduce hypertonicity. American Journal of Occupational Therapy 35:189-194.

McPherson J, Becker A, Franszczak N (1985). Dynamic splint to reduce the passive component of hypertonicity. Archives of Physical Medicine and Rehabilitation 66:249-252.

McPherson J, Kreimer D, Aalderks M, Gallager T (1982). A comparison of dorsal & volar resting hand splints in the reduction of hypertonus. American Journal of Occupational Therapy 36:664-670.

Mills V (1984). Electromyographic results of inhibitory splinting. Physical Therapy 64:190-193.

Neeman RL (1971). Technique of preparing effective orthokinetic cuffs. Bulletin on Practice (AOTA) 6(1):1.

Neeman RL (1973). Orthokinetic sensorimotor treatment. Australian Occupational Therapy Journal 20:122-125.

Neeman RL, Neeman M (1984). Comments on orthokinetics. Occupational Therapy Journal of Research 4:316-318.

Neuhaus B, Ascher E, Coullon B, Donohue MV, Einbond A, Glover J, et al. (1981). A survey of rationales for and against hand splinting in hemiplegia. American Journal of Occupational Therapy 35:83-90.

Peterson LT (1980). *Neurological Considerations in Splinting Spastic Extremities*. Menomonee Fall, WI: Rolyan Orthotics Lab.

Poole JL, Whitney SL, Hangeland N, Baker C (1990). Function in stroke clients. Occupational Therapy Journal Research 10: 360-366.

Poole JL, Whitney SL, Haworth PR (1992). Treatment for individuals with stroke. Physical and Occupational Therapy Geriatrics 11:17-27.

Rood M (1954). Neurophysiological reactions as a basis for physical therapy. Physical Therapy Review 34:444-449.

Rose V, Shah S (1987). A comparative study on the immediate effects of hand orthoses on reduction of hypertonus. Australian Occupational Therapy Journal 34(2):59-64.

Sammons-Bissell Health Care Corporation (1995). *Catalog*. Western Springs, IL.

Sammons Preston Roylan (2005). *Catalog*. Western Springs, IL.

Scherling E, Johnson H (1989). A tone-reducing wrist-hand orthosis. American Journal of Occupational Therapy 43(9):609-611.

Smith & Nephew Rolyan, Inc. (1998). *Catalog*. Menomonee Falls, WI.

Snook JH (1979). Spasticity reduction splint. American Journal of Occupational Therapy 33:648-651.

Switzer S (1980). The Switzer splint. British Journal of Occupational Therapy 43:63-64.

Takami M, Fukui K, Saitou S, Sugiyama I, Terayama K (1992). Application of a shape memory alloy to hand splinting. Prosthetic Orthotics International 16:37-63.

Tona JL, Schneck CM (1993). The efficacy of upper extremity inhibitive casting: A single subject pilot study. American Journal of Occupational Therapy 47(10):901-910.

Trombly C, Scott A (1989). *Occupational Therapy for Physical Dysfunction, Third Edition*. Baltimore: Williams & Wilkins.

Ushiba J, Masakado Y, Komune Y, Muraoka Y, Chino N, Tomita Y (2004). Changes of reflex size in upper limbs using wrist splint in hemiplegic patients. Electromyography Clinical Neurophysiology 4:175-182.

Wallen M, O'Flaherty S (1991). The use of soft splint in the management of spasticity of the upper limb. Australian Occupational Therapy Journal 38(15):227-231.

Zislis J (1964). Splinting of hand in a spastic hemiplegic client. Archives of Physical Medicine and Rehabilitation 45:41-43.

CHAPTER 15

Splinting on Older Adults

Marlene A. Riley, MMS, OTR/L, CHT
Helene Lohman, MA, OTD, OTR/L

Key Terms

Arteriovenous anastomosis
Ecchymosis
Integumentary system
Preformed splints
Soft splints
Working memory

Chapter Objectives

1. Describe special considerations for splinting older adults in different treatment settings.
2. Identify age-related changes and medical conditions that may affect splint provision.
3. Explain how medication side effects may affect splint design and care instructions for older adults.
4. Recognize how an older adult's occupational performance may influence splint use and design based on the following client factors:
    - Mental functions:
        - Affective
        - Cognitive
        - Perceptual
    - Sensory functions:
        - Vision
        - Auditory
        - Touch
        - Pain
    - Neuro-musculoskeletal functions:
        - Joint mobility
        - Strength
        - Muscle tone
    - Cardiovascular and hematological functions
    - Digestive, metabolic, and endocrine functions
    - Genitourinary functions
    - Skin functions:
        - Integrity of skin
        - Wound healing
5. Be familiar with a variety of prefabricated splint options and materials available to custom design splints.
6. Describe factors that influence methods of instruction for an older adult and caregiver.

The age of 65 has been used as the marker in establishing policies for the older adult [Chop and Robnett 1999]. According to the Administration on Aging, by 2030 (when the baby boomer generation reaches 65) the older adult population will double and represent 20% of the total population [DHHS 2003]. Although most older adults live independently, approximately 4.5% reside in nursing home facilities (with the percentage increasing with time).

Regardless of health status, 27.3% of community dwelling older adults and 93.3% of institutionalized Medicare beneficiaries have some limitation in function that prevents them from being fully independent in activities of daily living (ADL) [DHHS 2003]. Thus, approximately 7.2 million individuals aged 65 and older have chronic illnesses and disabilities that require supportive care for ADL [Binstock 2001]. Therapists often provide therapeutic interventions for older adults to improve functional status. Interventions include the design and fabrication of splints. Aging may affect hand dexterity [Lewis 2003], and older adults may benefit from splinting to improve occupational performance.

Note: This chapter includes content from previous contributions from Serena M. Berger, MA, OTR; Maureen T. Cavanaugh, MS, OTR; and Brenda M. Coppard, PhD, OTR/L.

Box 15-1 General Hints for Splinting Older Adults in Any Setting

- Label splints with person's name, right or left hand or foot, and additional landmarks that will help the splint to be positioned properly.
- Monitor for discharge plans to best prepare splinting instructions for the discharge setting.
- When the splint is not scheduled to be worn, it should be stored in the same place and kept within easy reach of someone with restricted mobility.
- Provide clear caregiver education on wear and care of splint, including precautions.
- Keep the splint design simple for easy donning and doffing; include attached straps.
- Follow privacy regulations and avoid public posting of information related to client's care.

Fundamental principles of evaluation, design, and fabrication of splints do not change as people age. Therapists do, however, need to be aware of special considerations necessary to accommodate unique needs of the older adult. When designing a splint for an older adult, the therapist should consider the special needs of the older adult, the goal of the splint, and the splinting supplies available. A splint for an older adult should (1) prevent undesirable motion while permitting normal motion, (2) provide adequate stability, (3) decrease energy expenditure when worn, (4) provide safe distribution of force, (5) be comfortable, (6) be applied and removed easily, (7) be economical, (8) be durable, (9) be easily modified [Good and Supan 1992], and (10) be easily cleaned.

Influence of Different Treatment Settings on Splint Design

The older adult's environment is also an important consideration for clinical decision making. Therapists treat older adults in multiple settings. Box 15-1 provides a summary of considerations for the design of splints for individuals in any treatment setting. Table 15-1 presents specific considerations for different settings. The older adult's living situation (e.g., independence in a community versus dependence in a long-term care setting) is important when the therapist determines the most appropriate splint. For example, an 80-year-old woman with osteoarthritis who performs her own self-care and requires the use of her hands throughout the day may benefit from a thumb carpometacarpal (CMC) immobilization splint to improve her daily function.

In contrast, a long-term care resident who has had multiple cerebrovascular accidents (CVAs) may require splints to maintain sufficient range of motion (ROM) to be dressed and bathed. Hand ROM is necessary to prevent skin maceration in the palm caused by sustained full-finger flexion. Therapists who treat older adults during the acute stage of an illness must be aware of risk factors toward preventing secondary complications such as loss of passive ROM, edema, and skin breakdown.

Table 15-1 Splint Design for Older Adults in Different Treatment Settings

TREATMENT SETTING	SPECIAL CONSIDERATIONS
Acute intensive care unit (ICU)	• Prevent secondary complications such as loss of passive range of motive and compromised skin integrity.
Subacute inpatient rehabilitation	• Awareness of potential risk factors, such as contractures, is important to determine appropriate early intervention to decrease the need for corrective splinting later in the recovery process. • Forward information related to the splint to the site where the client is being discharged.
Assisted living long-term care outpatient therapy	• Provide pictures and carefully written instructions discretely in the older adult's room or in the medical record to encourage follow-through with the splint program. • Provide pictures and carefully written instructions for home programs because outpatients may receive a great deal of new information in one session. • Provide a phone number where the older adult can ask questions between sessions. • Educate the older adult not to make own splint adjustments.
Home health	• Home-bound clients may have old splints in need of repair or replacement. • Provide clear education on splint wear and care. • Educate the older adult not to make own splint adjustments.
Geropsychiatry units	• Follow safety precautions such as keeping away toxic materials that older adults with cognitive problems may put in their own mouths or chew. • Follow safety precautions so that splints may not be used as weapons or cause physical harm to the client, another resident, or staff.

Age-Related Changes, Medical Conditions, and Splint Provision

Older adults' body systems are vulnerable to chronic medical conditions. For instance, someone who has been referred for a hand splint following a CVA may have other conditions prevalent with aging, such as diabetes and osteoarthritis. In addition to obtaining a thorough medical history to determine the appropriate goals for a splint, the therapist needs to be familiar with how different medical conditions concurrently affect hand function.

Table 15-2 provides a summary of age-related changes and medical conditions that affect the design and approach to splinting. The following client factors [AOTA 2002] are based on selected classifications from the World Health Organization's *International Classification of Functioning, Disability and Health* (ICF) [WHO 2001] as they relate to considerations for splinting older adults.

Mental Functions (Cognition)

The therapist assesses the cognitive status to determine the older adult's ability to follow a splint-wearing schedule and to be aware of splint problems. Working memory impairment may prevent the older adult from recalling the splint's storage location or application procedure. Sometimes a therapist can ascertain memory problems by noting how an older adult follows directions during splint fabrication. If memory is a problem, the therapist establishes a routine schedule for splint wear and care, fabricates a simple splint, and labels the splint for easy application.

If the older adult has significant cognitive impairments, the therapist recommends assistance. The therapist must educate any new caregiver about the splint's purpose, wearing schedule, care, correct application, and possible problems. Individuals with later-stage dementias often posture in flexed positions and thus the caregiver may require recommendations to maintain skin integrity. If there are cognitive

Table 15-2 Summary of Age-related Changes and Medical Conditions Impacting Splint Design or Provision

BODY FUNCTIONS AND AGE-RELATED CHANGES	DIAGNOSTIC CATEGORY	COMMON SPLINTS	SPLINTING HINTS
Mental Functions			
Cognition	Cognitive impairment	Splints to prevent contractures secondary to loss of mobility if bedridden or deconditioned	Recommend caregiver assistance. Consider alternative positioning options. Evaluate person's ability to understand the splint's purpose, schedule, and precautions. Establish routine schedules.
Sensory Functions			
Visual	Presbyopia, macular degeneration, cataracts, glaucoma		Use compensation techniques to find splint, such as visual scanning. Use simple, large-print instructions. Be sure the print is in high contrast to the color of the paper. Practice splint application and removal. Use magnification devices for reading instructions and performing skin inspections. Use contrasting colors for the splint and the straps.
Auditory	Loss of hearing (presbycusis)		Use the guidelines for talking to the hearing impaired (Box 15-2). Share guidelines for talking to the hearing impaired with appropriate staff, family, and caregivers.
Touch	Decreased sensibility		Perform visual skin checks, or if vision is also impaired, instruct a caregiver. Consider if a soft splint or padding will be an appropriate alternative to a rigid splint.

Table 15-2 Summary of Age-Related Changes and Medical Conditions Impacting Splint Design or Provision—cont'd

BODY FUNCTIONS AND AGE-RELATED CHANGES	DIAGNOSTIC CATEGORY	COMMON SPLINTS	SPLINTING HINTS
Pain	Variable etiologies	Resting or functional position of involved joints	Because pain tolerance may vary, an adjustable splint or adjustable straps may enable the older adult to control comfort levels.
Neuro-musculoskeletal Functions			
Skeletal (decreased bone mass and joint degeneration)	**Osteoporosis:**		
	• Wrist fractures	Wrist splints	Pre-pad bony prominences.
	Osteoarthritis:		
	• Heberden's and Bouchard's nodes	Distal interphalangeal immobilizaton splint	Make sure splint is easily donned and doffed.
	• Thumb trapeziometacarpal osteoarthritis	Hand-based thumb carpometacarpal splint	Use lightweight thermoplastic material.
General mobility			Keep the splint within reach or easy walking distance. Maintain a consistent storage location for the splint. Keep the splint simple so that the older adult can easily apply and remove it. Permanently attach one end of each strap to the splint to prevent the straps from falling to the floor. Use D-ring straps.
Neurologic			
Nervous system	**Parkinson's disease (tremors):**		
	• Idiopathic essential tremors	Use splint as a base to stabilize activities of daily living devices	
	• Cerebrovascular accident contracture risks	Hand immobilization splints, antispasticity splints and footdrop splints (see Chapter 17)	Instruct the person and caregiver about inhibition techniques that that assist in splint application.
	Peripheral compression neuropathies:		Provide instruction on proper positioning and ergonomics to prevent nerve compression.
	• Carpal tunnel	Wrist splint	
	• Cubital tunnel	Elbow splint or elbow padding	
Cardiovascular and Hematological Functions			
	Arteriosclerosis:		
	• Lower extremity amputations	Foot-drop splint, knee extension splint	Use stockinette because older adults may be less able to dissipate heat. Consider a design to float the heels.
Digestive, Metabolic, and Endocrine Functions			
	Diabetes:		
Decreased hormonal stimulation	• Peripheral neuropathies	Thumb opposition splint (median), metacarpophalangeal block splint (ulnar)	Frequent visual inspection of skin.

Continued

Table 15-2 Summary of Age-Related Changes and Medical Conditions Impacting Splint Design or Provision—cont'd

BODY FUNCTIONS AND AGE-RELATED CHANGES	DIAGNOSTIC CATEGORY	COMMON SPLINTS	SPLINTING HINTS
	• Carpal tunnel syndrome	Wrist splint	
	• Trigger finger	Finger MP flexion restriction	
	• de Quervain's disease	Long opponens thumb immobilization splint	
	• Palmar fascia contractures	Hand immobilization splint	
	• Lower extremity amputation	Knee extension splint	
	End-stage renal disease:		
	• Forearm AV fistula for hemodialysis	Wrist splint or splints for peripheral neuropathies	Splints should be used selectively because any source of pressure could cause skin breakdown in an insensate hand with compromised vascularity. Straps must be easily adjusted to avoid constriction with fluctuations in edema.
Genitourinary Functions			Provide instructions on safe removal and splint use at night if older adults frequent the bathroom.
Skin Functions			
Thinning of dermis and epidermis	**Fragile skin:** • Burn and skin tear risks, delayed wound healing	Soft splint lining	Apply stockinette before molding lightweight thermoplastic material on an older adult.

impairments, or if a caregiver is involved, the risks versus the benefits of a splint must be carefully weighed against alternative positioning (such as the use of pillows or dense foam wedges). In addition, the therapist may consider using D-ring straps for a person with dementia who is constantly trying to remove the splint.

Sensory Functions

Visual System

Of people over age 65, researchers found that 17.2% have some type of visual impairment related to developing functional limitations [Dunlop et al. 2002]. Decreased vision can also play a role in noncompliance of splint wear. For example, some older adults may be unable to apply their splints because of poor figure/ground discrimination. Older adults may also have difficulty seeing straps and Velcro as well as inspecting their skin. Using colored thermoplastic splinting material and contrasting colored straps may assist the older adult who has poor visual discrimination. Bright colors may prevent the splint from being easily lost or mistakenly sent to the laundry.

When receiving splint instructions by demonstration, older adults who have correctable vision should wear their glasses. The older adult demonstrates to the therapist proper splint application and removal. The therapist provides simple large-print instructions. A high contrast of the ink and paper is helpful. The use of magnification devices can also help with reading instructions and with performing skin inspection.

For older adults who have macular degeneration (e.g., blurred or loss of central vision), the therapist encourages the use of compensatory techniques during application and removal of the splint and during skin inspections. Compensatory techniques include eye scanning, head turning, and placement of the splint or hand into the field of vision.

Auditory System

Approximately 25% of older adults between 65 and 74 years of age, 50% of older adults age 75 or older, and 65% of those age 85 and older describe difficulty with hearing [American Federation for Aging Research 2004]. Hearing impairment influences verbal explanations and statements. Sometimes hearing problems can be detected during the initial interview or during splint fabrication. Therapists should not rely solely on printed information to relay instructions because some older adults may be unable to read or have visual impairments that make reading difficult or impossible. The therapist may need to use more tactile cues when positioning the person for splinting. When talking to a person who is hearing impaired, the therapist should use the guidelines outlined in Box 15-2.

Touch

Somatosensory research has demonstrated a decline in two-point discrimination with age [Stevens and Patterson 1995]. Because the decline is gradual over the life span, older adults may not be aware of their diminished sensibility. Because vision is the primary sense used to compensate for decreased tactile sensation, when both sensory functions have declined the older adult is at greater risk for compromised skin integrity.

Tactile sensation may become impaired secondary to poor positioning of older adults with limited mobility. Decreased sensation may contribute to compression neuropathies of the median or ulnar nerves. Cubital tunnel syndrome, a compression of the ulnar nerve at the elbow level, may result from constant pressure on flexed elbows while sitting in a wheelchair or from prolonged bed confinement. A well-padded elbow splint with the elbow flexed 30 to 60 degrees prevents further pressure to the nerve [Clark et al. 1998, Blackmore 2002].

Prefabricated soft elbow pads are another option. Compression of the median nerve at the wrist may be due to prolonged wrist flexion posturing or secondary to an associated medical condition, such as rheumatoid arthritis (RA) or diabetes. A prefabricated wrist splint with D-ring straps is easier to don and can be used to prevent nerve compression (Figure 15-1; and see Chapter 13 for further discussion of these conditions).

Pain

Perception of pain is variable among individuals regardless of age. A visual analog scale and careful history (including assessment of location and particular activities that increase or decrease pain) should be part of the initial evaluation.

Box 15-2 Guidelines for Talking to the Hearing Impaired

- Seat or position the hearing-impaired person to see the face of the person speaking.
- Whenever possible, face the hearing-impaired person on the same level during verbal communication.
- Before talking, gain the older adult's attention by using a touch, a gesture, and eye contact.
- Use visual aids when possible. Take a photograph or draw a diagram that shows correct splint application.
- Use demonstration as part of the instructions.
- Keep hands away from your face while talking.
- If the person misses statements, rephrase the statements rather than repeat the same words.
- Reduce background noises during verbal communication (e.g., turn off television or radio). When possible, work with the person one-on-one in a quiet room.
- Do not shout because doing so distorts voices. Talk in a normal voice but at close range.
- Avoid chewing gum during verbal communication because this makes speech more difficult to understand.
- Be aware that people hear better if they are vertical rather than horizontal. If a person is standing or sitting, sound waves are directed into the ears. If a person is lying on a bed, sound waves are dispersed over the head.
- Recognize that hearing-impaired persons may not hear as well if they are tired or ill.
- If hearing is better in one ear, direct speech toward that ear. Never shout directly into the ear.

Data from Lewis SC (1989). *Older Adult Care in Occupational Therapy*. Thorofare, NJ: Slack. Barlowe E, Siegal DL, Edwards F, Doress PB (1987). Vision, hearing, and other sensory loss associated with aging. In PB Doress, DL Siegal (eds.), *Ourselves, Growing Older*. New York: Simon & Schuster, pp. 365-379. Hills GA (2002). The changing realm of the senses. In BB Lewis (ed.), *Aging: The Health Care Challenge, Fourth Edition*. Philadelphia: F. A. Davis.

Neuro-musculoskeletal Functions

Skeletal System

One of the most impacted body systems affected by age is the skeletal system. Osteoporosis and osteoarthritis (OA) are common diagnoses that often require splinting as part of the intervention process. Osteoporosis is a gradual loss of bone density that begins as young as age 35 [Boughton 1999]. After menopause, the rate of bone loss for women increases [Barzel 2001], and the distal radius is especially vulnerable to fractures [Bostrom 2001]. A common fracture of the distal radius is called a Colles' fracture, which often occurs because of accidental falls [Nordell et al. 2003].

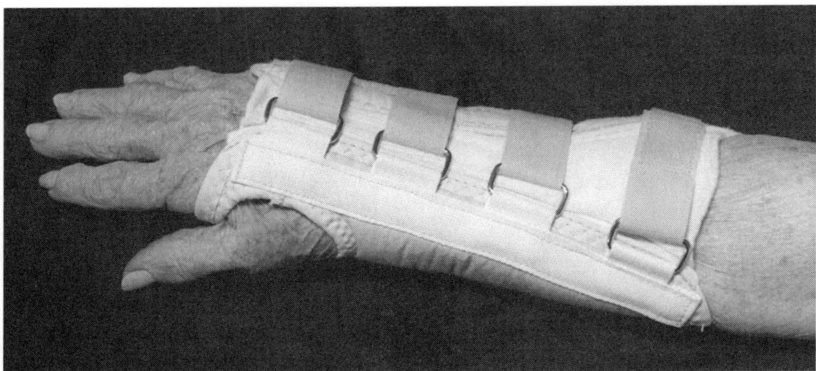

Figure 15-1 The D-ring wrist splint for positioning has a circumferential design that holds the splint in place during application.

Although wrist fractures are usually treated in an outpatient setting, older individuals may at the same time fall and sustain a hip fracture, which initially requires inpatient therapy. Sustaining a Colles' fracture can be associated with functional declines in physical performance in hand strength and walking speed [Nordell et al. 2003]. A volar wrist splint is generally indicated after removal of an arm cast or external fixator for immobilization (see Chapter 7). As the fracture heals, the splint goal may change to one of mobilization (which can be achieved by serial adjustments to improve wrist extension). It is also important to determine if there are other etiologies causing upper extremity impairments. For example, a thorough evaluation for a client referred with a wrist injury may reveal preexisting sensory loss in the digits due to compression of cervical nerve roots caused by OA. The sensory loss might otherwise have only been associated with the wrist fracture.

Another condition that affects the skeletal system is OA. Women are more frequently affected, and the initial onset typically occurs between ages 50 and 60 [Melvin 1989, Rozmaryn 1993, Hellman and Stone 2004]. Primary OA results from idiopathic or known causes. Secondary OA results from congenital joint abnormalities; genetics; infections; and metabolic, endocrine, or neurological disorders [Beers and Berkow 1999]. Most older adults have evidence of some cartilage damage [Bland et al. 2000]. Hand joints are more frequently affected by primary OA [Rozmaryn 1993, Bozentka 2002], which is characterized by enlarged distal interphalangeal (DIP) joints (Heberden's nodes) and enlarged proximal interphalangeal (PIP) joints (Bouchard's nodes). The nodes typically cause more discomfort in the index finger because of the demands placed on the joints during activities that require pinch. An immobilization splint for the DIP joint is a conservative measure to decrease pain (Figure 15-2). Surgical fusion may be warranted for more advanced cases.

OA of the thumb at the CMC joint is another common reason for a splint referral. Initial conservative management usually requires a hand-based thumb immobilization splint (see Chapter 8). Individuals with this condition must be educated in joint protection techniques and instructed with methods to balance activities throughout the day to break the pain cycle. As discussed in Chapter 8, there are different approaches to splinting arthritic hands. The most prevalent approach is to fabricate a removable hand-based splint to immobilize only the CMC joint.

Researchers evaluated the effectiveness of a short opponens splint (only the CMC is immobilized) compared to a long opponens splint (the wrist, CMC, and thumb metacarpophalangeal (MP) are immobilized). Researchers found that 42% of the subjects who wore the short opponens splint reported performance of ADL to be easier. Fifty-one percent of the subjects reported performance of ADL to be the same when wearing the short opponens splint. Some subjects

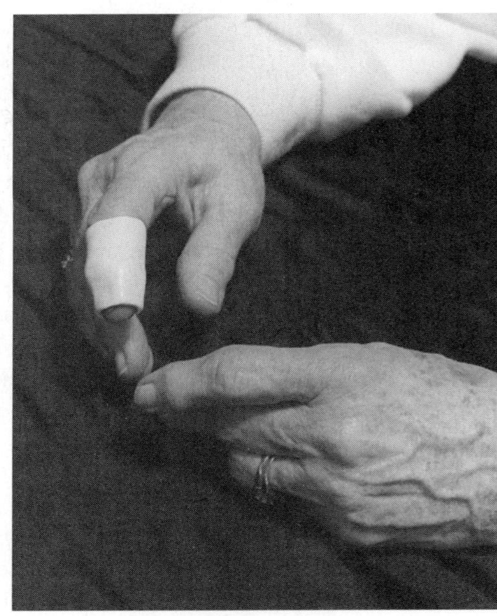

Figure 15-2 Enlarged DIP joints from osteoarthritis may become painful and benefit from immobilization to decrease pain.

(7%) found ADL performance more difficult while using the short opponens splint. Only 16% of subjects who wore the long splint found activities easier to perform [Weiss et al. 2000]. The researchers concluded that splinting is effective for pain reduction and helps to reduce subluxation in the early stages of OA.

Chronic flexion of the thumb MP joint, or an adduction contracture, can lead to a hyperextended interphalangeal (IP) joint. This can be conservatively treated with a figure-of-eight splint to improve stability and function of the thumb (Figure 15-3). If the older adult needs to use a walker and has thumb pain or a weak grip, a prefabricated walker splint can be used to decrease stress to the thumb (Figure 15-4).

OA may also affect the cervical spine and result in sensorimotor deficits in the hand. The therapist checks the older adult's medical history for cervical involvement in order to distinguish peripheral nerve from cervical nerve root compression. In older adults who have multiple medical conditions, the source of decreased sensorimotor function in the hand requires careful medical evaluation.

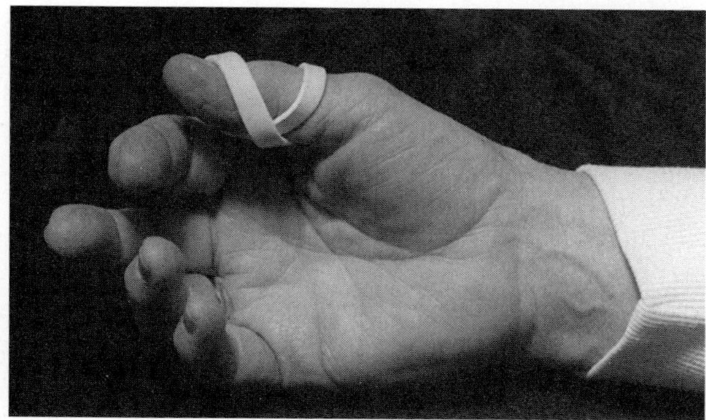

Figure 15-3 A tri-point figure-of-eight design can stabilize the thumb IP joint to prevent hyperextension during pinch.

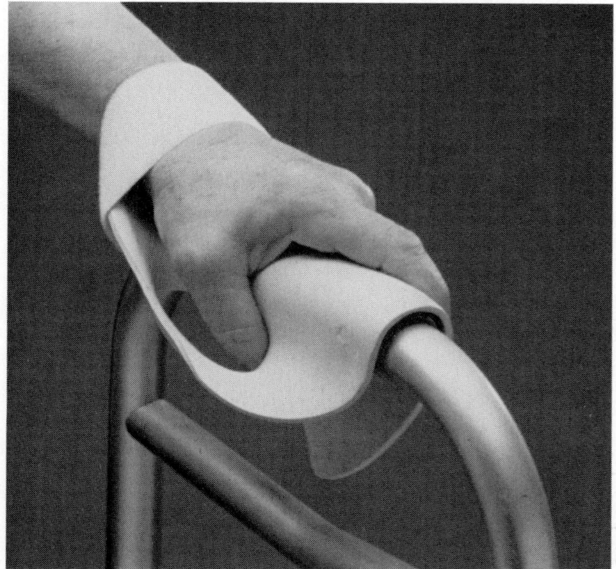

Figure 15-4 Walker splint: a functional splint for persons with limited or painful grasp. (Original design by Beth Beach, OTR.) [From Sammons-Preston Rolyan (2004). *Professional Rehab Catalog*. Bolingbrook, IL.]

Deformities that result from RA may be seen in older adults. However, the most common onset of this systemic condition is in women typically between the ages of 40 and 50 [Pincus 1996]. Mitt splints lined with Plastazote can be helpful for older adults who have residual painful deformities and fragile skin (Figure 15-5). Additional examples of splints for RA are included in the chapters on wrist, hand immobilization, thumb, and mobilization splints.

General Mobility

Many older people become sedentary, which decreases aerobic capacity, muscle strength, ROM, and coordination [Lavizzo-Mourey et al. 1989, Evans 1999]. The therapist should be cautious that splints do not result in unnecessary immobility or loss of engagement in activity. Among persons over age 65 living in the community, 30% fall each year [Gillespie et al. 2004]. Associated injuries include lacerations and bruising; scalds and burns; arm, wrist, hand, and hip fractures; and concussions [Lavizzo-Mourey et al. 1989, Daleiden 1990, Potempa et al. 1990, Carter et al. 2000].

The percentage of falls in institutions is even higher [Gillespie et al. 2004]. The risk for falls increases with age, with one out of two older adults over age 80 experiencing a fall every year [Crane 2002]. If a splint is out of reach, the older adult may not be able to reapply it because of difficulty with ambulation and reach. Maintaining a consistent storage location within reach and easy walking distance is important.

The splint design should be simple. The older adult may be unable to manipulate multiple straps to apply a splint by using one hand. Riveting one end of the strap to the splint or using adhesive straps prevents their removal and loss. Attached straps reduce the risk of the older adult falling while attempting to retrieve a dropped strap.

Neurologic System

Progression of cardiovascular disorders may lead to a CVA resulting in abnormal tone on one side of the body. When making a splint for an older adult with abnormal tone, it may be important to also consider principles involved with splint design related to a coexisting condition such as OA of the thumb CMC joint. In addition, orthokinetic properties of materials should be cautiously selected because they may affect tone (see Chapter 14).

Some neurologic conditions cause tremors. Tremors may be associated with Parkinson's disease, idiopathic essential tremors, or tremors secondary to medication side effects. Splints may be used as a base to hold assistive devices to

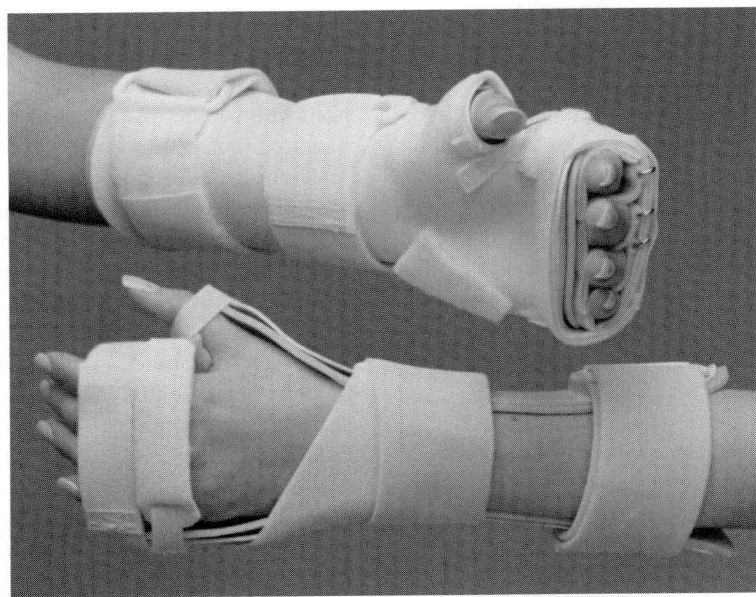

Figure 15-5 Rolyan Arthritis-mitt splint. This splint immobilizes the wrist at 20 degrees extension and 45 degrees of MP flexion, and allows movement of the PIPs. [From Sammons Preston Rolyan (2004). *Professional Rehab Catalog*. Bolingbrook, IL.]

improve self-care function in the presence of tremors. An adaptation may be made to a splint that is required for a coexisting diagnosis. A splint may be made solely to position a self-care utensil, such as a spoon, or to stabilize a pen to write (Figure 15-6).

Cardiovascular and Hematologic Functions

Many older adults who receive therapy have cardiovascular disease, which may be the primary or secondary reason for referral. For someone who has cardiovascular disease, the therapist should educate the older adult to store the splint in close proximity in order to conserve energy. When fitting someone with a lower extremity splint, precautions for peripheral vascular disease should be observed. Another age-related change is a decreased small vessel supply [Saxon and Etten 1994, Bottomley and Lewis 2003].

The temperature of the splint material should be carefully checked, and a double layer of stockinette should be considered instead of applying warm splint material directly to the skin. Older adults who have less ability to dissipate heat are vulnerable to burn or torn skin. If older adults have decreased

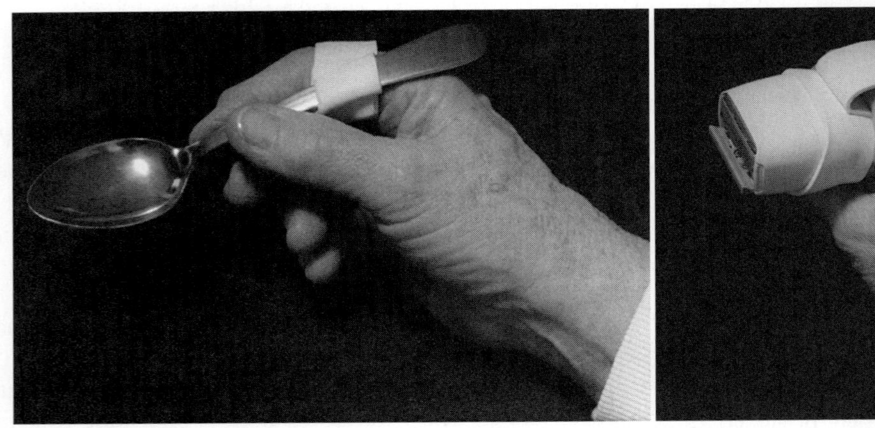

A

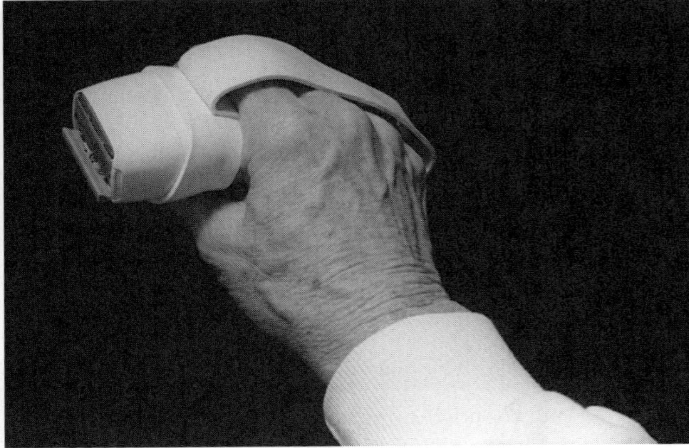

B

Figure 15-6 (A) Example of a hand-based splint used as a base for an ADL device. (B) Example of how splint material can be used to adapt an ADL device.

cognition and thin skin, they may not be aware of the potential for burns. Poor circulation also results in delayed wound healing after skin breakdown.

Digestive, Metabolic, and Endocrine Functions

Digestive System

Dehydration, alcohol abuse, chronic disease, or poor diet in older adults may cause nutritional deficiencies. Sensory testing is carefully completed with individuals who have digestive disorders and nutritional deficiencies, including pernicious anemia, because they may also present with impaired nerve function. Poor wound healing may be the result of a poor nutritional status. The condition of the skin and nails is observed to determine appropriate materials and splint care.

Endocrine System

Diabetes mellitus (DM), a disorder of the endocrine system, is a common secondary diagnosis affecting up to 15.1% of older adults [DHHS 2003]. There are two types of diabetes. Type 1 is insulin-dependent diabetes mellitus (IDDM), with onset before age 30. Type 2 is non-insulin-dependent diabetes mellitus (NIDDM), with onset more typically after age 30 [Beers and Berkow 1999]. Individuals with long-standing diabetes have an increased incidence of other conditions that must be considered before a splint is made.

A careful sensory evaluation will help determine whether there are peripheral neuropathies in the fingers or toes. If sensation is diminished, pressure caused by a splint may not be perceived by the older adult and may lead to skin breakdown. Straps must never cause constriction, especially if there is associated peripheral vascular disease. These considerations are particularly important when someone with diabetes is referred for a foot-drop splint, a knee extension splint after a below-the-knee amputation, or a finger flexion contracture secondary to a CVA.

Individuals with diabetes are at greater risk of associated conditions [Cagliero et al. 2002] that may require splints for the upper extremity [Chammas et al. 1995]. There is an increased incidence of carpal tunnel syndrome in persons who are diabetic. Conservative management includes a wrist immobilization splint with the wrist positioned in neutral. This splint is worn at night. Stenosing tenosynovitis may occur at the first dorsal extensor compartment on the radial aspect of the wrist. This is called de Quervain's tenosynovitis, which is managed with a thumb immobilization splint on the wrist and thumb (see Chapter 8).

Trigger finger is another form of stenosing tenosynovitis that occurs during middle age and that has an increased incidence associated with diabetes. Conservative management may include a splint to restrict MP flexion [Fess et al. 2005] to decrease inflammation in the distal region of the palm near the involved digit. The therapist may decide to (1) custom fabricate a splint (Figure 15-7A), (2) take measurements

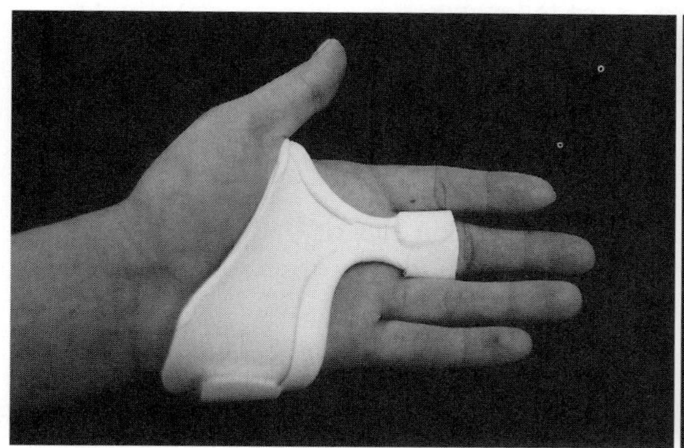

A

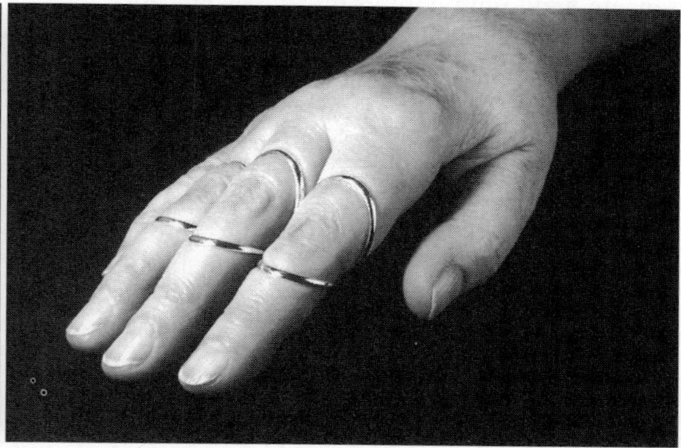

B

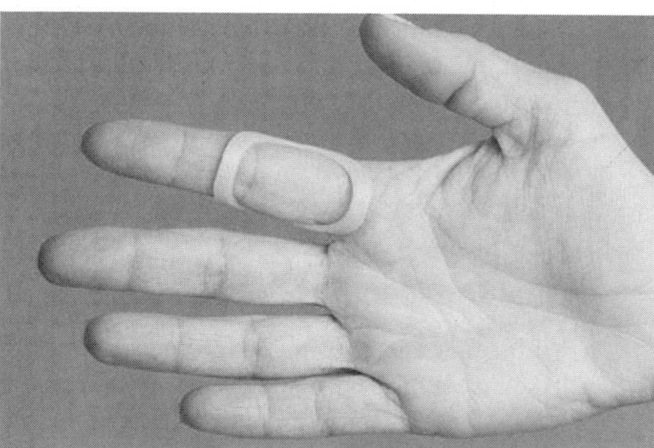

C

Figure 15-7 (A) A splint to restrict MP flexion for trigger finger. [From Fess EE, Gettle K, Philips CA, Janson JR (2005). *Hand and Upper Extremity Splinting: Principles and Methods, Third Edition.* St. Louis: Elsevier/Mosby.] (B) Siris™ Trigger Splint. [Courtesy Silver Ring Splint Company.] (C) Oval-8™ for trigger finger. [Courtesy 3-Point Products, Stevensville, Maryland]

for the purchase of a custom-manufactured silver ring splint (Figure 15-7B), or (3) order a prefabricated splint (Figure 15-7C). Considerations for this decision include the availability of materials, reimbursement source, and client input.

A flexion contracture of the palmar fascia may resemble Dupuytren's disease and is another example of a soft-tissue condition associated with diabetes [Cagliero et al. 2002]. Idiopathic Dupuytren's disease is most common in Caucasian men about 50 years of age with Northern European heritage [McFarlane and MacDermid 2002]. These individuals have limited extension of their fingers or thumbs, with nodules at the palmar base of the involved digits. A splint is not effective in preventing contractures because the contracted tissue of Dupuytren's disease does not respond to low-load prolonged stress. Splinting with a hand immobilization splint to regain extension of the digits is appropriate only after a surgical release of the fascia (see Chapter 9).

Kidneys are part of the urinary system but have an endocrine function. When treating individuals with end-stage renal disease (ESRD), it is important to carefully determine the location of the subcutaneous arteriovenous (AV) fistula (typically on the forearm) used for vascular access for hemodialysis. As a result of the radial artery anastomosis with the cephalic vein [Beers and Berkow 1999], vascularity distal to the AV is compromised and can result in edema and peripheral neuropathies that affect sensorimotor hand function [Liu et al. 2002]. Splints should be used selectively because any source of pressure could cause skin breakdown in an insensate hand with compromised vascularity.

Genitourinary Functions

If an older adult needs to wear a splint during sleep periods, the history should include urinary function. Older individuals often go to the bathroom two to three times per night due to medications such as diuretics, changes in sphincter function in females, or prostate conditions in men. With splint wear during sleep, it is especially important that the splint is easy to don and doff for bathroom hygiene.

Skin Functions

Aging of the integumentary system includes thinning of the epidermis and dermis. Older adults with little subcutaneous fat may be more susceptible to pressure sores. Fragile older adults are more likely to have skin tears. A soft splint or padding to line the splint should be considered.

Medications and Side Effects

Many older adults take medications that cause side effects [Skidmore-Roth 1997] that may affect splint provision. Corticosteroids are commonly prescribed for chronic conditions such as RA and chronic obstructive pulmonary disease (COPD). Long-term steroid use can lead to ecchymosis (bruising), osteoporosis, and thin skin that is vulnerable to skin tears. Long-term steroid use can also lead to delayed wound healing. Anticoagulants, such as heparin, are prescribed for collagen vascular disorders. Their side effects include increased risk of ecchymosis and edema from minor soft-tissue trauma.

Antihistamines for respiratory conditions and psychotrophic medications for depression can cause tremors. When designing a splint for older adults who take these medications, the additional risks of fragile skin, osteoporosis, bruising, edema, or tremors need to be factored into the splint design. In older adults, sleep medications may affect splint wear. For example, the person may not notice problems if the splint becomes uncomfortable during the night, thus increasing the possibility of skin breakdown. In addition, the older adult may be noncompliant with the wearing schedule and wear the splint too long [Knauf 1999].

Purposes of Splints for Older Adults

The splints prescribed for the discussed medical conditions are not unique to older adults. In the older population, however, there is an increase in the effects of chronic health problems. Neurologic and orthopedic problems are also more common in this group [Lewis 2003]. Therapists should obtain client input in order for the splint to maximize desired outcomes, including satisfaction and occupational performance [McKee and Rivard 2004]. The purposes of splinting an older adult may include, but are not limited to, the following:

- Prevent range of motion loss
- Reduce pain
- Improve occupational performance
- Manage contractures
- Decrease edema
- Protect skin integrity
- Substitute for loss of sensorimotor function

Range of Motion

The design of a splint should always allow full ROM of noninvolved joints. Serial mobilization splinting is generally the preferred method to improve decreased ROM for an older adult. A splint that is serially adjusted to improve ROM is easier to manage because the therapist has better control over the amount of force applied. For example, a volar wrist extension mobilization splint after a distal radius fracture may require several progressive adjustments to improve wrist extension [Laseter 2002] (see Chapter 7).

Pain Reduction

With acute and chronic conditions, one goal of splinting is to reduce pain by providing support and rest to the involved joints. For example, for an older adult who has RA the purpose of the splint is primarily to reduce pain by stabilizing the involved joints [Merritt 1987, Ouellette 1991]. The therapist uses different splint designs according to the stage of the arthritis and the joints involved. However, "the use of splints to rest the hands during periods of pain and inflammation is controversial" [Ouellette 1991, p. 68].

Intermittent periods of rest (i.e., three weeks or fewer) appear to be beneficial, but prolonged immobilization for longer periods may cause loss of ROM [Ouellette 1991]. In addition to the design of the splint to rest specific joints, the wearing schedule can provide the appropriate balance between rest and activity. The hand-based thumb immobilization splint worn for CMC osteoarthritis is an example of a splint removed periodically for ROM and reapplied during activities that otherwise cause pain and stress to the joint.

Improvement of Occupational Performance

A splint may improve or maintain an older adult's function. When possible it is preferable to adapt the environment rather than restrict ROM in a hand splint. For example, a figure-of-eight finger splint on a pen allows the older adult to continue writing. Rather than making a wrist splint for use during shaving, the therapist makes adaptations from thermoplastic material on an electric razor to allow an older adult to remain independent (Figure 15-6B). Using hand splints during ADL is extremely awkward when sensory input is impeded [Redford 1986].

Specially adapted splints that help promote function are available. Older adults who have RA may benefit from hand splints that immobilize joints rather than mobilize them. If the wrist is weak, a wrist immobilization splint provides external stability to improve distal finger function. If the functional deficit is due to tremors, as with Parkinson's disease or as a side effect of medications, the elbow can be stabilized on a table surface. Modification of an ADL device to decrease dexterity requirements can be used in addition to elbow stabilization to improve function.

Contracture Management

Loss of mobility and neurologic conditions place an older adult at increased risk of developing contractures [Portnoi and Ramzel 2001]. Changes in the older adult's connective tissue and cartilage increase the risk of contractures, especially during inactivity [Portnoi and Ramzel 2001]. Goals may be to prevent further contracture, decrease pain, or enable better skin care. It is important to weigh the risks of a splint that causes additional complications, such as contributing to skin breakdown.

If the splint is applied while passive ROM is still within normal limits, it may be possible to prevent a contracture. If the loss of passive ROM is recent, mobilization splinting may improve ROM and correct the contracture. An example is a foot-drop splint to gradually position the ankle at 90 degrees after a loss of active ankle dorsiflexion. In addition, therapists commonly use hand immobilization splints to prevent further deformity when there is a loss of active hand or wrist ROM.

Edema Management

When there is loss of active ROM combined with diminished circulation, edema can lead to secondary shortening of soft tissue. It is important to prevent edema when possible through such techniques as elevation and active ROM. The edematous hand is positioned in a splint to counteract adaptive tissue shortening and residual contractures. The position of deformity caused by edema results in thumb adduction, MP extension, and IP flexion. To prevent this deformity, the wrist is positioned in an intrinsic plus position.

The intrinsic plus position consists of 20 to 30 degrees of extension, the thumb in palmar abduction, and the fingers in MCP flexion with the PIP and DIP joints in extension [Strickland 2005]. Additional adjunctive techniques will be necessary to treat the edema unless active ROM returns. Wearing a pressure garment, such as an Isotoner glove, at the same time as the splint may assist in controlling edema. If the noninvolved side of an older adult also appears edematous, a systemic cause—such as congestive heart failure (CHF)—should be considered, in which case a physician may prescribe diuretic medications to decrease fluid retention.

Protection of Skin Integrity

The combination of impaired cardiovascular function and changes associated with aging, such as diminished sensation and thinning of the dermis and epidermis, creates the risk for loss of skin integrity. The heel is the most vulnerable area for skin breakdown in the lower extremity. Use of a foam positioning splint or foot-drop splint with the heel elevated from the splint surface may prevent pressure sores from developing on the heel. Older adults who hold their hands in a fist position or continually flex their elbows, knees, and hips also create an environment conducive to skin breakdown.

The accumulation of perspiration within the skin folds allows bacteria to grow [Redford 2000]. This constant posturing and the resulting bacteria growth may cause joint contractures, skin maceration, and possible infection. A splint made of molded thermoplastic, a hand roll, or a palm protector positions the involved joints in submaximum extension (allowing adequate hygiene of the hand). To accomplish any of these goals, the therapist obeys the following rules:

- A splint should not impede function unnecessarily. For example, the splint should not prevent an older adult from safely grasping an ambulation device or interfere with wheelchair propulsion.
- A splint should not exacerbate a preexisting condition. For example, an older adult who demonstrates a flexor-synergy pattern may wear a functional position splint at night for pain and contracture management. The older adult may also have CMC OA in the thumb. The functional position splint should therefore place the

thumb MP and IP joints in extension and the CMC joint in 45 degrees of abduction, midway between radial and palmar abduction. This thumb position differs from that of functional position splints in which the thumb is placed in palmar abduction and opposition to the pads of the index and middle fingers. This midway position may provide more comfort to the thumb CMC joint than palmar abduction [Mallick 1985].

- A splint should not limit the use of uninvolved joints. An example is the arthritis mitt (see Figure 15-5) splint, which immobilizes the wrist in 20 degrees of extension and the MCP joints in 45 degrees of flexion but allows movement at the PIP joints. When wearing these bilateral splints, older adults are able to complete tasks such as pulling up blankets, ringing doorbells, and holding glasses of water.

Substitution for Loss of Sensorimotor Function

When there is a nerve compression severe enough to cause loss of motor function, a splint may substitute for the lost function. In the case of median nerve compression, a splint may need to position the thumb in opposition to the index finger. If the ulnar nerve is affected, the fourth and fifth MCP joints need to be blocked in slight flexion to prevent a claw deformity with MCP hyperextension and IP flexion of the fourth and fifth digits [Fess et al. 2005]. (See Chapter 13 for more information on splinting for nerve conditions.) In the case of damage to the peroneal nerve, an ankle-foot orthosis can substitute for the loss of ankle dorsiflexion. (See Chapter 17 for more information on lower extremity splinting.)

Splinting Process for an Older Adult

Evaluation for an Older Adult

As with any person, the therapist completes a comprehensive rehabilitative assessment to determine whether splinting is indicated. All components of a therapy evaluation are essential for determining an effective treatment plan. (See Chapter 5 for a discussion of a hand examination.) The therapist pays special attention to the cognitive, sensory, physical, and ADL status of the older adult to determine the usefulness of splinting as part of the treatment plan. The results of the evaluation are used to develop a list of problems to be addressed by the treatment plan. Typical goals include those listed in the section "Purposes of Splints for Older Adults." The therapist documents functional goals in the treatment plan. Additional problems associated with aging (such as decreased visual discrimination, decreased cognition, and hearing impairments) are considered when providing splint instructions for the older adult or caregiver.

During the initial evaluation, the therapist notes any current use of adaptive devices and techniques. For example, an older adult may already have a splint for a chronic condition such as RA. The therapist evaluates the splint for its functional purpose, proper fit, and wearing schedule.

Observation during the assessment is vital to determine the purpose and to select the design of the splint. It is important to observe and assess movement of the extremities in relation to the trunk. For example, an older adult who has hemiplegia with a spastic upper extremity may be wearing a hand splint that is resting on the chest and causing pressure.

Material Selection, Instruction, and Follow-up Care

The choice of thermoplastic splinting material, straps, and padding varies and is based on the older adult's needs. For instruction and follow-up care, many factors influence the older adult's needs, including the following:

- Home, long-term care, hospital settings, assisted-living facilities, subacute, hospice, or adult day care
- Severity of contractures: mild, moderate, or severe
- Skin integrity: fragile skin, open wounds, or pressure areas
- Level of care: home health aid assistance, full- or part-time family or caregiver assistance, or independent functioning
- Other impairments: cognitive or sensory impairments

Environment

Older adults may reside in a variety of settings, including homes, condominiums, apartments, independent-living facilities, or assisted-living facilities. Other older adults may live permanently or temporarily in hospitals or in assisted-living or other long-term care facilities. The older adult's environment affects the selection of strapping and thermoplastic splinting material properties and follow-through. For example, persons responsible for their own splint follow-through receive complete instructions. For older adults in institutional settings, the therapist provides instructions to all caregivers responsible for the older adult's care.

Contracture Risk

The level of joint contracture risk affects the splint-wearing schedule. For example, an older adult with spasticity has a high risk of joint contractures and may frequently wear a splint. Older adults who have a low contracture risk with increasing active ROM may decrease wearing time, thus allowing the affected hand to engage in activities. The therapist uses clinical judgment to determine wearing schedules and completes frequent monitors to adjust wearing schedules according to the older adult's needs.

Skin Integrity

Skin integrity can influence the choice of splint materials. For example, the therapist uses soft, longer, and wider strapping for an older adult who experiences edema fluctuations. The therapist uses a splint made of soft material for a person who has fragile skin. In addition, the therapist may apply polypropylene stockinette under a splint to absorb perspiration because this type of stockinette material is more effective than cotton at wicking the moisture away from the skin.

Level of Care and Impairments

Anticipated older adult and caregiver compliance affects material choice and splint design. For example, the therapist uses a simple splint design for an older adult receiving care from various health care providers in a long-term care facility. The therapist uses a brightly colored thermoplastic material that has contrasting colored straps for an older adult who has difficulty with figure/ground discrimination. Older adults who have hearing loss need written directions. These approaches increase compliance with and tolerance of the splint-wearing schedule.

Selection of Splinting Materials

Depending on client considerations and the goal(s) of the splint, the optimal material may be rigid thermoplastic, lightweight, multiperforated, less rigid thermoplastic, or soft fabrics and foams. Selection of a low-temperature thermoplastic splinting material is determined by the following: (1) the extent to which an older adult's joint can assume and maintain a gravity-assisted position, (2) the size of the splint, (3) the performance requirements of the splint, (4) the padding requirements, (5) the weight of the splinting material, and (6) the therapist's skill level.

If the older adult is physically and cognitively able to hold the limb in the desired splinting position, the therapist uses a splinting material with high drapability and moldability to ensure an intimate fit. The therapist positions the older adult's extremity to ensure that gravity assists in the draping of the material over the extremity. Splinting material with a high degree of conformability allows detailed molding for a precise fit, thus increasing comfort and decreasing the risk of splint migration and friction over bony prominences.

Some older adults cannot assume positions that allow gravity to assist in the molding of splints. Older adults may be anxious and may respond to the stretch applied during splinting by exhibiting increased tone. In such situations, or during the fabrication of large splints, material with resistance to drape and memory is helpful. A material that lightly sticks to stockinette placed on the older adult facilitates antigravity splinting (see Chapter 3). Preshaping techniques are also helpful when splinting an older adult with diminished cognition or abnormal tone.

Thinner thermoplastic materials (e.g., $\frac{3}{32}$-inch, $\frac{1}{16}$-inch) are less rigid. The therapist should select the thinnest material that can perform effectively. Minimizing the weight of a splint increases comfort and enhances compliance (Figure 15-8). The more contoured the splint is to the underlying shape the greater the strength. Older adults usually appreciate lightweight splints. These splints may be perceived to be more comfortable.

Another option is to custom fabricate or purchase a prefabricated soft splint. Prefabricated splints may be made of soft material or foams such as Plastzote. An older adult's hand may be adequately positioned by sewing a soft splint with materials such as neoprene or Velfoam (Figure 15-9).

Strapping Material

Wide, soft, foam-like strapping material distributes pressure over more surface area than thin, firm straps. The softer strapping accommodates slight fluctuations of edema. In addition, fragile skin tolerates soft straps well. Neoprene or Velfoam materials are good choices for straps. Neoprene and Velfoam straps can be easily cut to the desired width. They can also be fringed to decrease pressure against skin. In order to prolong the durability of soft strapping material, it is beneficial to sew standard Velcro loop over the area where Velcro hook will attach. For older adults who have fragile skin, the therapist designs the Velcro loop strap to completely cover

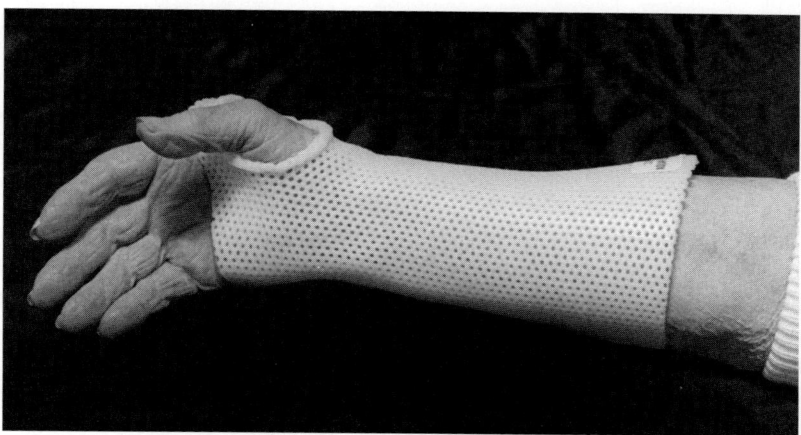

Figure 15-8 A lightweight volar wrist support splint.

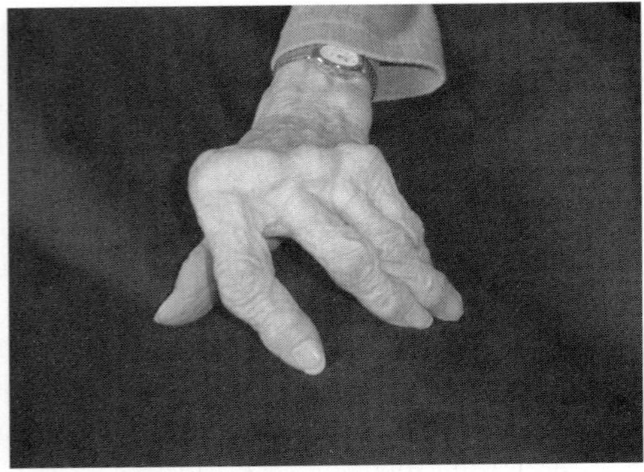

A

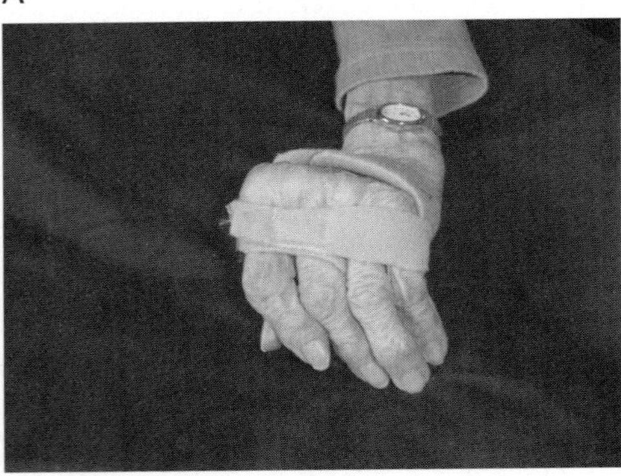

B

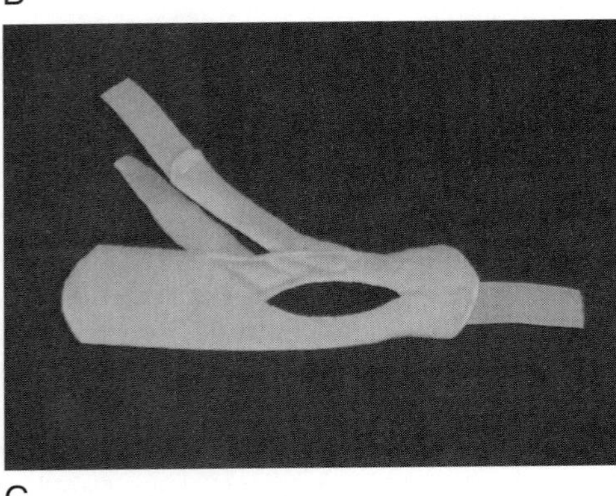

C

Figure 15-9 (A) Ulnar drift of MP joints. (B) A soft splint can provide sufficient positioning to improve occupational performance for ADL. (C) Soft splint pattern.

the Velcro hook on the splint surface. This prevents abrading the older adult's skin or catching the splint on clothing and blankets. The use of pre-sewn self-adhesive Velcro straps reduces the loss of the strap.

There are advantages and disadvantages of using D-ring straps. An advantage is that D-ring straps provide mechanical leverage to effectively tighten the strap. Using D-ring strapping may also be an advantage for an older adult who has dementia and does not understand the splint's purpose, and for similar situations in which the older adult has greater difficulty spontaneously removing the splint. A disadvantage of using these straps is that an older adult who has diminished dexterity may have difficulty threading the strap through the D-ring. However, if the ends of the straps are doubled over or looped the strap will not de-thread through the D-ring.

Padding Selection

The two basic types of padding are open-cell foam (which is absorbent) and closed-cell foam, which is nonabsorbent. Open-cell padding absorbs moisture, is more difficult to keep clean, and can become a breeding ground for bacteria. Before molding, the therapist may apply padding to the thermoplastic splinting material. This ensures a proper fit to accommodate the thickness of the padding.

If the therapist adds padding after the molding process, splint modifications must account for the thickness of the padding. The fabrication of a splint with the addition of 1/16-inch padding results in a splint that is 1/16 inches too tight. Open-cell padding should not be immersed in hot water. When using an open-cell padding (or when using a low-temperature thermoplastic that is pre-padded), the materials can be placed in a resealable plastic bag to keep the padding dry [Sammons-Preston Rolyan 2004].

Closed-cell padding does not hold moisture and is easily washed and towel dried. Plastazote is an example of a foam material available in various thicknesses. The thinner widths can be used to pad a splint, and the thicker widths can be used to fabricate an entire soft splint. Other materials (such as Gel shell pads) can be used if more pressure relief is needed.

Padding may also be required on the outside of a splint. The therapist provides cushioning to the outside of a splint if the splinted extremity rests against another body part. For example, an older adult who has hemiplegia and a flexed upper extremity may rest the splint against the rib cage, or a right ankle splint may press against the left leg when the older adult is side lying.

Choosing the correct thermoplastic, strapping, and padding material is important. Clinical judgment and the ability to make adaptations are important during the splinting of older adults because these clients are most prone to contractures and pressure sores with illness [Bliss and Bennett 2003]. The splint should fit well, achieve the clinical goal, and be acceptable to the older adult and the caregiver.

Technical Tips

Therapists acquire technical skills through practice. During the splinting of an older adult, one or more of the following technical tips may be helpful to the therapist.

- Choose a splinting material that has a slightly longer working time. For example, when fabricating a hand immobilization splint (see Chapter 9), partially pre-shape the hand portion of the resting pan before applying it to the older adult. Complete the pre-shaping on a hand of similar size.

- During the molding process, use Theraband or an elastic bandage to temporarily secure the forearm trough. This activity allows attention to be focused on the contouring of the hand and wrist parts of the splint.
- Pre-pad bony prominences by using circular pieces of adhesive-backed foam or gel padding. Mold the splint over the padding. When molding the splint, place the foam or gel pad inside the splint to ensure intimate congruous contact.
- Use tubular stockinette under the splint to maintain skin hygiene and prevent pressure areas. Loss of skin elasticity and adipose tissue make older persons prone to skin breakdown.
- Use uncoated and self-bonding material for splints if darts or tucks are necessary. Therapists often use this type of design for ankle, knee, and elbow splints.
- Use a coated material for thumb immobilization splints. Often the thumb IP joint is enlarged or deformed, thus making application and removal of a closed circumferential splint difficult or impossible. Use of a coated material allows circumferential wrapping around the proximal phalanx of the thumb. After hardening, the overlap on the proximal phalanx pops open. If self-bonding materials are preferred, use a wet paper towel between the overlapping surfaces to prevent bonding.
- During planning of serial repositioning, select a splint material that has memory.
- For an extremely deformed extremity, make the splint pattern on the opposite extremity and reverse it. If the older adult is unable to cooperate, draw the pattern while he or she is sleeping.
- To ease the splint fabrication process when working among multiple settings, therapists should carry splint boxes with all necessary supplies in them [Swedberg 1997].

Older Adult and Caregiver Instructions and Follow-through

Clear client and caregiver instructions and consistent follow-through are of paramount importance in successful splinting. Many factors influence compliance with a splint-wearing schedule. The person responsible for the splint's wearing schedule and care is the older adult or the caregiver. See Box 15-3 for more information on caregiver and client compliance.

Instructions to Caregivers

Older adults unable to care for themselves need caregiver assistance. Caregivers are family members or staff members from an agency or facility. When fitting a splint to an older adult, the therapist must provide thorough instructions to the caregiver. Instructions should include information regarding (1) the splint's purpose, (2) the wearing schedule, (3) the splint's care, and (4) splint precautions. The therapist should inform caregivers about whom to contact if a splint problem occurs. For example, for a client who has fluctuating edema, tone, and passive ROM, the caregiver would be instructed how to adjust the Comfy Wrist/Hand/Finger splint (Figure 15-10).

The therapist gives oral and written instructions to the caregiver and demonstrates any procedure the caregiver is to perform. The therapist asks the caregiver to demonstrate the application of the splint, corrects mistakes the caregiver makes, and asks the caregiver to repeat the demonstration until it is mastered.

The therapist labels parts of the splint for easier application (e.g., right/left, thumb/wrist/forearm). When possible, photographs of proper splint position, a written wearing

Box 15-3 Factors That Influence Compliance with Older Adults and Caregivers

Older Adult Responsible

- Explain the purpose and goals of the splint to the older adult and caregiver.
- Provide simple written and oral instructions.
- Use positive reinforcement for correct follow-through.
- Listen to the older adult's complaints and make splint adjustments as necessary.

Caregiver (Family and Staff) Responsible

- Provide simple written and oral directions.
- Explain the purpose of the splint.
- Demonstrate proper splint application.
- Encourage the caregiver to demonstrate the correct procedure several times.
- Use pictures to demonstrate correct application.
- In an institution, correlate the older adult's splint-wearing schedule with staff work shifts.
- In an institution, ensure that the splint-wearing schedule and hand hygiene are part of the older adult's care plan.
- Educate the caregiver about precautions and the way to contact the therapist to report splint problems.
- Label the splint for easy application.

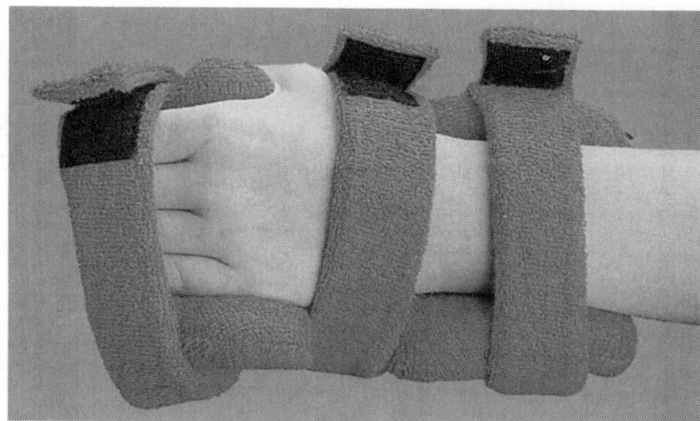

Figure 15-10 Comfy Wrist/Hand/Finger Orthosis is an example of an adjustable prefabricated splint. [Courtesy Sammons Preston Rolyan.]

schedule, a list of precautions, and a splint maintenance sheet should be readily available and consistently updated.

When splinting an older adult in a long-term care facility, the therapist includes instructions in the chart to ensure staff follow-through. In addition, the therapist speaks with the immediate caregivers to determine a realistic splinting program. If an older adult is to wear a splint for a portion of the day, evening, or night shift, all staff members involved with that older adult's care must receive instructions about the splint-wearing schedule and precautions. The splint-wearing schedule may require modification to match the staff schedule.

When appropriate, the therapist instructs caregivers about the use of inhibition techniques to facilitate proper splint application. The therapist also teaches the older adult and caregivers about the importance of intermittent passive ROM and active-assisted ROM to the immobilized joints [Dittmer et al. 1993].

Skin Care

Maintenance of skin integrity is important for older adults who need long-term splinting. The splint must be clean for application. A good cleaning method involves the use of isopropyl alcohol. Chlorine is appropriate for removal of stains. An autoclave cannot be used, and a machine is not appropriate for washing the splint. After removal of the splint, the hand requires thorough washing and drying. Stockinette worn under the splint absorbs perspiration, and powder may be helpful with moisture management.

Wearing Schedule

To determine a splint-wearing schedule, the therapist considers the goals of the splint. The purpose of the splint may be pain reduction during activity, maintenance of functional activities, prevention of skin ulceration, or prevention of a joint contracture. The goal determines whether a daytime, nighttime, or intermittent splint-wearing schedule is most beneficial. For example, an intermittent wearing schedule helps the palm or skin to dry and prevents potential skin maceration. A nighttime-wearing schedule is most appropriate if the older adult uses the extremity for functional assistance during the day.

SELF-QUIZ 15-1*

In regard to the following questions, circle either true (T) or false (F).

1. T F Observing the older adult's skin condition is important when the therapist is making splinting decisions.
2. T F The therapist should apply closed-cell foam after the formation of the splint.
3. T F To ensure intimate contour, the therapist should use a material with high drapability for an older adult who has spasticity.
4. T F The therapist should use wide straps on a splint for an older adult who has fragile skin.
5. T F A functional position splint is always appropriate to position the arthritic hand.
6. T F Older adults are more prone to joint contractures than younger persons who have similar diagnoses.
7. T F After splint completion for an older adult in a long-term care facility, there is little follow-up needed by the therapist.
8. T F A younger person is more prone to skin breakdown than an older adult.
9. T F The therapist may use splinting materials to adapt ADL devices.
10. T F Medication use does not affect splint design.
11. T F It is always important to initially evaluate the entire upper extremity for an older adult with any injury.
12. T F People with diabetes are at greater risk of associated conditions that may require splinting of the upper extremity.
13. T F Poor positioning of older adults with limited mobility may contribute to neuropathies of the median and ulnar nerves.
14. T F When fitting a splint on an older adult with cardiovascular disease, the therapist should consider precautions for peripheral vascular disease.

*See Appendix A for the answer key.

SELF-QUIZ 15-2*

CRITICAL-THINKING CASE SCENARIOS

1. You are fabricating a volar hand immobilization splint for an older adult who is unable to actively supinate the forearm. You choose a material that has high drapability and moldability. Is this the best choice? Why?

2. You are treating an 86-year-old woman one year after a CVA. Since that time she has held her left hand in a fisted position. Gentle passive extension is painful to her. The palm of her hand perspires, and the palmar skin is macerated. She does not have active motion in the left hand and does not use the hand for functional assistance during ADL. Which type(s) of positioning device(s) would be appropriate?

3. An older adult who has RA complains of pain in the wrists and MP joints. The therapist provides hand immobilization splints to rest all of the joints of the wrist and hand at night. What problems can you identify with this splint provision?

4. You fabricate a functional position hand splint for an older adult who has spasticity and hemiplegia and is in a flexor-synergy pattern. The older adult wears the splint at night for pain relief and contracture management. When the older adult is in bed, the splint is positioned against the rib cage. What can you do to relieve the pressure on the rib cage?

5. You have fabricated a hand immobilization splint for an older adult who has hemiplegia and congestive heart failure. You are concerned about the fluctuating edema you have noted in the hemiplegic hand. How would you modify the splint and straps?

*See Appendix A for the answer key

Laboratory Exercise 15-1*

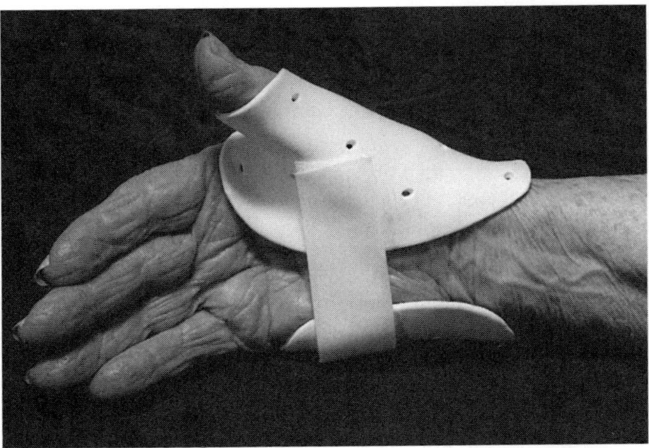

1. What problems are identified in the splint (previous figure) made for someone with thumb CMC OA?

____

____

____

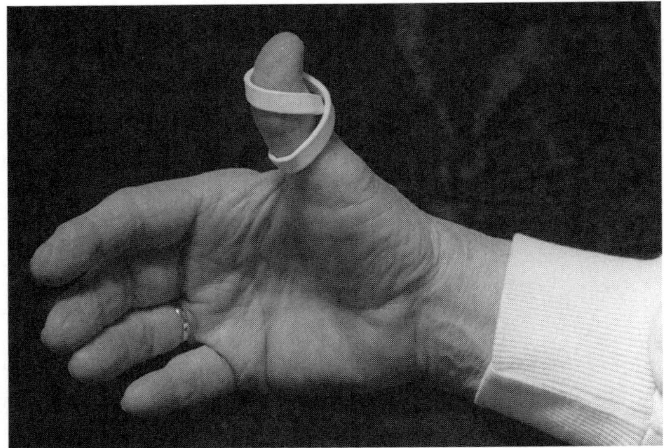

2. How would the splint shown in the figure above be modified for someone with hyperextension of the thumb IP joint?

____

____

____

____

*See Appendix A for the answer key.

CASE STUDY 15-1*

Read the following scenario and answer the questions based on information in this chapter.

Edna is a 90-year-old right-hand-dominant female who lives in an independent unit of a retirement community. She was referred to occupational therapy to be evaluated for a splint and interventions for ADL. She is two years status post a trigger finger release of the right middle finger and has right thumb CMC OA. She no longer experiences triggering of the middle finger. However, she does have some loss of active MCP extension. She reports enjoying painting with watercolors, but finds that she has progressively painted less due to pain in her thumb. Upon observation of self-care performance, due to loss of active MCP extension of the middle finger Edna is noted to use only index-to-thumb opposition for activities that require pinch.

1. The therapist needs to consider which of the following in order to determine the most appropriate splint? Circle all that apply.
   a. Postoperative trigger finger protocols
   b. Biomechanical principals of pinch with OA
   c. Materials for custom splint designs
   d. Prefabricated splints for trigger finger
2. The splint design should incorporate a combination of which of the following? Circle all that apply.
   a. Thumb CMC immobilization
   b. Thumb CMC mobilization
   c. Middle finger MCP extension assist
   d. Middle finger MCP flexion block
3. Goals for the splint should include which of the following? Circle all that apply.
   a. Thumb mobilization
   b. Improved occupational performance
   c. Pain reduction
   d. Substitute for loss of motor function
4. In order to promote occupational performance, which of the following is least significant?
   a. Self-care function
   b. Leisure interests
   c. Location and degree of pain
   d. Age

*See Appendix A for the answer key.

CASE STUDY 15-2*

Read the following scenario and answer the questions based on information in this chapter.

Samuel is a 74-year-old male who lives with his wife in a high-rise apartment building. He was recently discharged from an inpatient rehabilitation facility to his home. He receives home care services that include physical therapy, occupational therapy, and nursing. His referring diagnosis is left CVA with right hemiplegia. Medical history is also significant for CHF, and COPD. His chief complaints are limited endurance and decreased use of his right upper extremity.

Upon evaluation, Samuel presents with bilateral upper extremity tremors, good return of function at the shoulder and elbow, minimal active extension of the wrist, edema in his fingers and on the dorsum of his right hand, and enlarged DIP finger joints. Although he is referred for splinting at this time, he was not fitted with a splint during his inpatient stay because he was showing signs of motor return and was receiving daily treatment to prevent loss of motion.

1. Goals for the splint should include which of the following? Circle all that apply.
   a. Prevent loss of range of motion
   b. Substitute for loss of sensorimotor function
   c. Decrease pain
   d. Decrease edema
2. What splint do you recommend?
   a. Wrist immobilization splint with D-rings
   b. Thumb immobilization splint
   c. Soft neoprene prefabricated splint
   d. Prefabricated Comfy Wrist/Hand/Finger orthosis or similar adjustable prefabricated splint
3. What type of straps would you recommend?
   a. Soft, wide straps that are a little long
   b. Thin Velcro loop straps
   c. D-ring straps cut to the exact size
   d. Wide Velcro hook straps
4. What splint-wearing schedule would you recommend?
   a. Wear splint at all times
   b. Remove splint only for hygiene
   c. Wear splint only during the day
   d. Wear splint at night and periodically during the day to encourage motion
5. What is the most likely cause of the enlarged DIP joints?
   a. Rheumatoid arthritis
   b. Osteoporosis
   c. Osteoarthritis
   d. Peripheral vascular disease

*See Appendix A for the answer key.

REVIEW QUESTIONS

1. What are the accommodations a therapist can make for each of the following problems: edema, ecchymosis, fragile skin, contracture, ulceration, diminished cognition, sensory loss, and motivation?
2. What are four possible goals of splinting an older adult?
3. Why are older adults prone to develop contractures?
4. What are five medical conditions more prevalent in older adults? Describe implications for splinting.
5. What are common medication side effects for three medications commonly prescribed to older adults? Describe how they could affect splinting.
6. How do instructions and selection of splint materials vary with an individual living independently in the community versus an individual in an institution?
7. What are three specific splint adaptations for older adults who have impaired cognition, sensory function, and compliance?

References

Abrams WB, Beers MH, Berkow R (1995). *The Merck Manual of Geriatrics, Second Edition*. West Point, PA: Merck & Co.

American Federation for Aging Research (AFAR) (2004). Prevalence of hearing loss. URL: *http://www.infoaging.org/l-hear-01-loss.html*.

American Occupational Therapy Association (2002). Occupational therapy practice framework: Domain and process. American Journal of Occupational Therapy 56:609-639.

Barzel US (2001). Osteoporosis. In GL Maddox (ed). *The Encyclopedia of Aging, Third Edition*. New York: Springer, pp. 778-780.

Beers MH, Berkow R (1999). *The Merck Manuel of Diagnosis and Therapy, Seventeenth Edition*. Whitehouse Station, NJ: Merck & Co.

Binstock RH (2001). In BR Bonder, MB Wagner (eds.), *Functional Performance in Older Adults, Second Edition*. Philadelphia: F. A. Davis.

Blackmore SM (2002). Therapist's management of ulnar nerve neuropathy at the elbow. In EJ Mackin, AD Callahan, TM Skirven, LH Schneider, AL Osterman (eds.), *Rehabilitation of the Hand and Upper Extremity, Fifth Edition*. St. Louis: Mosby, pp. 679-689.

Bland JH, Melvin JL, Hasson S (2000). Osteoarthritis. In JL Melvin, KM Ferrell (eds.), *Rheumatologic Rehabilitation Series: Adult Rheumatic Diseases*. Bethesda, MD: AOTA.

Bliss MR, Bennett GJ (2003). Pressure sores. In RC Tallis, HM Fillit (eds.), *Brocklehurst's Textbook of Geriatric Medicine and Gerontology, Sixth Edition*. London: Churchill Livingstone, pp. 1347-1366.

Bostrom M (2001). Fractures. In MD Mezey (ed.), *The Encyclopedia of Older Adult Care: The Comprehensive Resource on Geriatric and Social Care*. New York: Springer, pp. 272-276.

Bottomley JM, Lewis CB (2003). *Geriatric Rehabilitation: A Clinical Approach, Second Edition*. Upper Saddle River, NJ: Prentice Hall.

Boughton B (1999). Osteoporosis. In D Olendorf, C Jeryan, K Boyden (eds.), *The Gale Encyclopedia of Medicine*. Farmington Hills, MI: Gale Research, pp. 2116-2120.

Bozentka DJ (2002). Pathogenesis of osteoarthritis. In EJ Mackin, AD Callahan, TM Skirven, LH Schneider, AL Osterman (eds.), *Rehabilitation of the Hand and Upper Extremity, Fifth Edition*. St. Louis: Mosby, pp. 1637-1645.

Cagliero E, Apruzzese W, Perlmutter GS, Nathan DM (2002). Musculoskeletal disorders of the hand and shoulder in clients with diabetes mellitus. American Journal of Medicine 112:487-490.

Carter SE, Campbell EM, Sanson-Fisher RW, Gillespie WJ (2000). Accidents in older people living at home: A community-based study assessing prevalence, type, location and injuries. Australian New Zealand Journal of Public Health 24(6):633-636.

Chammas M, Bousquet P, Renard E, Poirier JL, Jaffiol C, Allieu Y. (1995). Dupuytren's disease, carpal tunnel syndrome, trigger finger, and diabetes mellitus. The Journal of Hand Surgery (Am) 20(1):109-114.

Chop WC, Robnett RH (1999). *Gerontology for the Health Care Professional*. Philadelphia: F. A. Davis.

Clark CL, Wilgis EF, Aiello B, Eckhaus D, Eddington LV (1998). Hand Rehabilitation: A Practical Guide (2nd ed.). New York: Churchill Livingstone.

Crane M (2002). Preventing falls: New strategies for helping all of us stay on our feet as we age. URL: *http://www.infoaging.org/feat19.html*.

Daleiden S (1990). Prevention of falling: Rehabilitative or compensatory interventions? Topics in Geriatric Rehabilitation 5:44-53.

Department of Health and Human Services (DHHS) (2003). Profile of Older Americans. Washington, DC: US Department of Health and Human Services, Administration on Aging. *http://www.aoa.gov/prof/Statistics/profile/2003/2003profile.pdf*.

Dittmer DK, MacArthur-Turner DE, Jones IC (1993). Orthotics in stroke. Physical Medicine and Rehabilitation State of the Art Review 7(1):171.

Dunlop DD, Manheim LM, Sohn MW, Liu X, Chang RW (2002). Incidence of functional limitation in older adults: The impact of gender, race, and chronic conditions. Archives of Physical Medicine & Rehabilitation 83:964-971.

Evans WJ (1999). Exercise, nutrition and healthy aging: Establishing community-based exercise programs. In K Dychtwald (ed.), *Healthy Aging: Challenges and Solutions*. Gaithersburg, MD: Aspen, pp. 347-360.

Fess EE, Gettle K, Philips CA, Janson JR (2005). *Hand and Upper Extremity Splinting: Principles and Methods, Third Edition*. St. Louis: Elsevier/Mosby.

Gillespie LD, Gillespie WJ, Robertson MC, Lamb SE, Cumming RG, Rowe BH (2004). Interventions for preventing falls in older adult people. Cochrane Database Syst Rev 4:CD000342.

Good DC, Supan TJ (1992). Basic principles of orthotics in neurologic disorders. In M Aisen (ed.), *Orthotics in Neurological Rehabilitation*. New York: Demos, pp. 1-23.

Hellmann DB, Stone JH (2004). Arhritis and musculoskeletal disorders. In LM Tierney Jr., SJ McPhee, MA Papadakis (eds.), *Current Medical Diagnosis and Treatment, Forty-third Edition*. New York: Lange Medical Books/McGraw-Hill, pp. 778-832.

Knauf JJ (1999). Drugs commonly encountered in hand therapy. In N Falkenstein, S Weiss-Lessard (eds.), *Hand Rehabilitation: A Quick Reference Guide and Review*. St. Louis: Mosby.

Laseter GF (2002). Therapist's management of distal radius fractures. In EJ Mackin, AD Callahan, TM Skirven, LH Schneider, AL Osterman (eds.), *Rehabilitation of the Hand and Upper Extremity, Fifth Edition*. St. Louis: Mosby, pp. 1136-1155.

Lavizzo-Mourey R, Day SC, Diserens D, Grisso JA (1989). *Practicing Prevention for the Elderly*. St. Louis: Hanley & Belfus/Mosby.

Lewis SC (2003). *Older Adult Care in Occupational Therapy, Second Edition*. Thorofare, NJ: Slack.

Liu W, Lipsitz LA, Montero-Odasso M, Bean J, Kerrigan DC, Collins JJ (2002). Noise-enhanced vibrotactile sensitivity in older adults, clients with stroke, and clients with diabetic neuropathy. Archives of Physical Medicine and Rehabilitation 83:171-176.

McFarlane RM, MacDermid JC (2002). Dupuytren's disease. In EJ Mackin, AD Callahan, TM Skirven, LH Schneider, AL Osterman (eds.), *Rehabilitation of the Hand and Upper Extremity, Fifth Edition*. St. Louis: Mosby, pp. 971-988.

McKee P, Rivard A (2004). Orthoses as enablers of occupation: Client-centered splinting for better outcomes. Canadian Journal of Occupational Therapy 71:306-314.

Melvin JL (1989). *Rheumatic Disease in the Adult and Child: Occupational Therapy and Rehabilitation, Third Edition*. Philadelphia: F. A. Davis.

Merritt JL (1987). Advances in orthotics for the client with rheumatoid arthritis. Journal of Rheumatology 14(15):62-67.

Nordell E, Jarnlo G, Thorngren K (2003). Decrease in physical function after fall-related distal forearm fracture in elderly women. Advances in Physiotherapy 5(4):146-154.

Ouellette EA (1991). The rheumatoid hand: Orthotics as preventative. Seminar in Arthritis and Rheumatism 21:65-71.

Portnoi V, Ramzel P (2001). Contractures. In MD Mezey (ed.), *The Encyclopedia of Older Adult Care: The Comprehensive Resource on Geriatric and Social Care*. New York: Springer, pp. 161-163.

Pincus T (1996). Rheumatoid arthritis. In ST Wegener, BL Belza, EP Gall (eds.), *Clinical Care in the Rheumatic Diseases*. Atlanta: American College of Rheumatology.

Potempa K, Carvalho A, Hahn J, LeSage J (1990). Containing the cost of older adult falls: A risk management model. Topics in Geriatric Rehabilitation 6:69-78.

Redford JB (1986). *Orthotics Etcetera, Third Edition*. Baltimore: Williams & Wilkins.

Redford JB (2000). Orthotics and orthotic devices: General principles. Physical Medicine and Rehabilitation: State of the Art Reviews 14(3):381-394.

Rozmaryn LM (1993). The aging wrist: An orthopedic perspective. In CB Lewis, KA Knortz (eds.), *Orthopedic Assessment and Treatment of the Geriatric Client*. St. Louis: Mosby.

Sammons Preston Rolyan (2004). *Professional Rehab Catalog*. Bolingbrook, IL.

Saxon SV, Etten MJ (1994). *Physical Change and Aging: A Guide for the Helping Professions, Third Edition*. New York: The Tiresias Press.

Skidmore-Roth L (1997). *Mosby's Nursing Drug Reference*. St. Louis: Mosby.

Stevens JC, Patterson MQ (1995). Dimensions of spatial acuity in the touch sense: Changes over the lifespan. Somatosensory and Motor Research 12(1):29-47.

Strickland JW (2005). Biologic basis for hand and upper extremity splinting. In EE Fess, K Gettle, CA Philips, JR Janson (eds.), *Hand and Upper Extremity Splinting: Principles and Methods, Third Edition*. St. Louis: Elsevier/Mosby.

Swedberg L (1997). Splinting the difficult hand. WFOT-Bulletin 35:15-20.

Weiss S, LaStayo P, Mills A, Bramlet D (2000). Prospective analysis of splinting the first carpometacarpal joint: An objective, subjective, and radiographic assessment. Journal of Hand Therapy 13(3): 218-226.

World Health Organization (WHO) (2001). *International Classification of Functioning, Disability, and Health (ICF)*. Geneva, Switzerland: World Health Organization.

CHAPTER 16

Pediatric Splinting

Linda S. Gabriel, PhD, OTR/L

Key Terms

Occupation-based assessment
Client-centered approach
Contracture
Sensory system modulation
Neoprene
Wearing schedules
McKie thumb splint
Serpentine splint

Chapter Objectives

1. Identify the characteristics of children who need orthotic intervention.
2. Explain the impact of upper extremity splinting on the development of childhood occupations.
3. Describe the major features and purposes of a resting hand splint, wrist splints, thumb splints, serpentine splints, and weight-bearing splints.
4. Describe the process for fabricating each of these splints, as well as individual variations.
5. Identify resources for the purchase of prefabricated pediatric splints.
6. Explain precautions for these splints and their variations.
7. Justify an effective and reasonable wearing schedule.
8. Explain how to provide instructions to care providers to maximize correct application and usage of the splints.
9. Judge when a splint is fitting properly and identify and correct errors in the fit of a splint.
10. Examine evidence for splinting children and recommend future areas of needed research.
11. Apply knowledge of splinting children to a case study.

This chapter presents applications of general splinting principles to the selection, design, fabrication, or purchase of several basic hand splints. The splints presented in this chapter should be used as part of a comprehensive treatment program for children with a focus on children with developmental disabilities or congenital anomalies. Like splints for adults, splints for children may be used to prevent deformity, to increase function, or to do both. However, splinting children involves more than just making a smaller splint pattern. The purpose of this chapter is to guide the beginning therapist in applying splinting knowledge to the special needs of children with developmental disabilities or birth defects of a neurologic or orthopedic nature, such as cerebral palsy or arthrogryposis multiplex congenita.

The resting hand, weight-bearing, wrist, thumb, and serpentine splints represent basic designs that are the focus of this chapter. In practice, the therapist should consider modifying these designs or creating entirely new ones to ensure that they meet the needs of an individual child. The therapist may use a single splint for a child or fabricate two splints for a child, which are worn alternately. For example, this alternate schedule is appropriate for children who have some functional use of their hands but are also at risk of developing contractures.

It may not be possible or desirable to accomplish all of the splinting goals with one splint. Attempting to do so may not meet any of the stated goals [Exner 2005]. Children with severe or complex hand problems may require a series of splints that addresses the most pressing needs first or that is serial in nature, with each new splint coming closer to the desired end product.

Before splinting decisions can be made, the therapist must establish overall treatment goals based on a frame of reference appropriate to the child and the environment. The splint, if appropriate, then becomes a component of this treatment program—which also includes goals for improving function and the child's ability to participate in childhood occupations (including play, self-care, and such productive activities as schoolwork). Splint designs in this chapter are compatible with neurodevelopmental treatment, rehabilitative, and/or biomechanical frames of reference. Splinting decisions must also be compatible with the lifestyle, values, and culture of the child and the family—as well as with the child's home, day care, community, and school environments.

Because the purpose of this chapter is to introduce basic concepts to beginning splinters, there are many types and variations of pediatric hand splints that will not be covered. A number of children may respond best to a splint designed to reduce spasticity (see Chapter 14). Children with traumatic injuries or burns can be approached in a manner similar to adults [Hogan and Uditsky 1998], which is described in previous chapters. Other children may benefit from the use of plaster or pneumatic splints for the elbow or hand (see Chapter 14). Some splints are part of interventions in advanced areas of practice, such as the neonatal intensive care unit. These complex or specialized splints are beyond the scope of this chapter. Readers are encouraged to read articles cited in the references at the end of this chapter for more information. Those who desire additional skills in these areas should explore continuing education courses or arrange for advanced study.

The previous chapters have described basic splinting principles, designs, and fabrication techniques that need not be repeated here. However, examples and applications in previous chapters focused primarily on adults. Successfully splinting a child is different from splinting an adult in many respects, including the following:

- Abnormal muscle tone has been present since birth or infancy and may differ qualitatively from abnormal muscle tone acquired after disease or injury.
- The child experiences the dynamic process of maturational and neurologic development, which has a continuous effect on the acquisition of functional hand skills. It is also important to realize that because of the plasticity and immaturity of the child's systems inappropriate splints can result in harmful effects [Granhaug 2006].
- Muscles and tendons undergoing growth respond differently to stretch [Wilton 2003].
- Children experience continued growth of the upper extremities. As children grow, splints fit tighter and create pressure. During a growth spurt, the risk of deformity or skin breakdown may increase as a result of bone growth that exceeds growth or lengthening of muscles and soft tissues because of spasticity. Deformity may also occur secondary to a splint that has been outgrown and no longer fits properly.
- Many children must rely on adults, such as parents or teachers, to apply and remove their splints. Therefore, the level of understanding and cooperation of these adults is a factor.
- Children have a low tolerance for interference by adults and the imposition of a piece of equipment (splint) unfamiliar to them. Their cognitive level may be insufficient for them to understand abstract concepts such as prevention or to comprehend cause-and-effect relationships (*if* you wear this splint, *then* your hand will work better). They may resist holding still, become fearful and cry, or be able to cooperate only for brief periods of time because of a short attention span. Any or all of these factors may create greater challenges to the fabrication and application of the splint(s) for children. In addition, as the child asserts his or her autonomy, a power struggle may develop with adults and the child may resist donning or removal of the splint at home or school.
- The placement and molding of a splint on a child is more difficult than on an adult because the child's hand is much smaller in proportion to the therapist's hand.

Diagnostic Indications

The focus of this chapter is on splinting the child with a developmental disability or congenital anomaly. However, many of the principles and splints described also apply to adults with developmental disabilities. According to the Centers for Disease Control and Prevention (CDC), developmental disabilities are a diverse group of chronic conditions that result from a mental and/or physical impairment and interfere with major life activities [CDC 2006]. Many developmental disabilities, such as cerebral palsy, are accompanied by central nervous system dysfunction and abnormal muscle tone.

Central nervous system dysfunction can be the result of many types of brain injury, such as an intracranial hemorrhage, hypoxia, infections, tumors, or trauma. Abnormal muscle tone can include increased, decreased, or fluctuating tone and presents a number of splinting challenges. Lower motor neuron dysfunction may also occur at birth as the result of excessive stretch to the brachial plexus during delivery. Depending on the nature and extent of the nerve damage, this may result in developmental arm and hand dysfunction.

Other diagnoses in children for which splinting may be indicated include brachial plexus injury or congenital defects or anomalies of the hand or upper extremity, which are generally due to malformations of the musculoskeletal system. Malformations include finger flexion contractures, soft-tissue or bony fusion (syndactyly), and dysplasia of the ulna or radius. Children with brachial plexus injury (Erb's palsy) may require splinting or casting of the hand and the entire upper extremity, especially after surgery. Another congenital or birth defect that may require orthotic intervention is arthrogryposis multiplex congenita.

According to Banker, "Arthrogryposis multiplex congenita is not a specific disorder but rather a symptom complex of congenital joint contractures associated with both neurogenic and myopathic disorders....The main feature shared by these disorders appears to be the presence of severe weakness early in fetal development, which immobilizes joints, resulting in contractures" [Banker 1985, p. 30]. Programs that involve early passive stretching and serial splinting of contracted joints are recommended [Bayne 1986, Donohoe 2006, Palmer et al. 1985, Sala et al. 1996, Williams 1985]. Splints, such as a dynamic elbow flexion splint, have also been developed to compensate for lost muscle power [Kamil and Correia 1990].

Children with developmental disabilities or congenital anomalies often present with indwelling thumbs (thumbs held adducted into the palm). This may be the result of abnormal muscle tone, weakness, or abnormal anatomy of the hand. To effectively grasp and manipulate objects, it is crucial that the thumb be positioned in opposition. Splinting, along with active movement, is often required to effectively position the thumb in opposition for grasp and optimal hand function.

Juvenile rheumatoid arthritis (JRA) is a systemic rheumatic disease that causes major disabilities in children younger than 16 years. Children with JRA may present with pain, fatigue, and reduced range of motion (ROM). These symptoms often result in difficulty performing school tasks and activities of daily living. In addition to medical management and interventions to promote participation, treatment for JRA may include splinting and passive and active ranging of the joints [Rogers 2005]. In summary, a number of pediatric diagnoses may indicate a need for splinting. However, rather than strictly on a specific diagnosis the final splinting decision is made on the basis of the limitations in specific movements, the type and severity of abnormal muscle tone, the extent of soft-tissue and bony involvement, the child's functional level, the child's environment, and the frame of reference guiding therapy.

Assessment

Before fabricating a splint, the therapist must complete a comprehensive assessment. According to the American Occupational Therapy Association (AOTA) Occupational Therapy Performance Framework, the therapist should consider performance in areas of occupation first and then evaluate performance skills, performance patterns, context, activity demands, and client factors [AOTA 2002]. This chapter discusses areas of assessment in the categories of areas of occupation, client factors, performance skills, and context.

Areas of Occupation

Clinical observation of the child participating in his or her occupations, and/or an occupation-based assessment, is necessary to determine the overall direction of the intervention program—and more specifically whether and how a splint will contribute to that intervention program. Each child and family attaches meaning to different occupations, and it is participation in these valued occupations that ultimately determines the success of the intervention program.

When considering a splint, it is essential that the therapist consider the child's strengths and level of participation as well as musculoskeletal problems. Although the child may use an "abnormal pattern," this pattern may afford the child his or her only opportunity for participation in valued occupations. It may be necessary for a temporary loss of function in the short term in order to gain increased function in the long term. However, careful thought should be given to splinting choices before deciding on an option that will take away a child's ability to function in favor of "fixing" the problem. As Armstrong [2005, p. 481] stated, "Is an important action being taken away to gain something else? Which is more important?"

The decision about whether to splint, and what type of splint should be made, should be client centered—and the assessments used to determine the effectiveness of the splint should also be client centered [McKee 2004]. According to McKee, "An occupation-based approach ensures that the central therapeutic aim for splinting remains that of enabling either current or future occupation rather than the mere provision of a splint" [McKee 2004, p. 307].

Client Factors

Muscle Tone

The quality and distribution of muscle tone should be assessed at rest and during functional activity. The therapist should also determine whether the amount of tone varies according to the child's mood, physical health, amount of effort exerted, or state of alertness. Some children have greatly increased tone during active movement but minimally increased tone during rest or while asleep. If the child's muscle tone is not significantly increased at night, there may be no need for a night splint [Exner 2005]. Children with decreased tone may need a splint to stabilize or support joints. Children who are severely hypotonic and lack active movement may need splints to offset the constant pull of gravity that could lead to contractures.

Range of Motion

The therapist should measure both active and passive ROM and compare measurements with those taken previously to determine whether range is increasing, decreasing, or remaining the same. Before moving the joint, the therapist must be sure that the child is well positioned and is as relaxed as possible. The therapist should look for compensatory patterns the child may use to fixate or stabilize specific joints, because this will affect available joint range.

It may also be helpful to prepare the child's musculoskeletal system for movement before taking measurements. Because muscle tone and sometimes cooperation vary, it may be necessary to take measurements on several occasions to get the most accurate estimate. Goniometric measurements are more reliable when taken by the same therapist. Even so, measurement error can occur. The therapist should describe the child's position and the position of adjacent joints when measuring ROM to increase the likelihood that subsequent measurements are taken in the same manner.

Contractures

The therapist should discriminate between types of joint end feel. When tightness at a joint is primarily the result of muscle and soft-tissue shortening, with full passive range still possible with effort, this effect is known as soft end feel. When the joint cannot be moved to the end of passive range, it is said to have a hard end feel. The latter, where full passive range cannot be obtained, is known as a contracture [Hogan and Uditsky 1998, Yamamoto 1993].

A limb with a contracture is also said to have a deformity. One has only to tour a program, school, institution, or group home for individuals with developmental disabilities (especially those with more severe disabilities) to see multiple cases of contractures that restrict functional use of the upper extremities and that make caring (i.e., dressing, toileting, seating, bathing, and feeding) for these children and adults difficult. Never underestimate the deforming forces of spasticity, or lack of active movement, especially during the formative period of childhood growth and development.

Active orthotic management or splinting during childhood may prevent many contractures and resulting deformities and thus improve the quality of life for children and their families. Early orthotic intervention is usually less costly to the medical and educational systems than attempts to treat a deformity after the fact. Prolonged stretching of soft tissue (such as that provided with a splint) appears to be of greater benefit in reducing contractures than repeated briefer stretch typical of passive ROM exercises [Hogan and Uditsky 1998, McClure et al. 1994]. Provision of some passive ROM is still necessary to keep the splinted joints mobile. Passive ranging is also important for joints that are not splinted.

Understanding the possible physiologic mechanisms for the formation of a contracture can assist the therapist in splint design and establishment of wearing schedules. Hogan and Uditsky [1998], McClure et al. [1994], and Watanabe [2004] provided useful discussions of this topic. Briefly, when a joint is held in a fixed position (for example, wrist flexion) the result "is a decrease in the functional length of the periarticular connective tissues and associated muscles that have been held in this shortened position.... The muscle then accommodates to this shortened immobilized position through biological changes that take place such as a loss in the number of sarcomeres" [Hogan and Uditsky 1998, p. 71].

Preventing contractures, or minimizing their severity, is one of the most important functions of splinting for children with developmental disabilities or congenital anomalies. Even with ongoing intervention, prevention of all contractures in children who have severely increased tone can be difficult and may not be possible. However, even if an existing contracture cannot be improved splinting should be done to prevent the contracture from becoming worse. A moderate contracture is better than a severe contracture because the latter can result in problems with skin breakdown and can make care much more difficult. When working to decrease a contracture it is important to keep in mind that "soft tissue connective tissue responds better to low-load prolonged stress (LLPS) than high-load brief stress (HLBS)" [Granhaug 2006, p. 419].

Integrity of Skin, Bones, and Circulatory System

In severe cases, the therapist should use extreme caution when splinting a child with osteoporosis because stress to the bones could cause a fracture. Osteoporosis in children occurs as a result of lack of weight bearing while bones are growing. Children with tightly fisted hands are at risk of developing maceration or skin breakdown in the palms or between the fingers, and maintenance of skin hygiene becomes a priority.

Some children experience pain in certain positions or have very sensitive skin. Other children have poor circulation, which necessitates careful monitoring of the color and temperature of the skin during splint wear. Finally, some children who have developmental disabilities also have significant feeding problems and may be underweight. Children with little subcutaneous fat probably have more difficulty tolerating pressure on bony areas, thus affecting the splint's design and wearing schedule.

Performance Skills

The therapist should evaluate components of reach, grasp, manipulation, release, bilateral hand use, and tactile and proprioceptive reactivity and discrimination. It is important to evaluate upper extremity function in various positions, such as supported sitting, unsupported sitting, and prone, supine, and side lying. This gives crucial information about the proximal stability needed for effective distal function of the hand. Sensory system modulation should be observed. Hyperreactivity or hyporeactivity to sensory stimuli affects how the therapist approaches the child and influences splint selection and fabrication.

The child's level of cognitive ability also affects hand use, and the therapist should obtain information about the child's cognitive level. Because one of the most important determinants of a successful splint is the improvement of hand function, the therapist should use an objective measure of hand function such as a criterion-referenced assessment tool. This allows the therapist to periodically reevaluate and compare the child's performance over time. A qualitative description of how the child moves and performs should also be included to complete the functional assessment.

Context

Children with disabilities live, rest, play, and are productive in a variety of environments—including home, school, child care centers, and sometimes hospitals. The fabrication and monitoring of splints may occur in any of these environments. When selecting and designing a splint, persons who are responsible for donning the splint must be considered. Simplicity of design is desirable and may be a necessity in cases where the child interacts with multiple care providers in a variety of environments. Compliance with using the splint is likely to decline as the complexity with the donning and wearing schedule increases. In the hospital setting, care must be taken to obtain information from family members and the treating therapist (if applicable) about home and school settings that will influence splinting decisions.

Careful planning must be made when splinting in the intensive care units of the hospital because splints must be fabricated with minimal handling of the infant or child and while navigating carefully around life-supporting tubes and monitors. Consideration must be given to incorporation of the use of the splints in the daily medical care provided by nursing staff. The therapist must also be familiar with the child's medical condition and be able to recognize signs of stress that can be harmful to the child. Practice in the neonatal intensive care unit requires advanced competencies, and therapists considering practice in this environment should obtain training beyond entry level [Hunter 2005].

When a splint is used in the school environment, it must contribute to the child's ability to benefit from a specially designed program of instruction such as special education. It is important for a child to be able to reach, grasp, manipulate, and release learning materials and other objects in order to function in the classroom, lunchroom, playground, hallways, library, and gymnasium.

The therapist should include the purpose of a splint as a part of educationally related occupational therapy described by the individualized education plan (IEP) if the child is 3 to 21 years of age or the individualized family service plan (IFSP) if the child is under 3 years of age. Remember, the splint is a *means* to an end and not the *end* itself. Therefore, the IEP or IFSP goal would be a measurable statement describing the child's performance skills, patterns, or client factors and not the fabrication of the splint. The splint is part of the intervention that allows or facilitates participation in educational programming. This distinction is important if personnel at the school question whether splinting is an educational or a medical intervention.

Information about the home environment should be obtained from interviews with the parents and caretakers, and if possible via a home visit. Splints with wearing schedules incompatible with family schedules or splints that family members do not understand will not be used effectively. The family should not be expected to follow a "one size fits all" splinting protocol. Rather, the therapist must individualize the splint design and wearing schedule not only to fit the child's needs but to fit the family's strengths and needs. The therapist should always bear in mind that families are expected to carry out other therapeutic, educational, or medical interventions in addition to meeting the challenges of day-to-day life with a child who has a disability.

After an assessment is completed, the therapist can establish therapeutic goals and intervention strategies for the child. A splint may be a component of this treatment plan. According to Schoen and Anderson, orthotic devices (like adaptive equipment) are an important part of intervention because they reinforce neurodevelopmental treatment therapeutic goals: "If preventative measures such as adaptive equipment and orthotic devices are provided, then the child will receive consistent input to prevent or reduce the occurrence of deformities and limitations" [Schoen and Anderson 1999, p. 107]. Once a decision is made to provide a splint for a child, the splinting process is initiated.

Overview of the Splinting Process

Prepare the Child

Position the child so that the effects of abnormal tone and postural reflexes on the arm and hand are at a minimum. This position depends on the results of the assessment of the individual child and may be different from how the child is typically positioned. It is important to provide external stability through equipment or handling for children who have not acquired internal stability of proximal joints. This may involve a seating system or other adaptive equipment. For the infant or young child, it may be possible for the parent to hold the child and provide external stability with the therapist's instructions.

It is also important to reduce the child's fearfulness and maximize his or her cooperation. If the therapist does not already have a relationship with the child, time must be provided to allow the child to warm up to a stranger. Even if the child knows the therapist, a brief time should be provided to allow the child to acclimate to the equipment and setup for splinting. The therapist should have toys, music, books, stickers, or other materials to establish a reciprocal interaction with the child before starting the fabrication process. With an infant, the therapist can talk in a soothing voice and touch the child in a playful manner before fabrication. With an older child, the therapist can show the child what to expect by first fabricating a "splint" on a doll or stuffed animal or by making "thermoplastic jewelry" or other play objects.

When appropriate, the child should be given the opportunity to touch and feel the material while it is warm and soft and again after it becomes cool and hard. The child's response to tactile stimuli should be noted, and if signs of tactile defensiveness occur the therapist should follow sensory processing guidelines for improving sensory system modulation. If colored thermoplastic material is available, the child should be encouraged to select a color. Decorating the splint with stickers or leather stamps also encourages the acceptance of the splint for some children.

Giving children a role to play in the fabrication process may increase their cooperation. This could include keeping time by counting, holding the tail of the Ace wrap, or any other role the therapist can invent to keep them involved. However, if associated reactions are present it is best for the child to be involved without exerting effort—because this may increase tone. Although preparing the child may take a few extra minutes at the beginning of a splinting session, it can save hours of frustration in having to reschedule or remake a splint because of lack of cooperation.

Prepare the Environment

Thoughtful preparation is especially important when splinting children because of their short attention spans. In addition to having splinting and play materials close at hand, it is recommended that the therapist plan to have a second pair of adult hands to help with the fabrication process [Armstrong 2005]. This additional person might be a parent, teacher, paraprofessional, or another therapist. This is especially important if the child has increased tone, is not able to follow verbal instructions, or is likely to be uncooperative. The therapist must clearly explain the helper's role so that efforts assist the process and not hinder it. This usually involves maintaining the child's overall position, calming or entertaining the child, holding the arm just proximal to the joint being splinted, or stabilizing the material once in place and while it is cooling.

Selection of Splinting Materials

Pediatric splints may be made of many different types of materials, depending on the purpose of the splint and the age and needs of the child. Thermoplastic materials are commonly used for the fabrication of static splints or those that require restricting motion at certain joints. Soft splints are commonly made of materials such as neoprene. Soft splints may not totally immobilize a joint, but they provide support and allow greater freedom of movement. Children with athetosis or involuntary flailing movements should be protected from possible harm from the splint by selection of a soft material or by covering a thermoplastic material with a mitt or sock.

When splinting with neoprene, the therapist should be alert to the possibility of skin irritation or rash. According to Stern et al. [1998, p. 573], "skin contact with neoprene poses two dermatological risks: allergic contact dermatitis (ACD) and miliaria rubra (i.e., prickly heat)." Although neoprene hypersensitivity is rare, the authors recommend that therapists screen patients for a history of dermatologic reactions; instruct clients to discontinue use and inform the therapist if a rash, itching, or skin eruptions occur; and report cases of adverse skin reactions to the manufacturer of the neoprene material. They also recommend that therapists limit their own exposure to neoprene and neoprene glue because of the exposure to thiourea compounds that are thought to contribute to allergic reactions.

Thermoplastic materials range in conformability (and in stretch, thickness, and rigidity) and are described in Chapter 3. Generally, thermoplastic materials with a high plastic content have more conformability—whereas materials with a high rubber content have less stretch but are less likely to be indented with fingerprints during fabrication or stretch out of shape. When making a splint that counteracts the forces of spasticity, it is especially important to select a thermoplastic material that resists stretch (i.e., one with a high rubber content) because it is necessary for the therapist to apply considerable pressure to obtain the desired position of the wrist, thumb, and fingers [Armstrong 2005].

There are also products that combine the properties of plastic and rubber. Usually the rubberlike (or combination) thermoplastic material is necessary when one is splinting against spasticity, even though it is less rigid than the plastic type. If necessary, a reinforcement component can be added to the splint. Selecting a material with a high degree of memory is helpful when one is working with a child whose movements may be unpredictable and require the therapist to start over (sometimes more than once!). These plastics are elastic-like and self-adhere easily. This latter characteristic can also be problematic.

One way to reduce the stickiness is to add a tablespoon of liquid soap or shampoo to the hot water [Hogan and Uditsky 1998]. When splinting a neonate or young infant, the standard 1/8-inch material may be too thick and heavy. Rather, the therapist should use material that is 1/16-inch or 3/32-inch in thickness. The therapist's experience and preferences also affect the choice of thermoplastic material. (See Chapter 3 for a review of splinting material.)

Patterns

Patterns are made for each splint on each child, depending on the therapeutic goal of the splint and the child's characteristics. A pattern is essential. It not only determines the correct size and fit but allows the therapist to conceptualize the entire splinting process. The pattern can be revised through trial and error until the desired result is achieved. Patterns can be made from paper, such as paper towels, or from aluminum foil. Masking tape can be used to repair tears or reinforce contours. Many children with abnormal tone may be unable to lay their hands on a table surface for tracing. In this case, the pattern must be held under the extremity in whatever position is least stressful. The therapist may also consider using an uninvolved contralateral side to start a pattern, given there is some symmetry of anatomy.

It may be helpful to plan on extending the splint material a little beyond that of the finished product in order to give the therapist leverage to help hold joints in position. The extra can be cut away when the essential part of the splint is finished and hardened [Granhaug 2006].

Heating the Thermoplastic Material

The therapist should heat the water to the temperature range recommended by the manufacturer. After cutting out the splint, it may be necessary to reheat the plastic to obtain the desired degree of pliability before the molding process. Before placing the plastic on a child's extremity, the therapist should dry off the hot water and make sure the plastic is not too hot. Checking the thermoplastic material's temperature can be done by placing it against the therapist's face or anterior portion of the forearm. This is especially important when spot heating with a heat gun because this method tends to result in higher surface temperatures.

Some children may be hyperreactive to temperature and react negatively, even though the temperature does not feel hot to the therapist. Because many children cannot communicate that the plastic feels too hot, the therapist should watch the child's facial expressions and listen for vocalizations that indicate discomfort. The child's arm and hand can be moistened with cold water just before molding, or the therapist can wait longer for the plastic to cool. Some therapists use stockinette to protect the extremity. However, care must be taken that it does not wrinkle under the plastic during fabrication.

Hastening the Splinting Process

Time is of the essence when one is splinting a moving target, a rebellious little one, or a difficult-to-position extremity. Rubber-based plastics, which are necessary to resist stretch, are somewhat slower to harden. Once the plastic is in place on the extremity, an ice pack can be rubbed on the splint to hasten the setting process. A rubber glove filled with ice chips can easily serve the purpose. After partially hardened, the splint can be carefully removed and put into a pan of ice water or placed under a faucet of cold running water to finish hardening.

A spray coolant may be used, but only with great care to spray after the splint is off the child and with the spray directed away from the child. The use of coolant spray should be avoided with children who are unable to keep their heads turned away from the direction of the spray and those who have frequent respiratory problems.

A Theraband roll that has been cooled in a freezer can help form the splint, especially for the forearm. This will accelerate the cooling process at the same time. If not available, an Ace wrap can be useful to hold the forearm trough in place while the therapist works on the hand portion of the splint—although this maintains heat and may increase setting time. In either case, the therapist should not apply the wrap or Theraband too tightly and should flare the edges of the forearm trough away from the skin after formation of the splint.

Padding

Padding, or some form of pressure relief, may be necessary over bony areas to prevent skin problems. Padding does *not* compensate for pressure resulting from a poorly made splint. Padding takes up space, a factor the therapist must take into account before formation of the splint. Otherwise, the amount of pressure against the skin may increase. A variety of paddings exist, including closed- and open-cell foam and gel products. Pressure-relief padding with a gel center is useful in protecting bony areas for children with little subcutaneous fat.

To ensure a proper fit, the therapist should lay the padding on the child's extremity before molding the plastic or place it on the thermoplastic material before molding the splint. When molding with padding, the stretch of the thermoplastic material and the contourability may be compromised. Therefore, the therapist should add padding only if absolutely necessary. In addition, padding becomes soiled and needs to be replaced. For more information on padding, see Chapter 3.

Another way to create pressure relief around a bony prominence without using padding is to cover the prominence with a small amount of a firm therapy putty before forming the splint. The putty creates a built-in bubble and is removed from the splint after cooling [Hogan and Uditsky 1998]. Thin forms of padding may also be useful to create friction and reduce migration or shifting of splints, or for covering edges. Microfoam tape is useful for this purpose, especially on small splints.

Strapping

A variety of strap materials are available. The therapist should consider strength, durability, elasticity, and texture when the strap is against the skin. Strapping with sharp edges should be avoided with younger children and those with sensitive skin. The wider the strap the more force is dispersed, as long as the entire strap width is in full contact with the skin. Strap material may have to be cut narrower, especially around the wrist and fingers, to be proportionate to the size of the child's hand.

Straps can be secured at each end with hook Velcro, which is attached to the splint. This allows them to be easily replaced when they become soiled, which is important if the child drools on the splint or mouths it. However, loose straps easily become lost and many times are not placed on the splint at the correct angle or location. An alternative is to adhere the strap at one end with a rivet or strong contact adhesive. When soiled, straps must be removed by the therapist and a new strap reattached. See Chapter 3 for more detailed information about attaching straps.

Increasing the likelihood that the child will not remove straps and the splint requires knowledge of child development and creativity. Children at certain ages (such as 2- and 3-year-olds) are in the developmental stage of asserting their autonomy and may resist the parent's choice of clothing or food or splint application. In this case, using principles of behavior analysis (such as shaping or rewarding successive approximations, finding times during the day when the child is most likely to be compliant, and contingent use of praise and attention) may be helpful. Actively involving the child in the choice of colors and decorations may increase the child's willingness to wear the splint. Strap Critter patterns are provided by Armstrong [2005], along with suggestions for using decorative ribbon, fabric paints, or shoelace charms. She also suggested describing the splint as something cool to wear and providing the child with language to use to explain to peers, such as this is my Batman or scuba diver's glove.

If positive methods to prevent splint removal have not worked, therapists can use their creativity to keep the little "Houdinis" in their splints, especially young children who do not understand cause and effect. Some kid-proof methods include using shoelaces, buttons, or socks/stockinette/puppets. Lacing can be done by punching holes along the lateral edges of the splint and lacing with wide decorative shoelaces. The therapist should place padding under the laces against the skin. To secure the laces, the therapist can use a "bow biter" (a plastic device available in children's shoe departments) to hold the laces in place [Collins 1996]. Depending on the function of the splint, a sock puppet worn over the splint may be used as camouflage (Figure 16-1). Care must be taken not to provide any attachment the child could bite off and swallow.

Providing Instruction for Splint Application

Those responsible for applying the child's splint should have been part of the assessment process and should have already provided input on the splint design and have agreed with the need for the splint. They must understand the splint's purpose, the rationale for using the splint, precautions, and risks of incorrect usage. Although the correct application of the splint may seem obvious to the therapist, it may not be obvious to many teachers, nursing staff, or parents unfamiliar with splints.

The more complex the splint the more detailed and explicit the instructions should be. This is especially true when there are multiple care providers. The therapist should provide written instructions, along with a phone number and/or e-mail to contact with questions or concerns. A demonstration of the steps involved in putting the splint on correctly should be provided, followed by an opportunity for the caretaker to practice applying the splint under supervision. A photograph of the child's forearm and hand, showing the splint on the child in the correct position, is often an effective teaching tool if it does not conflict with policies regarding confidentiality.

Correct placement of straps can be facilitated by writing a number or placing a small design on the strap end and a corresponding number or design on the splint. The therapist should do everything possible to take the guesswork out of putting on the splint. It is also wise to instruct the caregivers to inspect the skin every time the splint is removed to assess the splint for signs of excessive pressure.

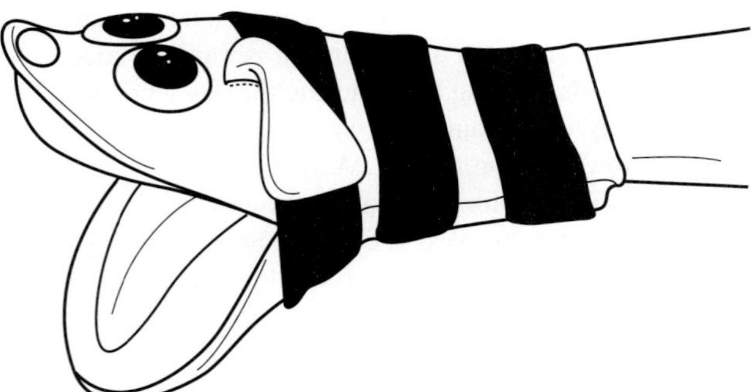

Figure 16-1 A sock puppet worn over a splint may be more appealing to a child and camouflage the splint.

Wearing Schedules

Wearing schedules vary according to the purpose of the splint, the child's tolerance for the splint, the child's musculoskeletal status, and the child's occupations and daily routines. Splints may be worn for long or short intervals during the day, at night, during functional activities, or a combination of these. It is necessary to gradually increase the wearing time initially to build up the child's tolerance for the splint and to make any modifications that become apparent with use.

When the purpose of the splint is to increase functional use of the hands, wearing the splint should occur *during* times when the child is engaged in occupations. If the purpose is tone reduction, the splint should be worn just *prior to* activities or occupations. When the purpose of the splint is to prevent a contracture, the splint should be worn when the child is *not engaged* in occupations. Finally, if the splint is used to treat an existing contracture it is necessary for it to be worn for prolonged periods of time.

The total time spent wearing the splint during a 24-hour period appears to be more important than whether it is worn continuously or intermittently [Hogan and Uditsky 1998]. The length of time a splint can be worn is also affected by how much force is being applied to achieve the splinted position, which causes stress on the joints, muscles, and skin. Ultimately, wearing schedule decisions are based on developing and maintaining clinical competence, clinical reasoning, and collaborating with the child and/or family members or care providers.

The wearing schedule will work only if the splint is placed on the child during the times recommended. Incorporating the splint schedule into the child's regular routine may increase compliance because it becomes less of a special chore for the parent, teacher, caregiver, or nursing staff. The therapist should document the agreed-upon wearing schedule (along with instructions for putting on the splint) and provide written copies to parents, caregivers, teachers, nurses, and child care providers. As the child's developmental or ROM status changes, the therapist must evaluate the wearing schedule and possibly the splint design to make necessary modifications.

Precautions

The skin should be inspected frequently during the initial wearing phase. A distinct red area or generalized redness that does not disappear within 15 to 20 minutes after splint removal indicates excessive pressure and the need for revisions [Hill 1988, Hogan and Uditsky 1998]. During periods of monitoring, the therapist should be aware of any problems associated with joint compression, pressure on nerves, compromised circulation, and dermatologic reactions. Children's growth spurts often come without obvious signals and during times of growth therapists and caregivers should be extra vigilant.

Evaluation of the Splint

A plan should be made for the therapist to reassess the splint on a regular basis to ensure proper fit and function. The therapist should consider having the care provider put the splint on an hour before the reassessment. This allows the therapist to observe how the splint is put on and whether the splint migrates out of position after initial donning. A poorly fitting splint can do more harm than good.

This overview applies to all pediatric splints. The following section provides information specific to several common splint designs used with children who have a developmental disability or congenital anomaly.

Resting Hand Splint

The purpose of a resting hand splint is to prevent a contracture or deformity, to prevent an existing deformity from becoming worse, or to gradually improve or reduce a deformity (deformity-reduction splint). Children who are at the greatest risk of developing a contracture are those with moderately to severely increased tone or those with severely decreased tone who have no active movement. For children with severely increased muscle tone and tightly fisted hands, an additional purpose may be maintenance of skin hygiene.

Features

The components of a resting hand splint for a child are the same as those described in Chapter 9, except for the shape of the thumb trough and C bar. Components include a forearm trough, a pan for the fingers, a thumb trough, and a C bar (Figure 16-2). If spasticity is present in the thenar muscles, the thumb should be positioned in partial radial abduction in order to elongate the opponens muscle. Sustained stretch of tight thenar muscles may also inhibit tone in the hand [McKie 1998].

For children with moderately to severely increased tone, the ideal position of the wrist, fingers, and thumb may not be possible. Because its purpose is to prevent or reduce joint deformity, the splint should provide as much elongation of the tight muscles as possible without causing excessive stress.

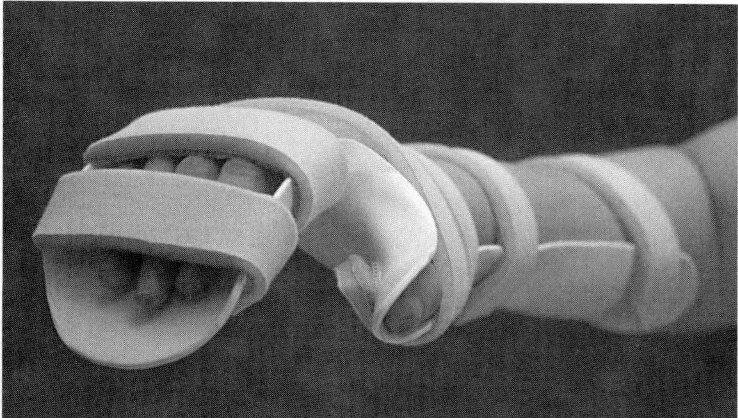

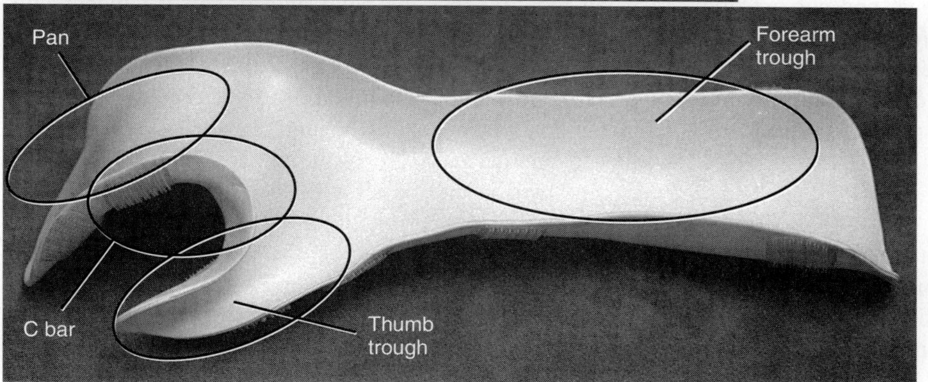

Figure 16-2 A resting hand splint.

The child should also be able to tolerate wearing the splint for several hours at a time to obtain the maximum benefit.

If the splint places the hand into the maximum range of passive motion, the forces generated may compromise circulation, cause skin breakdown, elicit pain, or reduce the length of time the child can tolerate wearing the splint. Therefore, the splint should place the wrist joint in submaximum range [Exner 2005, Hill 1988]—a position especially important at the wrist to allow for extension of the fingers. Low-load prolonged stretch provided by casts or splints is the best conservative way of increasing passive ROM [Duff and Charles 2004]. When flexor spasticity is severe, serial splinting may be necessary [Duff and Charles 2004, Exner 2005].

The therapist can usually determine the best splinting position by handling the child's extremity and feeling the amount of passive resistance. After achieving the desired position manually, the therapist should note the angles of the joints involved and where pressure is being applied to obtain this position. Handling the joints and feeling the resistance from muscles helps the therapist determine the most therapeutic position and the location of force application during splint fabrication and strap application.

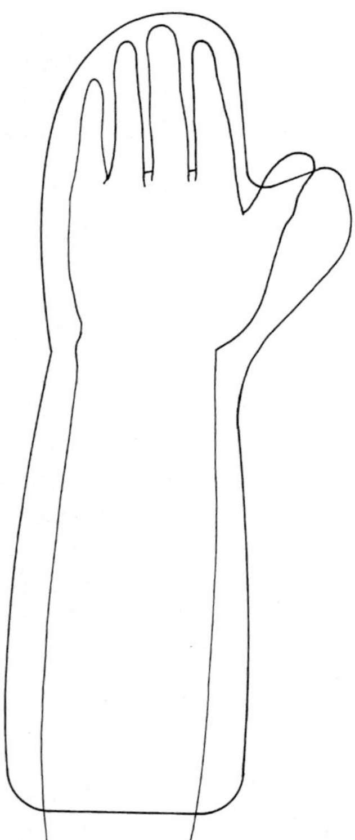

Figure 16-3 A pattern for a resting hand splint.

Process to Fabricate a Resting Hand Splint

Thermoplastic Material Selection

When making a splint that counteracts the forces of spasticity, the therapist should select a low-temperature thermoplastic that resists stretch. A considerable amount of pressure is applied against the splinting material while the therapist obtains the desired position of the wrist, thumb, and fingers. This pressure can indent and inadvertently stretch materials that have conformability. Usually a thermoplastic material containing a higher rubber content will have the desired working characteristics. (See "Overview of the Splinting Process.")

Pattern

The pattern should include the measurements and markings of landmarks (see Chapter 9). Because the thumb position of this splint is different from the traditional resting hand splint, the thumb trough and C bar are shaped differently (Figure 16-3). After the pattern is drawn and cut out, the therapist fits it to the child and makes further modifications as necessary. While making the pattern and molding the splint, the therapist should position the child to minimize the effects of abnormal tone and postural reflexes on the body and the extremities.

Padding

Before forming the splint, the therapist should consider the need for padding to allow the additional space necessary. Because padding places some restrictions on forming the splint and keeping it clean, it should not be used unless the assessment shows the child to be at risk of skin problems. Creating bubbled-out areas over bony areas may be sufficient to avoid skin problems. If used, follow guidelines described in the section headed "Overview of the Splinting Process."

Forming the Splint

Before placing the plastic on the child's extremity, the therapist should prestretch the edge of the splint that forms the C bar (Figure 16-4A). The therapist should then place the soft plastic on the child's upper extremity so that it conforms to the web space of the thumb (Figure 16-4B). If available, an assistant stands beside the child and secures the forearm trough. The therapist should form the splint into the palmar arches and around the wrist and thumb. To obtain the desired contour and fit, the therapist may need to be aggressive when molding into the palm and around the thenar eminence—especially if working against spasticity.

The therapist must form the splint so that the bulk of pressure positioning the thumb is directed below the thumb metacarpal phalangeal (MP) joint and distributed along the thenar eminence. This formation is necessary to avoid hyperextension and possibly dislocation of the thumb MP joint [Exner 2005]. The thumb trough should cradle the thumb and extend about ½ inch beyond the end of the thumb. The interphalangeal (IP) joint of the thumb should be slightly flexed, and the C bar should fit snugly into the web space and contour against the radial side of the index finger (Figure 16-4c).

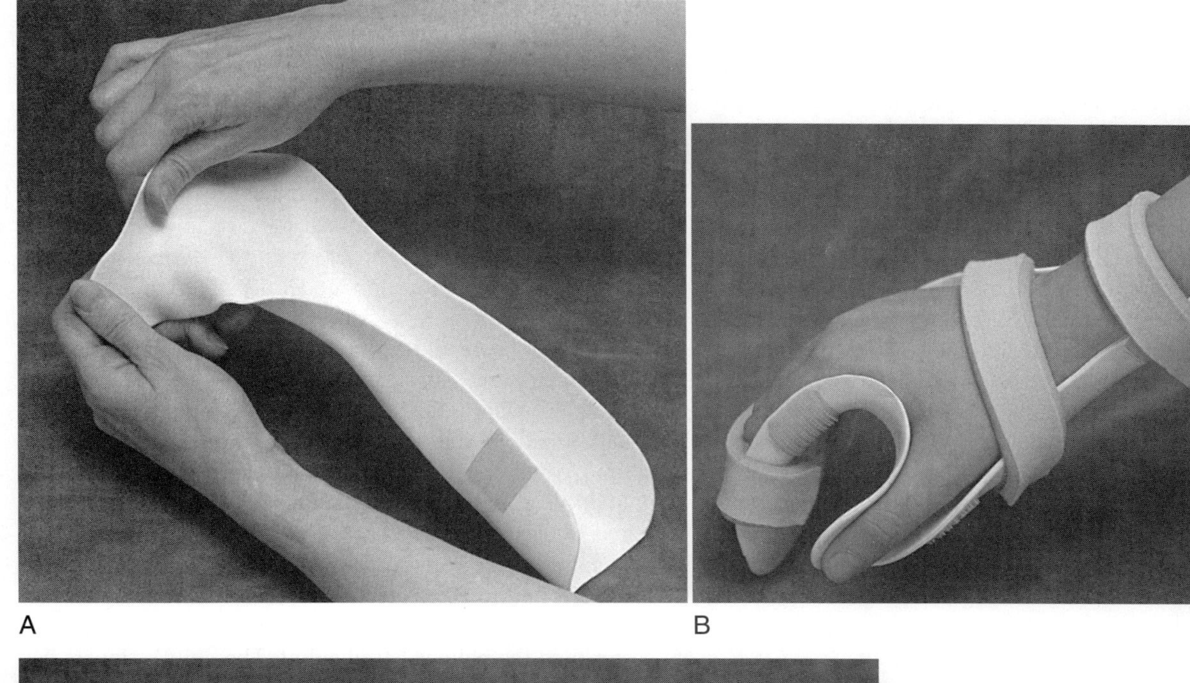

A B

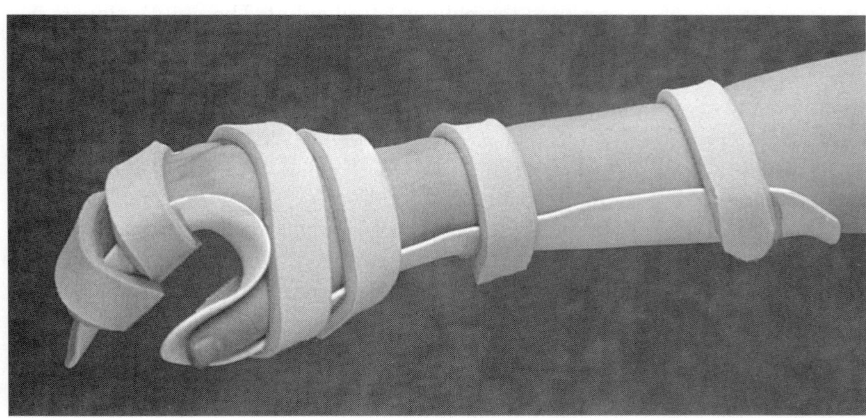

C

Figure 16-4 (A) Prestretching of the C bar. (B) The fit of the C bar into the web space. (C) The contour of the C bar.

Forearm Trough

After completing the wrist, palm, and thumb portion, the therapist can finish forming the forearm trough. (See Chapter 9 for guidelines on securing the forearm in the trough and avoiding pressure points.) If the edges of the trough are too high, the straps will bridge (i.e., the straps are raised from the skin's surface and do not follow the contour of the forearm, thus losing skin surface contact). To keep the forearm securely in place, the straps should have maximum surface contact. If not secure, the forearm may rotate in the trough or the splint may shift distally and the position of the wrist, fingers, and thumb will be compromised.

Pan

Finally, the therapist forms the finger pan to position the fingers. The pan may require reheating because controlling all joints at the same time is often difficult. (See Chapter 9 for the correct width and height of the pan.) In addition, the distal portion of the pan should extend about ½ inch beyond the fingertips to allow for growth. When forming the curve of the pan, the therapist should follow the proximal and distal transverse arches.

Straps

The correct placement of straps is as important as correct formation of the splint, especially when the splint is holding against increased muscle tone. The straps and splint must work together to create the necessary leverage and to distribute pressure. If the forearm, palm, fingers, and thumb do not stay in the correct position in the splint, the benefit of the splint is greatly reduced. The optimum location and angle of each strap should be determined in relation to the forces being applied by abnormal muscle tone.

The forearm trough requires two straps for an older child. However, for a smaller child or an infant one wide strap across the forearm may be sufficient. Stability should be provided at the proximal and distal areas of the forearm. If considerable wrist flexion is present, two straps will be necessary to provide three points of pressure to secure the wrist.

One strap should extend directly across the wrist just distal to the ulnar styloid, and a second strap should be angled from the thumb web space across the dorsum of the hand and secured proximal to the metacarpophalangeal (MCP) joints on the ulnar side. Otherwise, one strap across the dorsum of the hand may be sufficient. If there is considerable finger flexion, straps may be needed across each of the three phalanges. Finally, the therapist should add a strap between the MP and IP joints of the thumb. When making a small splint for a young child, the therapist should make the straps narrower. (See Figure 16-5 for an illustration of strap placements, although not all of these may be necessary on every splint.)

Adaptations

The resting hand splint provides a basic form for positioning the child in good alignment and may serve as an inhibitor of hypertonicity. However, often the therapist must deviate from the basic form to truly meet the needs of the child. One way the splint can be adapted is by the addition of finger separators (also described in Chapter 9) to abduct the fingers and assist in tone reduction. This can be done by bubbling the material between digits or by simply attaching a roll of thermoplastic material between the digits. Finger separators can also be made from thermoplastic pellets or elastomer.

With pellets, the therapist softens them in hot water and kneads them together to the shape and size required. The pellets have 100% memory and are attached in the same way as any other thermoplastic material. Because of the puttylike consistency, these pellets work well when the therapist needs to make individualized finger separators—such as for children who have arthrogryposis and different deformities in each finger [Hogan and Uditsky 1998].

Elastomer is a silicone-based putty that can be used in pediatric splinting for thumb positioning or finger spacers. Pellets and elastomers are available from many splinting product catalogs. The putty types of elastomers "with a gel catalyst or the 50/50 mix are probably the easiest to work with because they can be mixed in the hand and varied in stiffness by adding more or less catalyst" [Armstrong 2005, p. 485]. Another option for modeling is Permagum, a silicone rubber dental-impression material [Bell and Graham 1995]. Elastomers and pellets may also be used to maintain the palmer arches or as a base for a small hand splint [Granhaug 2006].

The therapist may choose to use a dorsal-based resting splint [Armstrong 2005, Snook 1979] as an alternative to the palmar-based splint already described. This design is illustrated in Chapter 9. The dorsal-based splint will avoid sensory input to the forearm flexors, although it is somewhat more difficult to fabricate. For a child with very tight wrist flexors, donning the dorsal-based resting splint may be easier than the palmar-based splint. The child's fingers can be placed into the finger slot (with the fingers sufficiently through the slot to support the MP joints), pressure can be placed across the wrist flexors, and slowly the forearm trough can be levered down onto the dorsum of the forearm. Armstrong [2005] is a good source of information on fabricating this splint for children.

Infants with congenital finger contractures often need resting hand splints. However, when all digits are not affected the splint may be altered to free nonaffected digits to engage in movement and sensory experiences. Resting hand splints may be made with alternative materials, especially for infants. The therapist may select a semirigid pliable material when splinting neonates, as it is less likely to cause abrasions. Bell and Graham [1995] describe the use of Permagum, a silicone rubber dental impression material, to mold into shape for neonatal splints. Several layers of adhesive cloth tape may also be an effective semirigid support.

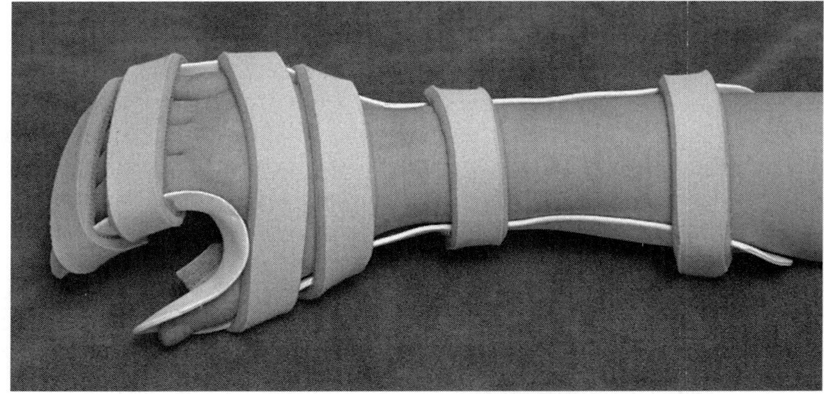

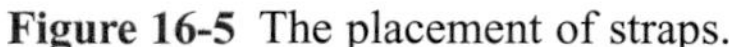
Figure 16-5 The placement of straps.

Precautions

When splinting against increased muscle tone, the therapist must consider biomechanical principles of force distribution. The therapist should monitor for any undesired lateral forces on the fingers or wrist that may result in poor anatomic alignment or dislocation or deformity. In addition, the therapist should be aware of any circulation compromise or pressure on nerves. The therapist must make astute observations and elicit important information from the child, parent, or caregiver—especially when assessing very young children or those with communication dysfunction.

Precautions for this splint are the same as those for any splint. (See Chapter 6 for guidance in determining problems with skin, bone, or muscles.) When applying these precautions to a child who has increased tone, the therapist should shorten the initial wearing time to 15- to 20-minute intervals on the first day. The therapist should then carefully inspect the skin. A distinct red area or generalized redness on the skin that does not disappear within 15 to 20 minutes after splint removal indicates excessive pressure and the need for revisions [Hill 1988, Hogan and Uditsky 1998]. If no pressure areas are present, the therapist may increase the wearing time to 30-minute intervals. The therapist may then increase the wearing time by adding 15 to 30 minutes of wearing time until the maximum wearing period for the child is reached.

An additional precaution to consider when making a resting hand splint for a child who has moderately to severely increased tone is maintaining the integrity of the MP joint of the thumb. The therapist must direct pressure below the MP joint of the thumb. Exner [2005] cautions that distal force to the spastic thumb can result in hyperextension and dislocation of the MP joint.

Wearing Schedule

The wearing schedule is determined on an individual basis, as are all other aspects of the treatment plan. In general, the more serious the threat of deformity the longer the splint is worn each 24 hours. If tone continues to be increased at night, this may be a good time for extended wearing unless it interferes with the child's sleep or presses against another part of the child's body. During the day, the splint is removed for periods of passive ranging, active movement, and opportunities for sensory experiences.

McClure et al. [1994] provide a flow chart or algorithm for making clinical decisions regarding wearing schedules for splints. They describe the biologic basis for limitations in joint ROM and increasing ROM. This information is especially helpful in cases in which contractures already exist. According to these authors, "the primary basis for using splints to increase ROM is that by holding the joint at or near its end-range over time, therapeutic tensile stress is applied to the restricted periarticular connective tissues (PCTs) and muscles. This tensile stress induces remodeling of these tissues to a new, longer length, which allows increased ROM" [McClure et al. 1994, p. 1103]. McClure et al. [1994, p. 1102] define remodeling as "a biological phenomenon that occurs *over long periods of time* rather than a mechanically induced change that occurs within minutes."

It is also beneficial for the child to participate in occupations immediately after removal of the resting hand splint to capitalize on increased hand expansion and elongation of tight muscles. If developing or improving functional hand skills is a primary goal, the splint should be removed more frequently or for longer periods of time.

Providing Instruction for Splint Application

It is imperative that those individuals responsible for applying the child's splint know how to do so correctly. In addition, caregivers should understand the purpose of the splint, precautions, risks of incorrect usage, and how to reach the therapist with questions or concerns. See "Overview of the Splinting Process" for a description of instructing others in splint application and uses.

Evaluation of the Splint

The self-evaluation described in Chapter 9 can be used to evaluate the finished splint. In addition to evaluating the splint after fabrication, the fit of the splint should be reviewed at regular intervals. The splint's effectiveness in accomplishing stated goals and outcomes should be reevaluated on an ongoing basis.

Laboratory Exercise 16-1* Recognizing Problems in Splint Fabrication No. 1

What problems in splint fabrication are present in the following picture?

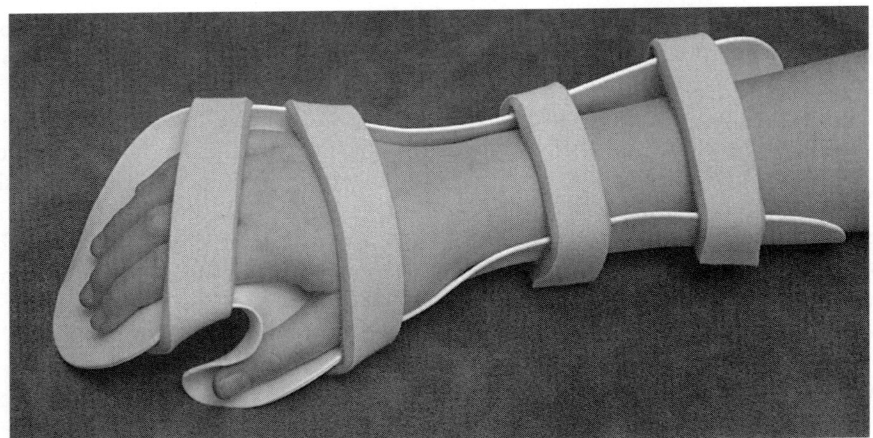

*See Appendix A for the answer key.

Laboratory Exercise 16-2* Recognizing Problems in Splint Fabrication No. 2

What problems in splint fabrication are present in the following picture?

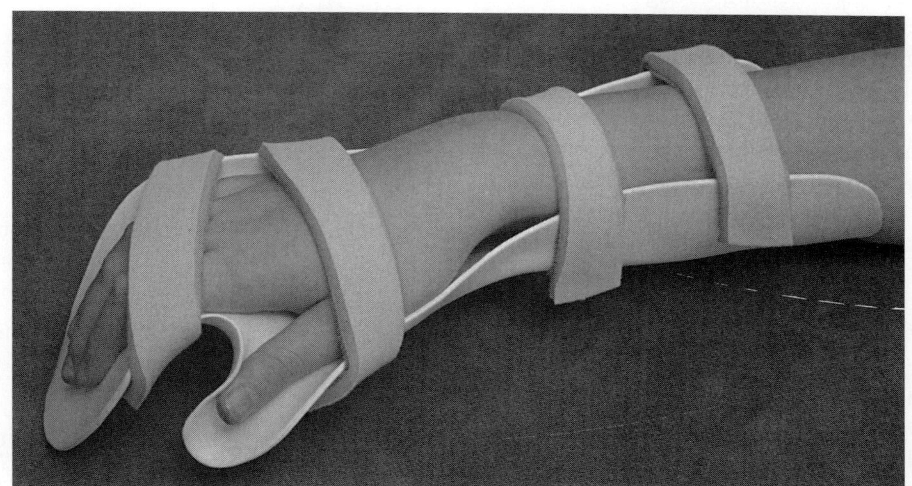

*See Appendix A for the answer key.

Weight-Bearing Splint

The weight-bearing splint (Figure 16-6) positions the hand in the most effective position for weight-bearing activities [Kinghorn and Roberts 1996, Lindholm 1986]. The splint requires significant wrist extension for effective use. The weight-bearing splint is used as a therapeutic tool, generally with children who have mild to moderate spasticity in their upper extremities. It is worn only during intervention. According to Lindholm [1986], the splint positions the wrist in extension to counteract the usual position of wrist flexion resulting from spasticity.

This position allows weight bearing through the heel of the hand. The splint positions the hand to allow normal weight bearing through the lateral borders of the hand and the fingertips. An effectively positioned hand allows the child to work on more proximal control. The splint serves as an assist for positioning the hand while the child is performing weight-bearing activities. During therapy, the splint allows the therapist to focus less on the hand and fingers and more on facilitation or inhibition techniques of the upper extremity.

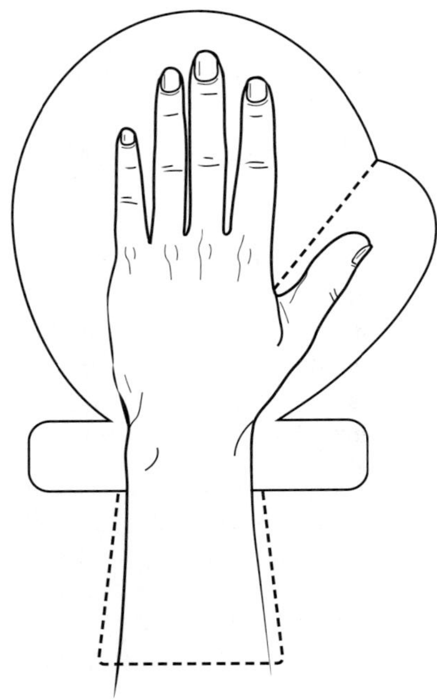

Figure 16-7 A pattern for the weight-bearing splint.

Features

The weight-bearing splint was originally designed as a hand-based splint. However, more stability is provided when the splint is fabricated with a forearm trough. The weight-bearing splint is similar in design to the aforementioned resting hand splint. However, there is more extension at the wrist and the thumb is in more radial abduction.

Pattern

The pattern for the weight-bearing splint (Figure 16-7) is similar to that for the resting hand pattern. However, extra space is provided when tracing around the fingers and thumb. The web space is not tapered. The pattern should look like a mitt for the hand. If a forearm trough is added to the splint design, it should extend two-thirds the length and half the circumference of the forearm.

Forming the Weight-Bearing Splint

Mold the splint on the volar surface of the hand. The proximal interphalangeal joints and distal interphalangeal joints should be in slight flexion and the thumb in radial abduction (Figure 16-8). The wrist should be in 45 to 50 degrees of extension. Much attention should be given to the palmar arches by positioning the hand in a cupped position. A small ball that fits comfortably in the child's hand can be used to reinforce the arches. A wide strap over the IPs will aid in keeping the fingers on the mitt. A diagonal strap over the wrist reinforces the wrist position. Straps should be placed proximally and distally on the forearm trough.

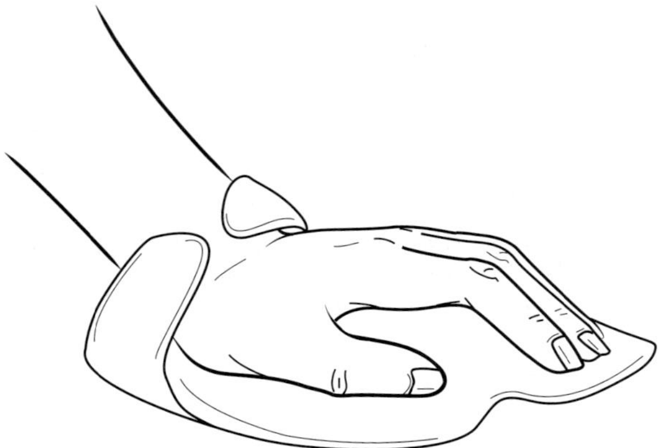

Figure 16-6 Weight-bearing splint.

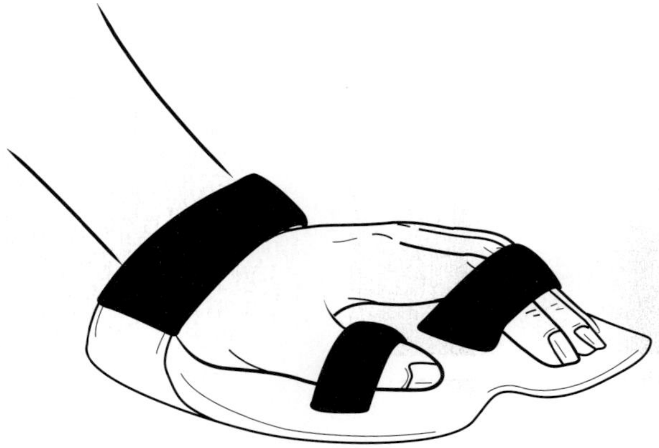

Figure 16-8 Positioning the straps over the fingers.

Precautions

This splint requires adequate wrist extension. ROM must be obtained before it is fabricated. When the wrist is in extension, the fingers often attempt to curl into flexion. Attention should be given to stabilizing the fingers in slight abduction.

Adaptations to the Weight-bearing Splint

To maintain stability of the fingers, slits may be made in the hand portion of the splint. This is accomplished by threading the strapping material through the slit and looping it over each joint (see Figure 16-8). To ensure stability at the hand, a dorsal hood may be fabricated by draping thermoplastic material over the dorsum of the hand. If additional concerns exist with respect to stabilizing the wrist and dorsum of the hand, the wrist and the forearm may be covered with thermoplastic material. This will create a clam shell type of splint (Figure 16-9). Because considerable pressure may be present, the dorsal piece of the splint may require padding.

Wrist Splints

A therapist usually selects a wrist splint to improve functional use of the hand rather than to prevent or manage a deformity. Providing proximal stability at the wrist, the splint allows for improved control of distal finger movement for grasp and release. When a therapist uses a wrist splint for a child who has tightness of the long finger flexors, the splint may have to position the wrist in slight flexion.

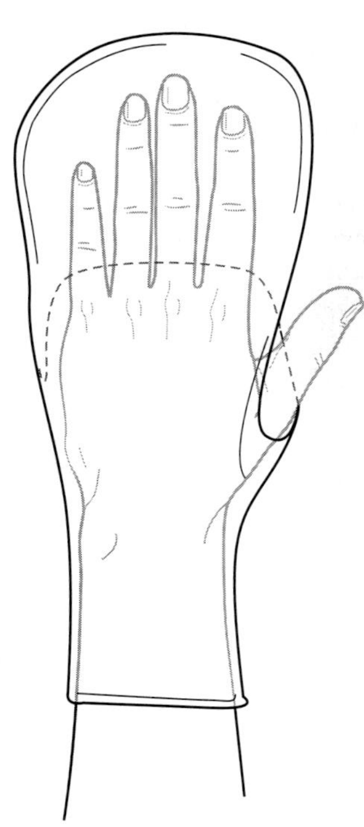

Figure 16-9 Weight-bearing clam shell splint.

Otherwise, the child may be unable to actively extend the fingers—thus restricting participation in occupations.

Because of the tenodesis effect, the wrist splint may not be appropriate if the finger flexors have severe tightness causing a fisted hand posture. If the child has only mildly increased tone or is hypotonic, a soft wrist splint with a reinforcement component under the wrist may be preferable. If tightness is also present in the opponens muscle, a splint that includes a thumb trough may be indicated.

The thermoplastic wrist splint can be either volarly or dorsally based. The volar design is more effective if wrist flexion is difficult to control. However, it covers the palm of the hand—thus reducing sensory input and creating more bulk in the hand. The dorsal design allows more sensory input to the palm but may be more difficult to construct when the child has wrist and finger flexor spasticity. If the palmar bar is too narrow, it can be dangerous and painful. It is also more difficult to add attachments, such as a pointer, to the dorsal wrist splint. This chapter describes the process for the volar design. See Chapter 7 for a description of the dorsal design.

The wrist splint may be used alone or alternately with a resting hand splint. This combination would be appropriate for a child who has some functional use of the hand but is at risk of developing contractures.

Features

The features of a wrist splint for a child are the same as for an adult (see Chapter 7).

Process to Fabricate a Volar Wrist Splint

Materials

The selection of tools and materials is essentially the same as that described previously for the resting hand splint. A thermoplastic material that resists stretch is frequently desirable when the therapist positions the wrist of a child with spasticity. However, when the purpose of a wrist splint is to serve as a base for attaching pointers or holders the thermoplastic material's surface must be properly prepared for self-bonding. It is preferable to select a thermoplastic that has a high degree of self-adherence (see Chapter 3).

Pattern

After tracing the child's extremity, the therapist makes the splint pattern. Use the guidelines presented in Chapter 7 to locate landmarks and determine how the splint should fit in the palm. (See Figure 16-10 for a sample pattern.)

Forming a Wrist Splint

The fabrication process is essentially the same as described in Chapter 7. The splint should follow the contour of the palmar arches as they are configured during grasp [Hill 1988]. The splint should not interfere with MCP flexion or thumb opposition. The therapist rolls the edges around the thenar eminence and MP bar. Occasionally, rolling an edge

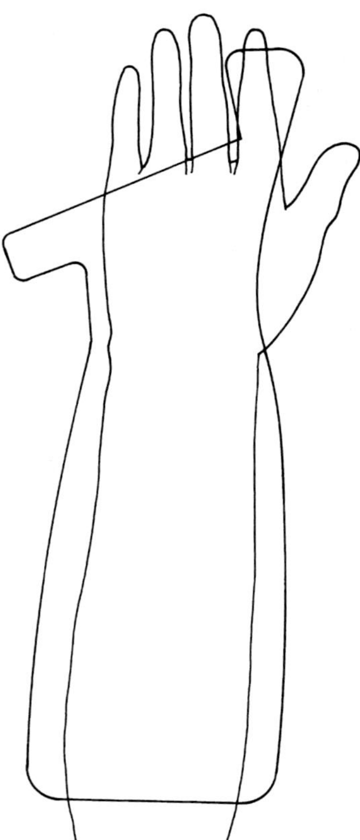

Figure 16-10 A pattern for a volar wrist splint with a pointer.

can cause the splint to become too bulky. Minimally, the edges should be contoured to prevent pressure areas from the edges. The ulnar side of the splint may require a bubble to accommodate the ulnar styloid.

Straps

The needs of the child determine the number and angles of straps. Usually two straps secure the forearm trough (although in some cases this can be accomplished with one wide strap) and one strap secures the hand. The hand strap is angled from the ulnar side of the metacarpal bar to the hypothenar bar. The therapist may have to cut the strap material narrower for small children.

Precautions

The precautions for the application of the wrist splint to children are essentially the same as those for the adult (see Chapter 7). The splint should distribute pressure to avoid skin irritation. In addition, the splint must stabilize the forearm so that the splint does not shift during use. The splint should not interfere with thumb opposition or MCP flexion of the fingers.

Wearing Schedule

The therapist should consider the child's therapeutic goals, occupations, and the extent of functional hand skills with and without the splint. In general, the child wears the splint during activities that require grasp and release that can be accomplished more easily while wearing the splint.

Evaluation of the Splint

The therapist can use a self-evaluation form to determine whether the fabrication of the splint is correct (see Chapter 7). The therapist should also perform frequent, ongoing reevaluation of the splint's effectiveness and the child's functional hand skills.

Adaptations to the Splint

Adaptations to the wrist splint include the attachment of pointers, crayon holders, or other assistive devices (Figure 16-11). When designing a pointer, the therapist should angle it so that the pointer is within the child's visual field. When possible, the therapist makes a finger trough to position the index finger for pointing—thus allowing sensory feedback to the tip of the index finger after contact is made with the target.

A spiral finger trough allows for more sensory input. Some children may benefit from the addition of a spiral strap to facilitate partial supination while wearing the wrist splint. This can be accomplished by attaching a strap to the palm of the hand and wrapping it radially across the dorsum of the hand over the wrist and forearm and attaching it to itself just proximal to the elbow.

Thumb Splints

Increased muscle tone frequently pulls the thumb into palmar adduction. The purpose of a thumb splint is to improve functional use of the hand by stabilizing the thumb in a functional position of opposition. The therapist uses this splint for a child who has some active wrist and finger extension but has difficulty actively moving the thumb out of the palm because of increased tone. If tone is moderate to severe, a splint made out of thermoplastic material may be more effective.

If tone is mild to moderate, a splint made from a more pliable material such as neoprene is recommended. Thumb splints can be hand or forearm based. This section describes hand-based thermoplastic splints and neoprene thumb splints that are hand and forearm based. Fortunately, prefabricated thumb splints for children have become much more common in recent years. They are discussed in the material following.

Thermoplastic Thumb Splint

Features

The hand-based thumb splint can be of a palmar or dorsal design. The dorsal design results in less bulk in the palm, but

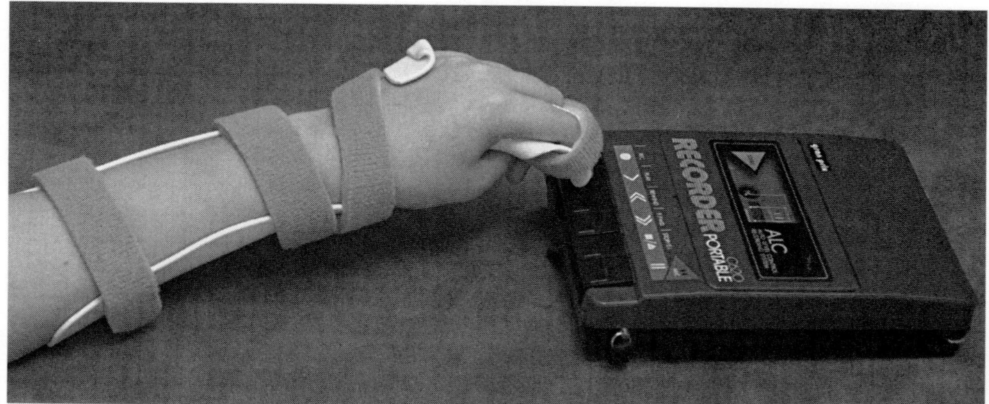

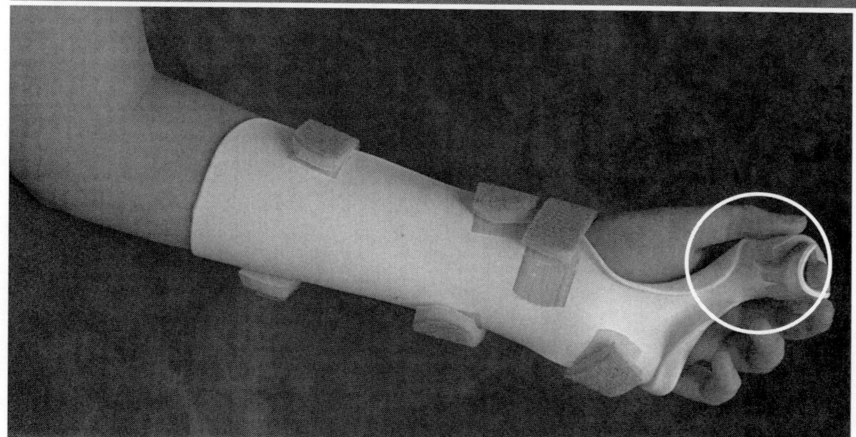

Figure 16-11 Volar wrist splint with an index finger pointer allows for more sensory input.

the splint may not apply adequate pressure against spastic thenar muscles and can be difficult to don. The palmar design includes a metacarpal bar, a thumb trough with a C bar, and a hypothenar bar (Figure 16-12).

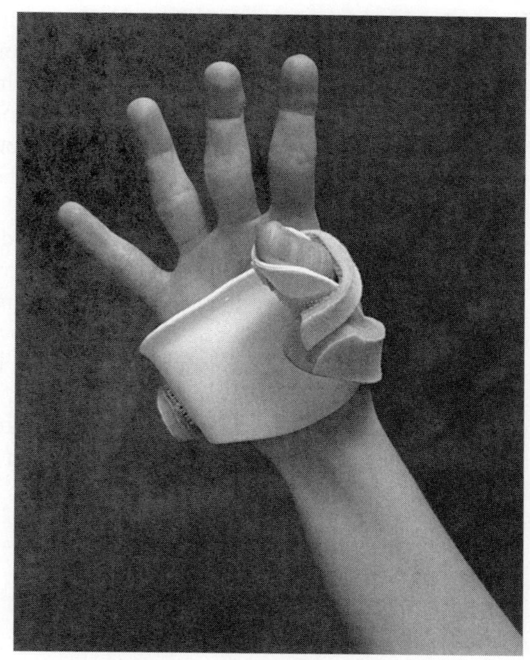

Figure 16-12 A thermoplastic thumb splint.

Process to Fabricate a Thermoplastic Thumb Splint

Materials

The selection of tools and materials is essentially the same as previously described for the resting hand splint.

Pattern

A sample pattern is shown in Figure 16-13.

Forming the Splint

After cutting out the splint and reheating the material, the therapist places the material on the child's hand and carefully molds the C bar to the thumb web space. The hypothenar bar wraps around the ulnar border of the hand far enough to secure the hand, and the metacarpal bar is rolled proximal to the distal creases to allow finger flexion.

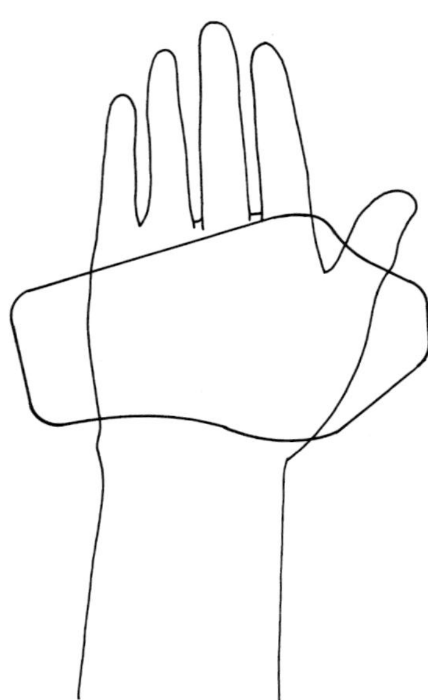

Figure 16-13 A pattern for a thermoplastic thumb splint.

The body of the splint should conform to the palmar arches as they occur during grasp and should extend proximally far enough to adequately position the carpometacarpal joint of the thumb but not so far that it interferes with wrist flexion. The therapist should ensure that the splint does not position the wrist in radial or extreme ulnar deviation.

The therapist forms the thumb trough by positioning the thumb in palmar abduction and stretching the plastic to form the C bar. The therapist should distribute pressure along the thenar eminence, thus providing optimal positioning of the thumb and avoiding hyperextension of the MP joint. The thumb trough should extend just past the IP joint of the thumb but should leave the tip of the thumb free for sensory contact during grasp (Figure 16-14). The finished splint should allow the index and middle fingers to contact the tip of the thumb. The therapist should place a strap across the dorsum of the hand. If necessary, the therapist should also place a strap across the thumb trough.

Sometimes during fabrication it is necessary to modify a small area. This can be especially challenging when one is working on a small curved splint. If the therapist wants to use hot water but does not want to risk losing the overall shape, a kitchen baster or eye dropper can be used to draw up hot water and place it repeatedly over the target area [Hogan and Uditsky 1998]. A device called the Ultratorch (available through UE TECH) is a fine spot heater that allows pinpoint modifications, even with 1/16-inch material [Armstrong 2005].

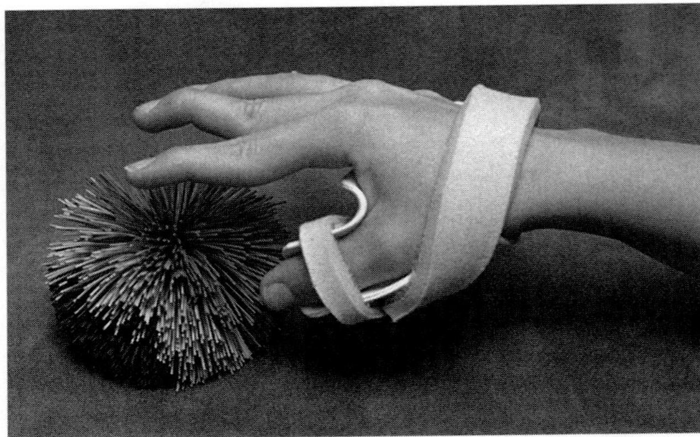

Figure 16-14 The thermoplastic thumb splint should allow the index and middle fingers to contact the tip of the thumb during grasp.

Precautions

The pressure to position the thumb should be directed below the MP of the thumb to prevent stress and possible dislocation of this joint. The splint should also fit snugly into the thumb web space. The therapist must watch for signs of skin irritation and pressure, a problem that is most likely to occur in the thumb web space or at the MCP joints of the fingers. In addition, the therapist should monitor the child for circulation and nerve compression problems caused by an ill-fitting splint.

Wearing Schedule

The child should wear the thumb splint while participating in occupations and activities that require grasp, manipulation, and release. Although it is primarily a functional splint, the thumb splint can also be worn during the day to prevent the opponens muscle from remaining in a fully shortened position. If contractures are a concern, the child may also need to wear a resting hand splint to provide further stretch of the thenar muscles.

The therapist should give the child opportunities to use the thumb actively, especially just after the splint is removed to take advantage of the elongation of the thenar muscles. As the child gains active control of thumb abduction, the therapist should reduce wearing time of the splint so that the child's own muscle strength increases. Activities should be planned while the splint is off that will provide opportunities to practice active thumb movements so that motor learning can occur.

Laboratory Exercise 16-3* Recognizing Problems in Splint Fabrication No. 3

What problems in splint fabrication are present in the following picture?

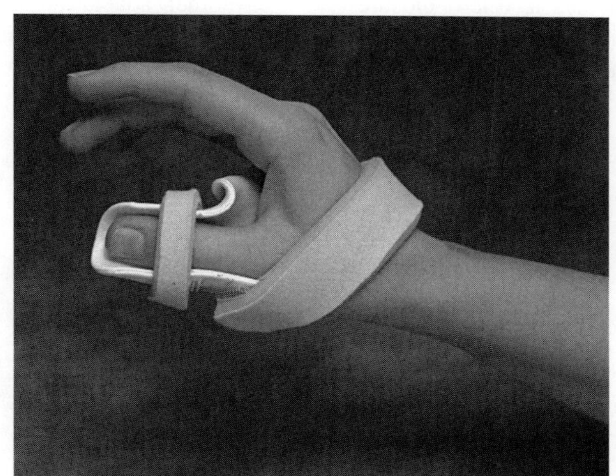

*See Appendix A for the answer key.

Soft Thumb Splints

Features

The soft thumb splint allows more movement of the intrinsic muscles of the hand and active movement of the thumb. The soft thumb splint restricts palmar adduction of the thumb but does not prevent it. The therapist can fabricate the splint from neoprene or purchase a prefabricated neoprene splint available in sizes ranging from infancy to youth (Figure 16-15). A thumb splint made of neoprene has the advantage of providing neutral warmth, which may have an inhibitory influence on hypertonicity.

If purchasing a neoprene thumb splint, the therapist should consider whether the splint has a Velcro closure. A thumb splint that slides over the fingers and thumb may be more difficult to apply. The tone and positioning splint (*www.sammonspreston.com*) is made of neoprene for thumb positioning and forearm supination. It provides constant low-level stretch to the forearm pronators.

Adaptations

Some children have difficulty maintaining an open thumb web space with a neoprene splint because of moderate to severe hypertonicity. The therapist can make a web space opener out of elastomer, thermoplastic pellets, or Permagum that is worn under the neoprene splint. Elastomer, thermoplastic pellets, and Permagum are described under the "Adaptations" section earlier in this chapter. Hogan and Uditsky [1998] provide a detailed description of the application of elastomer.

Another adaptation is the attachment of a crayon or marker to the neoprene thumb splint. The marker should be positioned so that the tip will contact the paper while the

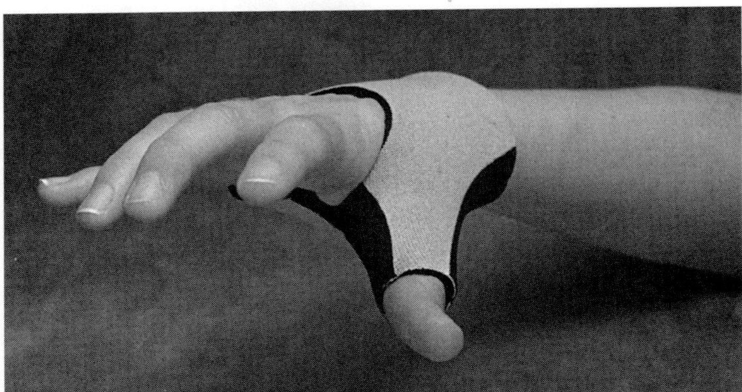

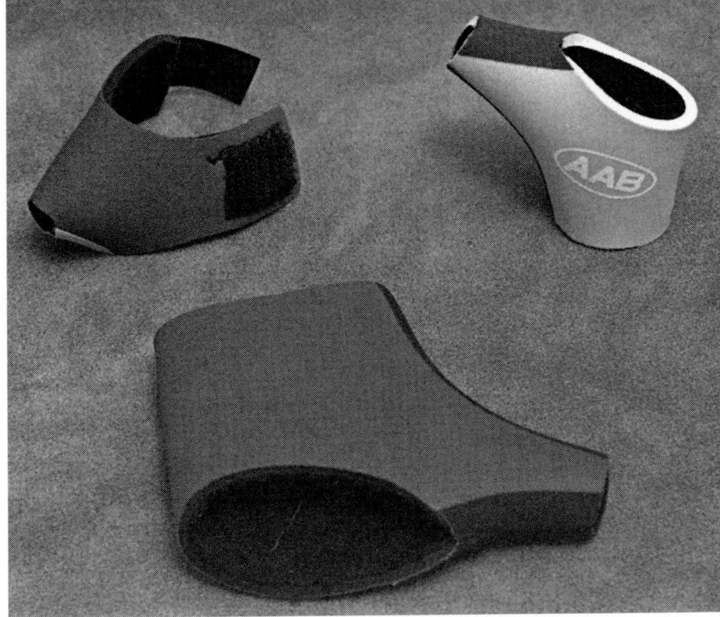

Figure 16-15 Neoprene thumb splints. (One supplier of such splints is the Benik Corporation, 11871 Silverdale Way Northwest, Suite 107, Silverdale, WA 98383 [1-800-442-8910].)

forearm is in neutral or slight supination (not pronated). A Velcro strap can secure the marker, and Sticky Tac (for mounting pictures on walls) or rubber bands above and below the attachment can keep the marker from sliding. A separate holder could also be made of thermoplastic material if necessary. One such adaptation to a Benik glove is described by Thompson [1999].

Process to Fabricate a Soft Thumb Splint with Thumb Loop

Materials

The therapist makes the wrist band and thumb loop from neoprene (Figure 16-16). The strap that forms the thumb loop should be wide enough to support the thumb but not so wide that it buckles or wrinkles in the thumb web space. The strap that forms the wrist band should be wide enough to secure the thumb loop, remain in place on the wrist, and distribute pressure. This strap should be long enough to form an adequate overlap to secure the Velcro. The therapist can determine the specific dimensions by placing strap material on the child's arm and hand to measure lengths and widths and determine the desired angle of pull.

Pattern

The therapist should make the wrist band to overlap on the volar side of the wrist. The length of the thumb loop should be the distance from the proximal edge of the wrist band, around the thumb, and back around to the point of origin.

Forming the Splint

Neoprene heat-sensitive tape can be used to bond the pieces because it is very difficult to sew. (With the proper needle, thread, and variable-tension sewing machine, sewing neoprene can be done.) First, the therapist should attach hook-and-loop Velcro to each end of the wrist band that is designed to overlap on the volar side of the forearm. To form the thumb loop, the therapist should attach one end of the thumb loop to the dorsal portion of the wrist band. The therapist then attaches loop Velcro to the free end of the thumb loop and hook Velcro to the dorsal portion of the wrist band (partially covering the origin of the thumb loop).

The thumb loop is directed up across the web space, around the thenar eminence, and pulled diagonally to attach to the dorsal portion of the wrist band. The amount of tension on the thumb loop and the attachment location of the free end to the wrist band influence the amount of radial and palmar abduction of the thumb. If the wrist band does not fit snugly the splint shifts distally on the wrist, thus reducing the amount of tension on the thumb loop. The wrist band must avoid circulatory restrictions.

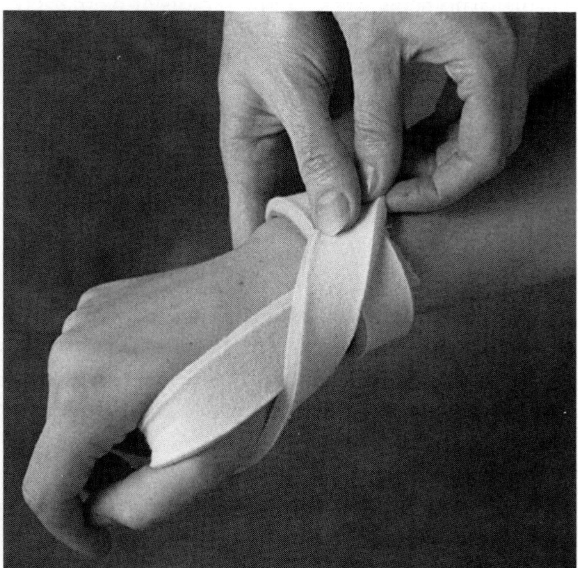

Figure 16-16 A soft thumb splint with a thumb loop.

Variations

Currie and Mendiola [1987] described a cortical thumb orthosis for children with spastic hemiplegic cerebral palsy. The splint was fabricated out of LTT, moleskin, Velcro, and super-glue. The LTT formed a ring around the base of the thumb and it was held in position using a Velcro strap.

Precautions and Wearing Schedule

The precautions and wearing schedule are similar to those for the thermoplastic thumb splint, although the soft thumb splint presents less danger of pressure-related problems because of the softer material. Care should be taken that the wrist band is not so tight it interferes with circulation. Persons applying the splint should be sure the thumb loop fits snugly into the web space with pressure against the thenar muscles.

If the thumb loop is applying pressure above the MP joint of the thumb, there is risk of deviating, hyperextending, or dislocating this joint. The therapist must also monitor the amount of tension on the thumb loop to prevent excess stress to the thumb MP joint. If the child is active and wears the splint often, it is likely to become soiled and worn. The splint then requires washing and eventual replacement.

Prefabricated Soft Thumb Splints

Several companies offer prefabricated soft thumb splints for children, such as the McKie thumb splints (*http://www.mckiesplints.com*), thumb splints by Benik Corporation (*www.benik.com/pediatrics.html*), and thumb splints by The Joe Cool Company (*www.joecoolco.com*).

The McKie thumb splint can be worn with or without a supinator strap. It is sized for children as young as 3 months of age, thus assisting young children develop a more normal grasp during the critical first year of life [McKie Splints 2006].

The McKie thumb splint is one of the very few splint designs that has been studied empirically. McKie [1998] used a multiple baseline technique to measure three types of grasp in four children with cerebral palsy, ages 24 to 42 months, when wearing the McKie thumb splint with supinator strap. The children were videotaped 15 times over a 10-week period. Videotapes were made pre- and during intervention and were rated by two independent raters using a modified version of the Erhardt Developmental Prehension Assessment.

Children were evaluated while grasping food items or developmentally appealing objects. Results showed that the means increased in every instance in the "splints on" phase. Furthermore, "the statistical analysis of mean differences across subjects should a significant improvement in grasp scores associated with using the splint" [McKie 1998, p. 42]. Differences between scores while wearing the splint and the nonsplint condition were analyzed using the Koehler-Levin nonparametric procedure. The differences were =.005 for the cylindrical and circumferential grasps and =.015 for the pincer grasp. This study used a well-conceived design, excellent implementation, and carefully planned data analysis, and thus is one of very few studies demonstrating the effectiveness of a thumb splint intervention with young children with cerebral palsy.

Serpentine Splint

The serpentine splint (Figure 16-17) is a hand-based splint to position the thumb out of palmar adduction (Hogan and Uditsky 1998). The serpentine splint allows the thumb to move within radial and palmar abduction for opposition. The splint may be used with children who have hypertonicity, hypotonicity, muscle weakness, or decreased ROM. Although its primary focus is on positioning the thumb, it has some inhibitory effect on finger flexion. The serpentine splint is often well received by children because it is less bulky and more appealing than a thermoplastic thumb opponens splint.

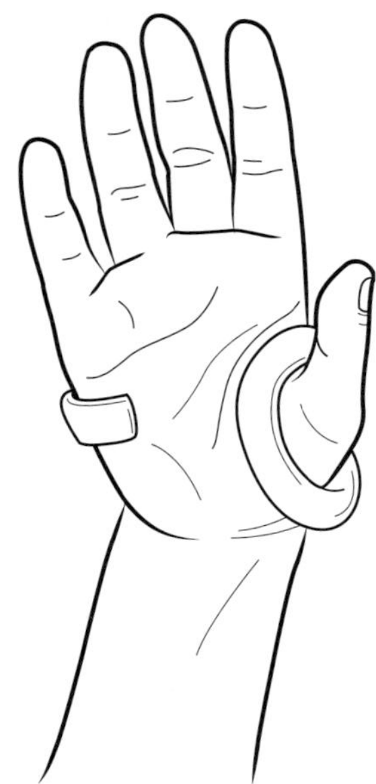

Figure 16-17 Serpentine splint.

Features

The serpentine splint is relatively easy to make. It is made of a spiral wrap, and its fabrication does not require a significant amount of skill. The thermoplastic material opens up the web space and provides good support to the thumb, while allowing for some mobility. The splint allows the child to move the thumb within a specified range.

Process to Fabricate a Serpentine Splint

Materials

A small rectangular piece of thermoplastic material may be used. A thermoplastic material with some stretch is helpful for making the tube. A pattern is not necessary. However, measuring to determine the length of the splint as described next is helpful.

Forming the Splint

Measure from the hypothenar area just below the distal palmar crease, across the dorsum of the hand just below the metacarpal joint, through the web space around the thenar eminence, and to the dorsum of the hand. Cut a piece of thermoplastic material one-half to three-fourths the length of the measured length just described and 1 inch in width. The width will vary according to the size of the child's hand and the size of the thumb web space. Heat the material and roll the piece into a smooth tube.

While the tube is still soft, wrap it around the hand, starting at the hypothenar area, below the distal palmar crease, and proceed to wrap as indicated with measuring for the tube (Figure 16-18). Straps may be added for additional support. However, typically this splint may be worn without straps. The splint should be labeled to orient the caregiver on how to don the splint. Once the splint has been removed, it can be perceptually confusing to reapply.

Wearing Schedule

This splint was designed to facilitate function. Thus, it should be worn during functional activities. It also serves to minimize thumb palmar adduction contractures and thus may be worn at intervals during the day and night.

Precautions

The splint should not exert excessive pressure into the hypothenar area that may cause skin irritation.

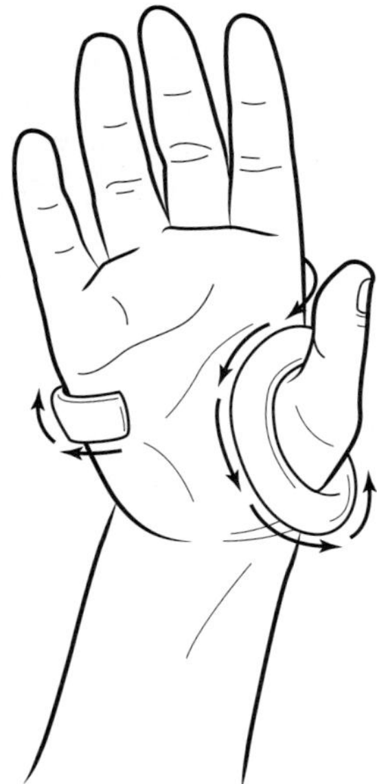

Figure 16-18 Wrapping the thermoplastic material for the serpentine splint.

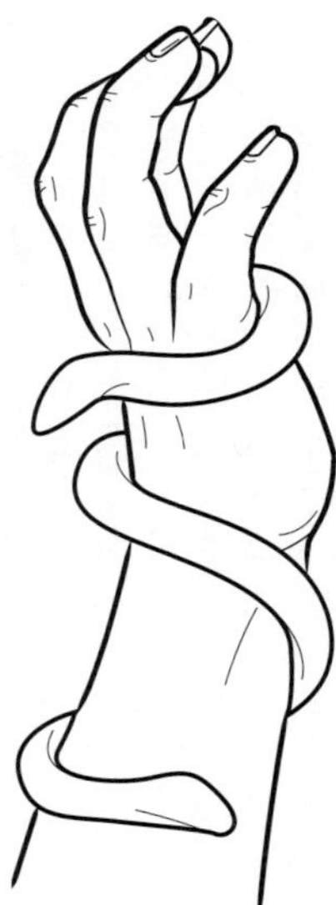

Figure 16-19 Serpentine splint for increased wrist stability.

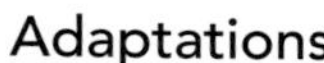

Adaptations

The splint may be fabricated to continue the spiral tube over the wrist and onto the forearm. This adaptation provides wrist support (Figure 16-19). The splint may also be fabricated with a flat piece of thermoplastic material. A flat piece can allow more molding and additional stabilization and support of the thumb.

Evidence-Based Research

Table 16-1 summarizes the studies done since 1990 that evaluated the effectiveness of hand splints in children.

Summary

This chapter described the use of several types of hand splint in the management of children who have developmental disabilities as a result of central nervous system damage, lower motor neuron injury, or upper extremity congenital malformations. Splint designs for a child differ from many of the adult designs. In addition to the dynamics of development, children differ from adults in the types of environments in which they live, learn, work, and play. Published case reports and research studies are needed to determine the effectiveness of pediatric splint designs and optimal wearing schedules. This will allow therapists to make decisions based on clinical reasoning and evidence from the literature.

Table 16-1 Studies Evaluating the Effectiveness of Hand Splints in Children

CITATION	DESIGN	NO. OF PARTICIPANTS	DESIGN	RESULTS	LIMITATIONS
Goodman G, Bazyk S (1991). The effects of a short thumb opponens splint on hand function in cerebral palsy: A single subject study. American Journal of Occupational Therapy 45:726–731.	AB single subject design	1	Dependent variables included active ROM, grip strength, pinch strength, scores on the Box and Block Test of manual Dexterity, the average number of 1-inch cubes stacked in three trials, and observation of qualitative aspects of prehension with the Erhardt Developmental Prehension Assessment using photographs. The independent variable was a volar short opponens splint made of low-temperature thermoplastic. The splint was worn for 6 hours during the day and all night for 4 weeks. The dependent variables were measured twice weekly for 4 weeks.	Data analysis was primarily through visual inspection of the slopes of the lines (computed from means) during baseline and treatment for each dependent variable. "A clinically significant change in slope was defined when the slope changed in a positive direction from the baseline phase to the treatment phase. We used clinical judgment in this analysis in considering the variable being measured, the units of change across phases, and the significance of the changes in relation to normative data, or how the change affects hand function. All of the dependent variables except palmar pinch and tip pinch were judged as being clinically significant for change in slope" (p. 729).	"Although none of the dependent variables showed stable baseline (stability was defined as 80% of the scores within 15% of the mean), the decision was made to begin treatment after the forth week due to the subject's limited availability" (p. 728–729). This compromises the AB design, which is already limited because it does not rule out the possibility of other factors that may have accounted for changes. Instrumentation limitations include lack of sensitivity to grip and pinch strength scores, lack of stability in ROM scores, lack of norms for 4-year-olds for the Box and Block Test, and difficulty conveying the need to go fast (speed) to the subject.
McKie A (1998). Effectiveness of a neoprene hand splint on grasp in young children with cerebral palsy. University of Wisconsin.	Multiple baseline across subjects	4	Dependent variables were three types of grasp (pincer, radial, and cylindrical), and the thumb splint with supinator strap was the independent variable. Measures of the dependent variables were derived from videotapes and rated by two independent raters. Raters scored each grasp pattern using a modified Erhartdt Developmental	Graphic analysis was done for the visual inspection of scores over time. Although baselines were generally stable, there was some variability between children and between some grasp patterns for a given child. In general, improvements of grasp occurred as soon as the splint was introduced. Means and standard deviations were calculated	The raters could not be blind to the conditions, as the child was wearing a splint during intervention. Compliance with splint wear was not monitored carefully enough and a power struggle between one child and his mother may have affected his wearing schedule. While generalizability is always limited with a

			Prehension Assessment (EDPA) during a therapy session. They had five attempts per type of grasp. Once the intervention phase began, children were to wear the splint for at least 8 waking hours per day. Children were randomly assigned to be child A, B, C, or D. Measurements were taken twice weekly over the next 10 weeks. There was 1 week of baseline for Child A.	for each type of grasp for each child (over the 10-week period) during the "no splint" and the "splint" phases. A nonparametric procedure (Koehler-Levin) was applied to the difference between the mean scores for each grasp. The two-tailed *p* value obtained for each type of grasp was .016 for pincer, .005 for cylindrical grasp, and .005 for circumferential grasp, indicating significantly higher scores on the modified EDPA during the splint condition.	single-subject design study, this study was an excellent example of a carefully planned, designed, implemented, and analyzed study. It invites replication.
Reid DT, Sochaniwskyj A. (1992). Influences of a hand positioning device on upper extremity control of children with cerebral palsy. International Journal of Rehabilitation Research 15:15–29.	Prospective outcome study	10	The independent variable was a hand positioning device designed by the first author. Based on its description, it sounds similar to the MacKinnon splint. It consisted of a hard post in the hand, with an elastic cord to provide dynamic action at the wrist. "The goal of the device was to facilitate a better hand position for enhancing upper-extremity movement patterns and functional use" (p. 18).	The results of paired *t*-tests comparing the differences between splint on and off did not reach statistical significance. Significance was defined as *p* value = 0.0001 due to the number of comparisons. Seven out of 10 subjects showed better scores with the splint on, and subjective analysis revealed an increase in quality of performance. Furthermore, with the splint on the subjects showed activation of the anterior deltoid first—whereas with the splint off the extensor carpi radialis was activated first. This indicates a pattern of muscle activation that is more normal with the splint on.	One limitation was the use of a small sample size with a parametric test for analysis. It is likely that there was variability among the children, which could also decrease the finding of significant results. Combining data into a single score for comparison may have resulted in losing some valuable information.

CASE STUDY 16-1*

Read the following scenario and answer the questions based on information in this chapter.

Aaron is a 10-year-old boy who has cerebral palsy and is moderately mentally handicapped. His family includes parents, a younger sister, and an older brother. Both parents work outside the home. There is supportive extended family, and parents have been actively involved in programming decisions. Aaron is in an educational program that includes special education, physical and occupational therapy, and speech and language therapy for augmentative communication. He has moderate to severely increased muscle tone in all four extremities, with reduced tone in his trunk. Tone in the extremities remains increased at night and tends to increase further during the day when he is excited, upset, or exerting effort. Aaron's functional use of his upper extremities is limited because of both increased tone and delayed development.

You have been Aaron's therapist for the past two years. Among team goals are increasing opportunities to play; improving his ability to indicate choices in the classroom, at home, and for purposes of communication by eye or hand pointing; and increasing his active participation in dressing and eating. Specific objectives include increasing speed and accuracy of reach of the right upper extremity, improving functional gross grasp and release of the right hand, and facilitating any active movement of the left upper extremity. You have selected neurodevelopmental treatment and biomechanical frames of reference to guide your intervention.

Splinting has not been a part of his program to date. Over the past year, however, you have noted a decrease in the amount of wrist and finger extension bilaterally—with more loss on the left side, which is more involved. You find that there is more resistance to passive movement of his hands and arms when you are assisting Aaron in functional activities. Aaron's left hand is frequently tightly fisted, with the thumb in the palm. His right hand is often loosely fisted, and although he can actively extend his fingers the right thumb remains in the palm. You are concerned about maintaining passive ROM but are hesitant to encumber his hands with splints that might interfere with the development of grasp and release on the right side.

You are modifying Aaron's treatment program to address your concern about increased tightness in the upper extremities. Which of the following options would you select, and why?

- *Option A:* Increase the frequency of passive and active ROM activities for both upper extremities and fabricate bilateral thermoplastic thumb splints.
- *Option B:* Fabricate resting hand splints for both hands and a thermoplastic thumb splint for the right hand. Recommend wearing both resting hand splints at night and the left splint periodically during the day (depending on status of ROM). Recommend wearing the right thumb splint during functional grasp activities.
- *Option C:* Fabricate resting hand splints for both upper extremities. Recommend that they be worn both at night and during the day except during scheduled activities involving reach, grasp, and release.
- *Option D:* Fabricate resting hand splints for both upper extremities. Because you are not sure the splints would be put on correctly at home, recommend that they be worn only during the day at school. Both splints will be removed during scheduled activities involving reach, grasp, and release.

____
____
____
____

*See Appendix A for the answer key.

CASE STUDY 16-2*

Read the following scenario and answer the question based on information in this chapter.

Maria is a 3-year-old girl with left hemiparesis resulting from an intracranial hemorrhage secondary to prematurity. She has full passive and active ROM in her left upper extremity, but there is mildly to moderately increased tone. She has a fairly well controlled reach with the left arm, but her hand tends to close before reaching the object she is trying to grasp. Her thumb is almost always adducted into her palm, which makes manipulation of objects difficult.

Maria can release objects with her left hand, but this is slow, and she frequently flexes her left wrist by pressing on it with her right hand to assist with finger extension. Which of the following orthotic interventions would you consider as a component to her overall treatment program?

- *Option A:* Fabricate a resting hand splint for the left upper extremity.
- *Option B:* Fabricate a standard wrist extension splint for the left wrist.
- *Option C:* Order or fabricate a neoprene thumb abduction splint for the left hand and consider adding a C bar made from elastomer.

____

____

____

____

*See Appendix A for the answer key.

REVIEW QUESTIONS

1. Describe five ways in which splinting a child with developmental disabilities is different that splinting an adult with an acquired impairment.
2. How would you prepare the room and the child to increase the probability of a successful splinting session?
3. How does an occupation-based assessment approach influence your decision to splint or to decide which type of splint to fabricate?
4. What factors should you consider in deciding on a wearing schedule for a resting hand splint for a child?
5. Describe the purpose of the McKie thumb splint.
6. When splinting the thumb into radial abduction or opposition, where should the bulk of the force be directed?
7. Name the pros and cons of using a rubber-based low temperature thermoplastic when splinting a child with significant spasticity.
8. What should you consider when reevaluating the effectiveness of a thumb splint for a child?
9. How would you provide instructions to parents, teachers, and other care providers to maximize correct application and usage of a splint?

References

Anderson LJ, Anderson JM (1988). Hand splinting for infants in the intensive care and special care nurseries. American Journal of Occupational Therapy 42(4):222-226.

AOTA (2002). Occupational therapy practice framework: Domain and process. American Journal of Occupational Therapy 56: 609-639.

Armstrong J (2005). Splinting the pediatric patient. In EE Fess, K Gettle, C Philips, R. Janson (eds.), *Hand and Upper Extremity Splinting: Principles and Methods, Second Edition*. St. Louis: Elsevier Mosby 480-516.

Banker BQ (1985). Neuropathologic aspects of arthrogryposis multiplex congenita. Clinical Orthopedics and Related Research 194:30-43.

Bar K (1994). The use of air bag splints to increase supination and pronation in the arm. American Journal of Occupational Therapy 48(8).

Bayne LG (1986). Hand assessment and management of arthrogryposis multiplex congenita. Clinical Orthopedics and Related Research 194:68-73.

Bell E, Graham HK (1995). A new material for splinting neonatal limb deformities. Journal of Pediatric Orthopedics 15(5).

Bellefeuille-Reid D (1984). Ideas exchange: Aid to independence, hand splint for cerebral palsied children. Canadian Journal of Occupational Therapy 51(1):37-39.

Carmick J (1997). Case report: Use of neuromuscular electrical stimulation and a dorsal wrist splint to improve the hand function of a child with spastic hemiparesis. Physical Therapy 77(6):661-671.

Casey CA, Kratz EJ (1988). Soft splinting with neoprene: The thumb abduction supinator splint. American Journal of Occupational Therapy 42(6):395-398.

Centers for Disease Control and Prevention: Developmental Disabilities, 2006. Retrieved September 12, 2006, from *www.cdc.gov/ncbddd/dd/default.htm*.

Collins LF (1996). Splinting survey results. OT Practice 42-44.

Currie DM, Mendiola A (1987). Cortical thumb orthosis for children with spastic hemiplegic cerebral palsy. Archives of Physical Medicine and Rehabilitation 68:214-216.

Donohoe M (2006). Arthrogryposis multiplex congenita. In SK Campbell, R Palisono, DW Vander Linden (eds.), *Physical Therapy for Children*. Philadelphia: Saunders 381-400.

Duff SV, Charles J (2004). Enhancing prehension in infants and children: Fostering neuromotor strategies. Physical and Occupational Therapy in Pediatrics 24:129-172.

Exner CE (2005). Development of hand skills. In J Case-Smith (ed.), *Occupational Therapy for Children, Fifth Edition*. St. Louis: Elsevier Mosby 347-350.

Exner CE, Bonder BR (1983). Comparative effects of three hand splints on bilateral hand use, grasp, and arm-hand posture in hemiplegic children: A pilot study. Occupational Therapy Journal of Research 3(2):75-92.

Flegle J, Leibowitz JM (1988). Improvement in grasp skill in children with hemiplegia with the MacKinnon splint. Research in Developmental Disabilities 9(2):145-151.

Goodman G, Bazyk S (1991). The effects of a short thumb opponens splint on hand function in cerebral palsy: A single subject study. American Journal of Occupational Therapy 45(8):726-731.

Granhaug KB (2006). Splinting the upper extremity of a child. In A Henderson, C Pehoski (eds.), *Hand Function in the Child: Foundations for Remediation, Second Edition*. St. Louis: Mosby Elsevier 401-431.

Hill SG (1988). Current trends in upper extremity splinting. In R Boehme (ed.), *Improving Upper Body Control*. Tucson: Therapy Skill Builders 131-164.

Hogan L, Uditsky T (1998). *Pediatric Splinting: Selection, Fabrication and Clinical Application of Upper Extremity Splints*. San Antonio: Therapy Skill Builders.

Hunter JG (2005). The neonatal intensive care unit. In J Case-Smith (ed.), *Occupational Therapy for Children, Fifth Edition*. St. Louis: Elsevier Mosby 688-770.

Kamil NI, Correia AM (1990). A dynamic elbow flexion splint for an infant with arthrogryposis. American Journal of Occupational Therapy 44(5):460-461.

Kinghorn J, Roberts G (1996). The effect of an inhibitive weight-being splint on tone and function: A single case study. American Journal of Occupational Therapy 50:807-815.

Lindholm L (1986). Weight bearing hand splint: A method of managing upper extremity spasticity. Physical Therapy Forum 5(3).

McClure PW, Blackburn LG, Dusold C (1994). The use of splints in the treatment of joint stiffness: Biological rationale and an algorithm for making clinical decisions. Physical Therapy 74(12): 1101-1107.

McKee P (2004). Orthoses as enablers of occupation: Client-centered splinting for better outcomes. Canadian Journal of Occupational Therapy 71:306-314.

McKie A (1998). Effectiveness of a neoprene hand splint on grasp in young children with cerebral palsy. Master's Thesis. University of Wisconsin.

McKie Splints: Features, 2006. Retrieved September 12, 2006, from *www.mckiesplints.com/features.htm*.

Palmer PM, MacEwen GD, Bowen JR, Mathews PA (1985). Passive motion therapy for infants with arthrogryposis. Clinical Orthopedics and Related Research 194:54-59.

Reid DT, Sochaniwskyj A (1992). Influences of a hand position device on upper-extremity control of children with cerebral palsy. Int J Rehabil Res 15(1):15-29.

Rogers SL (2005). Common conditions that influence children's participation. In J Case-Smith (ed.), *Occupational Therapy for Children, Fifth Edition*. St. Louis: Elsevier Mosby 160-215.

Sala DA, Rosenthal DL, Grant AD (1996). Early treatment of an infant with severe arthrogryposis. Physical and Occupational Therapy in Pediatrics 16(3):73-89.

Schoen S, Anderson J (1999). Neurodevelopmental treatment frame of reference. In P Kramer, J Hinojosa (eds.), *Frames of Reference for Pediatric Occupational Therapy, Second Edition*. Philadelphia: Lippincott Williams & Wilkins 83-118.

Sheridan RL, Baryza MJ, Pessina MA, et al. (1999). Acute hand burns in children: Management and long term outcome based on a 10-year experience with 698 injured hands. Annals of Surgery 229(4):558-564.

Snook J (1979). Spasticity reduction splint. American Journal of Occupational Therapy 33(10).

Staley M, Richard R, Billmire D, Warden G for the PT/OT Forum (1997). Head/face/neck burns: Therapist considerations for the pediatric patient. Journal of Burn Care and Rehabilitation 18(2): 164-171.

Stern EB, Callinan N, Hank M, Lewis EJ, Schousboe JT, Ytterberg SR (1998). Neoprene splinting: Dermatological issues. American Journal of Occupational Therapy 52(7):573-578.

Thompson T (1999). "La Victoria" makes drawing a reality for one little girl. Advance for Occupational Therapy Practitioners 12(14):26.

Tona JL, Schneck CM (1993). The efficacy of upper extremity inhibitive casting: A single-subject pilot study. American Journal of Occupational Therapy 47(10):901-910.

Watanabe T (2004). The role of therapy in spasticity management. American Journal of Physical Medicine and Rehabilitation 83:S45-S49.

Williams PF (1985). Management of upper limb problems in arthrogryposis. Clinical Orthopedics and Related Research 194:60-67.

Wilton J (2003). Casting, splinting, and physical and occupational therapy of hand deformity and dysfunction in cerebral palsy. Hand Clinics 19:573-584.

Yamamoto MS (1993). Developmental disabilities. In RA Hansen, B Atchison (eds.), *Conditions in Occupational Therapy*. Baltimore, MD: Williams & Wilkins 52-78.

UNIT THREE

Topics Related to Splinting

CHAPTER 17

Lower Extremity Orthotics

Deanna J. Fish, MS, CPO
Michael Lohman, MEd, OTR/L, CO
Dulcey G. Lima, OTR/L, CO
Karyn Kessler, OTR/L

Key Terms

Basic biomechanical principles
Orthotic design principles
Orthotic terminology
Orthotic treatment objectives

Chapter Objectives

1. Describe the general purposes and basic functions of lower extremity orthoses.
2. Understand normal gait and pathological gait.
3. Describe the biomechanical principles of lower extremity orthoses.
4. Describe the basic design principles of lower extremity orthoses.
5. Understand the relationship between structure (i.e., anatomic alignment) and function (i.e., walking ability).
6. Understand basic terminology used in lower extremity orthotic prescriptions.
7. Describe various components and materials commonly used in the fabrication of lower extremity orthoses.
8. Recognize commonly prescribed foot, ankle/foot, knee, knee/ankle/foot, hip, and hip/knee/ankle foot orthoses.
9. Outline the role of the occupational therapist in the orthotic treatment program.
10. Summarize short- and long-term orthotic treatment objectives.
11. Understand the importance of a multidisciplinary team approach.

Role of the Occupational Therapist

Historically, occupational therapy has primarily been involved in the provision of upper extremity orthotic services. However, with increased emphasis on the multidisciplinary team approach the scope of occupational therapy practice has expanded to include lower extremity orthotic care as it impacts the acquisition of occupational performance. It is important to delineate the role of occupational therapy in lower extremity, as opposed to upper extremity, orthotic treatment programs. In upper extremity orthotic practice, occupational therapists typically design, fabricate, fit, and supervise functional training. In effect, occupational therapists provide seamless delivery of orthotic services. Occupational therapists manage every stage of the upper extremity orthotic delivery process and are therefore able to adapt each step to individual needs and specific functional requirements.

In contrast, occupational therapists are not direct providers of lower extremity orthotic care. Typically, orthotists design, fabricate, and fit lower extremity orthotic devices and physical therapists provide functional gait training with lower extremity orthoses. Occupational therapy collaborates in the delivery of lower extremity orthotic services to ensure that the orthosis is designed to facilitate occupational performance at each stage of development.

Any given lower extremity device may address a biomechanical goal such as providing a stable base of support. The device may also address a functional gait training goal such as decreasing knee hyperextension during stance. However, if the orthosis does not also address the occupational performance goal (such as donning and doffing the device independently) the person may discard the orthosis. It is the occupational therapist's role to anticipate such performance issues and initiate effective intervention before design and fabrication decisions have been completed. Occupational therapy clinicians are clearly the strongest advocate of advancing occupational performance goals.

Biomechanical and gait considerations are irrelevant when the lower extremity orthosis is rejected because it is too difficult to apply, interferes with activities of daily living, or is designed without consideration of individual strengths and weaknesses. With pediatrics, lower extremity orthoses can impact occupational performance differently and may be focused on the development of balance and equilibrium as a foundation for skill development and motor milestone acquisition. A lower extremity orthosis to position the hips may provide a stable base of support and help the child sit for longer periods of time to facilitate independent eating or writing skills. The same orthosis may not provide sufficient mobility for crawling and transitional movements unless it is designed to address these functional skills as well.

This chapter does not describe specific criteria used to design and fabricate orthoses, as do other chapters in this text. As the orthotist exclusively manages the fabrication process in lower extremity orthotics, it is not necessary or appropriate to cover this topic. However, if the occupational therapist is to be involved as part of the clinical team making decisions regarding lower extremity orthotics he or she must have a working knowledge of basic principles and terminology used by both physical therapists and orthotists in the decision-making process. This chapter is designed to provide a basic understanding and is not intended to be definitive or comprehensive in nature. Those with an interest in developing further expertise in this area should invest in additional educational seminars and reference texts.

Definition and Historical Perspective

An orthosis is generally identified as any orthopedic device that improves the function or structure of the body. Evidence of orthotic applications has been found as early as 2750 BCE [Bunch and Keagy 1976]. Excavation sites have uncovered mummies with various splints still intact. Historically, increased focus and advancements in orthotic design have centered on civil strife and periods of war. Today, continued advancements in the ever-expanding world of technology promote the development of new orthotic designs, materials, and components.

Purpose and Basic Function

The four basic functions of an orthosis include support and alignment, prevention or correction of deformity, substitution for or assistance of function, and reduction of pain. An orthosis is designed to address any one or all of these basic functions. Additional indications for lower extremity orthotic intervention are listed in Box 17-1.

General Applications

In the lower extremity, orthoses are prescribed for a variety of reasons and may be used on a temporary or permanent basis. For example, knee orthoses are often prescribed postoperatively to restrict joint motion while healing of soft-tissue structures occurs. After the rehabilitation phase, the knee orthoses are then either discontinued or used only during periods of increased physical activity.

In contrast, the young child with a diagnosis of spina bifida may require extensive orthotic designs to enable him or her to stand and walk. Such systems will be adjusted and replaced with growth but will play an ongoing role in maximizing and maintaining the child's ambulation skills. In both instances, orthoses play a critical role in maintaining the structural integrity of the anatomy and the functional ability of the person. The relationship between structure and function is discussed in detail later in the chapter.

Box 17-1 Indications for Lower Extremity Orthotic Intervention

- Relief of muscle and/or joint pain
- Rest or immobilization of affected joint(s)
- Promotion of joint protection
- Support of weakened muscles
- Contracture management
- Support of body weight
- Reduction of axial loading
- Correction or prevention of joint deformities
- Limitation, restriction, or enhancement of available joint motion
- Control of planar motion
- Joint instability
- Control of undesirable or ineffective motions
- Improvement of motor coordination and joint proprioception
- Enhancement of normal movement patterns
- Suppression of spasticity
- Improvement of body alignment
- Improvement of activities of daily living (ADL)
- Improvement of instrumental activities of daily living (IADL)
- Reduction of metabolic cost of walking
- Improvement of efficiency of movement patterns
- Transfer of movement from one joint to another (e.g., tenodesis)
- Promotion of circulation and tissue recovery (e.g., fractures)
- Improvement of functional ADL

Data from Bunch WH, Keagy RD (1976). *Principles of Orthotic Treatment*. St. Louis: Mosby; Kraft GH, Lehmann, JF (eds.), (1992). Physical Medicine and Rehabilitation Clinics of North America 3(1); and Braddom RL (1996). *Physical Medicine and Rehabilitation*. Philadelphia: W. B. Saunders.

Basic Biomechanical Principles

Individual Evaluation

Prescription criteria for lower limb orthoses are based on a thorough pre-orthotic evaluation of the person. Components of this evaluation process are listed in Box 17-2. Observational gait assessment (OGA) is performed with the

Box 17-2 Pre-orthotic Individual Evaluation Procedures for Lower Extremity Orthotic Intervention

- Personal history
- Medical background (i.e., current medications, previous orthopedic procedures, and so on)
- Functional manual muscle test
- Grading of spasticity
- Range of available joint motion(s)
- Static and dynamic alignment of joints
- Functional deficits
- Contractures
- Individual goals and expectations
- Current and previous orthotic use
- Exercise/therapy program
- Neurologic profile
- Sitting and standing balance
- Sitting and standing posture
- Sensation (i.e., light pressure, deep touch)
- Proprioception
- Daily activity level (current and anticipated)
- Specific functional challenges
- Cognitive abilities
- Potential for progression of joint deformities
- Observational gait assessment
- Areas of pain/discomfort

Data from Fish DJ, Kosta CS, Dufek JS (1997). Functional Walking: An EPIC Approach. Oregon Orthotic System course manual, unpublished manuscript.

person wearing shorts and a snug T-shirt. This allows the observer to relate the function of the lower limbs to the stability of the upper torso. Walking trials are performed with the person barefoot and then with any existing orthosis or ambulation aids being used. Biomechanics laboratories can offer a detailed analysis to assist in evaluation of the person's gait deviations with the use of force plates and high-speed cameras. However, these facilities are sparse and the cost of such a procedure is often prohibitive. Individual goals, motivation, and available social support contribute to the success of any orthotic program.

Walking Requirements

Walking is a complex series of muscular interactions that manipulate the skeletal structures in specific sequential and reciprocal patterns. As a result, normal walking occurs in a mechanically effective and energy-efficient manner (Figure 17-1). The gait cycle consists of heel-strike to ipsilateral heel-strike of the same limb, covering periods of double and single limb support as well as swing. The gait cycle can be further divided into eight specific phases: initial contact, loading response, mid-stance, terminal stance, pre-swing, initial swing, mid-swing, and terminal swing [Perry 1992]. Critical events occur at each phase of gait to enhance stability and encourage functional mobility. Extensive texts are available on this topic, which is not the focus of this chapter. Therefore, a brief summary is presented in the following as it relates to lower extremity orthotic treatment programs.

Normal Gait

Limb stability is one of two basic components of walking. Each lower limb, in turn, must be effectively aligned and controlled to accept the transfer of body weight, support and balance the entire body mass independently, and then transfer the weight to the contralateral limb as it comes in contact with the ground. Sixty percent of the gait cycle is spent in periods of single and double limb support, when one and then both lower limbs support the body weight. Limb advancement is the second basic component serving to help translate the body mass forward and is dependent on the support provided by the contralateral stance limb. Swing phase accounts

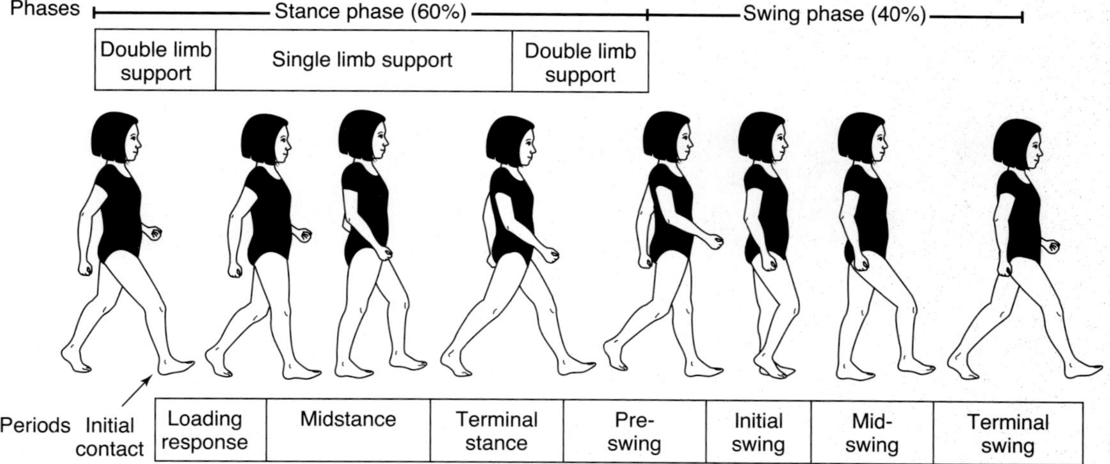

Figure 17-1 Gait cycle: normal gait. The normal gait cycle consists of swing and stance phases, with periods of double and single limb support.

for 40% of the gait cycle. These actions occur reciprocally while maintaining forward momentum of the body through space with minimal metabolic costs.

Although most lower limb joint motions occur in the sagittal plane (i.e., hip and knee flexion and extension, ankle dorsiflexion and plantar flexion), motions also occur in the coronal and transverse planes. This serves to streamline the gait cycle and limit the translation of the center of mass (COM) to minimal vertical and horizontal excursions. As a result, a decrease in the displacement of the top-heavy trunk segment is evidenced and energy is conserved. The most efficient gait pattern for each individual occurs at a self-selected walking speed, when the person is trying neither to increase nor decrease normal walking speed.

Pathologic Gait

A pathologic gait pattern often develops secondary to neuromuscular deficits, joint instabilities, pain, disease processes, congenital involvements, and many other conditions (Figure 17-2). Excessive or insufficient joint motions occur and lead to exaggerated or inhibited movements of the body throughout the gait cycle. The normal walking speed of the individual will also be affected. Increases in energy costs tend to promote decreased walking speeds and further increases in energy costs.

Clinical training in observational gait assessment ensures the identification of all pathologic gait deviations in need of orthotic intervention. Commonly observed deviations include drop-foot, hyperextension or genu (knee) recurvatum, lateral trunk lean, anterior knee instability, genu varum or genu valgum, pelvic instability, increased lordosis, tone-induced equinovarus, pes planus, and so on. Observational gait assessment also evaluates many factors, such as overall symmetry, step lengths, loading patterns, width of the base of support, weight transfer, terminal stance stability, swing phase function, and trunk alignment, just to name a few. Other pathologic factors include joint contractures, muscle weakness, and disturbed motor control programs.

Functional Motions (Compensations)

Most persons acquire a pattern of walking that serves a *functional* rather than an *efficient* purpose, when compared with normal parameters. For example, when dorsiflexion capabilities at the ankle are lost, a person experiences a drop-foot condition. The toes drag on the ground during swing phase and contact first with the ground during the loading phase. Persons will adopt a gait pattern that provides ground clearance for the plantar-flexed foot during swing phase. This is accomplished by excessive hip and knee flexion (i.e., steppage gait) or by excessive hip circumduction (Figure 17-3). Both of these compensations achieve a functional result; specifically, ground clearance during swing phase. Although these compensations occur without conscious thought and may allow for ambulation, the need for an orthosis is supported by increased energy costs and safety concerns.

Dysfunctional Motions (Detractors)

Although such clinically observable gait deviations detract from effective and efficient gait, some dysfunctional motions are more notably difficult to compensate for in a functional manner. Hyperextension (or "back knee") is such a condition. This occurs as the knee moves in the posterior direction

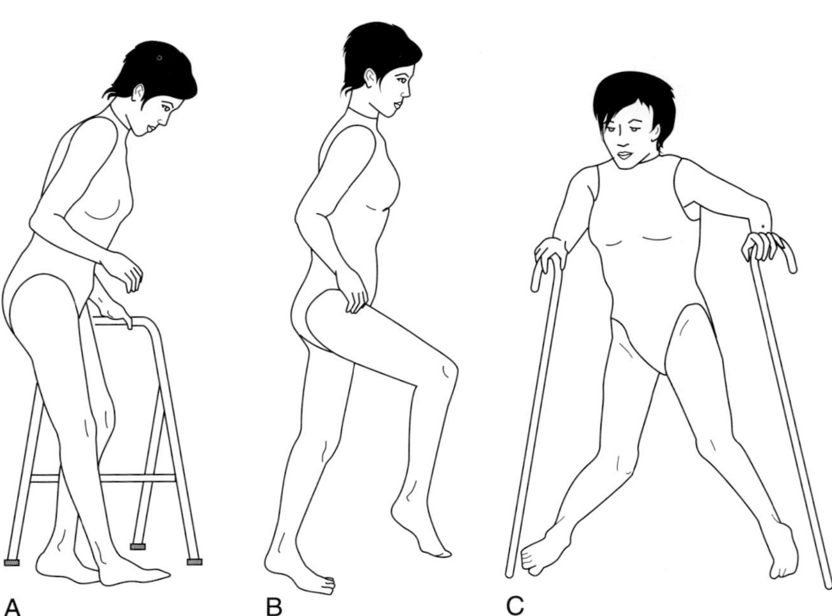

Figure 17-2 Pathological gait: various individual profiles: (A) anterior knee instability with forward trunk lean, (B) steppage gait with excessive hip and knee flexion to compensate for drop-foot, and (C) crouched gait.

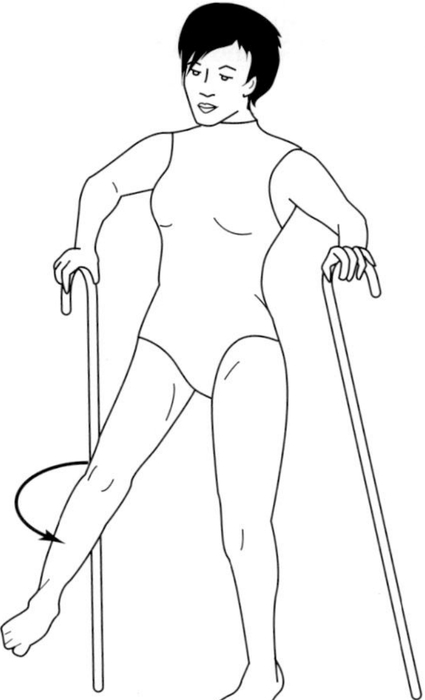

Figure 17-3 Functional motions (compensations): hip circumduction. Circumduction is a functional hip joint compensation for a drop-foot condition. The hip is externally rotated and abducted, moving through an arc from initial to terminal swing.

during mid-stance, often secondary to weakness of the quadriceps and/or posterior calf muscle groups. Without hyperextension, the person experiences uncontrolled knee flexion and collapse.

As a side note, a plantar-flexion contracture is often noted upon examination as either the primary cause or result of the posterior knee moment and serves to limit tibial advancement over the base of support during stance phase. Genu recurvatum (Figure 17-4) is the long-standing result of hyperextension, when permanent damage to the posterior soft-tissue structures of the knee has occurred. This gait disruption affects the efficiency of gait because the lower extremity is forced posteriorly as the body mass is attempting to move anteriorly over the limb. Working at odds, large truncal deviations are noted and energy costs increase dramatically.

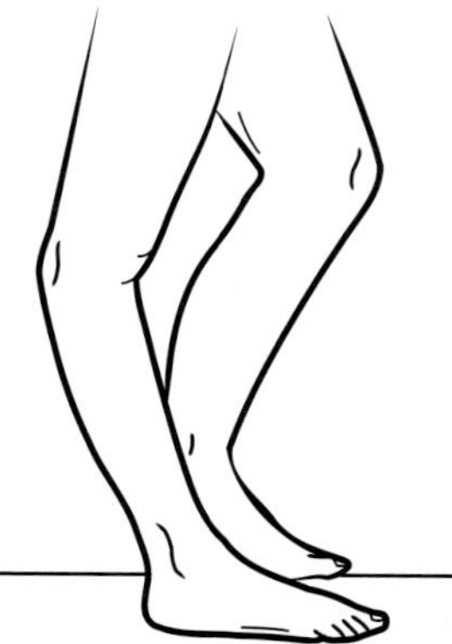

Figure 17-4 Dysfunctional motions (detractors): genu recurvatum. Genu recurvatum is a progressive deformity identified from initial contact through terminal stance. The knee joint alignment is angled posteriorly, serving to disrupt forward momentum and functionally shorten the limb during loading.

Orthotic Design Principles

General Concepts

Principles of lower extremity orthotic design consider the interaction of anatomic and mechanical structures. The mid-tarsal, subtalar, talocrural, knee, and hip joints are evaluated in regard to the individual joint alignment and range of motion (ROM), as well as the interaction of these five major joints during the task of walking. Application of mechanical joints can serve to encourage, restrict, or eliminate potential joint motion.

Considerations of joint position, relief of pain, restriction of motion, or relief of weight bearing relate to the effect of the application of forces. Force is applied to effect an angular change at a specific joint in one or more of the three planes of motion. As a result, care is taken to apply forces over pressure-tolerant areas (i.e., soft tissue or adequate surface areas), with relief of force over pressure-sensitive areas (i.e., bony prominences). Mechanical leverage is another important concept, as specific force is increased with shorter lever arms and decreased with longer lever arms. Properly applied forces over adequate surface area with long lever arms exert less force for effective joint control than do orthotic designs with short mechanical lever arms.

Additional orthotic considerations include weight, cost, adjustability, ease of application, cosmesis (appearance), maintenance, and the necessary training required to ensure successful outcomes [Bunch et al. 1985, Kottke and Lehmann 1990]. These factors should be discussed thoroughly by the rehabilitation team and the individual before a final orthotic design is determined.

Relationship of Structure and Function

Structure and function are two important concepts to keep in mind during the individual evaluation and orthotic design processes. Structure relates to stability by realigning or maintaining the skeletal structure in a mechanically effective position through the application of externally applied forces. Function relates to mobility with controlled motion at anatomic joint structures. Both concepts have unique requirements and yet are extremely interdependent. Structural stability can eliminate function, just as altered function can lead to deterioration of joint structures. Compromises based on unique personal attributes are identified and addressed by the rehabilitation team.

Joint Alignment

All five major joints (mid-tarsal, subtalar, talocrural, knee, and hip) of the lower extremities exhibit triplanar joint

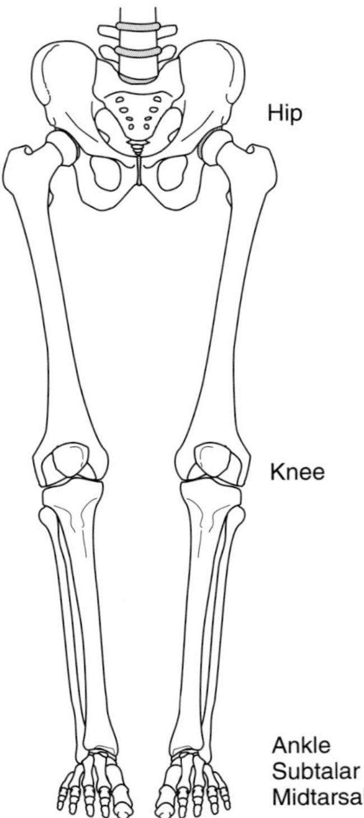

Figure 17-5 Five major joints of the lower extremity. The hip, knee, ankle, subtalar, and mid-tarsal joints work in unison to produce a streamlined and energy-efficient gait.

motion (Figure 17-5). Still, they work together during walking to allow progression of the body in the desired direction. These motions occur largely through the sagittal plane, specifically hip and knee flexion with ankle dorsiflexion and plantar flexion. Alignment of skeletal joint levers is a critical component of efficient and effective ambulation.

Mechanically speaking, the foot can be divided into anterior and posterior portions, with the mid-tarsal joint serving as the connection (Figure 17-6). Through mechanical leverage, the long anterior lever is used to control ankle dorsiflexion, knee flexion, and hip flexion. The short posterior lever limits ankle plantar flexion, knee extension, and hip extension. Medially, the first metatarsal ray and the medial heel act as medial levers to support proximal joint structures and prevent subtalar valgus and genu valgum, limit hip adduction, and discourage excessive internal rotation of the entire limb. The fifth metatarsal ray and the lateral heel serve as lateral levers to prevent subtalar varus and genu varum, limit hip abduction, and discourage excessive external rotation of the entire limb.

Joint Stability

The base levers of the foot are similar in concept to the foundation of a house. A square and true foundation always provides the best support. An unstable base of support has the potential to create larger moments of instability at proximal joint structures. For example, a pronated (flat) foot has clinically observable features: hind-foot valgus, mid-foot collapse,

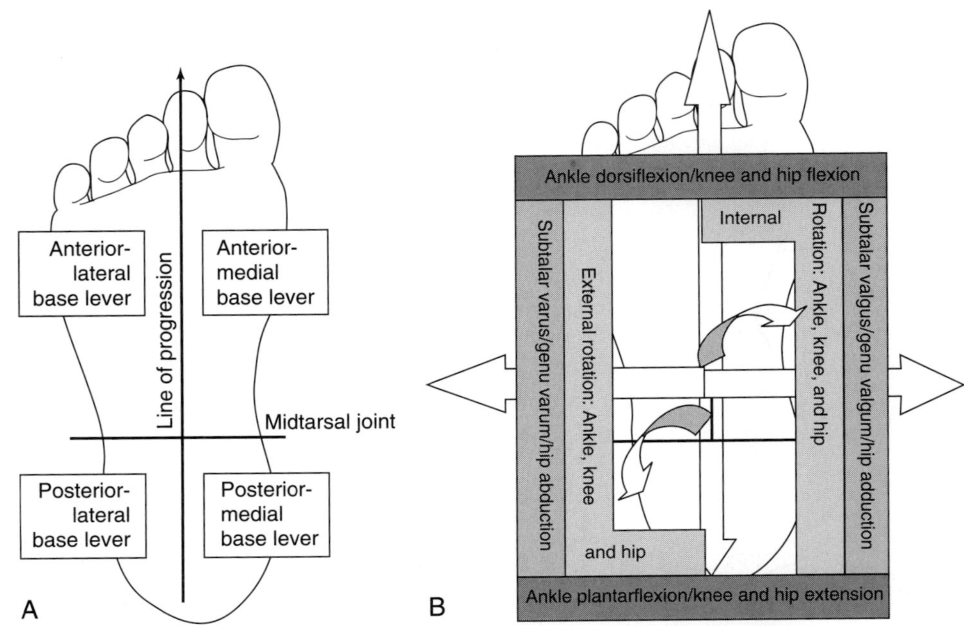

Figure 17-6 (A) The foot can be divided into anterior and posterior base levers, each with a medial and lateral component. (B) Anterior base levers resist dorsiflexion and flexion, posterior base levers resist plantar flexion and extension, medial base levers resist subtalar valgus and knee valgum, and lateral base levers resist subtalar varus and genu valgum. Anterior-medial base levers resist internal rotation and posterior-lateral base levers resist external rotation.

and forefoot abduction. Mechanical assessment reveals a loss of the anterior-medial forefoot and posterior-medial hind-foot base levers. Therefore, the ankle joint is subjected to excessive dorsiflexion, internal rotation, and medial displacement; the knee is subjected to flexion, internal rotation, and valgum moments; and the hip joint is subjected to flexion, internal rotation, and adduction moments. An effective orthotic design that returns joint stability and proper alignment to the mid-tarsal and subtalar joints will serve to effect positive alignment changes at the ankle, knee, and hip joints.

Three-point Force Systems

As mentioned earlier, the application of force is used to effect angular changes at deviated joints. A three-point force system (Figure 17-7) effects an alignment change with two forces working in opposition to a counterforce (or fulcrum). The counterforce is positioned on the convex side of the joint deviation, close to the joint requiring an angular change. The opposite two forces are positioned proximal and distal to the counterforce, on the side of the joint concavity. The greater the linear distance between opposing forces the less pressure is required to maintain the angular correction.

Components and Materials

A wide variety of mechanical joints and materials are now used in orthotic designs. Mechanical joints are designed to mimic anatomic joint function, and care is taken to approximate anatomic joint alignments. Orthotic joints are manufactured in a variety of metals and plastics, with unique design features to control available ROM. Special strapping is often used to enhance alignment and control.

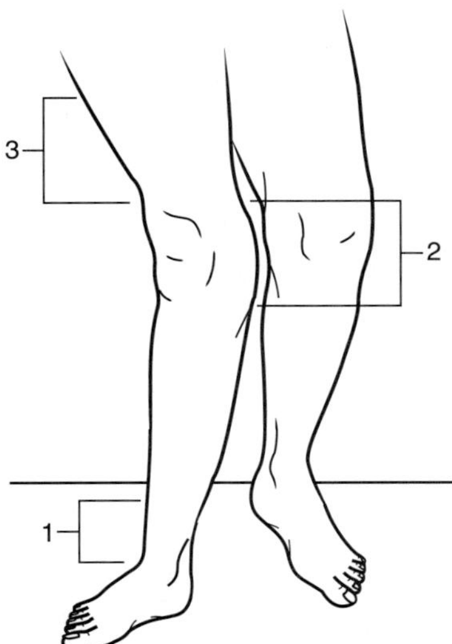

Figure 17-7 Three-point force system to correct genu valgum. Pictured is a three-point force system applied in the coronal plane to effect an angular change at the knee joint (i.e., resistance to genu valgum).

Material selection is based on the desired design characteristics of the orthosis. Material properties range from extremely flexible to extremely rigid. Different types of foam padding are available in variable thickness, density, and durability to meet different mechanical design requirements. Keep in mind that an orthosis is a mechanical device that requires periodic checkup and maintenance to ensure proper mechanical functioning and to extend the longevity of the orthosis.

There are a number of questions that need to be answered before selecting the appropriate material. Does the material need to be flexible or rigid? Lightweight or heavy duty? Inexpensive? Temporary or permanent? What is the length of time required for preparation? Can the materials be easily cleaned? Can the material be maintained easily? Can the material allow for easy donning and doffing? Although all concerns are usually not met at the first orthotic fitting, much frustration on the part of the team and the client can be avoided if all are involved early in the process and share the same end-product outcome goals.

Material selection is based on the desired design characteristics of the orthosis. Material properties range from flexible to rigid, lightweight to heavy-duty, inexpensive to costly, limited to prolonged durability, and minimal to extensive fabrication preparation. Each of these factors must meet the client's anticipated activity level as well as demands of aesthetics, ease of cleaning, maintenance, and don/doff procedures. These various, at times conflicting, considerations compound the difficulty of clinical decision making in orthotic selection. Appropriate choices lead to acceptance and independence, whereas unwise selection may cause not only rejection of a device but unintended injury to the client.

The process of material selection weighs each of these factors in consideration of the client outcome or goal. The selection process can be relatively apparent. If the desired outcome is to gradually increase active motion of a postoperative knee joint over several weeks, the clinician selects an orthosis that is lightweight, inexpensive, adjustable, of limited durability, and easily fabricated. If, however, the desired outcome is to protect the same knee joint from ACL tear reoccurrence during a contact sport such as soccer the material selection process focuses on an orthosis that is highly durable, of rigid construction (probably involving extensive/costly fabrication), very low profile in design to minimize interference during the activity, easily cleanable to reduce skin irritation, and cosmetically appealing (as the orthosis would be highly visible).

More challenging material selection processes involve competition between factors. The client may desire a lightweight, flexible, inexpensive, easily fabricated device to reduce foot drop. These material selections, however, will not address the underlying problems of a severe osteoarthritic ankle, which may necessitate selections the client finds unacceptable. At times, material selection focuses on a single factor that supercedes all other considerations. To reduce hypertrophic scarring that accompanies severe burns, it is essential that a continuous hard smooth surface be applied 24/7 to achieve the clinical outcome of scar prevention/reduction.

All other factors of comfort, aesthetics, ease of don/doff procedures, fabrication procedures, and costs are subservient to the factor of material texture in the determination of the clinical outcome. For some conditions, hand function is severely limited. No matter how effective any knee/ankle/foot orthosis (KAFO) functions are in improving gait, if the client is unable to don/doff the device efficiently and consistently it will be rejected as not practical for their daily routine. It is imperative that therapists communicate their concerns during the material selection process, during the orthotic evaluation.

Orthotic Classifications

Three main types of orthoses are available. Prefabricated (or over-the-counter) designs are manufactured in a variety of sizes and offer immediate application, reduced cost, and simplicity. They are generally used as evaluative tools or for temporary use because the fit/function and the durability of these products are limited. Custom-fitted designs require a more involved measurement and fitting procedures to obtain better fit and function. Used for moderate involvements, custom-fitted designs are prescribed on both a temporary and definitive basis. Custom orthotic designs are the most sophisticated, requiring extensive measurements, castings, fitting, and follow-up procedures from a skilled orthotist. Most often prescribed on a permanent (or definitive) basis, a custom orthotic design is made to specifically fit the individual and is therefore more expensive to manufacture. The result, however, is a more intimately fitting device with greater joint control, limb stability, and improved function and mobility.

Another aspect to consider is whether a static or dynamic splint is warranted. The most common uses of static splints are (1) to support joints that need to be immobilized, (2) to help prevent further deformity, and (3) to prevent soft-tissue contractures. As an immobilizing force, these rigid devices place and maintain a joint or joints in one position while allowing healing of a fracture or an inflammatory condition. It is optimal to place and hold joints in a position of function. Static splints prevent further deformity by maintaining a controlled stretch on the affected joint.

Conversely, dynamic splints allow motion of a joint within a prescribed range while supporting other joints. Primary uses of dynamic splints include (1) to act as a substitute for lost motor function, (2) to correct a deformity, (3) to provide controlled motion, and (4) to facilitate fracture alignment and wound healing. The dynamic action comes from hinges or springs placed in line with the joint to be acted upon. The tension of the hinge/spring can be set at a prescribed ROM and tension can be based on the use and desired outcome. Dynamic splints are more complex in their design and fabrication than static splints. Understanding the functions and uses of the static and dynamic splint will lead to the most effective choice.

Orthotic Terminology

The terminology for lower extremity orthoses is based on the anatomic area affected by the orthosis. An arch support or shoe insert is called a foot orthosis (FO). An orthosis designed to address drop-foot is called an ankle/foot orthosis (AFO). The orthoses may be further defined by descriptive terms such as *rigid FO* or *thermoplastic AFO*, or may be designated by the function performed such as *ground reaction AFO* or *stance-control KAFO*. Consistency in terminology ensures effective communication within the rehabilitation team. Standard abbreviations for lower limb orthoses are listed in Table 17-1.

Duration of Use

Therapists and orthotists both make devices intended to support, align, stretch, control, and replace the function of compromised joints and muscle groups. Often the decision of whether the device is made by a therapist or orthotist is based on the amount of time the device is expected to be used. Splints that are usually made by therapists are fabricated from low-temperature splinting materials with a life span of 3 to 6 months. These splints can be technically demanding but the duration of time in the orthosis is limited. Low-temperature thermoplastic splinting materials do not require a scan or cast of the body part to be fabricated, and are contoured directly over the client's skin or stockinette-covered skin.

Lower extremity splints, fabricated using components that are easily assembled, may also have metal attachments. They are assembled using hand tools normally available in the splinting lab. Splints used for smaller body parts such as the arms, hands, neck, and sometimes the lower leg can be changed fairly easily as the client moves through the

Table 17-1 Standard Abbreviations for Lower Limb Orthoses

ABBREVIATION	NAME
O	Orthosis
F	Foot
A	Ankle
K	Knee
H	Hip
FO	Foot orthosis
AFO	Ankle/foot orthosis
KO	Knee orthosis
KAFO	Knee/ankle/foot orthosis
HO	Hip orthosis
HKAFO	Hip/knee/ankle/foot orthosis

rehabilitation process. Some rehabilitation centers use low-temperature materials to fabricate full body splints for post-operative positioning. However, working with large sheets of plastic that easily stick together is quite cumbersome and technically demanding.

Orthotists, on the other hand, use high-temperature thermoplastic material that is heated to 325° F or more. These devices (usually referred to as orthoses) are ordered when the orthosis is expected to be worn for more than 6 months or to withstand greater forces as in weight bearing. High-temperature thermoplastic material is too hot to be contoured directly over the client's skin, and thus a scan or cast is taken of the affected body part to acquire a detailed mold. The mold is closed and filled with plaster. The high-temperature thermoplastic is then heated and draped over the mold under a vacuum to create the orthosis. After cooling, trim lines are drawn, and the plastic is removed using a cast cutter.

Edges are finished and buffed using grinders and routers, and any metal hinges or hardware are applied before the straps are attached. The high-temperature plastic and metal components are made to last for years, and can withstand the forces of spasticity and muscle weakness for longer periods of time than low-temperature splinting materials. A variety of high-temperature thermoplastic choices is available and these are chosen based on needed characteristics. Lower extremity orthoses have to withstand the repeated forces of weight bearing over long periods of time. Spinal orthoses are often made of more flexible high-temperature thermoplastic materials with full foam liners. Orthotic designs intended for high activity over long periods of time are best fabricated by an orthotist from high-temperature materials.

Foot Orthoses

A functional FO is designed to redistribute weight-bearing pressures over the plantar surface of the foot. Relief to painful areas, reduced stress to proximal joint structures, equalization of a limb length discrepancy, support to arches of the foot, and limiting motion at specific joints are some of the problems addressed by a foot orthosis [Goldberg and Hsu 1997]. Foot orthoses are available in prefabricated, custom-fitted, and custom designs, each yielding variable results relative to fit, function, comfort, sizing, cost, adjustability, personal acceptance/satisfaction, and effectiveness.

Biomechanical Function

Most FOs are biplanar designs, addressing joint deviations and providing support in the sagittal (i.e., mid-foot depression) and coronal planes (i.e., hind-foot and forefoot varus or valgus). More involved FO designs, such as the University of California Biomechanics Laboratory (UCBL) FO, offer triplanar support with additional control for transverse plane deviations (i.e., forefoot abduction or adduction). A thorough individual evaluation procedure is the basis for design and selection of the most appropriate FO.

General Indications and Contraindications

Prescription criteria for FOs are based on three main principles: accommodation, support, and correction. Accommodative FOs are generally fabricated of soft materials and are designed to provide additional padding, relief of pressure, and protection for insensate or deformed feet. Supportive orthoses are fabricated from semirigid materials, offering a greater degree of alignment control. Corrective orthoses tend to be manufactured from rigid materials and require extensive fitting procedures to obtain maximum joint alignment/correction and acceptance. A variety of orthotic designs are shown in Figure 17-8.

Design Options

FOs are measured in a variety of ways. Foam impressions, hand casting, or computerized mapping of the foot are the first steps in obtaining an accurate impression of the person's foot. Material selection offers the greatest variety of design options. Open- and closed-cell foams, leather, cork, plastics, laminates, and other materials serve to create a flexible, semirigid, or rigid orthotic design. Joint alignment is altered via posting, where additional material is placed in a particular area of the plantar surface of the orthosis to limit ROM or to "tilt" the foot into the correct alignment. Maximum joint alignment is achieved in designs offering triplanar control.

Specific Applications

Pronated conditions are effectively treated with custom orthotic designs. Runners often experience an excessive and sustained pronation moment, which may involve excessive joint ROM or sustained pronation throughout the stance phase. An FO is helpful in reducing the hind-foot valgus deviation, depression of the longitudinal arch, and excessive forefoot flexibility and supination. A semirigid orthosis allows a normal pronation moment to occur from heel-strike through the loading response, and then encourages the foot to become rigid for improved forward progression and propulsion.

Diabetic and insensate feet require daily inspection to prevent pressure sores and ulcerations from the stresses incurred during normal daily activities. Ulcerations develop in areas of excessive pressure, when joint deviations and bony prominences are susceptible to skin breakdown. Accommodative orthoses can be effectively designed to provide sufficient padding, redistribution of weight-bearing pressures, and slow and gradual healing (Figure 17-9).

Role of the Occupational Therapist

It is recommended that the therapist provide personal education (visual skin inspection) for individuals with insensate feet. Handheld skin inspection mirrors are indicated for

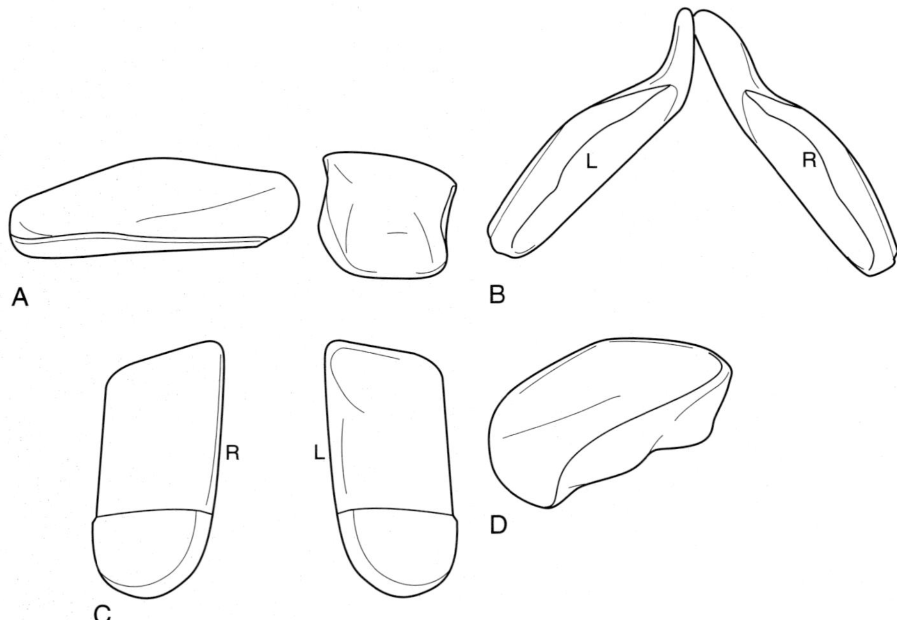

Figure 17-8 Various foot orthoses (note posting). (A) Soft insert. (B) Cork and leather arch support. (C) Rigid arch supports with coronal plane heel posting. (D) Rigid triplanar arch support. [University of California Biomechanics Laboratory (UCBL) type.]

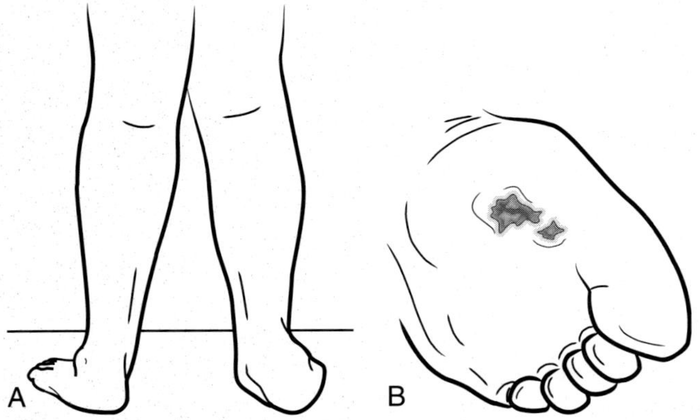

Figure 17-9 Pronated diabetic foot with ulceration. (A) Person with rheumatoid arthritis and severely pronated foot conditions. (B) Person with diabetic ulceration at the first metatarsal head.

some clients with reduced lower extremity ROM to ensure full inspection of the plantar surface of the foot. Selection of appropriate shoes is an important consideration with FOs. Slip-on flats or loafers are not recommended because they allow heel pistoning (sliding up and down in the shoe) and do not provide adequate counterpressure over the dorsum of the foot to maintain the foot securely in the shoe. Lace-up or Velcro-closure shoes are preferable because they provide added security.

Other shoe features that assist in accommodating the bulk of FOs include removable insoles, padded heel collars, and higher heel counters. Some athletic shoes feature nylon heel loops to assist in donning and doffing with ease. Long-handled shoehorns may be indicated for people with limited ROM.

Ankle/Foot Orthoses

AFOs are designed from metal and leather, thermoplastics, and laminates. Most AFO designs incorporate a foot plate to control the foot and ankle complex, a solid or jointed ankle (depending on the desired control), and a calf section to provide mechanical leverage for ankle and knee control. Metal and leather designs can be attached externally to a shoe or can incorporate a foot plate to fit within the shoe. Thermoplastic and laminated AFO designs use a molded foot plate to improve mid-tarsal and subtalar joint control, as well as to improve aesthetics and allow different shoes to be worn with the orthosis. It is important to note that when changing shoes a common heel height must be maintained. As with most orthotic designs, AFOs are available in prefabricated, custom-fitted, and custom designs.

A basic AFO is diagrammed in Figure 17-10, which shows the standard components. The proximal trim provides leverage for foot control during swing and is contoured to provide appropriate pressure around the soft tissue of the calf. The anterior opening allows for donning and doffing while the anterior closure secures the orthosis to the limb. The closure mechanism may vary, depending on the manual dexterity of the person. The anterior and ankle trim lines relate to the flexibility or rigidity of the orthosis. Specifically, wider trim that covers more anatomic area generally creates

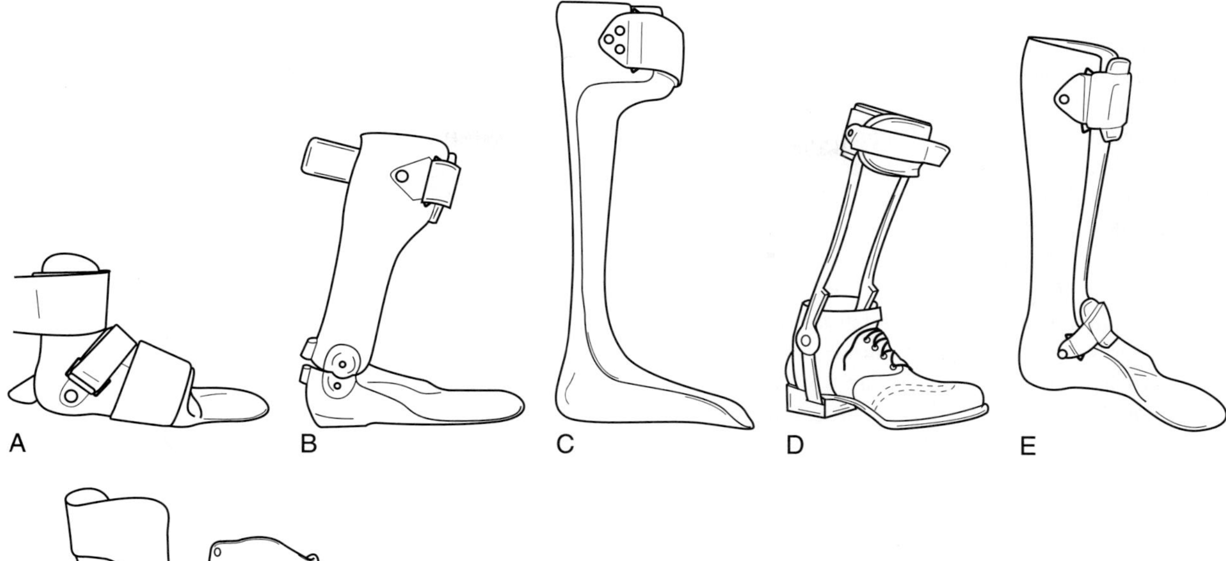

Figure 17-10 Various ankle/foot orthosis designs. (A) Supramalleolar orthosis. (B) Jointed AFO with posterior plantar-flexion stop and full-length foot plate. (C) Posterior leaf spring. (D) Double-upright design with medial T-strap and dorsiflexion-assist ankle joints. (E) Solid ankle AFO with instep strap. (F) Laminated AFO with double-action ankle joints and pretibial shell. (G) Patellar tendon-bearing orthosis (PTBO) for load-bearing relief of the foot and ankle complex with carbon fiber reinforcements at ankle.

a more rigid orthosis and narrower trim creates a more flexible orthosis. The trim lines can be adjusted throughout the course of the rehabilitation program. Finally, the length of the distal trim line contributes to the mechanical function of the orthosis by allowing or delaying rollover as needed.

Biomechanical Function

AFOs are designed to structurally bridge the ankle joint, providing a stable base of support at the foot and control of the alignment of the distal leg segment. Direct control of the ankle joint and indirect control of the knee joint are achieved with the use of various ankle joint designs. AFOs can be used to enhance, limit, or negate ankle joint ROM, depending on the individual requirements of the person and the person's unique gait pattern. Some AFOs are designed to encompass the foot and ankle complex only and are termed *supramalleolar AFOs* (SMOs).

General Indications and Contraindications

Lehmann and De Lateur [Kottke and Lehmann 1990] noted the primary reasons for AFO application: mediolateral stability of the foot and ankle during stance, dorsiflexion assistance during swing, plantar flexion assistance for propulsion during terminal stance, maintenance of knee alignment through stance, approximation of a more normal gait pattern, decrease in energy costs, and prevention of the development of associated joint deformities [Kraft and Lehmann 1992]. Personal safety is another important reason for AFO prescription, especially for the person with a changing pattern of neuromuscular control. Temporary or permanent use of an AFO may very well prevent an unnecessary fall for the person who has poor balance or even mild functional deficits (i.e., foot drop).

Design Options

As noted, material choices for AFO designs are numerous. Metal and leather AFOs require a tracing and a series of exact measurements for fabrication. Attachment to a shoe limits shoe wear options but can improve ease of donning for a person with lesser cognitive or lesser upper extremity functional abilities. This type of AFO contacts the foot (via the shoe) and the calf (via the calf band). Such limited anatomic contact may be indicated for the person with periods of fluctuating edema, although the potential application of force for joint correction is also limited. Metal AFOs may incorporate a leather T-strap to assist in coronal plane control of the ankle joint. Various metal ankle joints offer free, limited, or restricted ankle joint ROM (Figure 17-10).

Thermoplastic and laminated AFOs are fabricated from a mold of the person's limb. The casting material is applied to the limb while the orthotist maintains and holds proper joint alignment of the mid-tarsal, subtalar, and ankle joints. Proper hip and knee alignment is also important during this procedure to obtain correct anatomic relationships. Removal of this cast provides a negative mold, which is then processed into a positive mold ("statue") of the person's limb. Careful and specific modification procedures enhance the effectiveness of the desired three-point force systems and relief of pressure to bony prominences. The thermoplastic material or liquid laminate is then vacuum-molded over the positive mold to create a unique and individual orthosis. (*Note:* The casting, modification, and fabrication procedures are similar for all thermoplastic and laminated custom orthotic designs.)

Ankle joints are now available in a variety of sizes, functions, and materials (Figure 17-11). Specially designed straps may be added to the orthosis to help maintain the foot within the orthosis or to shift the joint alignment. The flexibility or rigidity of the orthosis is determined primarily by the biochemical properties of the selected plastic. It is possible to create an orthosis with areas of rigidity and flexibility by altering the thickness of the plastic during the fabrication process. As always, a skilled orthotist can provide the necessary expertise in this area.

Specific Applications

A person with a recent cerebrovascular accident (CVA, or stroke) can present with a varied neuromuscular picture. Generally, the involved limb presents with complete flaccidity (i.e., hypotonic) or extreme rigidity (i.e., hypertonic), but the tone may fluctuate with periods of both throughout the day. An orthotic prescription recommendation is often difficult for this group, as the tendency is to prevent "overbracing" of a person with expected functional return. However, delay of bracing often promotes the development of compensatory and inefficient gait patterns as well as deformities that are often difficult to resolve, even after some functional control has returned. An appropriate orthotic design is one that provides immediate stability and safety, with ongoing adjustability to substitute for only those functions that are still lost (Figure 17-12). An effective orthosis should not prevent functional muscle groups from returning to their normal roles.

A person with cerebral palsy requires an intensive and integrated rehabilitation team approach from a very early age. Effective stretching and strengthening exercises maintain ROM and enhance potential ambulation abilities. Functional orthoses will be designed to help promote delayed age-appropriate activities, such as knee standing and pull-to-stand. Once the child is standing, functional abilities and walking patterns are evaluated and new orthotic prescriptions may be required. Effective biomechanical alignment and stability are balanced against functional mobility to prevent joint deviation and ligamentous laxities while allowing the child to explore the environment. It is often very difficult to achieve maximum outcomes in both structural stability and functional mobility. Compromises must be understood and discussed by the rehabilitation team.

Role of the Occupational Therapist

AFO design options can positively or negatively influence occupational performance tasks. Although rigid ankle designs provide biomechanical alignment and maintain joint corrections, this design also completely restricts ROM. Such activities as operating an automobile gas pedal, kneeling, bending at the waist, or using stairs can be difficult to achieve with a rigid ankle AFO. Conversely, an articulated AFO design provides obvious advantage in functional mobility, but it may compromise some individuals' sense of balance and security. Often, a person is required to stand for long periods of time at work or meal preparation, and low endurance may contribute to knee buckling and loss of balance. Articulated AFO designs do not provide the plantarflexion/knee-extension couple that rigid ankle designs offer, thus affecting knee stability.

For those people concerned with professional dress standards, the cosmetic appearance of the AFO may make a critical difference in acceptance of the orthosis. Although both metal and thermoplastic AFOs are designed to be worn under clothing, metal AFOs are wider at the ankle, offering a higher profile with metal ankle joints that are visible to others when the person is sitting. Plastic AFOs contour intimately at the ankle, offering a lower profile, and are not as obvious to others (especially when a translucent thermoplastic is used for fabrication).

Knee Orthoses

Knee orthoses generally fall into three categories: prophylactic, postoperative, and functional [Bunch et al. 1985, Kottke and Lehmann 1990, Goldberg and Hsu 1997]. Prophylactic knee bracing focuses on the prevention of injury or the reduction of the severity of injury for those persons involved in high-impact or contact sports. Postoperative or rehabilitative knee orthoses are prescribed after a surgical procedure, usually ligament reconstruction, to limit ROM while soft-tissue structures are allowed to heal. Functional knee orthoses are designed to provide mechanical stability to the chronically unstable or reconstructed knee joint.

Biomechanical Function

Knee orthoses are designed according to the mechanical principles of hydrostatics, levers, and force systems.

Hydrostatics refers to tissue containment. In other words, the orthosis must contain (or "hold") the flexible thigh and calf tissues so as to stabilize the knee joint and limit excessive stresses to the ligamentous structures. Fit, joint alignment, and suspension are critical factors in the effectiveness of any knee orthosis. It is extremely important for the mechanical joint of the orthosis to closely mimic the alignment and function of the anatomic joint. If the orthosis is not suspended and maintained in the proper position, joint alignment is sacrificed and often a discrepancy is created between the anatomic and mechanical joint axes. Specially designed straps, supracondylar pads, or inner sleeves help prevent distal slipping of the orthosis during daily activities.

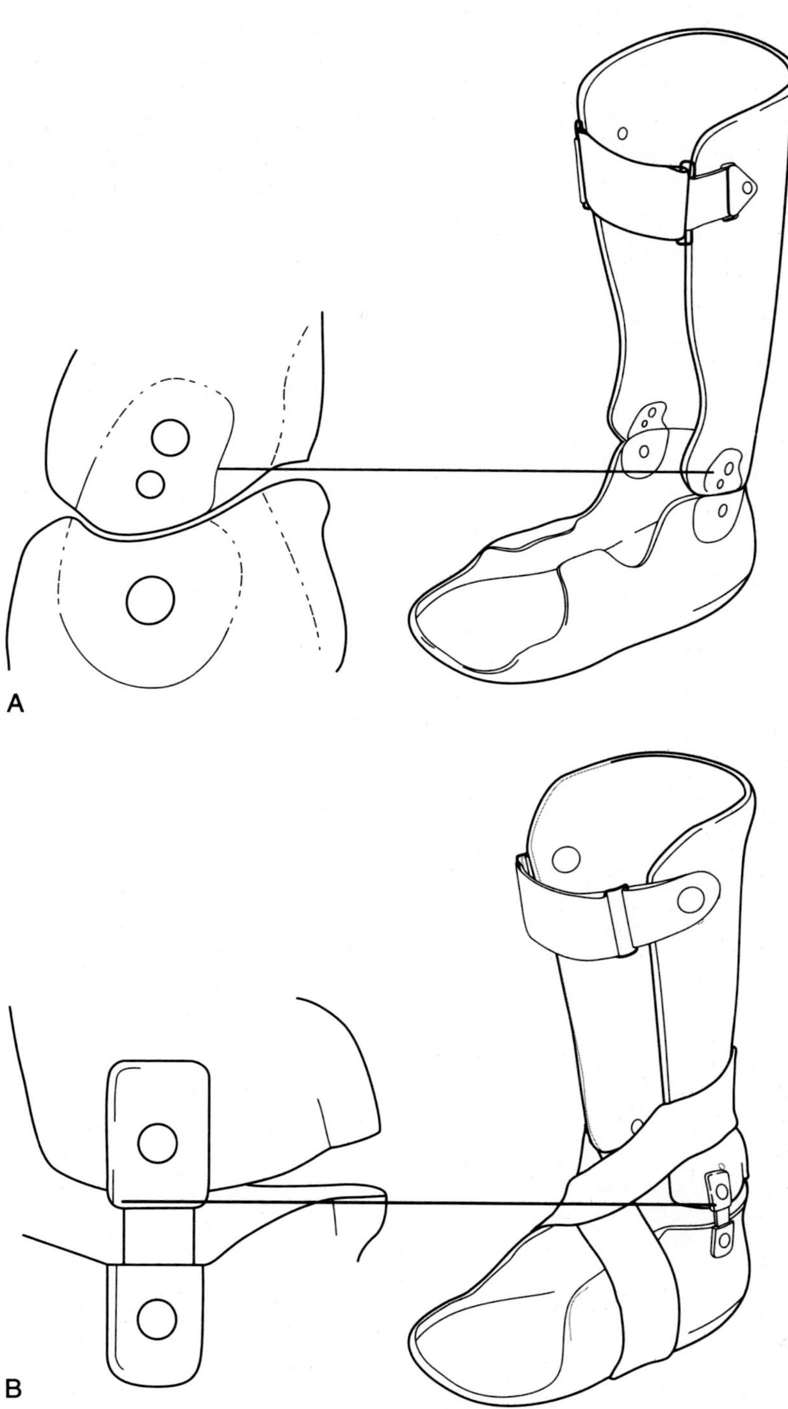

Figure 17-11 Various orthotic ankle joints. (A) Ninety-degree plantar-flexion stop, free dorsiflexion AFO with Oklahoma ankle joints. (B) Ninety-degree plantar-flexion stop, free dorsiflexion AFO with Gillette ankle joints.

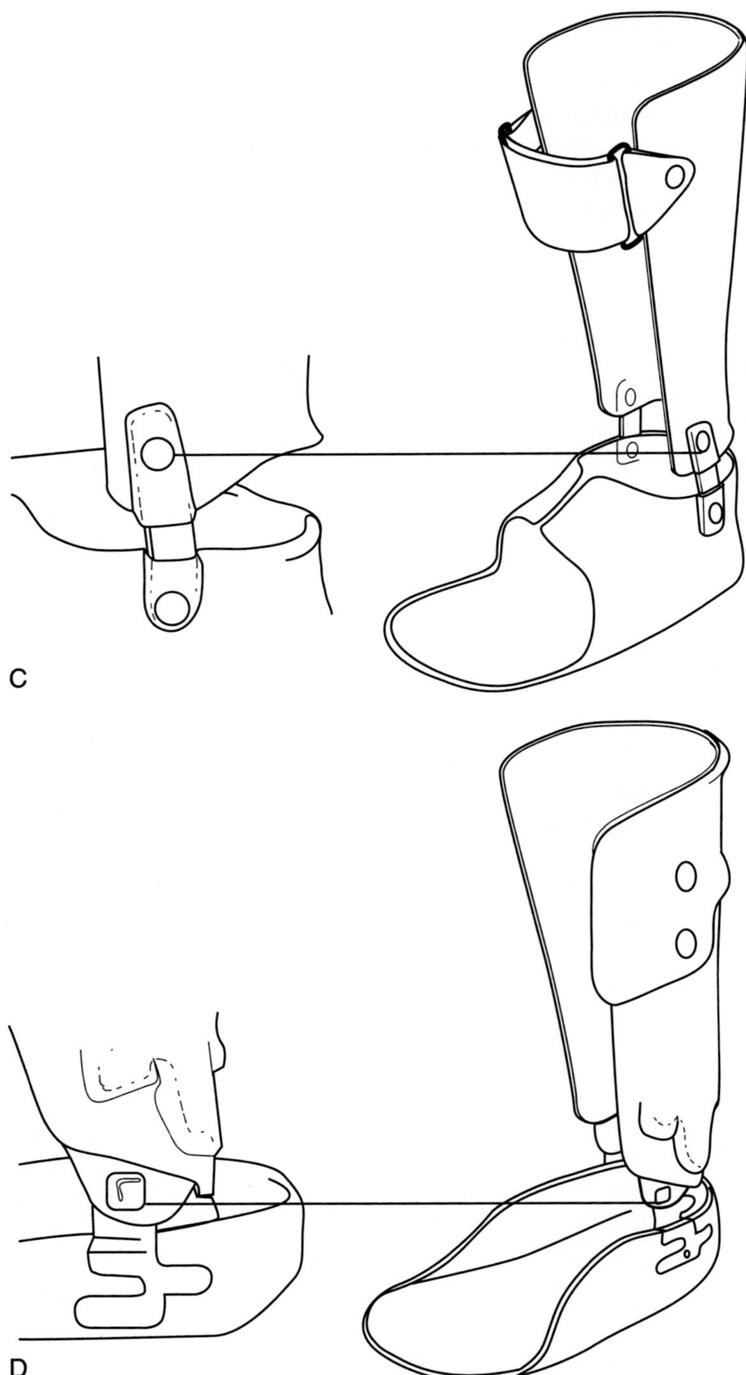

Figure 17-11, cont'd (C) Free-motion AFO with Gaffney ankle joints. (D) Dorsiflexion-assist AFO with Wafer ankle joints.

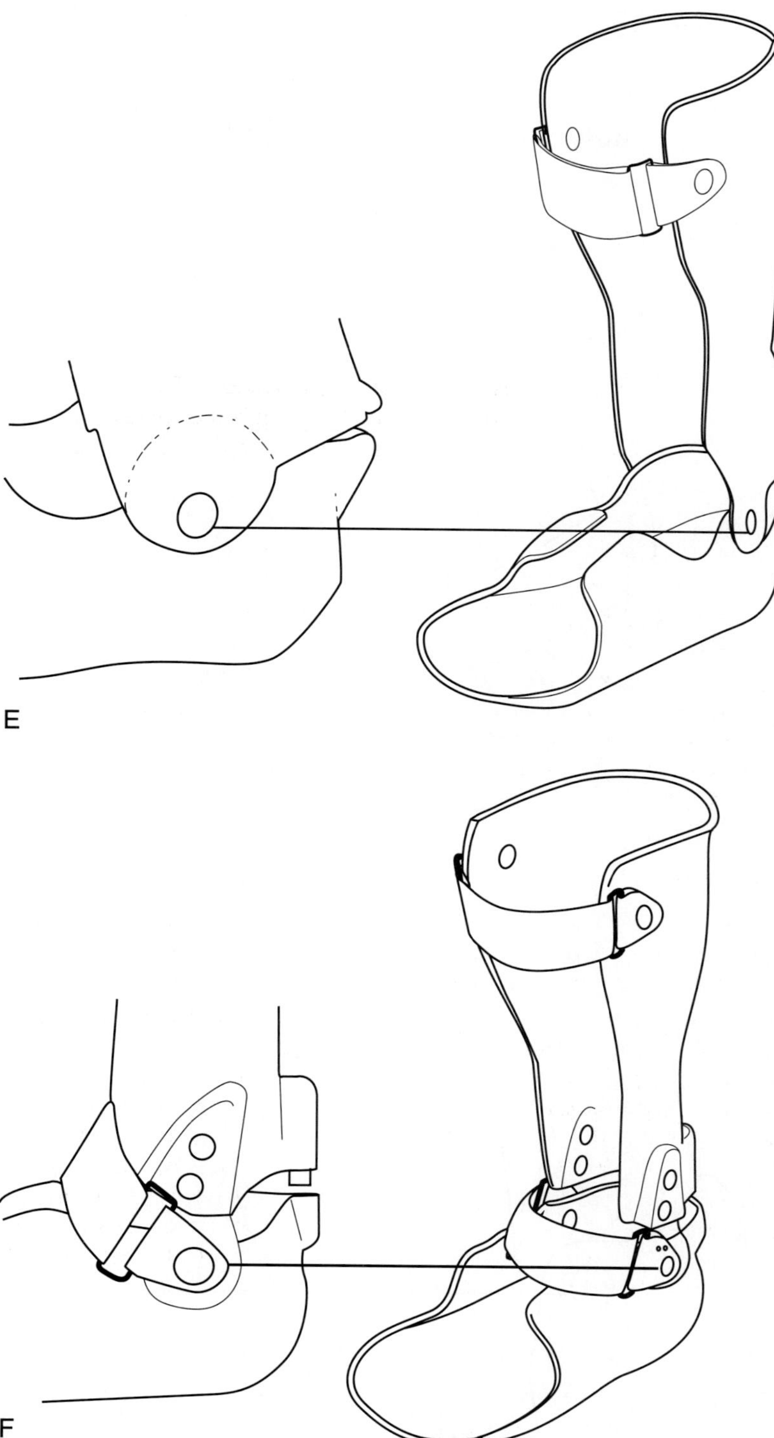

Figure 17-11, cont'd (E) Dorsiflexion-assist AFO with overlap ankle joints. (F) Adjustable posterior stop AFO with Oklahoma ankle joints.

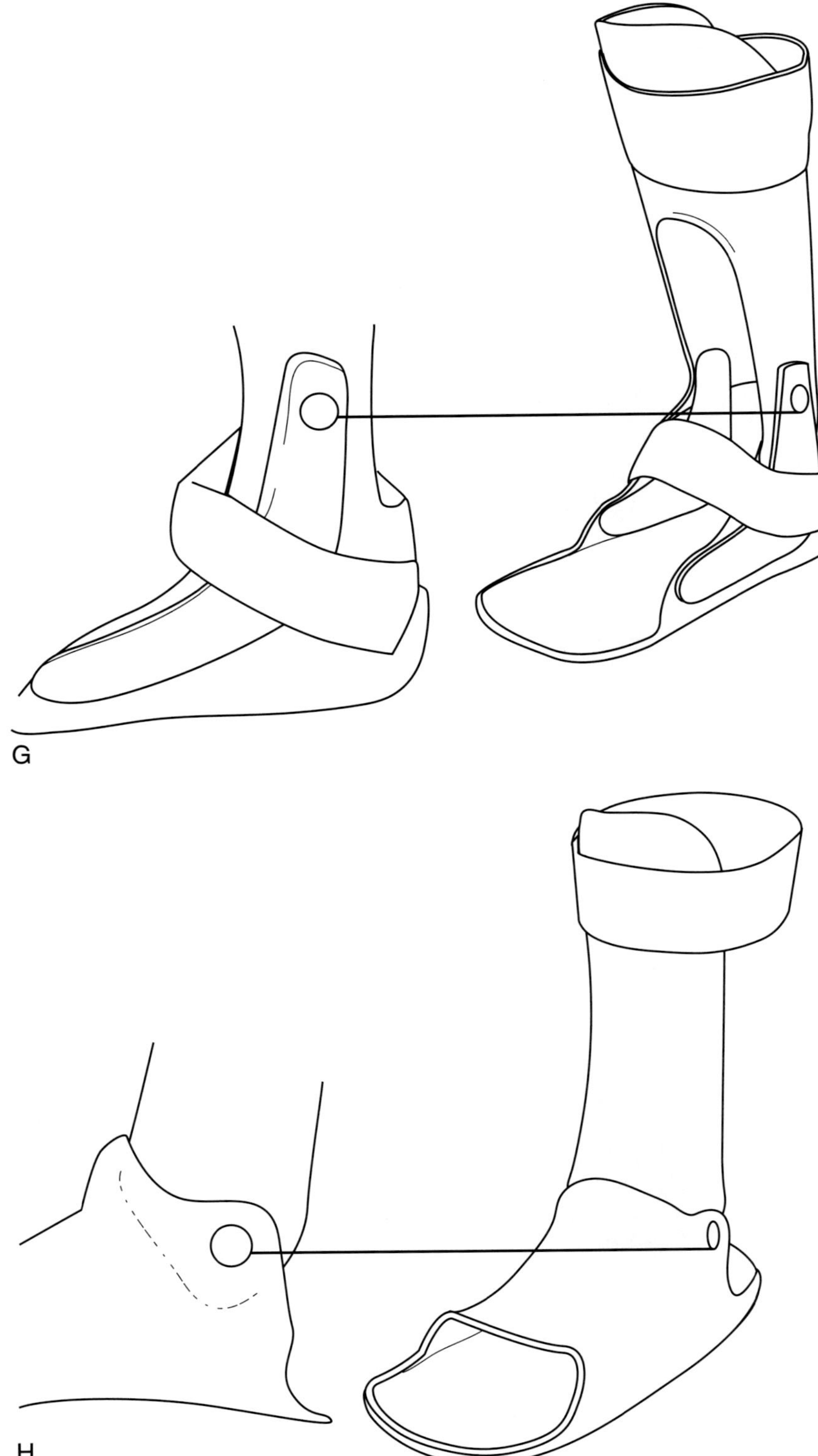

Figure 17-11, cont'd (G) Floor reaction AFO with carbon inserts for ankle reinforcement. (H) Posterior-entry 90-degree dorsiflexion stop, free plantar-flexion AFO with overlap ankle joints.

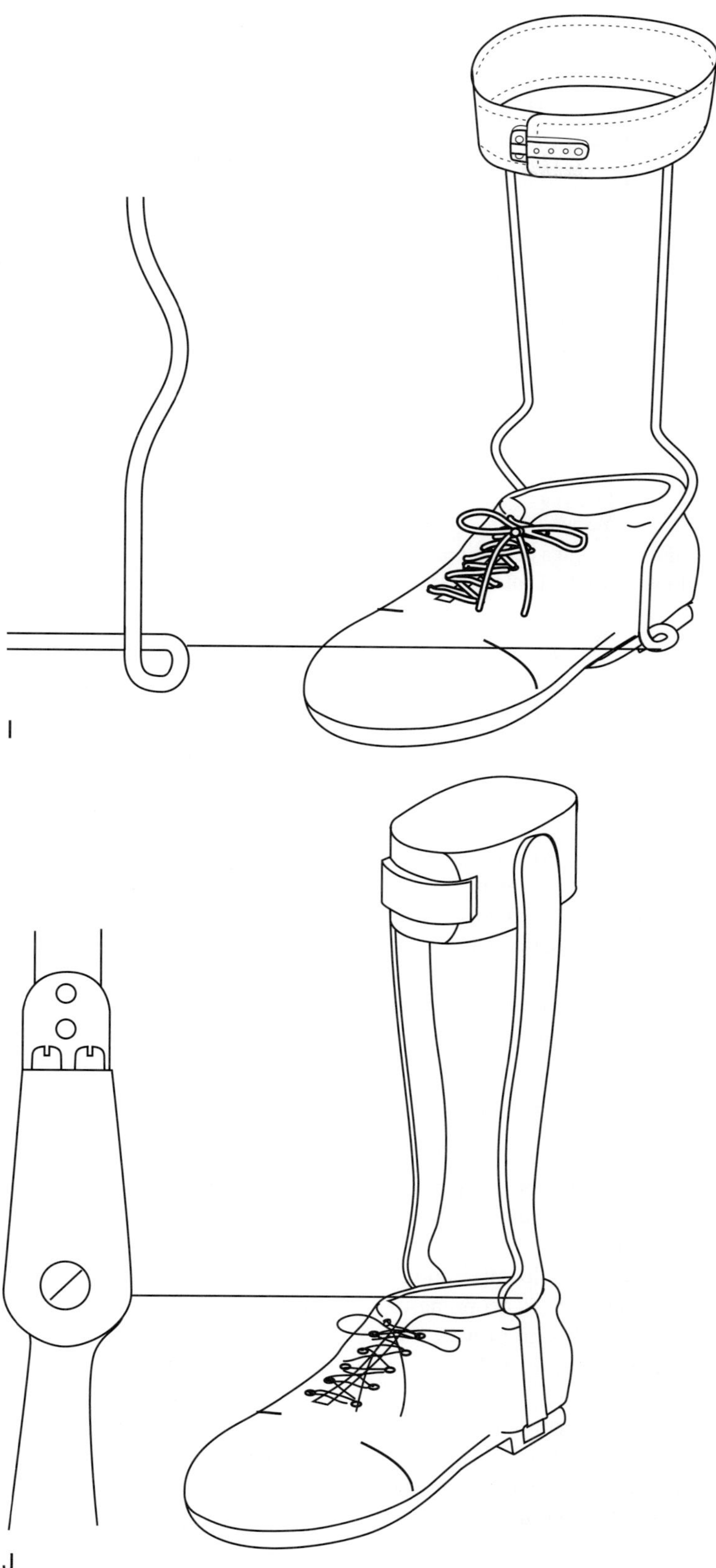

Figure 17-11, cont'd (I) Metal dorsiflexion assist. (J) Metal double action for dorsiflexion and plantar-flexion control.

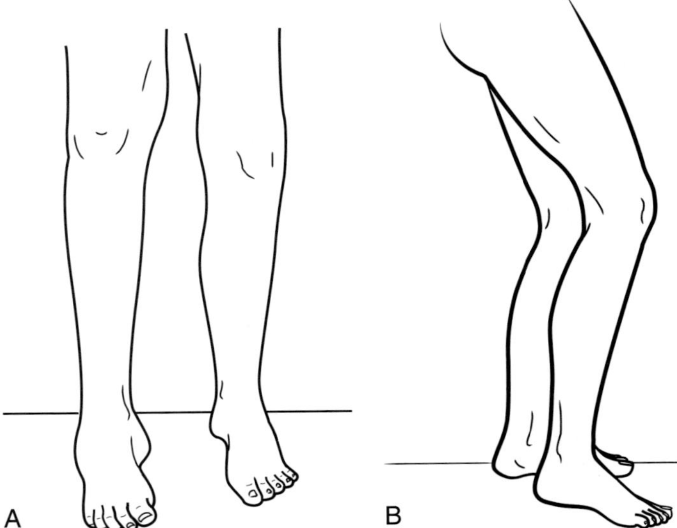

Figure 17-12 CVA person with equinovarus and a cerebral palsy child with crouched gait. (A) Person recovering from a CVA presents with tone-induced equinovarus. (B) Child with cerebral palsy presents with mild crouching, drop-foot, and poor balance.

Levers and force systems also play an important role in this process. As noted previously, the farther the points of force application are from the joint the longer the mechanical levers and the greater the mechanical effect of the three-point force systems. (See Figure 17-7 for an effective three-point force system to resist genu valgum.) If the orthosis slips distally during normal wearing, the length of the proximal levers has been shortened and the anatomic and mechanical knee joint discrepancy is dramatic. To receive maximum benefit from the orthosis, the person must perform proper donning techniques and periodic checking of the alignment of the orthosis throughout the day.

General Indications and Contraindications

Prophylactic knee orthoses are intended to prevent injury to the knee or to reduce the severity of injury for competitive athletes. Postoperative orthoses control ROM and encourage early weight bearing and limited activity. Functional knee orthoses are prescribed for chronically unstable knees and as an adjunct to many surgical procedures. Soft neoprene or elastic knee sleeves are generally prescribed to provide circumferential compression of the knee, warmth, and minimal medial/lateral stability.

Knee orthoses provide support in the coronal plane by preventing genu varum and genu valgum. Mechanical joint design and joint settings limit the available range of flexion and extension in the sagittal plane. Limited transverse plane control is available for attempts to "grasp" the thigh and calf sections through soft-tissue containment. Most important, the foot and ankle complex remains free to transmit internal and external rotation proximally to the knee during weight bearing. The hip joint also has available joint motion in all three planes and most often follows the alignment imposed distally at the base of support.

The knee is a complex joint with the motions of flexion and extension occurring about a changing anatomic axis. The exact motion of the knee joint has yet to be duplicated in mechanical joint designs, although many joints are quite sophisticated in their function. Mechanical joint options are discussed further in the knee/ankle/foot orthosis section of this chapter.

Design Options

Over the past 20 years, increasing awareness in the prevention and support of the injured knee has led to the development of many orthotic designs. Each custom knee orthosis is measured, casted, designed, and fitted to meet the unique requirements of the person's knee (i.e., anterior cruciate instability, medial collateral instability, hyperextension, and so on). Design features include reduced weight, colors and fabrics, and variable joint functions. Other options include specific sports applications for skiing and motocross. Despite the flood of orthotic designs and claims by the various manufacturers, no specific knee orthosis or brand has demonstrated clear superiority over any other design. An effective orthosis is selected according to the unique mechanical and functional needs of each person (Figure 17-13).

Specific Applications

Osteoarthritis is a degenerative condition that commonly affects the knee joint. Deterioration of the medial or lateral knee joint structure leads to genu varum and genu valgum deformities, respectively. People with severe joint deviation

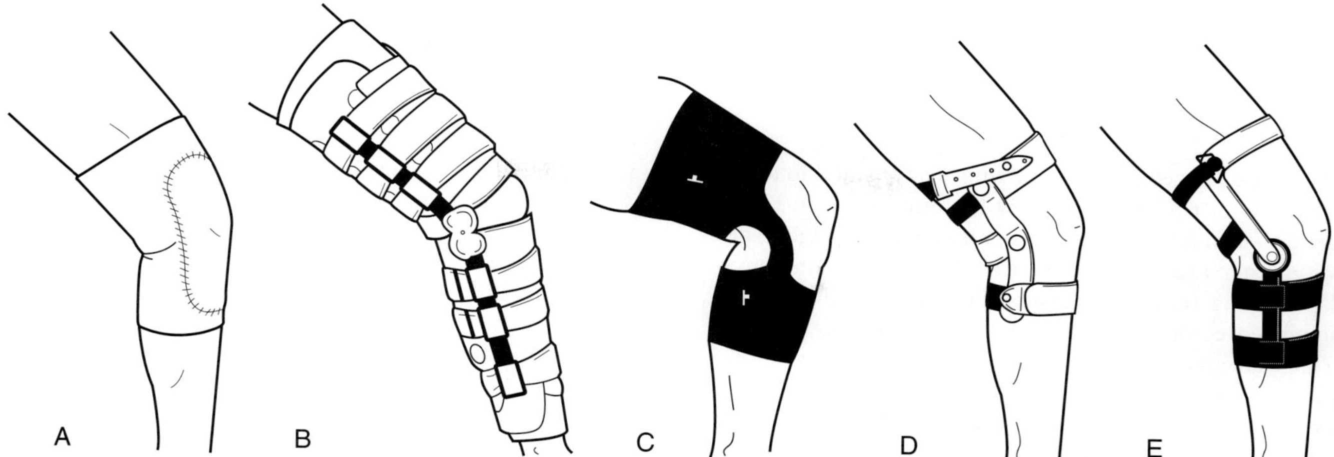

Figure 17-13 Various knee orthoses. (A) Soft neoprene knee sleeve. (B) Postoperative knee orthosis controls flexion ROM and extension ROM with adjustable joints. (C) Prophylactic knee orthosis with lateral joint. (D) Rehabilitative design to control knee hyperextension. (E) Custom knee orthosis to stabilize injured knee.

are considered for total joint replacement. Still, some people are not surgical candidates or may present with the early stages of the disease process. Such people may benefit from functional knee orthoses. These orthoses incorporate long mechanical lever arms to apply corrective forces to the affected knee joint. When a valgum or varum stress to the knee is induced, the medial or lateral compartments can be unloaded. Decreased pain and prevention of continued deformity are obvious benefits of this type of orthotic treatment program until such time as surgery is warranted (Figure 17-14).

Competitive athletes and active individuals enjoy the challenge of various levels of physical activity. Unfortunately, when created circumstances subject the knee joint and soft-tissue structures to repetitive high-load stresses injuries can occur. Knee orthoses serve as an adjunct to surgical restoration and rehabilitation programs by limiting ROM and excessive stresses postoperatively.

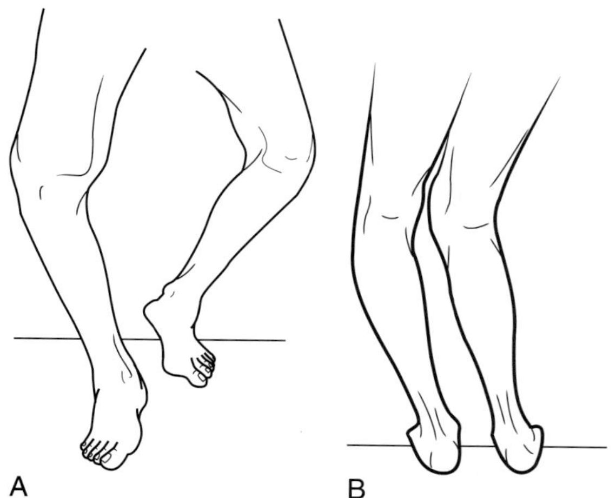

Figure 17-14 Osteoarthritis. (A) Persons with diagnosis of osteoarthritis and genu varum may benefit from a custom knee orthosis. (B) Person with diagnosis of osteoarthritis and left-side genu varum and right-side genu valgum.

Role of the Occupational Therapist

People receiving functional knee orthoses to prevent further knee deformity may also suffer from upper extremity degenerative changes that limit hand function. Although most knee orthosis designs use Velcro closure systems as opposed to traditional strap and buckle systems, medial or lateral placement of closure system loops is critical to enhance available functional dexterity. Closure systems that include a wider chafe opening allow the person with impaired hand function to feed Velcro straps through the opening with less difficulty.

Knee orthoses are generally designed to provide a total surface contact and are worn as close to the skin as possible. Don/doff procedures should be reviewed with the person to ensure that the most effective dressing routine has been established. Knee orthoses typically restrict anatomic knee flexion by 20 to 30 degrees because of the thickness of the posterior calf shells or straps. This ROM loss may impede certain work or leisure activities that require deep knee bends or squatting.

Knee/Ankle/Foot Orthoses

KAFOs are built on the same concepts that have been covered for ankle/foot orthoses. Structurally, KAFOs continue proximally by bridging the knee joint and containing the thigh tissues. Most KAFOs are custom made from measurements or casts and are fabricated from metal and leather, thermoplastic, or laminate materials. Hybrid designs incorporate a variety of materials to achieve the desired orthotic control. Some prefabricated designs are available for temporary use.

Biomechanical Function

KAFOs are successful in improving stability and functional mobility for persons with lower limb involvement. KAFOs are designed for persons with significant genu valgum, genu varum, genu recurvatum, or genu flexion (i.e., anterior collapse). As a result of structural bridging of the knee joint, improved coronal and sagittal plane control are achieved. Transverse plane control is determined distally by the foot plate design. Skeletal joint alignment of the knee is achieved by applying corrective forces through the soft-tissue structures of the thigh. Therefore, a well-molded and well-fitted thigh shell is an important component of the orthotic design. Excessive gapping reduces the mechanical effect of the design and reduces potential stability and function.

General Indications and Contraindications

When an AFO is ineffective in maintaining the knee over the base of support throughout the gait cycle, consideration of KAFO application is required. The knee is identified as the primary joint of instability, usually in combination with any number of neuromuscular involvements or functional deficits. Ideally, externally applied forces realign the knee over a stable base of support and normal joint motion is provided through mechanical joint structures.

In some cases, however, full correction or "ideal alignment" is not possible because of the long-standing nature of the deformity. Bony changes and musculoskeletal contractures at the hip, knee, and ankle present unique challenges for orthotic intervention. Donning and doffing abilities and individual functional activities must be evaluated to develop the most appropriate orthotic prescription.

Design Options

As with the AFO, there are many material and component choices available for KAFO designs, and material selection is generally based on the height, weight, activity level, and functional requirements of the person (Figure 17-15). Metal and leather, thermoplastic, laminated, and hybrid designs offer a variety of design options for the person with significant knee joint instability. Because the knee is the primary

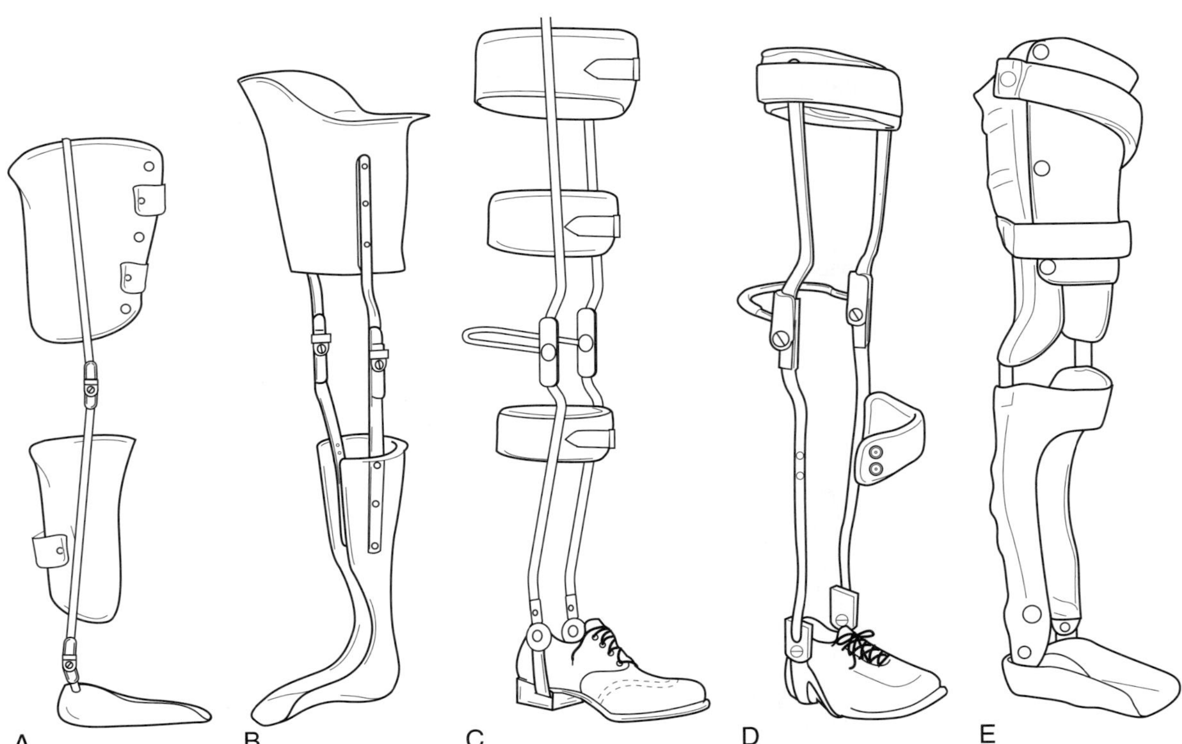

Figure 17-15 Various knee/ankle/foot orthoses. (A) Thermoplastic orthosis with molded foot plate, jointed ankle, long anterior tibial shell, drop locks, and circumferential thigh shell. (B) Thermoplastic orthosis with molded foot plate, solid ankle, drop locks, and quadrilateral thigh shell. (C) Double-upright orthosis attached to shoe, with jointed ankle, posterior calf band, bail lock knee, and two posterior thigh bands. (D) Scott-Craig orthosis with double-action ankle joints, pivot anterior tibial band, bail lock knee, and posterior thigh band. (E) Laminated orthosis with molded foot plate, double-action ankle, pretibial shell, free knee, and posterior thigh shell with long anterior tongue.

joint of involvement, mechanical joint selection warrants attention at this time.

Knee joints come in a variety of sizes and functions that provide free, limited, or restricted joint motion. Common locking mechanisms include the drop lock and bail lock designs. Drop locks are designed to fall into place over the mechanical hinge when the person stands. These locks must be lifted by hand before sitting (or any activity that requires knee flexion). Bail locks are designed to snap into place and lock the knee once the knee is extended. The joints must be unlocked before sitting and can be disengaged by bumping the posterior lever mechanism on the seat of a chair.

The person does not have to bend over and manually unlock the joints. Step-lock joints provide a variable range of motion and locking capability. This joint design can be used with a progressive stretching program to reduce a knee flexion contracture. It is important to note that energy costs increase approximately 20% when one walks with a locked knee [Kraft and Lehmann 1992], and therefore locked knee KAFOs should be used cautiously. Orthotists are well versed in the various designs and can provide specific pros and cons relative to the individual person.

Single-axis, polycentric, and offset joint designs refer to the pivoting motion and alignment of the mechanical joints. A single-axis joint functions as it is named, with a single hinged action. Polycentric joints produce a shifting axis in an attempt to mimic the functional motion of the knee joints. Offset knee joint designs shift the mechanical axis posteriorly to the anatomic joint axis. This provides improved stance-phase stability and resistance to anterior knee collapse. Size, weight, function, and durability are important factors in knee joint selection.

The most proximal component of the KAFO is the thigh section. Thigh designs are critical to the success of the orthosis. Posterior shells with anterior straps, anterior shells with posterior straps, and full circumferential shells are common thigh section designs. The thigh shells may be fabricated of rigid or flexible material. Narrow medial/lateral (M/L) and quadrilateral-shaped thigh sections are the most common designs, but all thigh sections are contoured to the unique characteristics of each individual. The thigh shell may also be designed to "unweight" or "unload" the lower limb by providing a shelf for the ischium to sit on in combination with soft-tissue containment of the thigh muscles. This is similar to the prosthetic socket design for above-knee amputees.

Recent technological advancements in orthotic componentry have introduced stance-control orthoses (SCOs), which are mechanical knee joints for use with knee orthoses and knee/ankle/foot orthoses. These mechanical joints are available in several designs. Common features are free motion during swing phase and flexion control during stance phase. These stance-control knee joints allow a more normal gait pattern because the knee is not required to be locked during both swing and stance to prevent stance-phase flexion.

This design has a significant effect on the reduction of energy costs during walking because the swing-phase flexion negates the need to circumduct and/or hip hike on the involved side or vault on the contralateral side in order to obtain ground clearance. The *ideal candidate* for a SCO presents with isolated unilateral quadriceps weakness, a relatively sound contralateral side, minimal contractures, minimal spasticity, and good hip and ankle musculature. People should be thoroughly evaluated by the rehabilitation team for potential application of the SCO.

Specific Applications

Genu recurvatum is a common involvement for KAFO application. Specifically, knee joint laxity allows the anatomic knee center to move posteriorly during weight bearing. This is usually an acquired deformity that develops secondarily to weakness of the quadriceps or posterior calf muscle groups. It may also develop secondarily to a plantar-flexion contracture at the ankle. With associated muscle weakness, anterior collapse of the knee would occur. Therefore, the person learns to compensate by maintaining the knee posteriorly and shifting the body weight anteriorly through hip flexion and anterior trunk lean. The effect is to place the body weight in front of the knee joint to prevent collapse and falling. A plantar-flexion contracture forces the knee posteriorly during initial loading and continues to disrupt forward progression throughout stance phase. In either case, load-bearing stresses cause permanent damage to the posterior capsule and soft-tissue structures of the knee, the deformity continues to progress over time, and energy costs increase dramatically. The potential for the development of a severe deformity with permanent damage to the knee requires prompt attention.

The objective of a KAFO varies for persons with genu recurvatum (Figure 17-16). In some orthotic designs, complete sagittal plane correction is the goal as long as there is

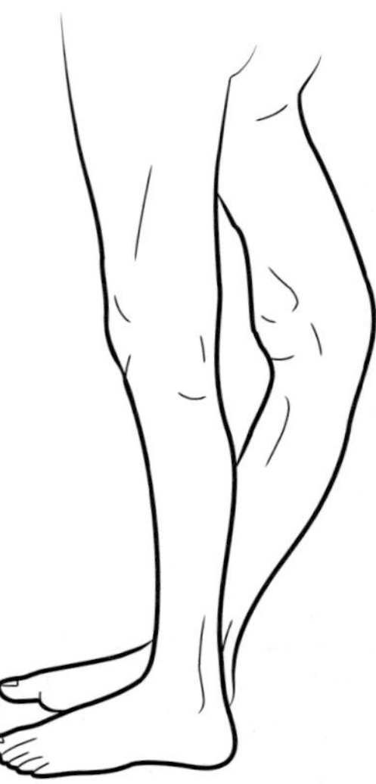

Figure 17-16 Genu recurvatum. A person with severe genu recurvatum is a candidate for a KAFO design.

a mechanical means of providing stance-phase stability to prevent anterior knee collapse when weakness is noted. For other persons, partial correction will reduce the deforming forces to the knee and limit progression of the deformity. Individual evaluation and assessment determine the appropriate design criteria.

Coronal plane deviations of the knee have been shown in Figure 17-14 and examined in the discussion of knee orthoses and osteoarthritis. If the mechanical leverage provided by the knee orthosis is not sufficient, it may be necessary to consider a KAFO design. By crossing the ankle and subtalar joints and encompassing the foot, it is possible to achieve greater coronal plane control and stability of the knee joint. Several knee joint options are shown in Figure 17-17.

Role of the Occupational Therapist

The choice of a KAFO knee extension locking mechanism is perhaps the most significant threat to occupational performance in lower extremity orthotics. Although locking of the knee during walking should be avoided whenever possible to reduce increased energy expenditure, it may be unavoidable for many persons who require stability and are at risk of falling because of weakness or imbalance. For improved cosmetic appearance and to maintain total surface contact, it is recommended that KAFOs be donned under clothing. However, manipulation of locking mechanisms, specifically drop locks, is infinitely more difficult when the mechanism is visually hidden under a layer of clothing and tactile feedback is reduced.

For the person who wears the KAFO only for specific tasks during the day and removes the device to be more comfortable, wearing the KAFO on the outside of clothing may be advisable. Care should be taken that such a person accepts the cosmetic ramifications and that biomechanical design is not compromised. It is important that occupational therapy evaluation of occupational performance be completed before the orthotist begins fabrication, as KAFO measurements will differ significantly over as opposed to under clothing.

Knee extension locking mechanisms include drop locks, bail locks, and trigger locks. Drop locks are the most commonly used mechanisms and are disengaged by using palmar or lateral pinch just before sitting. This task requires the person to bend forward, reach down, and use significant pinch strength to unlock mechanisms on both the medial and lateral aspects of the knee. Poor balance, limited upper extremity range, or reduced hand function may prevent independent operation of the unlocking mechanism. This population would be at a significantly higher risk of falls when using a KAFO with drop lock mechanisms.

Bail locks do not require the person to bend forward, reach down, or use any hand involvement to manipulate the mechanism because the knee lock is released by the application of slight pressure to the posterior knee loop of the KAFO from the front edge of a chair. Bail lock designs are dependent on a stable chair with a hard front edge to operate efficiently. The height of the chair is also an important factor if the person is to reach the lock effectively. It is not practical to disengage this type of lock against soft-surface furniture, such as sling wheelchair seats, couches, beds, or recliners. This limits the bail lock's scope of usefulness within the home environment. Tight clothing donned over the KAFO with bail locks may interfere with secure operation of the mechanism.

Trigger locks are a hybrid design that includes elements of both drop lock and bail lock mechanisms. This design employs medial and lateral locks connected to a common cable mounted on the proximal lateral aspect of the thigh. Minimal reaching, bending, and hook hand strength is required to operate this type of mechanism. This device is not dependent on furniture for efficient operation, and safe operation of the device is not impaired by clothing.

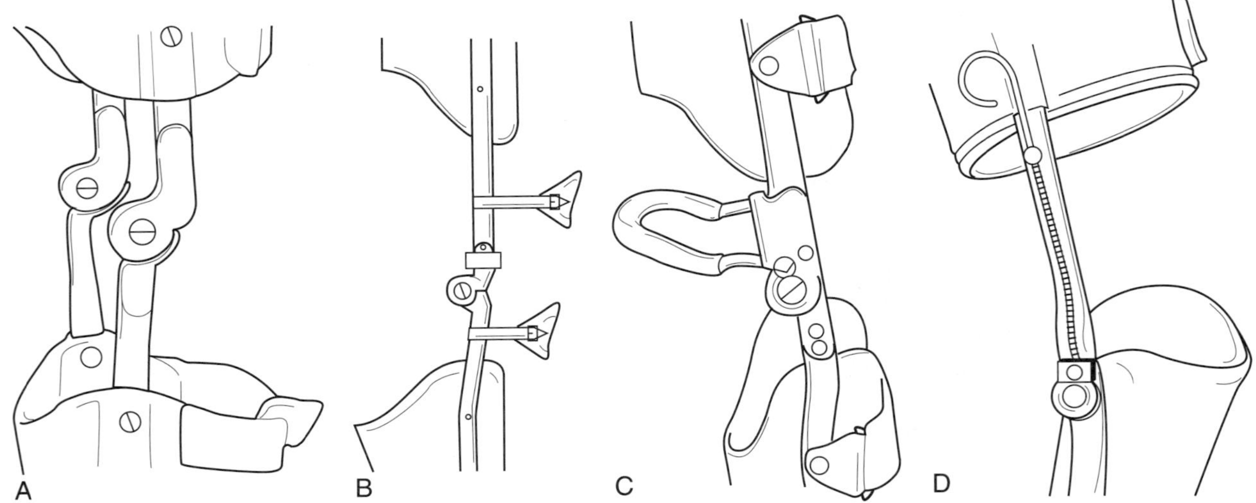

Figure 17-17 Various knee joint options. (A) Free posterior offset. (B) Posterior offset with drop locks. (C) Bail lock. (D) Trigger lock.

Each person should be carefully evaluated by the therapist in concert with other team members before a final decision is made regarding which knee extension locking device is employed. Occupational performance factors often play a key role in selection criteria.

Hip Orthoses

Hip orthoses are prescribed for problems associated with the femoral head or acetabulum. Custom-fitted and custom-molded orthoses consist of a pelvic section, hip joint(s), and thigh cuff(s) to control ROM and alignment. Occasionally a shoulder strap is used to assist with suspension of the orthosis. Orthoses may be designed to provide unilateral or bilateral control of the hip and are most often used to promote healing postoperatively. Hip orthoses are also used to provide a wider and more normal base of support for sitting, standing, and walking. This creates increased stability for functional activities and aligns the lower limbs for more effective biomechanical function.

Biomechanical Function

The hip joint is a universal ball-and-socket joint with available motion in all three planes. Many orthoses control abduction/adduction and flexion/extension. If internal and external rotational control is needed, a long leg extension may be included in the orthotic design. Congenital hip disorders are frequently diagnosed at or soon after birth and require proper positioning to encourage normal bone development and alignment and proper angulation of the head, neck, and shaft of the femur. Acquired or degenerative disorders may require precise positioning and control to decrease pain and limit excessive forces transferred through the joint. As the hip joint is the dynamic link between the trunk and leg segments, misalignments and dysfunctions at this joint affect pre-positioning of the limb for stance and exacerbate large truncal deviations throughout the gait cycle.

General Indications and Contraindications

Hip orthoses may be used for congenital, dysplastic, traumatic, degenerative, or post-surgical procedures [Goldberg and Hsu 1997]. The Pavlik harness, Ilfeld orthosis, Von Rosen orthosis, and Frejka pillow are all used for developmental problems associated with dysplastic hip joints (Figure 17-18). These designs are used to realign the femoral head in the acetabulum to prevent continued dislocation and developing laxities. Legg-Perthes disease is a disorder presenting with osteochondrosis of the head of the femur and several orthotic

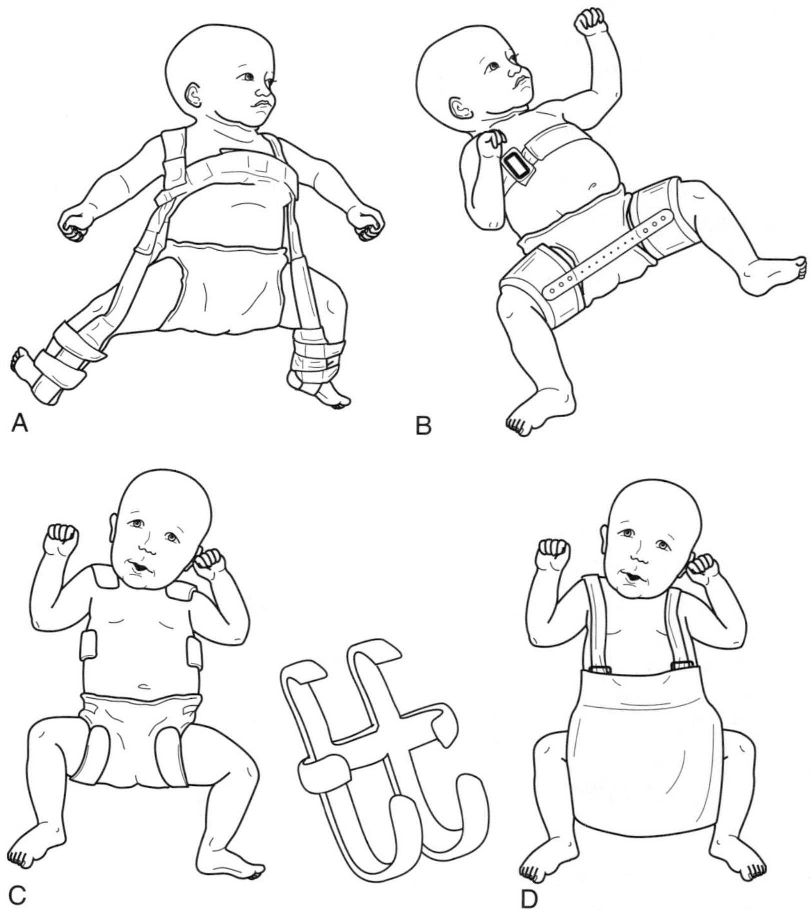

Figure 17-18 Various hip orthoses (note options). (A) Pavlik harness. (B) Ilfeld orthosis. (C) Von Rosen orthosis. (D) Frejka pillow.

designs have been developed to treat the affected pediatric population. Hip orthoses may also be used postoperatively after total hip replacement to control ROM and often to serve as effective "reminders" to maintain proper positioning during daily activities (Figure 17-19).

Many children with spasticity develop hip instability and pain, requiring either soft-tissue release of the adductors, flexors, and internal rotators of the hip or more complicated bony osteotomies of the pelvis or femur. Often hip spica casts are used postoperatively to maintain the surgical correction. Recently, pediatric hip orthoses have been used in some cases to replace hip spica casts. Hip orthoses are usually equipped with two sets of liners that can be washed daily to eliminate odor and improve hygiene. When the hip orthosis is no longer used 24 hours per day, it is sometimes used as a functional orthosis during the day or a positioning orthosis at night.

Design Options

Pediatric and adult populations require different orthotic approaches. In pediatrics, orthoses are designed to maintain good alignment during the normal growth processes of bone modeling. Controlled forces through the hip joints promote normal development of the head of the femur and the acetabulum. Hip orthoses for adults usually address the degenerative effects of joint deterioration. Clients with degenerative conditions are usually placed in orthoses that limit ROM in order to support and control compromised muscles and to prevent dislocation following primary or revision surgery.

Specific Applications

Although recurrent hip joint dislocation after surgical repair is rare, occasionally external support may be required for complicated procedures, revisions, or poor surgical outcomes. The joint of the hip orthosis is designed to provide variable alignment options as the person progresses through the rehabilitation process. Usually, the joint is aligned to maintain the hip in 10 to 20 degrees of abduction [Goldberg and Hsu 1997]. This helps to hold the head of the femur in the acetabulum.

Flexion and extension ranges are limited to prevent anterior or posterior dislocation while allowing the person to sit and walk. Internal and external rotation control is limited to some degree by "grasping" the soft tissue of the thigh. Proper fitting and adjustment and proper donning of the orthosis are critical to maximize function and effect. A shoulder strap is sometimes used to suspend the orthosis and maintain proper mechanical and anatomic joint congruency. A hip orthosis may also be ordered if the client has already dislocated the hip. The orthosis is usually worn for 3 to 6 months at all times to allow the soft tissue to heal and to serve as an effective kinesthetic reminder to maintain proper positioning during daily activities.

Dysplastic joints in the pediatric population present in varying degrees of severity. Legg-Perthes disease occurs more commonly in young boys and is identified as osteochondrosis of the femoral head. In the beginning of the disease process, occlusion of blood supply to the head of the femur promotes necrosis. Revascularization eventually occurs within the plastic bone. However, the bony contouring of the femoral head does not develop normally. Continued weight-bearing stresses increase the deformation of the hip joint and can result in permanent disability. Various hip orthoses have been designed to specifically treat this disease (Figures 17-18 and 17-19). As with most hip orthoses, this type of orthotic treatment program is temporary.

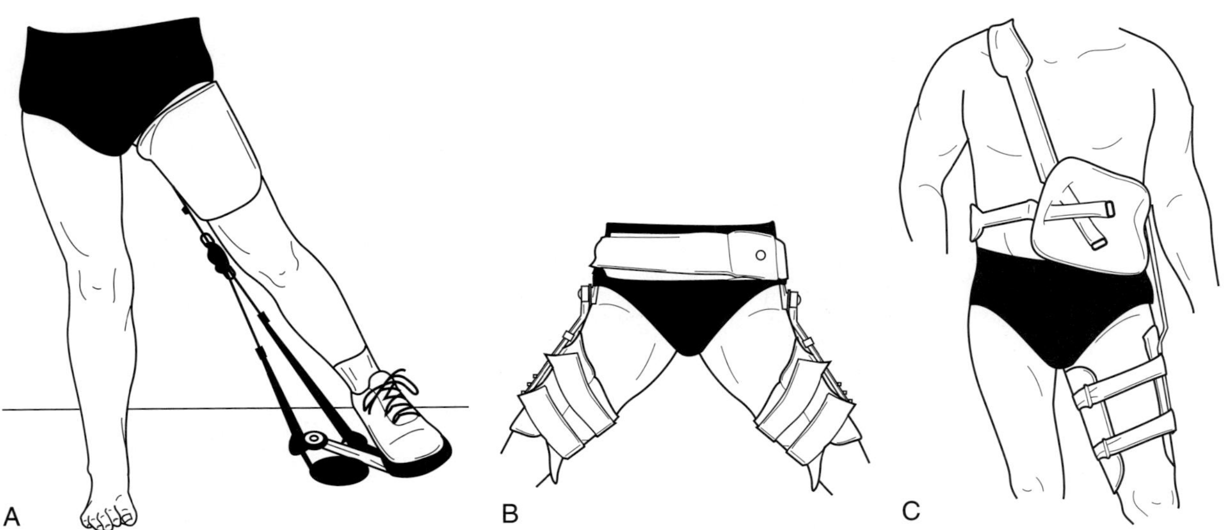

Figure 17-19 Legg-Perthes orthosis and total hip replacement orthosis. (A) Legg-Perthes orthosis. (B) Bilateral hip abduction orthosis with pelvic band. (C) Unilateral hip abduction orthosis with pelvic girdle and shoulder strap.

Role of the Occupational Therapist

After total hip arthrodesis (THA), hip abduction orthoses are commonly prescribed to limit ROM and promote healing. These devices are usually worn 24 hours per day for several weeks after surgery. Clothing is worn over the orthosis so that the client's hip is controlled at all times. Posterior dislocation is the most common type of dislocation and is most apt to occur with the hip positioned in flexion greater than 90 degrees internal rotation and adduction. Occasionally, the hip may dislocate in an anterior direction (<15% of dislocations). An anterior dislocation will also require a different set of hip precautions and a hip orthosis that has a long leg component attached to control rotation and hip extension.

Typically, persons require training in self-care activities such as dressing, bathing, toileting, and hygiene. Adaptive equipment (such as a reacher, sock-aid, extended bath sponge, extended shoe horn, and raised toilet seat) may reduce excessive hip flexion during hygiene and self-care. Most hip orthosis designs feature removable thigh and pelvic pads. These can be washed and hand dried quickly on a regular basis to prevent skin rash and breakdown.

Hip/Knee/Ankle/Foot Orthoses

Hip/knee/ankle/foot orthoses (HKAFOs) build upon the basic concepts outlined for KAFOs. A mechanical hip joint(s) and pelvic band or pelvic/trunk section is added to provide additional control and stability. These are very complex orthotic designs that require the skills of an experienced orthotist (Figure 17-20). Evaluation, casting, measuring, fitting, and follow-up are keys to the success of such extensive orthotic designs. HKAFOs can be used for both daily activities and therapeutic treatment programs. Energy costs may prohibit use of this type of orthosis for all instrumental activities of daily living, and wheelchair mobility may be a better option for some persons. Still, young persons with congenital deformities desire the opportunity to socialize with their peers "eye to eye," just as almost all persons with acquired trauma desire the opportunity to "walk" again.

Biomechanical Function

HKAFOs provide varying levels of mechanical control. Most simply, the KAFO is attached to the pelvic band with a single axis joint used to control rotational alignment of the limb during swing. This allows proper positioning of the limb for stance. More complex hip joint designs promote a reciprocal gait pattern so that extension of one limb promotes flexion of the contralateral limb, and vice versa. These reciprocating gait orthoses (RGOs) are used in both pediatric and adult populations, primarily for persons with flail bilateral lower limb involvement. Good upper extremity strength and adequate trunk control are prerequisites for this type of complex orthotic design.

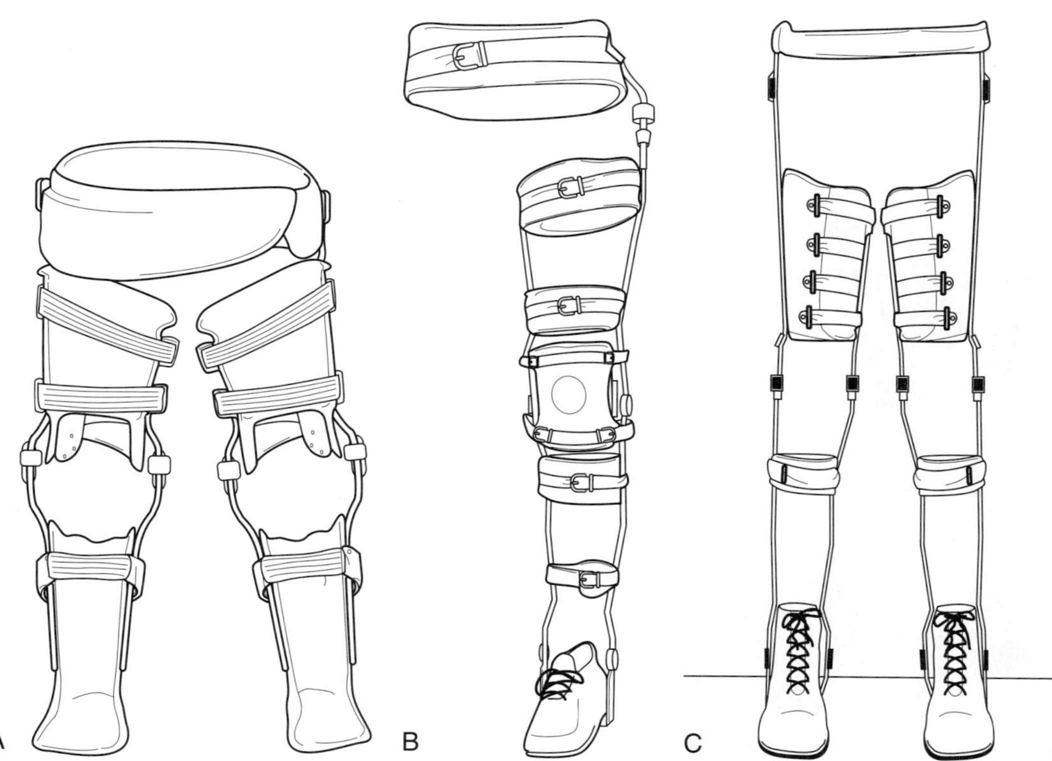

Figure 17-20 Various hip/knee/ankle/foot orthoses. (A) Bilateral thermoplastic HKAFOs. (B) Unilateral double-upright HKAFO. (C) Bilateral double-upright HKAFOs.

General Indications and Contraindications

HKAFOs control the hip joint alignment to pre-position the lower limb for weight acceptance. The hip or pelvic section may consist of a narrow band, or it may completely enclose the pelvis and trunk with a spinal orthosis that is then attached to the lower limb orthoses. The amount of bracing on the trunk segment depends on the functional abilities, control, and upper body strength of the person. HKAFOs are commonly prescribed for persons with spina bifida or spinal cord injury, or for any person presenting with a flail lower limb and limited hip control. Individual height, weight, strength, endurance, motivation, physical assistance requirements, donning abilities, and psychosocial situations must be evaluated with regard to the potential success of the orthotic program.

Design Options

The RGO is a unique design that makes ambulation possible for many persons who are unable to walk with the conventional HKAFO designs (Figure 17-21). The functions of the hip joints are coordinated and interdependent through a mechanical linkage. While standing, the person leans somewhat anteriorly to place the hip anterior to the distal base of support. Walking is initiated as the person pushes down with the ipsilateral arm while shifting the body weight toward the contralateral limb. As the limb is unloaded, it swings anteriorly, creating a slight forward momentum.

Through the mechanical linkage, ipsilateral hip flexion encourages contralateral (or stance side) extension. At this point, the contralateral hip is positioned anterior to the distal base of support and the cycle begins in the opposite direction. With training, this gait pattern can be smoothed considerably and an effective means of walking can be developed for those persons with few or no other options. Mechanical maintenance of the orthosis is extremely important to maintain the components in good working order, thus effecting the smooth transfer of momentum from side to side.

Specific Applications

Persons with spina bifida and spinal cord injury may benefit tremendously from this type of orthotic intervention. Upright weight bearing is associated with improved cardiopulmonary function, bowel and bladder function, circulation, and bone density [Kraft and Lehmann 1992]. Children benefit from the social interaction with their peers and can alternate with wheelchair mobility as needed. Almost all adult persons with traumatic spinal cord injury retain the desire to walk as a primary goal throughout their rehabilitation program.

Unfortunately, not all persons are candidates for this type of orthotic intervention. Modular RGOs are now available to be used as evaluative tools in determining the appropriateness of orthotic application at this level. Adjustable units are custom fitted and loaned to the person on a temporary basis. This allows the person to receive gait training, improve

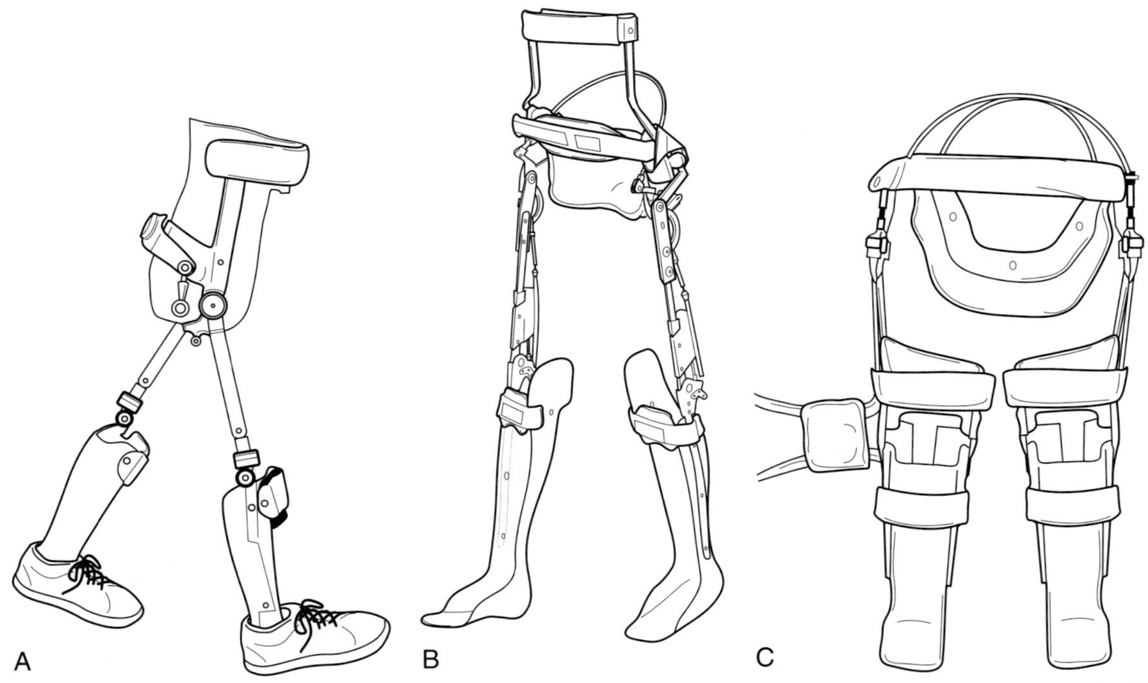

Figure 17-21 Reciprocating gait orthoses (note options). (A) Isocentric RGO. (B) Steeper advanced RGO (ARGO). (C) Fillauer cable design RGO.

upper body strength, and improve cardiovascular endurance. This is especially helpful in the person with questionable walking abilities who remains very motivated to pursue his or her walking potential. After a few weeks of training, definitive RGOs are then made to provide a more intimate fit and better control for the person.

Role of the Occupational Therapist

The potential success of the HKAFO program is dependent on many physical and biomechanical factors. The person's occupational performance potential may well be of critical importance in the team's decision to pursue HKAFO intervention. As previously stated, most persons identify ambulation as their primary rehabilitation goal. During intensive therapy, persons are likely to share their level of psychosocial acceptance with members of the rehabilitation team. The occupational therapist has ample opportunity to develop a level of trust during evaluation and training that allows the person to share feelings regarding the practicality of orthotic intervention.

HKAFO systems require much higher levels of energy expenditure, upper extremity strength, and endurance than many persons are able to maintain on a regular basis. Although it may be apparent to members of the multidisciplinary rehabilitation team that the person achieves much higher levels of functional independence when using a wheelchair for mobility, the person may still prefer to focus on ambulation as the primary goal. For many persons, the process of acceptance of the residual effects of disability may take many months or even years. The occupational therapist is in a unique position to help persons resolve these difficult issues in a supportive and encouraging manner.

Adding a pelvic component, hip joint, knee joint, or ankle control to an orthosis increases the difficulty of dressing and undressing. Difficulty with dressing tasks is magnified when the client is at work or school, and will require loose-fitting clothing and adaptive strategies for donning and doffing clothing. In addition, the occupational therapist may need to provide consultation for proper seating for toileting, desk work, or transportation. If the individual uses a wheelchair, it should be reassessed whenever a new orthosis is introduced to facilitate the best possible positioning.

Designing the Orthosis

The occupational therapist works closely with the orthotist during the design phase. All aspects of a comprehensive occupational therapy evaluation must be discussed and incorporated into the design of the orthosis. Because the HKAFO crosses and supports all lower extremity joints, considerations must be made based on the person's sensory, motor, psychosocial, and occupational performance. The person's strength should be considered in relation to the weight and force required to use the device. Fine motor strength and coordination will also impact the design and materials of the strapping system. Skin integrity and sensation will influence the material choice. The status of the activities of daily living must also be considered according to the donning and doffing of the device and the person's functional capabilities while using the device.

Overall, the occupational therapist's input related to the person's treatment goals, objectives, expectations, and living environment all impact the design decisions for the HKAFO. The orthotist has many options in designing the orthosis. Orthotists take all clinical information into consideration during this phase to help decide on each component of the design. Some examples include final materials, location of the openings for donning and doffing, and points of contact with the extremity. The distribution of the forces of contact falls within a continuum of total contact to that of multiple areas of contact. The complexities of the orthosis warrant discussion with the person and all members of the rehabilitation team. The more collaborative the team the better it will be for the person using the device.

Occupational Performance

Some adults find that donning an RGO over the head and sliding the device down the trunk to the hips while sitting on a bed is an energy-efficient method. Once the device is positioned at the hips, each lower extremity KAFO is donned. Tennis shoes that open to mid-foot are easier to slide into using the rigid-ankle AFO selection as a type of shoehorn. By pushing on top of the knee, people can usually put their heels into AFOs with shoes attached.

Once the pelvic band is secure, most people will be able to cross their legs to tie shoes. At times a rocker sole is added for balance assistance for the heel off phase of gait. As the center of gravity moves anterior on the stance side, the rocker will assist in initiation of knee flexion. Overall, people must persevere through a tedious process of skill acquisition to don and doff their RGO independently. Many find the process frustrating and time consuming. Learning to don and doff the orthosis requires the trial of many techniques before the most effective one is identified.

Summary

Short- and Long-term Treatment Programs

Orthotic treatment programs have both short- and long-term effects on persons fitted with assistive devices. The short-term benefits often include the relief of pain, support and alignment of the skeletal system, functional substitution, and correction of deformity. Long-term benefits relate to increased metabolic efficiency as the person acclimates to a more mechanically effective alignment. Correction and prevention of joint deformity is critical in maintaining long-term ambulation abilities. Keep in mind that any new orthosis will alter the mechanical profile of the person and affect his or her habitual walking pattern. It may take several days or

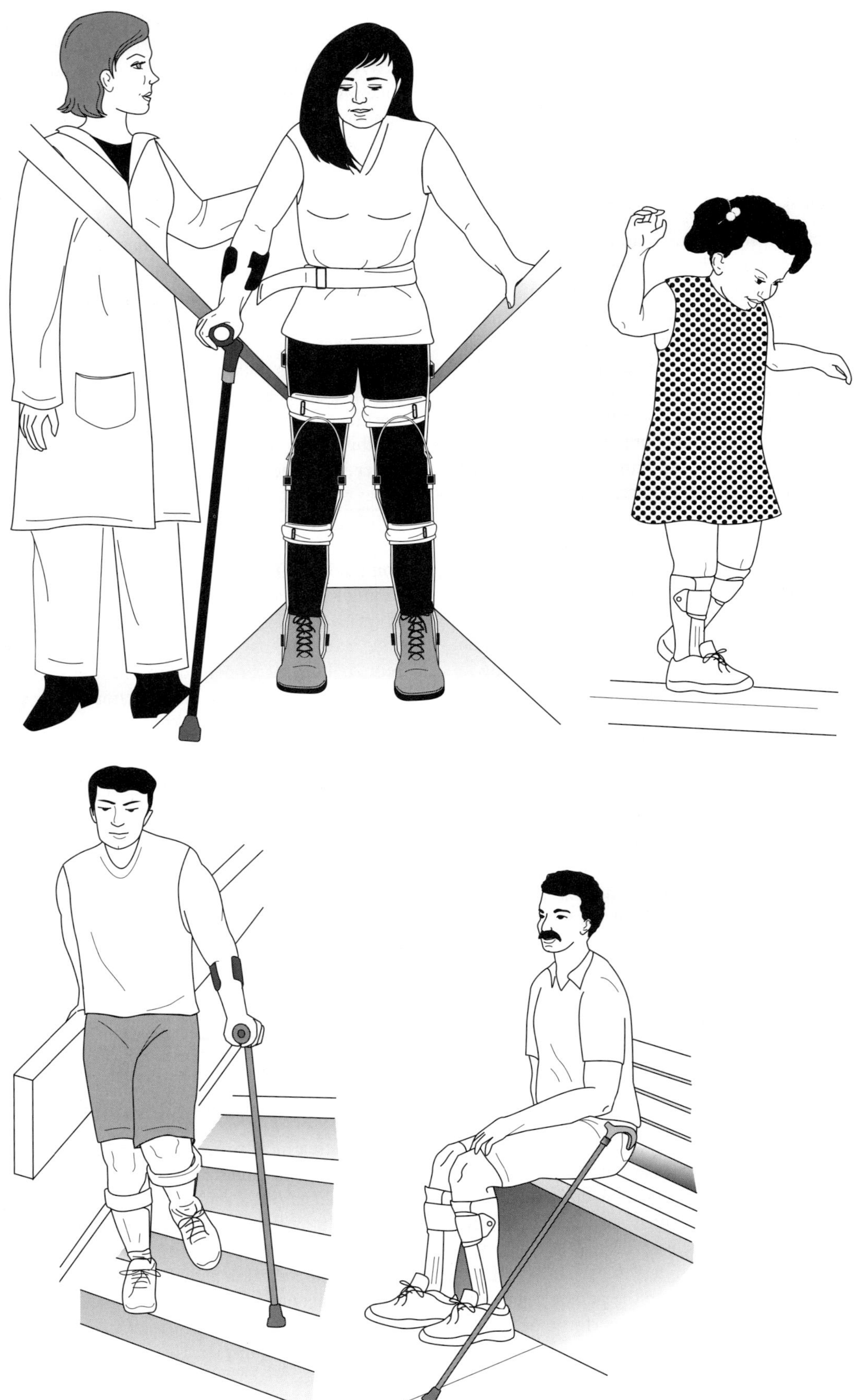

Figure 17-22 Functional activities and quality of life. With an effective orthotic treatment program, persons are able to return to their former life or to learn many functional activities and enjoy an improved quality of life.

even weeks of attention and concentration to adapt to a new orthosis, depending on the mechanical, functional, or alignment changes that have been made.

A graduated wearing schedule should be provided to each person, even if the new orthosis is a replacement. Acclimation should occur over a period of 1 to 2 weeks in most cases, although insensate limbs or limbs with severe deformities may require a longer period of time to get used to the corrective forces being applied. The person or caregiver is given specific wearing instructions, often starting with just 15 to 20 minutes of wearing time. Each time the orthosis is removed, careful inspection of the skin is required.

Immediately upon removal of the orthosis, the skin will appear slightly pink in areas of pressure application (i.e., relative to the three-point force systems used for alignment corrections). The discoloration of these areas should dissipate within 20 to 30 minutes. Discontinuation of the orthosis is recommended if dark or bright red areas are discovered (especially over bony prominences), if the discoloration continues for extended periods of time, or if excessive discomfort is experienced. The orthotist should be contacted and an appointment made for updated evaluation and adjustment to the orthosis.

It will be necessary to maintain a strict follow-up schedule with the orthotist, especially during the first two to three months after fitting. This ensures that proper alignment of the lower limb is maintained and allows for periodic maintenance of the orthosis. It may be necessary to make changes or adjustments to the orthosis during this initial wearing period. It is not uncommon to add or remove padding as changes occur in the skeletal alignment and walking pattern. Ultimately, the orthosis will be adjusted to provide maximum structural alignment and functional ability in the most comfortable manner possible. An annual or semiannual checkup routine is recommended thereafter.

Periodic reevaluation of the person is a necessary component of the orthotic treatment program. Functional abilities, muscle strengths and control, balance, and cognitive abilities can all change over time. The purpose of "minimal orthotic intervention" is to provide only the necessary stability or functions and to challenge the person's neuromuscular system to function at the most appropriate level. Depending on the person's physical condition, it may be necessary to downgrade or upgrade the orthosis over time.

Interprofessional Team Approach

The greatest advantage of the interprofessional team approach is the extensive background the team presents. Each member of the rehabilitation team brings with him or her specific skills and knowledge relative to care of the individual. It is important that information be shared among the members of the team so that the most appropriate treatment plan can be formed. Within a group, the exchange of information, experiences, and ideas allows the development of an individualized and effective rehabilitation program for each person. Keep in mind that the orthotic user is the most important member of the rehabilitation team, with important insight into medical condition, goals, motivations, and abilities. Involvement of all team members maximizes communication and increases the potential acceptance, satisfaction, and success of the orthotic treatment program as well as an improvement in the quality of life for the person (Figure 17-22).

Occupational therapist's unique training and skills enhance the treatment of individuals receiving lower extremity orthoses. By focusing treatment on motor performance, positioning, and function, the occupational therapist can impact on the success of orthotic programs. Therapists' treatment plans should incorporate techniques that increase ROM, strength, muscle control, and coordination. Skin desensitization and sensory reeducation strategies should also be employed. Furthermore, therapists' concentration on activities of daily living maximizes the person's functional performance. In general, as members of the interprofessional team occupational therapists support team goals and objectives during the treatment process. A collaborative team effort leads to the increased acceptance, utilization, and functional capacity of the orthotic user.

Rehabilitation Treatment Program

The field of orthotics is in a period of rapid change. The introduction of new materials, products, and computer-assisted design processes continues to evolve new and useful orthotic designs for persons requiring external support. Still, an orthosis is only a tool. The potential usefulness of an orthotic tool relies on the effectiveness of the therapy service or training program.

The coordinated efforts of the multidisciplinary team combine product (i.e., orthosis) and service (i.e., therapy) to create a successful rehabilitation program. Individual benefits include consistent information, cohesive protocols, improved outcomes, and improved satisfaction. The interdependence of the product and the service cannot be overemphasized. Rehabilitation team members must work together to maximize the functional skills and abilities of each individual. Ultimately, success is achieved with an improvement in the overall quality of life for each person served.

CASE STUDY 17-1*

Read the following scenario and answer the questions based on information in this chapter.

A. B. experienced a CVA six months ago. Initial evaluation reveals moderate spasticity and extensor tone of the right lower extremity. The foot and ankle complex is aligned in an equinovarus posture but can be realigned manually with moderate force. A 10-degree plantar-flexion contracture is present. A. B. reports occasional falling secondary to anterior knee collapse. Weakness is noted in the quadriceps, dorsiflexors, and gastrocnemius-soleus muscle groups. Observational gait assessment identifies the following: drop-foot during swing phase, circumduction to obtain ground clearance, sustained equinovarus posturing during swing and stance phases, knee hyperextension during stance phase, minimal weight transfer over the involved limb, and a step-to gait pattern in which the left uninvolved limb is never advanced beyond the right during walking. A. B. currently uses a cane for additional support and stability.

1. Which of the following orthotic designs is most appropriate for A. B.? Explain your answer.
   a. A UCBL-type foot orthosis designed to align the mid-tarsal and subtalar joints in a mechanically effective alignment during stance phase.
   b. A flexible thermoplastic AFO that provides dorsiflexion assistance during swing phase, free plantar-flexion and free dorsiflexion ROM during stance phase, and minimal foot and ankle alignment during stance phase.
   c. An articulated thermoplastic AFO that provides dorsiflexion assistance during swing phase, limited plantar-flexion and dorsiflexion during stance phase, and controlled alignment of the foot and ankle complex during stance phase.
   d. An articulated double-upright AFO that provides dorsiflexion assistance during swing phase, limited plantar-flexion and free dorsiflexion during stance phase, and minimal mediolateral foot and ankle alignment during stance phase.
   e. A locked-knee KAFO that provides dorsiflexion assistance during swing phase, limited plantar-flexion and dorsiflexion during stance phase, and controlled alignment of the foot and ankle complex during stance phase.

   ____
   ____
   ____

2. A. B. is resistant to the use of an AFO. He believes that if he continues to exercise and walk daily he will regain strength and control of the left lower limb. How would you address A. B. to persuade him to use the support and stability offered by an AFO?

   ____
   ____
   ____

A. B. received an orthosis from his orthotist 2 days ago. He received a graduated wearing schedule to help him acclimate to the forces and corrected alignment provided by the new orthosis. He reports a slight discoloration of the skin over the medial forefoot and medial heel after removal of the orthosis. The color fades completely within 10 minutes.

3. What is the best course of action at this time?
   a. A. B. is instructed to continue with the graduated wearing schedule and is to continue to inspect his skin after removal of the orthosis.
   b. A. B. is instructed to proceed to full-time wear of the orthosis.
   c. A. B. is instructed to discontinue use of the orthosis and return immediately to the orthotist.
   d. A. B. is instructed to place a Band-Aid or pad over the discolored areas before donning the orthosis.
   e. A. B. is instructed to wear extra socks before donning the orthosis.

A. B. has been wearing the orthosis for 6 months. He reports full-time wear of the orthosis, donning the orthosis in the morning upon rising and removing the orthosis each evening after dinner. He would like to regain some independence by learning to drive again but is concerned about the restricted ankle motion available in the orthosis, as it limits his ability to push down on the accelerator.

4. What is the best course of action for A. B.?
   a. Instruct A. B. to loosen the screws at the ankle joint until he can plantar-flex the foot freely.
   b. Instruct A. B. to return to his orthotist for a new orthosis to be used for driving purposes.
   c. Instruct A. B. that he will not be able to drive with the orthosis.
   d. Instruct A. B. to use right-side hip and pelvic motion to depress the accelerator, in that any adjustments to the orthosis will detract from his walking abilities.
   e. Instruct A. B. to purchase a bus pass.

5. A. B. reports enhanced walking abilities with the AFO. He now walks approximately 1 to 2 miles a day. With cold weather approaching, he is concerned about walking outdoors but is worried that he will lose all he has gained over the last six months. What advice can you give A. B. that will allow him to continue his walking program safely throughout the winter months?

   ____
   ____
   ____

---

*See Appendix A for the answer key.

CASE STUDY 17-2*

Read the following scenarios and answer the questions based on information in this chapter.

Case A

M. H. has osteoarthritis and has received a knee orthosis that was prescribed by her physician. M. H. returns to you for follow-up, reporting minimal use of her knee orthosis because she thinks it is unsightly and bulky.

1. How would you address the cosmetic concerns presented by M. H. and convince her of the need to wear the orthosis?

____

____

____

Case B

T. F. was involved in a car accident and sustained a closed head injury. He has been wearing an ankle/foot orthosis for the last 6 months after being discharged. T. F. has achieved functional walking with the AFO but wants to get back to a "normal" life and discontinue use of the orthosis. His motor profile is unchanged since discharge, still presenting with residual weakness of the lower limb and drop-foot.

1. What issues and concerns would you raise with this client, and how would you explain the need for long-term use of the AFO?

____

____

____

Case C

D. F. was fitted with bilateral foot orthoses to provide relief of plantar fasciitis and heel pain. She wears the foot orthoses occasionally, perhaps once or twice a week. She does not like them and thinks they have provided little relief of her discomfort.

1. How would you manage this client? What course of treatment would you outline so that D. F. receives maximum benefit from the existing foot orthoses?

*See Appendix A for the answer key.

REVIEW QUESTIONS

1. What health care professionals provide custom orthotic services to persons?
2. What are the four basic functions of a lower extremity orthosis?
3. What are the two basic components of walking?
4. What is one functional compensation used during walking?
5. Who should be involved in the development of the orthotic treatment program?
6. What are the five major joints of the lower extremity?
7. What are three classifications of orthoses?
8. What skin inspection techniques can be taught to the person with insensate feet?
9. What are some differences between metal and plastic AFOs?
10. What are some reasons for prescription of an AFO?
11. What are the three classifications of knee orthoses?
12. What are the names of some of the commonly used locking mechanisms at the knee?
13. Which type of knee joint lock requires the greatest balance, upper extremity range, and hand function?
14. What types of training would a person wearing a postoperative hip orthosis require?
15. Should all persons be fitted with RGOs? Why?

References

Braddom RL (1996). *Physical Medicine and Rehabilitation.* Philadelphia: W. B. Saunders.

Bunch WH, Keagy RD (1976). *Principles of Orthotic Treatment.* St. Louis: Mosby.

Bunch WH, Keagy R, Kritter AE, Kruger LM, Letts M, Lonstein JE, et al. (eds.), (1985). *Atlas of Orthotics, Second Edition.* St. Louis: Mosby.

Goldberg B, Hsu JD (eds.), (1997). *Atlas of Orthoses and Assistive Devices, Third Edition.* St. Louis: Mosby.

Kottke FJ, Lehmann JF (eds.), (1990). *Krusen's Handbook of Physical Medicine and Rehabilitation, Fourth Edition.* Philadelphia: W. B. Saunders.

Kraft GH, Lehmann JF (eds.), (1992). Physical Medicine and Rehabilitation Clinics of North America 3(1).

Perry J (1992). *Gait Analysis: Normal and Pathological Function.* Thorofare, NJ: Slack.

CHAPTER 18

Upper Extremity Prosthetics

Kris M. Vacek, OTD, OTR/L
Omar Aragón, OTD, OTR/L

Key Terms

Biofeedback machine
Body powered
Componentry
Compression socks
Contralateral limb
Dual site
Electrodes
Externally powered
Functional envelope
Grip force
Harness
Hook rubbers
Lamination
Myoelectrics
Nerve entrapment
Overuse syndrome
Phantom pain
Phantom sensation
Residual limb
Single site
Socket
Suspension systems
Terminal device
Transhumeral amputation
Transradial amputation

Chapter Objectives

1. Identify the characteristics of various upper extremity prosthetic devices.
2. Define the various causes and levels of amputation.
3. Differentiate between various levels of amputation.
4. Identify advantages and disadvantages of passive (semiactive), body-powered, externally powered, and recreational prostheses.
5. Differentiate the roles of the prosthetic team members.
6. Describe the sequence of training in prosthetic rehabilitation.
7. Explain the unique role of the occupational therapist in upper extremity prosthetic rehabilitation.
8. Identify psychosocial aspects of clients with amputations.
9. Describe upper extremity prosthetic intervention in children.
10. Discuss new updates in prosthetic technology and research.

Some readers may question the compatibility of a prosthetics chapter in this orthotics text. Several chapters in this text address needs of specific populations. This text is designed as a resource for those therapists interested in developing orthotic skills to address the needs of these populations. Therapists who treat persons with orthotic needs will naturally be called upon to provide services to persons with upper extremity amputations.

Orthotics and prosthetics are closely interrelated fields. Forty percent of American Board for Certification (ABC) certified practitioners hold credentials in both orthotics and prosthetics. This chapter is designed to serve as a resource for those therapists who serve this historically underserved population. Approximately 40,000 amputations occur each year in the United States. Thirty percent involve the upper extremity [Leonard and Meier 1988, Muilenburg and LeBlanc 1989], and upper extremity amputations represent approximately 10,000 people per year [Malone et al. 1984, Centers for Disease Control and Prevention 1996].

Approximately 50% of individuals are fitted with prostheses [Muilenburg and LeBlanc 1989]. Of the 50% fitted with a prosthesis, only half actually wear the device. Experts cite numerous reasons for this trend [Shurr and Cook 1990].

Fit and prosthetic training appear to be the most salient factors that affect prosthetic wear [Bennett and Alexander 1989]. The role of the prosthetist is to provide a well-fitting prosthetic device. It is the role of the occupational therapist to assist the individual to become an independent user of the device. The prosthesis is often heavy and awkward to use. If the fit is not tolerable, or if the potential wearer has not been properly trained to use the device, the prosthesis may end up on the closet shelf.

Unfortunately, only a small number of health care providers have extensive knowledge of the rehabilitation of the person with an upper extremity amputation. The typical therapist may encounter few individuals with upper extremity amputations. Thus, it is difficult to remain abreast of the current prosthetic trends and technologic developments that affect how therapists promote the maximal level of independence for the client with an upper extremity amputation. However, occupational therapists can make a substantial difference in the lives of individuals with amputations if they possess knowledge of the various factors that impact the life of a person with an amputation.

This chapter provides the therapist with general knowledge on upper extremity amputations and their impact on function. Next, the chapter delineates roles of the team members and discusses the various prosthetic options and componentry. Goals for occupational therapy (OT) throughout the prosthetic rehabilitation process are described. Finally, this chapter describes marketing strategies and recommendations for a therapist wanting to increase the number of prosthetic referrals received.

Amputation Levels and the Impact on Function

Figure 18-1 provides an outline of the various amputation levels, along with abbreviations associated with them [Santschi 1958]. The more distal the amputation the greater the degree of natural function retained. Consequently, less is demanded of the prosthesis [Law 1981]. For example, an individual who has an amputation at the midhumeral level may be functionally able to use shoulder internal and external rotation along with other shoulder motions. However, the person lacks elbow flexion and extension and forearm supination and pronation. This is a disadvantage. If an individual with a midhumeral amputation wants to receive money from a cashier, more effort is required.

First, positioning and locking the elbow in flexion is necessary. Next, the person manually rotates the terminal device to the palm-up position with the sound side. Finally, the person is ready to perform the act of receiving the money. Conversely, an individual with an amputation at the wrist level is functionally able to pronate and supinate, flex and extend the elbow, and retain full shoulder function in the completion of activities of daily living (ADL).

The ability to pronate and supinate serves as a substantial advantage, enabling the person with the amputation to turn the prosthetic hand palm up as if to receive money from a cashier without the substitution movements of shoulder external rotation. Whether or not an individual chooses to wear a prosthesis, the level of amputation directly impacts function. The estimated frequencies of levels of amputation of the 50% who wear a prosthesis are presented in Table 18-1, indicating which level is most common [Muilenburg and LeBlanc 1989]. It is apparent that most amputations occur at the transradial level.

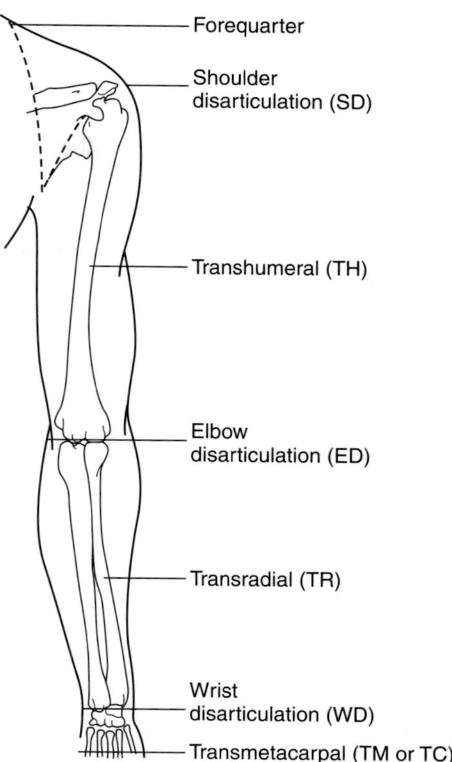

Figure 18-1 Levels of upper extremity amputation.

Causes of Upper Extremity Amputations

The causes of upper extremity amputations differ from the causes of lower extremity amputations. Lower extremity amputations are largely a result of disease. The majority of

Table 18-1 Percentage of Amputation Level for Prosthetic Users

AMPUTATION LEVEL	PERCENT
Shoulder disarticulation	5
Transhumeral	23
Elbow disarticulation	3
Transradial	57
Wrist disarticulation and partial hand	12

upper extremity amputations result from trauma [Leonard and Meier 1988]. Other causes include disease, tumors, elective surgery, and genetic anomaly [Bennett and Alexander 1989]. Commonly, therapists work with individuals who before injury used their hands extensively in their daily occupations. Often these persons hope to regain a similar level of independence. A power-line worker describes his experience in the following words.

The 7,200-volt power line was approximately five feet from where I came in contact with it. It's a strange thing, but I don't remember touching it. According to my co-workers, I started screaming and there was a bright electrical arc between my hands for about 10 seconds. The foreman shut off the power and got the boom truck to get me down. . . . I noticed there was no flesh on my hands anymore. Both hands were charcoal black! I knew they would have to be amputated, but the only thing I was concerned with was getting to a hospital to relieve some of the unbearable pain. . . . I've had four major operations at St. Elizabeth for amputations. I didn't know for sure at the time how much they would have to take off. They amputated just above the elbow the first time. And I remember that the stumps looked pretty long the first time, but the second time they got a little shorter, and then the third time they really got short. On the fourth operation they removed an infected area from my right stump and armpit. I was given medication to help build tissue to fill those holes back in [Crane 1979, p. 10].

The Team Members

The team treating a person with an amputation is instrumental in the prosthesis-fitting process. The team consists of the person with the amputation, the prosthetist, and the therapist. The primary goal of therapy is to provide the individual with the proper tools and techniques to regain independence. A team approach combines expertise and experience, creating a synergy of professionalism, with team members working together and promoting the maximal level of independence for the individual with the amputation. The best results in upper extremity rehabilitation include interdisciplinary teamwork [Baumgartner and Bota 1992].

The Client

The primary member of this team is the person with the amputation. Individual goals, desires, and needs establish the foundation for which the team develops the action plan. Clients' priorities for rehabilitation can vary. Common concerns include cosmesis, function, weight, maintenance, and funding for the prosthesis [Atkins et al. 1996]. For example, the needs of an individual with a transradial amputation who works full-time and desires to return to work may vary from those of an individual who is a stay-at-home parent. The type of prosthesis selected would vary, depending on a precise analysis of the client's work, leisure activities, and ADL.

An important aspect to the client is early postoperative prosthetic fitting. The advantages of early fitting are decreased edema, reduced postoperative and phantom pain, accelerated wound healing, improved rehabilitation, and decreased length of hospital stay [Malone et al. 1984].

The Prosthetist

The prosthetist has knowledge of the technology and componentry available. The prosthetist specializes in componentry, fit, and prosthesis fabrication. It is the responsibility of the prosthetist to understand the client's primary diagnosis as it relates to the need for prosthetic services [Billock 2003]. The prosthetist must introduce, educate, and orient the client to the controls and functions of the prosthesis. Daily care and maintenance of the prosthesis are taught to the client by the prosthetist and should be reinforced by the therapist. The prosthetist and the therapist may collaborate when exploring the prosthetic options with the client.

The Occupational Therapist

A well-rounded rehabilitation program is advised because the quality of training will directly determine how the individual uses the prosthesis for the rest of his or her life [Lake 1997]. The therapist has many responsibilities. It is important that therapists know the basic differences in prostheses to make proper recommendations of components to the team. Therapists should also recognize the importance of collaboration with skilled upper extremity prosthetists, with the purpose of maximizing the training process and the degree of independence [Atkins and Alley 2003]. Without proper therapy, the benefits of prosthetic use may be limited.

The therapist reinforces and builds on residual movement, developing functional applications of the prosthesis to address the distinct ADL (e.g., brushing teeth) and instrumental ADL (e.g., driving) of each individual [Toren 2002]. The therapist is responsible for ensuring the client knows how to clean and maintain the prosthesis. In addition, the therapist provides opportunities for the client to practice using the prosthesis in specific daily activities. The therapist focuses on bilateral activities. Often, after amputation the individual becomes successful in performing some ADLs unilaterally. Thus, therapy must begin early in the rehabilitation process to facilitate use of the prosthesis in bilateral activities.

Initial prosthetic training begins with a reorientation to the prosthesis and basic open-and-close control. Training then includes controlled grasp, such as opening in small increments to grasp small items and then more fully to grasp larger items. Training emphasizes grasping objects of varied texture and density to be handled. Sessions incorporate work on prehension and timing of release. Functional and appropriate tasks are encouraged and require the client to use the prosthesis for gross and fine motor activities. Training also emphasizes tasks to achieve all of these components in a variety of planes [Patterson et al. 1991, Keenan 1995]. With the combined efforts of the team members, the appropriate prosthetic components are chosen so that the individual can achieve goals through therapy, practice, and education.

Prosthetic Options

Generally, four categories of prosthetic options are available for the person with an upper extremity amputation. The options include (1) no prosthesis; (2) a passive (semiactive), cosmetic prosthesis; (3) a cable-driven body-powered prosthesis; and (4) an externally powered, electrically controlled prosthesis with either myoelectric sensors or specialized switches. Table 18-2 outlines the pros and cons of each prosthetic option [Law 1981, Muilenburg and LeBlanc 1989].

A prosthetic device cannot mechanically duplicate the amount of function, reliability, and cosmesis the human hand naturally provides. Therefore, it is important for the health care provider to possess knowledge of the various options continually being developed for future selection of prostheses. A fundamental understanding of these five components is necessary. These five components include the harness, socket, cable, terminal device, and glove.

No Prosthesis

Wearing no prosthesis is one option, and for some individuals it is the best option. For example, an individual may not be able to tolerate the prosthesis for reasons such as residual limb hypersensitivity, soft tissue adhesions, and excessive scarring [Atkins and Meier 1989]. Individuals who choose not to wear a prosthesis may find advantages and disadvantages with their decision, which are found in Table 18-2.

Advantages include increased proprioceptive and sensory input. Disadvantages include limited functional ability, difficulty in completion of bimanual tasks, and possibly the development of overuse syndrome and nerve entrapment in the contralateral limb [Reddy 1984]. Additional reasons an individual may not wear a prosthesis include not knowing the prosthetic options, having a bad first prosthetic experience, lack of funding, or reluctance to undergo revision surgery necessary for prosthetic fit and reduction of hypersensitivity [NovaCare 1991].

Passive Prosthesis

A passive (semiactive) prosthesis option is common for individuals who have had amputation distal to the elbow, in that they may maintain elbow flexion and extension and forearm pronation and supination. In this case, the obvious purpose is cosmetic. However, a passive prosthesis provides some degree of function. A passive prosthesis has many benefits, including its light weight, minimal (if any) harnessing, no cables, and low maintenance. Disadvantages include lack of prehensile abilities and difficulty in performing some bimanual tasks. Functionally, the digits of a passive prosthesis can be adjusted to assist with such activities as carrying a purse or a document or operating the gearshift in an automobile [Law 1981].

Body-powered Prosthesis

A body-powered prosthesis is a type of functional prosthesis most commonly used by clients with upper extremity amputations [Law 1981]. The body-powered prosthesis may not be cosmetically pleasing to everyone, but it is sturdy and

Table 18-2 Advantages and Disadvantages of Prosthetic Options

PROSTHETIC OPTION	ADVANTAGES	DISADVANTAGES
No prosthesis	• Maintain full proprioception and sensation	• Limited functional ability • Difficult to perform bimanual tasks
Passive prosthesis	• Light weight • Minimal (if any) harnessing • No cables; low maintenance	• Prosthesis has no prehension abilities • Difficult to perform bimanual tasks
Body-powered prosthesis	• Heavy-duty construction and function • Reduced maintenance cost • Proprioception	• Restrictive/uncomfortable harness • Poor cosmesis • Restrictive functional work area • Limited grip force
Externally powered prosthesis	• Unlimited work area • Function cosmetic restoration • Increased grip force • Harness system reduced or absent • Increased comfort • More modern, high-tech appeal • Interchangeable components • Development of technology to provide for individual custom fabrication	• Battery maintenance • Increased weight • Susceptible to damage from moisture • Increased cost

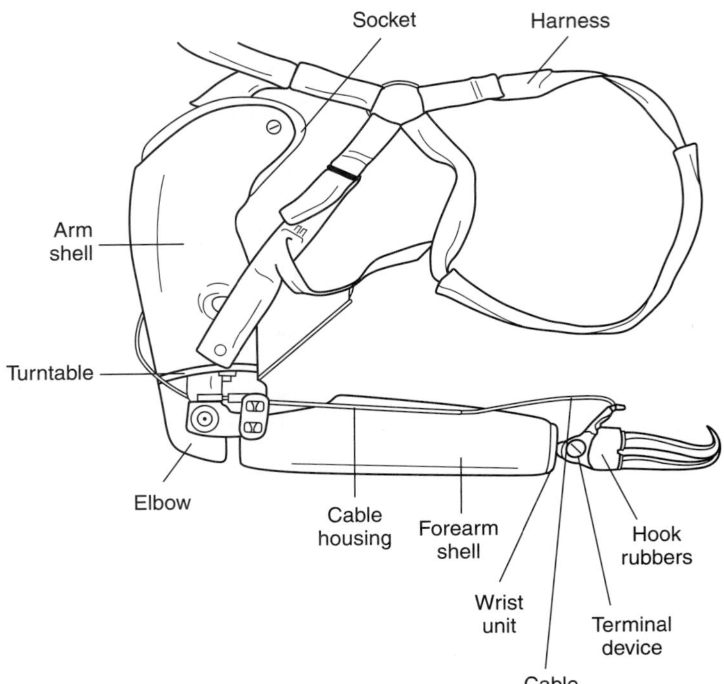

Figure 18-2 Components of a body-powered prosthesis.

allows for prehension. Body-powered upper limb prostheses are actuated by body motion, which generates tension in a cable. The cable courses from a shoulder harness through a helical coiled housing to a prosthetic component, such as a hook or elbow [Carlson et al. 1995]. In other words, the active movements of the shoulder and arm cause the tension in the cable to open and close the hand or handlike component (hook). The device is illustrated in Figure 18-2.

Benefits of a body-powered prosthesis include its heavy-duty function and construction, decreased maintenance cost, and increased proprioceptive input. Disadvantages may include the restrictive uncomfortable harness, potential for nerve entrapment or compression, decreased cosmetic appearance, restricted functional work area, and limited grip force. Body-powered terminal devices generally weigh less than the externally powered prostheses because they lack the heavy motors and circuitry placed within them to operate the myoelectric signals [Atkins and Meier 1989].

Body-powered Prosthetic Components

The Harness. The purpose of the harness is to suspend the prosthesis on the residual limb. It transmits force from the body to the prosthesis for independent operation of the prosthetic components [Muilenburg and LeBlanc 1989]. The body-powered prosthesis always requires harnessing. There are two primary types of harness: a figure-of-eight and a chest strap. The figure-of-eight harness passes over the shoulder, across the back, and under the contralateral axilla. "The ring lies flat in the back, inferior to C-7 and just to the sound side of the center of the spine" [Shurr and Cook 1990].

The standard figure-of-eight shoulder harness (Figure 18-3A) for the upper extremity has an axilla loop on the sound side that is commonly uncomfortable and can cause numbness and nerve damage [Collier and Le Blanc 1996]. The chest strap offers an alternative method of harnessing. It travels across the back, under the contralateral axilla, and across the chest (Figure 18-3B). It is important that the harness, either figure-of-eight or chest strap, be tight enough to activate the terminal device (TD) without excessive effort and loose enough to be comfortable and allow freedom of movement of both arms and shoulders.

Long-term wear and inappropriate fit may cause discomfort or physical damage. The harness has been found to limit the functional work envelope, which is the space in front of the person who is able to use the prosthesis successfully for functional tasks. Harness systems limit successful prehension when the TD is outside the functional work area. With the body-powered prosthesis, function is limited above the head, behind the back, and near the ground, primarily because of the restricting harness (Figure 18-4). The prosthesis functions as a result of the ability to move in these planes.

Discomfort and neurologic and musculoskeletal disorders can result from inefficient harness design [Carlson et al. 1995] and long-term wear. After years of wearing a harness, the axilla of the sound side experiences increased force and pressure to operate the prosthesis repetitively throughout the day. This can result in neurologic damage. A strong case can be made for providing a myoelectric or externally

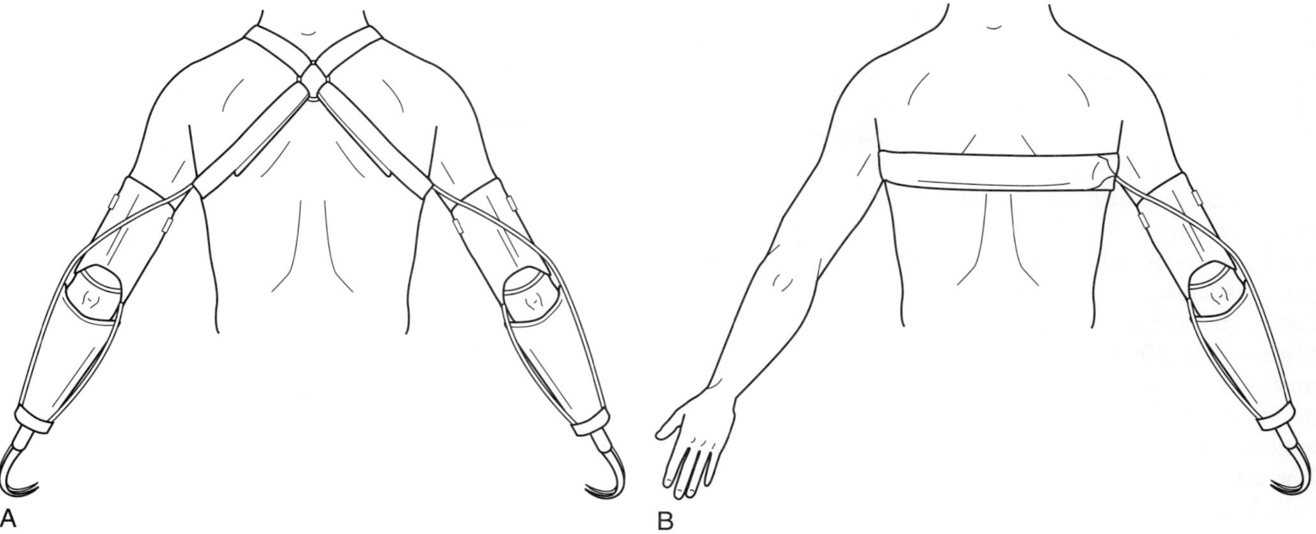

Figure 18-3 (A) A standard figure-of-eight harness. (B) A chest strap harness.

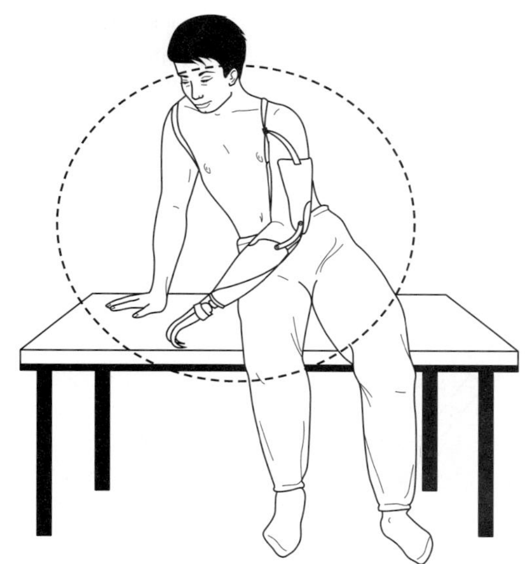

Figure 18-4 Functional work area (body-powered prosthesis).

powered prosthesis that either eliminates or reduces the harnessing. This prevents the risk of long-term nerve damage on the sound side.

The prosthetist is responsible for fabrication of the harness, and the therapist occasionally may make minor adjustments to improve function. Sometimes several harness options are attempted to find the type of system that best fits the amputee. It is often a trial-and-error process. Another important factor is the awareness of the increased workload in the remaining arm, which may produce symptoms ranging from minor aches to serious conditions such as nerve entrapment and overuse syndrome [Jones and Davidson 1999].

The Socket. The socket is the part of the prosthesis that intimately fits over the individual's residual limb. It is the connection between the prosthesis and the individual's body. The socket is fabricated from an exact mold of the residual limb, and it is fabricated from various types of laminate or thermoplastic material. Development of high-temperature rigid plastic materials has made it possible to have total contact on the skin and allow decreased weight and increased durability. The use of carbon graphite and the introduction of flexible thermoplastics are more comfortable, lighter, and durable and have made soft sockets with windows possible. The prosthetist makes modifications over bony prominences and areas susceptible to torque and shear forces [Andrews and Bouvette 1996]. Typically, three to four sockets will be fabricated before the final one is delivered.

Intimate socket fit provides a stable foundation of support necessary to transfer forces from the TD. It provides evenly distributed pressure on the residual limb, which prevents skin breakdown or pressure sores. In the last decade, a multitude of design innovations have been incorporated, which have resulted in developing better comfort, suspension, stability, and range of motion. The new fitting techniques and socket designs appear to be more efficient for force of transmission and motion capture and more functionally consistent than traditional sockets [Alley 2002]. Occasionally, the prosthetist instructs the individual to wear the socket before all components are attached. This increases wearing tolerance and facilitates reshaping of the residual limb.

As the person with the amputation ages, physical and physiologic changes occur. The person may experience weight loss or gain or muscle bulk increase or decrease. These changes have an impact on the size and condition of the residual limb, and the socket may no longer fit as it should. A new socket must be fabricated to fit the exact shape of the residual limb when changes occur. When a new socket is fabricated, it replaces the poorly fitting one in the individual's current prosthesis. An entirely new prosthesis is not needed because the socket is removable and replaceable.

This saves on cost. The wearer of a body-powered prosthesis may benefit from using a second sheath or sock made of either a fabric or a gel-like substance to manage poor skin integrity, prevent breakdown, absorb moisture, or provide padding.

The Cable. The harness allows placement of the cable, which is the transmitting force that operates the prosthesis. Body-powered prostheses are operated by body motion that generates tension in the cable. The cable is routed from the harness through a housing to the terminal device or elbow [Carlson et al. 1995]. The primary movement to operate the prosthesis is glenohumeral flexion. As the individual flexes the humerus, the TD opens. As the individual returns the humerus to neutral, the hook rubbers cause the TD to close. When the individual wishes to open the TD closer to the body, biscapular abduction is used and adduction or retraction of the scapula allows the TD to close (Figure 18-5). The following quotation from a client with an upper extremity amputation highlights the importance of the cable system for functional tasks.

The rubber bands on my hooks regulate tension I put on objects. To force the hook open, I first lock the elbow in the desired position. Then I proceed to bring my shoulder forward, putting tension on the cables. After I have grasped the desired object, I bring my shoulder back to the original position [Crane 1979, p. 12].

Cables need periodic replacement when they fray or break. Cable replacement is generally the most common repair need for the body-powered prosthesis wearer [Crane 1979]. The occupational therapist and the client should know how to replace an old cable with a new one. The process is fairly simple, involving removal of the old cable and reattachment of the new cable to the TD and the harness. It is beneficial for the client to have two or three spare cables at home so that replacement is convenient.

Terminal Device. The TD is the hand component and appears in the form of a hand or a hook. Most body-powered prosthetic hands open and close in a three-point prehension pattern. The prosthetic hooks open and close in a lateral or tip pinch prehension pattern, depending on positioning of the TD. In addition, a variety of TDs are available for certain recreational activities, such as bowling, skiing, baseball, golfing, and volleyball [Radocy 1987] (Figure 18-6). Therapists should be familiar with TD options because they

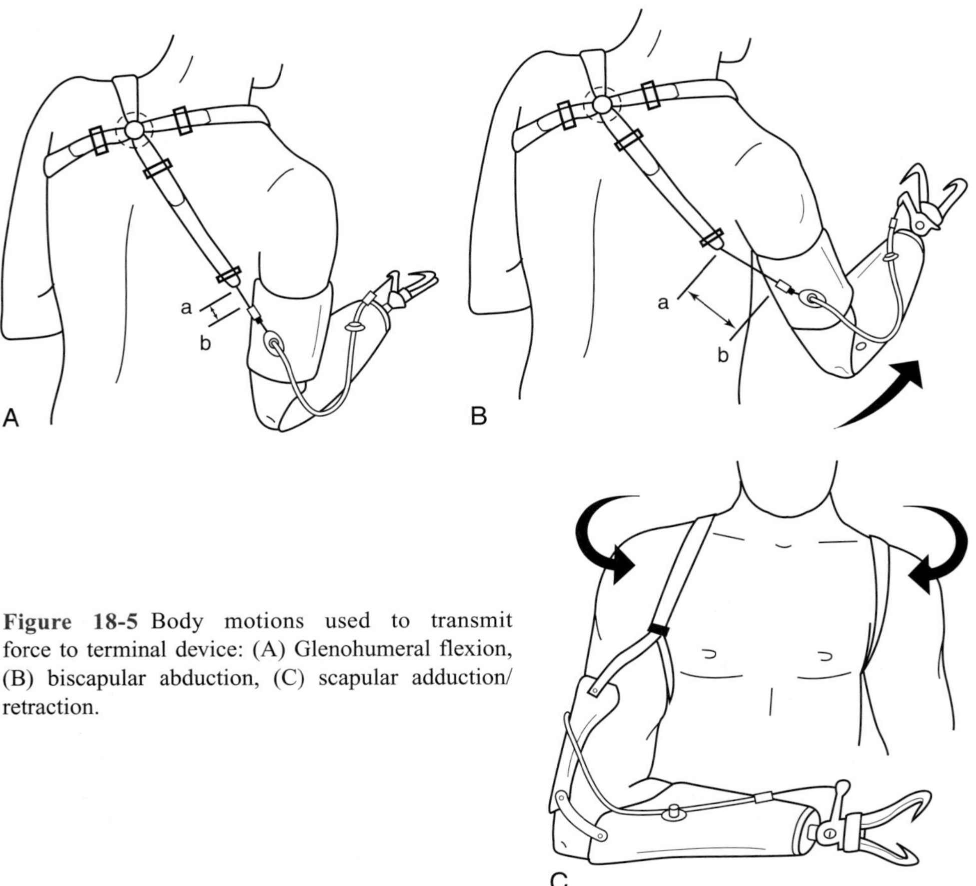

Figure 18-5 Body motions used to transmit force to terminal device: (A) Glenohumeral flexion, (B) biscapular abduction, (C) scapular adduction/retraction.

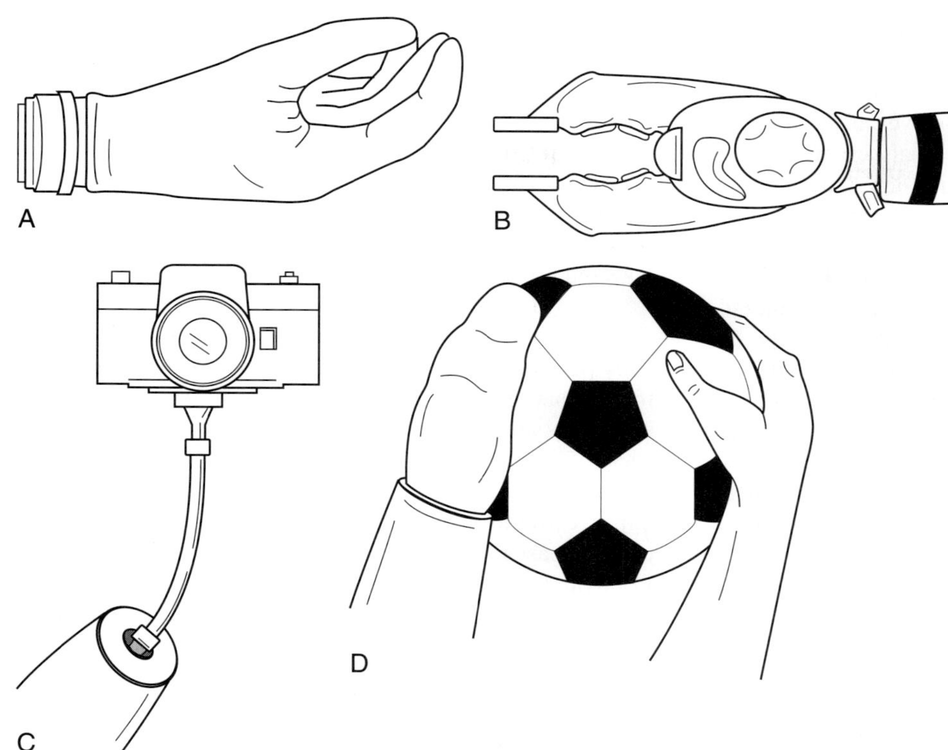

Figure 18-6 Terminal device options: (A) Hand, (B) greifer, (C) photography terminal device, (D) volley ball/soccer terminal device.

Table 18-3 Advantages and Disadvantages of the Hand and Hook Terminal Devices

TERMINAL DEVICE	ADVANTAGES	DISADVANTAGES
Hand	• Cosmetically appealing	• Digits 3, 4, and 5 are nonfunctional • Tendency to impair fine motor manipulation
Hook	• Superior fine motor prehension • Less bulky • Durable	• Cosmetically unappealing

will most likely introduce the person with the amputation to the available options and provide education in their use.

Generally, the initial goals of the prosthetist are to fit the person who has had an amputation with a standard prosthesis. The person with the amputation then requires time to adjust and become an independent user of the prosthetic device. This individual may not be visiting the prosthetist for some time but is interested in completing a specific activity. Sometimes the occupational therapist can fabricate a tool of thermoplastic or other material that can be attached to the TD to serve a specific function. At other times, collaboration with the prosthetist may be necessary to obtain a specific TD or a sophisticated adaptation.

Some individuals benefit from two TD options. Typically, an individual has some form of a hand and a hook, which are interchangeable. For example, the client uses the handlike TD for basic ADL and uses the hooklike TD for more challenging activities such as quilting or changing a tire. Every terminal device has its pros and cons. Differences exist between the hand and hook TDs (Table 18-3). The handlike TD seems to be more cosmetically pleasing. However, digits 3, 4, and 5 are nonfunctional, often impairing function and providing increased bulk. The hooklike TD allows for successful fine motor prehension, is less bulky, and is more durable. However, it may be less cosmetically appealing than the handlike TD.

Grip Strength of Body-powered TD. The body-powered grip can vary from 5 to 20 pounds, depending on the number of hook rubbers used. Hook rubbers are similar to thick, wide rubber bands providing resistance to the grip of the TD. Each rubber band provides 1 pound of grip force, consequently increasing the amount of pressure placed in the axilla on the contralateral side.

The Glove. The glove is the cosmetic covering of the handlike TD. Gloves are made of either latex or silicone substances and are removable and replaceable. Differences exist between the two types of glove. Latex gloves are sturdy and come in 10 to 15 shades of color. Individuals are matched to the shade that corresponds to their skin tone. Latex gloves easily absorb stains that do not wash off. However, latex gloves are more durable than silicone gloves.

A silicone glove is custom fabricated to match the individual in terms of shape, size, and coloring. It is difficult to differentiate between a silicone glove and a human hand by sight. Such a glove is truly a work of art. Silicone gloves are more costly and fragile than latex gloves. It is more difficult to permanently stain a silicone glove. However, they tear easily. Persons who have had an amputation generally request the silicone glove because of its lifelike appearance. Because silicone gloves are more expensive, funding for a silicone glove is difficult to obtain.

Externally Powered Prosthesis

The externally powered prosthesis is another prosthetic option. The externally powered prosthesis is also called a myoelectric prosthesis because it operates from the electromyographic (EMG) signal transmitted from the muscles of the residual limb. An externally powered prosthesis has several differences from the body-powered prosthesis, which are outlined in Table 18-2. Beneficial characteristics of a myoelectric prosthesis include an unlimited work area, functional cosmetic restoration, increased grip force, elimination of harnessing, increased comfort, interchangeable componentry, and individualized custom fabrication. Disadvantages of a myoelectric prosthesis include increased weight, increased cost, increased maintenance, and increased risk of damage.

Externally Powered Prosthetic Components

The externally powered prosthesis comprises various components, as shown in Figure 18-7. The components include a socket, a forearm shell, electrodes, battery, glove, and TD.

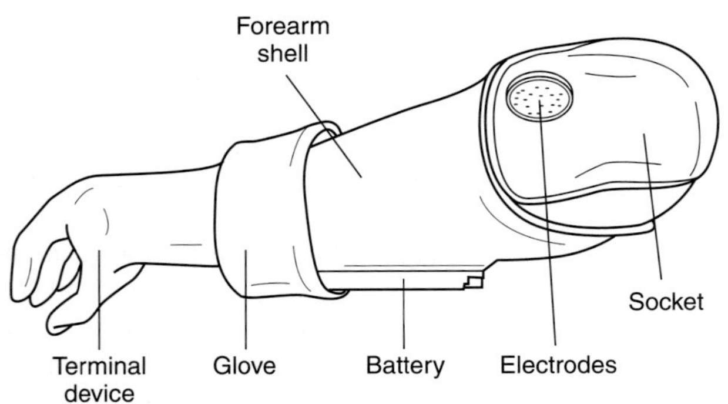

Figure 18-7 Components of an externally powered prosthesis.

The Harness. Most myoelectric prosthetic devices do not require a harness. Occasionally, a harness system is required if it is difficult to fit and maintain contact between the electrodes and the muscle signal or if the socket is loose because of weight loss or other factors. Because the harness system is either eliminated or reduced, the functional work area is expanded to include the areas above the head, behind the back, and near the ground compared with the body-powered prosthesis (Figure 18-8).

Externally Powered Prosthetic Socket. The externally powered prosthetic socket is unique in that it has electrodes that detect the EMG signals of the muscle. The electrodes are mounted directly in the walls of the flexible socket. The EMG signal stimulates the motor in the prosthesis to produce a desired motion. Prosthetics for clients with upper extremity amputations have dramatically changed over the past several years. The main changes have occurred in components, socket fabrication, fitting techniques, suspension systems, and sources of power and electronic controls [Esquenazi et al. 2002].

There are a variety of electrodes available. Some are more sensitive than others in detecting the muscle EMG and controlling the movement of the TD. Through the collaborative effort of the team, the best-suited electrodes are determined. Single- or dual-site control systems are available. A single-site system is used if the client cannot differentiate and isolate control of two separate and opposing muscles for electrode sites. This may be beneficial for persons who are cognitively unable to control the dual site system, such as with pediatrics. For example, the TD would remain in the

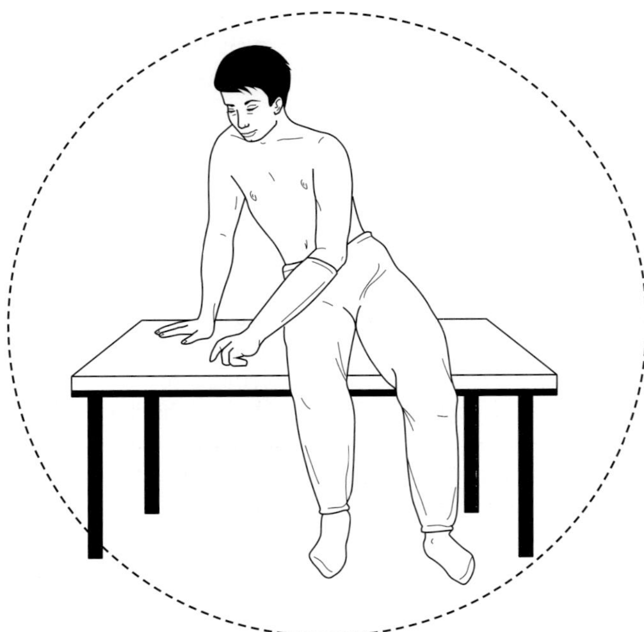

Figure 18-8 Functional work area (externally powered prosthesis).

closed position when the individual's muscles are relaxed and open when the muscle contracts. Thus, if the individual wanted to grasp an object he or she would contract the muscle to open the TD, position it around the desired object, and relax. Upon relaxation, the TD automatically closes and remains closed until the next muscle contraction.

Commonly, a dual-site control system is preferred over a single-site system. The dual-site control system is activated by two separate muscle contractions. For example, the individual with a transradial amputation will most likely contract the wrist extensor muscle group to open the TD and the wrist flexor muscle group to close the TD. The TD has the ability to remain in any position as long as the muscle signals are absent. For example, the same individual can open the TD with contraction of the wrist extensors. Once the muscles are relaxed, the TD will stay open as if to shake the hand of a friend. As soon as the wrist flexors are contracted, the TD will close. With this system, a sheath or sock cannot be worn because it would interrupt the connection between the muscle and the electrode. As a precaution, it is important to remember that the externally powered TD has a grip strength greater than that of the normal individual.

Externally powered terminal devices have a greater opening range, allowing for the ability to grasp objects of larger size. The externally powered prosthesis provides the ability to use prehension capabilities in all planes. This contributes to the expansion of the functional work area to include space above the head, behind the back, and near the ground.

Grip Strength of Externally Powered TD

There are differences between an externally powered TD and a body-powered TD. An externally powered TD presents with increased grip strength compared to the body-powered terminal device. The externally powered TD generally provides grip strength of approximately 20 to 30 pounds, compared with the 5 to 20 pounds of grip strength of the body-powered TD.

The Battery

Lithium-polymer battery technology advancements have improved the ease of externally powered prostheses. The lithium-polymer batteries are 80% lighter, 70% smaller, and offer 30% more storage capacity than nickel-cadmium batteries [Billock 2003].

Prosthetic Rehabilitation

The educational background of occupational therapists includes motor control, motor learning, and movement as they relate to the upper extremity function required for occupational performance. Education in the psychologic adjustment to disability is also the occupational therapist's area of expertise. These strengths are vital because postsurgical therapy often incorporates wound care and contracture management. In addition, occupational therapists assist persons in adjusting to the amputation. Post-surgical goals include scar management, desensitization, pain management, swelling reduction, and limb shrinkage. Psychological intervention related to phantom pain and phantom sensation should be implemented as soon as possible.

The sooner therapy is initiated the faster the client will be prepared for prosthesis fitting and the chances of engaging in bimanual activities will increase. Note how one individual describes part of his post-surgical therapy. This range of motion deficit possibly could have been prevented with early intervention from therapy.

During the first three weeks in therapy, I didn't have movement in my stumps. They were frozen solid. I just couldn't believe it. They stood straight out, and that was about it. It took a long time to break this loose to where I could get movement in my stumps again. . . . It was a very painful experience [Crane 1979, p. 11].

Effective communication is vital between the prosthetist, the therapist, and the individual with the amputation to ensure that everyone is striving to best meet the goals of the client.

Phases of Rehabilitation

Prosthetic rehabilitation can be categorized into two phases: the pre-prosthetic phase and the post-prosthetic phase. The pre-prosthetic phase prepares the client for prosthesis wear and usage. The post-prosthetic phase primarily teaches the client to maintain and use the prosthesis in daily activity.

Pre-prosthetic Phase

The pre-prosthetic period begins when the individual with the amputation becomes a prosthesis candidate. The phase concludes upon prosthesis delivery. Time during the pre-prosthetic phase is crucial for reinforcement of realistic expectations. Individuals with amputations may be under the assumption that they will perform all activities at the same level of independence they had before the amputation. This assumption needs to be discussed with the client. Therapists should explain that the prosthetic device will not replace the arm. Rather, it is an assistive tool used to stabilize, support, and hold objects during bimanual activities [Doolan 2001].

Clients may experience disappointment when the prosthesis is delivered and they are unable to use it as they imagined. It is the duty of the team to inform individuals of the advantages and disadvantages of the various components to provide a realistic picture of rehabilitation. Clients are usually surprised when they realize that the prosthesis is hard, cold, heavy, and not a true replacement for the hand. With establishment of realistic expectations and acceptance, use of the device greatly improves [Atkins et al. 1996].

During the pre-prosthetic phase, individuals frequently visit the prosthetist for fittings and modifications of the socket. Clients also see the therapists for rehabilitation services. Individuals receiving body-powered prostheses move much quicker through the fabrication and rehabilitation process because electrodes are not required and muscle sites and signals do not need to be identified.

Electrode Training

If an individual is receiving an externally powered prosthesis, the best muscle sites are identified and trained to operate the prosthetic features. Finding the sites and training the muscles for electrode placement are primarily the responsibility of the therapist. During this phase, the occupational therapist provides extensive training, using biofeedback to teach the individual to contract the identified muscle or muscles on command. The therapist facilitates the improvement of muscle site control and focuses on isolated muscle contraction, strength, and endurance. Special biofeedback machines are often available from the prosthetist. It is important for the client to practice muscle contractions in a variety of positions, including lying, standing, and sitting. Practicing muscle contraction in different positions, with the extremity in various planes, enhances maximal success after delivery of the prosthesis.

Once electrode sites are established in therapy, the prosthetist is informed of the exact and most appropriate electrode location for the individual to obtain the most function. Locating and training for electrode sites is often a lengthy, rigorous, trial-and-error process. Once the socket and electrode sites are sufficient to work the prosthesis, the prosthesis is ready for final fabrication. There may be a period of time after the pre-prosthetic phase when the individual is discharged from occupational therapy with a home program until the prosthesis is ready for delivery and therapy can resume.

Additional goals of occupational therapy during this phase include preparation of the individual to tolerate wearing the prosthesis and using it independently for daily activities. Specifics include promoting wound care and preventing infection; maintaining range of motion and eliminating contractures; desensitizing the residual limb to pressure, pain, and weight; edema control; and unilateral independence.

Promoting Wound Care and Preventing Infection

Specific goals of the treatment include the client's independence in dressing changes and good hygiene [Keenan 1995]. This may include instruction in dressing change techniques and scar mobilization to prevent adhesions and hypersensitivity.

Maintaining Range of Motion and Eliminating Contractures

By focusing on the residual joints of the affected extremity, the therapist prevents loss of motion. In some cases the therapist provides necessary stretching or joint mobilization to ensure adequate range of motion, and therefore successful function during use of the prosthesis. Home exercise programs are necessary. In addition, positioning or splinting techniques may be used if necessary.

Desensitizing the Residual Limb to Pressure, Pain, and Weight

It is common for the client to experience residual limb sensitivity. The occupational therapist can intervene by teaching and implementing the following desensitization techniques: wrapping, massage, weight bearing, and pain management.

Phantom sensation and phantom pain are normal experiences most clients who have had an amputation encounter [Omer 1981]. The role of the team is to prepare clients and assure them that these sensations and pain are expected and are a normal phenomenon. Phantom sensation occurs when the individual feels as if the nonexistent limb is still present. The amputated extremity may feel exactly like the original limb in terms of shape, size, position, and ability to move. Rings or watches that were previously worn may be part of the sensation [Omer 1981]. Phantom sensation is described as a pins-and-needles or tingling sensation. Phantom sensation diminishes over time. It has been reported to persist from 6 months to 20 years [Frazier and Kolb 1970].

Phantom pain is different from phantom sensation. The phenomenon of phantom pain is not completely understood. Phantom pain is generally described as pain that does not follow nerve distribution patterns [Omer 1981]. The pain is extreme and can be managed through alternative medicine techniques, therapeutic modalities, and medication. The following statement from a person with an amputation describes his experience with phantom pain.

I never realized it before, but there is a type of pain called phantom pain. It felt like my hands were in rubber gloves and the rubber gloves were filled with water all the time. I was afraid if I told the doctor, he probably wouldn't let me out of the hospital, or to go on to rehabilitation—he would think that I was nuts. When I got home it felt like a cigar butt had been put out in my hand, and it burned. . . . the first few days I walked the floor at nights with phantom pain. I couldn't sleep at night. I walked and I walked. Finally, I told [my doctor] about my problem. He told me that it wasn't unusual at all and prescribed some medicine. The pain didn't go away entirely, but it became bearable [Crane 1979, p. 11].

Desensitization and pain management are additional components of the therapy. The therapist may provide modalities for pain as well as educate clients to manage the pain independently. Each client presents with different complaints, and the treatment is individualized.

Edema Control

Edema can be controlled through wrapping the residual limb in a diagonal design, so as not to compromise circulation.

Another technique includes the use of compression socks. Compression has a direct impact on residual limb shrinkage and shaping. Elevation and retrograde massage are also useful alternatives to decrease edema. It is important for the therapist to reinforce the importance of edema management because it has a direct impact on socket fit and comfort.

Unilateral Independence

Unilateral independence involves using environmental adaptations and one-handed techniques, which are in an occupational therapist's area of expertise. It may be necessary to teach the client to switch hand dominance if the dominant hand was amputated. Generally, the occupational therapist works to promote the maximal level of independence for the individual. Often therapists issue adaptive equipment. For the client with an amputation, it may promote better prosthetic success if the therapist does not issue adaptive equipment until after prosthetic training because the client may become efficient with the adaptive equipment and may not be motivated to learn to use the prosthesis.

Post-prosthetic Phase

Post-prosthetic training can be divided into four general phases: orientation, control training, use training, and daily living skills training [Keenan 1995]. The post-prosthetic phase is initiated once the prosthesis is delivered. This phase is the most important to the occupational therapist. A client's visits to other members of the team decrease, and the occupational therapist acts as the team liaison. The following is a client's perception of the post-prosthetic phase.

It took a lot of practice and patience to learn how to manipulate my new arms. For example, as a normal individual would reach for that first cup of coffee in the morning, I would ask myself, "How should I hold that cup of coffee? Shall I lock my elbow in at a 90-degree angle and put my hook around the cup, or should I grab the cup through the handle?" If I want to move my arm up, I have to extend my shoulder forward or my stump forward. In order to reach a certain direction, I have to lock my elbows in the desired height, whether it's 45, 90, or 115 degrees, and then I lower my elbow to where the cable tightens up [Crane 1979, p. 12].

Orientation

Upon delivery of the prosthesis, the prosthetist educates the client about the prosthesis and its components. It is the responsibility of the therapist to reorient the client to the prosthesis. A prosthesis is a very complex tool, and it cannot be mastered in one instruction session. The client will not be independent with the prosthesis unless there is a complete understanding of all of the components.

Orientation for the client includes education on how to don, doff, operate switches and batteries, and care for the prosthesis. The therapist ensures that the fit and function of the prosthesis are adequate. This includes evaluation of the client's independence with donning and doffing. The client must know how to properly care for the prosthesis so as to promote success and prevent unnecessary damage.

Control Training

This phase is the longest portion of post-prosthetic rehabilitation for the client because it is repetitive and difficult. During this time, the client learns to operate the controls of the prosthesis and practices until becoming proficient. Depending on the features of the prosthesis, this includes such tasks as opening and closing the terminal device, elevating and lowering the elbow, and rotating the wrist on command. Activities can be graded (for example, controlling the TD to open in 3, 4, or 5 separate steps).

Use Training

Use training involves applying the mechanics of operation to repetitive tasks to facilitate eventful functional use and endurance. This portion of rehabilitation includes using the prosthesis to grasp and release objects of various sizes, textures, and weights in different planes and positions. It can be difficult to grasp an object above the head because the individual must relax the wrist extensors and contract the flexors while the hand is elevated. This is difficult to accomplish because of the weight of the prosthesis. Examples of other activities practiced during this portion of the rehabilitation include holding and placing a tomato on a shelf without crushing it or playing a card game with the cards held by the TD.

Daily Living Skills and Functional Training

This phase of rehabilitation should be the most familiar and comfortable phase for the occupational therapist because the focus is on function of the individual. During this time, the therapist and the client address the specific skills gained and apply them to the client's individual functional requirements, lifestyle, and interests. Training may include grooming and hygiene, meal preparation, dressing, child care, or other required tasks. The client may choose to work on any pertinent tasks that are meaningful.

Tasks may include preparation for return to employment or recreation. The primary focus of therapy with the prosthesis in rehabilitation should include bilateral activities, in which the individual is required to use the prosthesis in a functional manner because the primary advantage of a prosthesis for a unilaterally independent individual is the ability to complete bilateral activities never completed before. Individuals with amputations usually do not realize the functional benefits of the prosthesis until they experience success with bilateral tasks. This can be difficult for clients, especially if they have become proficient with one-handed techniques.

As stated earlier, the client is an active participant in the rehabilitation process. The therapist designs a home program for the client. The program is continually updated as the individual progresses to greater function and independence. It is important to schedule periodic follow-up visits with the client to review progress and prosthesis function. Often therapy will be reinitiated when clients find new skills they need help in learning. The occupational therapist serves as a resource for clients, enabling them to achieve maximal function and independence during the course of their lifetime.

Psychosocial Insights from Clients with Amputations

Having an amputation can impact many psychosocial dimensions of one's life.

Family Dynamics

The dynamics of the family may be altered when a family member looses a limb. Significant others or direct family members of the injured person experience a series of losses and adjustments. Family members may fear that the individual is suffering and at risk of dying. Fear and anxiety may become overwhelming at times. Family members may worry about how the individual will adjust to his or her changed body. Issues about intimacy and dependency are common concerns. The therapist should encourage a reconnection between the person who has sustained an amputation and his or her partner [Kohl 1984a, 1984b].

Impact on Rehabilitation

The rehabilitation team should become knowledgeable about the individual's response to the injury. Psychosocial aspects include change in self-image and body image, acceptance of the residual limb, and feeling comfortable in society as a person with an amputation. Some clients may be medically prepared to begin rehabilitation, but they are not psychologically ready. Health providers should not label the client as uncooperative and unmotivated. Rather, they should facilitate and reinforce good communication among the client and health care team. The client should be an active partner to establish rehabilitation goals.

Counseling People Who Have Amputations

According to Price and Fisher [2002], issues addressed during counseling sessions include depression, distress, sleeplessness, anxiety, changed body image, effects on relationships and intimacy, and feelings of anger and resentment. According to Kohl [1984a, 1984b], complaints of emotional distress in the early stages of rehabilitation seemed to be most apparent from 6 to 24 months after surgery.

Upper Extremity Prosthetic Intervention for Children

Early gross motor movements in children such as prone and sitting emerge between four and six months [Cronin and Mandich 2005]. These movements directly involve the use of hands in order to balance, support, and stabilize the trunk. As a result, fitting children with a prosthesis is considered necessary in order to maintain and preserve normal development [Shaperman 2003]. Exner [1989] stated that "The development of visual perception and eye-hand coordination skills in conjunction with cognitive and social development allow the child to engage in increasingly complex activities."

Early Fitting

According to Hanson and Mandacina [2003], "The single most important advantage of early fitting is the immediate acceptance of the prosthetic arm by the child." The most beneficial age range to receive a prosthesis is from two months to two years [Fisher 1976, Scotland and Galway 1986, Stark 2001]. Children fitted with a prosthesis at a young age and who wear their prostheses regularly will demonstrate spontaneous use in daily activities.

Children fitted at later ages are less spontaneous and more inclined to use the prosthesis passively [Atkins 2002, Bowers 2003, Hanson and Mandacina 2003]. In addition, because hand skills develop gradually children should be fitted early so that the prosthesis becomes naturally integrated with bilateral activities. While wearing their prostheses, children must practice activities that require crossing midline, hand position in space, grasping, bilateral tasks, and bringing hands to midline [Hubbard et al. 1991]. Table 18-4 suggests types of prostheses, goals, assessments, and interventions for children of different age groups.

Family Involvement

Acceptance of the prosthesis will involve the family. The family should be involved in donning and doffing the prosthesis, playing with the child while the prosthesis is on, and developing wearing schedules. The family should be educated about the importance and advantages of early and consistent prosthetic use. Futhermore, children who have myoelectric prostheses will require substantial one-to-one training and attention [Atkins 1997].

Marketing Strategies and Recommendations

To specialize in upper extremity prosthetic rehabilitation, the therapist must be motivated and persistent, as in any area of practice. There are many avenues for gathering basic information on upper extremity prosthetics, such as journals, books, agencies, other therapists, and the Internet. (See Appendix D.) Important information can be gathered from these resources to augment basic prosthetic knowledge. Next, the therapist should establish relations with a prosthetist who specializes in upper extremity prosthetics.

Table 18-4 Suggestions for Age Appropriate Prostheses, Goals, Assessment, and Interventions

AGE	TYPE OF PROSTHESIS	GOALS	ASSESSMENTS	INTERVENTION
2-18 months	Passive fitting suspension socket with no harnessing	• Weight bearing in sitting and standing • Crawling and pulling to stand • Rolling front to back • Stabilizing toys • Bilateral activities	• UNB Test of Prosthetic function • PUFI • Bennet Hand tool • Krebs • Southhampton • Hand Test	• No different than reaching all appropriate developmental milestones • Gross motor skills using the prosthesis • Fine motor skills with unaffected upper extremity • Typical screening assessments for age range
12 months to 2 years	Cookie Crusher Myoelectric Prosthesis (system discontinued at age 4)	• Using prosthesis as an assist • Discovering that the device opens and closes • Opening hand upon request • Placing toys in the myoelectric hand	• Carrying large balls • Weight bearing on the prosthesis while playing • Stabilizing the body while completing table top activities • Holding objects • Riding toys	

Data from Shaperman J, Landsberger SE, Setoguchi Y (2003). Early upper limb prosthesis fitting: when and what do we fit. Journal of Prosthetics and Orthotics. 15(1):11-17. Stocker D, Caldwell R, Wedderburn Z (1996). Review of infant fittings at the Institute of Biomedical Engineering: 13 years of service. ACPOC News 2:1-5.

Much valuable information can be learned from spending a week with a prosthetist learning about the process of reimbursement, fabrication, and orientation to various options. The funding process can take much time, depending on the source of reimbursement and the insurance company's specific benefits regarding prostheses. It is important to remain focused on the client and to serve as an advocate for the individual with the amputation. Phone calls and letters from health care professionals may expedite approval. Therapy can proceed without approval for the prosthetic device in order to accomplish goals from the pre-prosthetic phase.

In addition, it is important to locate area case managers and physicians who work with this population. Case managers and physicians will assist in establishing a referral base for those requiring therapy. It has been the experience of the author that physicians, prosthetists, and case managers are happy to know that a therapist exists who wants to work in upper extremity prosthetic rehabilitation. They are also often happy to refer their clients. The area of upper extremity prosthetics is a rewarding field.

SELF-QUIZ 18-1*

In regard to the following questions, circle either true (T) or false (F).

1. T F A myoelectric prosthesis uses the EMG of a muscle for operation.
2. T F One disadvantage of the externally powered prosthesis is that it is more prone to damage than a body-powered prosthesis.
3. T F One benefit of the body-powered prosthesis is the increased grip force (20 to 30 pounds).
4. T F Externally powered and body-powered prosthetic devices are operated by a cable.

In regard to the following questions, circle the letter corresponding to the correct answer.

5. Approximately 50% of all individuals with an upper extremity amputation are fitted with a prosthesis. What percentage of these individuals actually wear their prostheses?
   a. 10%
   b. 50%
   c. 75%
   d. 99.9%

6. An OTR receives an order to evaluate and treat an individual with a BE amputation (you know that BE stands for "below elbow"). Another term for this amputation level is:
   a. Transcarpal
   b. Transradial
   c. Transulnar
   d. Transhumeral
7. An OTR receives an order to evaluate and treat an individual with a transhumeral amputation. The prosthetist indicated that the individual received his prosthesis one week ago. Rank in order the steps of your treatment.
   a. Control training — Step 1 ______
   b. Use training — Step 2 ______
   c. Orientation — Step 3 ______
   d. Functional training — Step 4 ______
8. An OTR receives an order to evaluate and treat an individual with an AE body-powered prosthesis. During your evaluation, the therapist notices his harness seems to fit improperly. What is the proper way a figure-of-eight harness should fit?
   a. The ring of the harness should lie over the scapula of the amputated side.
   b. The axilla loop should pass under the amputated side.
   c. The ring of the harness should lie flat on the anterior side of the sound-side shoulder.
   d. The harness should be tight enough to activate the TD without excessive effort.

Matching (indicate the letter of all that apply):

   a. Body-powered hook
   b. Myoelectric hand

9. Offers increased grip strength: ____
10. Preferred when fine and gross motor function are more important: ____
11. Preferred when appearance is more important: ____
12. Has decreased grip strength: ____

*See Appendix A for the answer key.

REVIEW QUESTIONS

1. How are levels of amputation differentiated?
2. What are the roles of the client, prosthetist, and occupational therapist when treating a person with an amputation?
3. What are four prosthesis options available for people with upper extremity amputations?
4. What are the advantages and disadvantages of passive, boy-powered and externally powered prostheses?
5. What psychosocial impacts may an amputation impose upon the client who has an amputation?
6. When treating a child with an amputation, what assessments and interventions can be used?

References

Alley RD (2002). *Admancement of Upper Extremity Prosthetic Interface and Frame Design.* Institute of Biomedical Engineering, University of New Brunswick, MEC'02, "The Next Generation."

Andrews KL, Bouvette KA (1996). Anatomy for fitting of prosthetics and orthotics. Physical Medicine and Rehabilitation 10(3):489-507.

Atkins DJ (1997). Pediatric prosthetics: A collection of considerations. In Motion 7(2):7-17.

Atkins DJ (2002). Early fitting is key to success. First Step Magazine 2:29-30.

Atkins DJ, Alley RD (2003). Upper extremity prosthetics: An emerging specialization in a technologically advanced field. Journal of Prosthetics and Orthotics 2:1-8.

Atkins DJ (2003). A many-sided approach to kids with limb differences. In Motion 7(2):12-19.

Atkins DJ, Heard SCY, Donovan WH (1996). Epidemiologic overview of individuals with upper-limb loss and their reported research priorities. Journal of Prosthetics and Orthotics 8(1):2-11.

Baumgartner R, Bota P (1992). Upper extremity amputation and prosthetics. Medicine Orthotic Technology 1:5-51.

Bennett JB, Alexander CB (1989). Amputation levels and surgical techniques. In DJ Atkins, RH Meier (eds.), *Comprehensive Management of the Upper-limb Amputee.* New York: Springer-Verlag, pp. 28-38.

Billock JN (2003). Clinical evaluation and assessment principles in orthotics and prosthetics. Journal of Prosthetics and Orthotics 8(2):41-44.

Bowers R (2003). Facing congenital differences. First Step Magazine 4:23-26.

Carlson LE, Veatch BD, Frey DD (1995). Efficiency of prosthetic cable and housing. Journal of Prosthetics and Orthotics 7(3):96-99.

Centers for Disease Control and Prevention (1996). National Health Interview Survey by the Office on Disability on Health. National Center for Environmental Health, Centers for Disease Control and Prevention, Atlanta, GA.

Collier M, LeBlanc M (1996). Axilla bypass ring for shoulder harnesses for upper-limb prostheses. J Prosthet Orthot 8(2):130-131.

Crane V (1979). Amputee adjusts. Probe Magazine 4:10-14.

Cronin A, Mandich MB (2005). *Human Development and Performance Throughout the Lifespan*. New York: Thomson/Delmar Learning, pp. 139-164.

Doolan K (2001). Use and training of cosmetic and functional arm prostheses. Inside Case Manager 7(10):12-15.

Esquinazi A, Meier R, Sears H (2002). The state of upper limb prosthetics. Presentation at Orlando, FL. National Prosthetic and Orthtotic Conference.

Exner CE (1989). Development of hand functions. In PN Pratt, AS Allen (eds.), *Occupational Therapy for Children, Second Edition*. St. Louis, MO: CV Mosby, pp. 235-259.

Fisher A (1976). Initial fitting of the congenital below-elbow amputee: Are we fitting early enough? Inter-Clinic Information Bulletin 15:7-10.

Frazier SH, Kolb LC (1970). Psychiatric aspects of pain and the phantom limb.

Orthopedic Clinics of North America 1:481-495.

Hanson WJ, Mandacina S (2003). Microprocessor technology opens the door to success. The O&P Edge 5:36-38.

Hubbard S, Bush G, Kurtz I, Naumann I (1991). Myoelectric prostheses for the limb deficient child. Physical Medicine Rehabilitation Clinical North America 2:847-866.

Jones LE, Davidson JH (1999). Save the arm: a study of problems in the remaining arm of unilateral upper limb amputees. Prosthetics and Orthotics International 23:55-58.

Kohl SJ (1984a). Emotional coping with amputation. In DW Krueger (ed.), *Rehabilitation Psychology: A Comprehensive Textbook*. New York: Aspen, pp. 272-281.

Kohl SJ (1984b). The process of psychological adaptation to traumatic limb loss. In DW Krueger (ed.), *Emotional Rehabilitation of Physical Trauma and Disability*. Spectrum Publications, pp. 113-119.

Keenan DD (1995). Myoelectric prosthesis protocol. American Occupational Therapy Association Physical Disabilities Newsletter 18(1):1-4.

Lake C (1997). Effects of prosthetic training on upper-extremity prosthetic use. Journal of Prosthetics and Orthotics 9(1):3-9.

Law HT (1981). Engineering of upper limb prostheses. Orthopedic Clinics of North America 12(4):929-951.

Leonard JA, Meier RH (1988). Prosthetics. In JA DeLisa (ed.), *Rehabilitation Medicine Principles and Practice*. Philadelphia: J B Lippincott.

Malone JM, Fleming LL, Roberson J, Whitesides TE, Leal JM, Poole JU, et al. (1984). Immediate, early and late postsurgical management of upper limb amputation. Journal of Rehabilitation Research Development 21:10-39.

Muilenburg AL, LeBlanc MA (1989). Body-powered upper limb components. In DJ Atkins, RH Meier (eds.), *Comprehensive Management of the Upper-limb Amputee*. New York: Springer-Verlag.

NovaCare Orthotics and Prosthetics (1991). Client Information Packet. 1-800-522-4428.

Omer GE (1981). Nerve, neuroma, and pain problems related to upper limb amputations. Orthopedic Clinics of North America 12(4):751-761.

Patterson DB, McMillan PM, Rodriguez RP (1991). Acceptance rate of myoelectric prosthesis. Journal of the Association of Children's Prosthetic-Orthotic Clinics 25(3):73-76.

Price EM, Fisher K (2002). How does counseling help people with amputation. Journal of Prosthetics and Orthotics 14(2):102-106.

Radocy B (1987). Upper-extremity prosthetics: Considerations and designs for sports and recreation. Clinical Prosthetics and Orthotics 11(3):131-153.

Reddy MP (1984). Nerve entrapment syndromes in the upper extremity contralateral to amputation. Archives of Physical Rehabilitation 1(65):15-17.

Santschi WR (1958). *Manual of Upper Extremity Prosthetics, Second Edition*. Los Angeles: University of California Press.

Scotland TD, Galway HR (1986). Long-term review in children with congential and acquired upper limb deficiency. Journal of Bone and Joint Surgery 65:346-349.

Shaperman J, Landsberger SE, Setoguchi Y (2003). Early upper limb prosthesis fitting: when and what do we fit. Journal of Prosthetics and Orthotics. 15(1):11-17.

Shurr DG, Cook TM (1990). *Prosthetics and Orthotics*. Norwalk, CT: Appleton & Lange.

Stark G (2001). Upper-extremity limb fitting. In Motion 12(4):47-52.

Toren S (2002). Upper extremity. First Step Magazine 3:7-9.

CHAPTER 19

Ethical Issues Related to Splinting

Amy Marie Haddad, PhD

Key Terms

American occupational therapy code of ethics
Autonomy
Beneficence
Care-based ethics
Duty
Ethics
Justice
Morality
Nonmaleficence
Principles
Self-determination
Values
Virtue

Chapter Objectives

1. Compare and contrast the various sources of moral guidance.
2. Define three traditional approaches to applied ethics: principle, care-based, and virtue.
3. Apply one of the traditional approaches to ethics to a complex case to reach a morally justifiable resolution.

Health care is fraught with ethical issues, including questions about whether to tell clients disturbing and potentially harmful news, how to deal with impaired or incompetent colleagues, and how to distribute scarce and valuable resources. As one of the health professions, occupational therapy cannot help being involved in ethical problems and their resolutions. In fact, occupational therapists often find themselves caught between two moral goods. First is the desire to assist the client to function better with independence, and second is the client's right to self-determination that may lead to noncompliance and less-than-satisfactory outcomes.

The purpose of this chapter is to define applied ethics and its application to occupational therapy practice, with a specific emphasis on the special types of problems encountered in splinting. Sources of moral guidance and values are explored, along with three traditional approaches to ethics. The three approaches (principles, care-based ethics, and virtue) are applied to complex clinical situations involving splinting in the latter sections of the chapter. Resources to assist in the resolution of ethical problems are also noted.

Ethics and Health Care

Ethics itself is hardly a new area of study. Its application to the practical problems of health care is a relative newcomer, beginning approximately in the late 1960s with questions about research on human subjects, vital organ transplantation, and hemodialysis [Jonsen 1998]. What was needed at that time was a detailed study of professional ethics aimed at establishing standards of conduct and moral behavior. The need for the guidance ethics provides continues to the present day.

Normative ethics is that branch of ethical inquiry that considers general ethical questions whose answers have a relatively direct bearing on practice [Solomon 1995]. The results of applied ethics have immediate consequences for action and policy. In recent years, this definition of normative or applied ethics has been expanded. Now it includes concerns about relationships and the particular experiences of those who are ill or injured, as opposed to abstract universal approaches.

These types of concerns fall under the heading of care-based reasoning. Thus, a complete definition of normative ethics encompasses an examination of principles and virtues. It also includes what we should nurture and sustain as human beings to achieve the most of what is best in human life. The focus of this chapter is on the moral life in occupational therapy, particularly in the area of splinting. To arrive at a clearer understanding of ethics, it is helpful to have a baseline of key terms. Three terms underlie the discussion in this chapter: *ethics*, *morality*, and *values*.

Ethics

Ethics, as has already been explained, is the exploration of moral duty, principles, human character or virtue, and human relationships. In effect, ethics involves the study of right and wrong, good and evil, moral conduct on an individual and societal basis, rules, promises, principles, and obligations. Taken together, these constitute the important concerns of ethics.

From this broad definition of ethics, it might appear that all human interactions on some level involve ethics. Although this is true, it is important to be able to sort out and differentiate the ethical issues central to the question at hand from those that are merely the underpinning or backdrop for daily experience. A simple guide to determining whether a situation involves ethics involves answering the following three questions [Chater et al. 1993].

- Is there more than one morally plausible resolution?
- Is there no clear-cut best resolution?
- Is there direct reference to the welfare or dignity of others?

If the answer to any of these questions is yes, the situation in question involves ethics.

Morality

Human behavior or actions that are judged as either good or evil fall in the domain of morality. Although ethics can be thought of as the more formal and prescriptive of the two, many ethicists use the words *morality* and *ethics* synonymously. When we make a judgment about a person's conduct, saying "That action is bad or wrong," we are actually including a judgment about the act itself, the values attached to the action, and accountability for the action. If a therapist were to tell a lie, the very word we use to describe the action (*lie*) indicates that the action is wrong or at least opposed to the action of telling the truth. For example, suppose a client asked a therapist if she has any prior experience in fabricating a particular type of splint. Although the therapist has never made the specified splint before, she tells the client that she has made them on several occasions.

We can claim that the action is wrong only if we explore the values that support the worth or goodness of truth telling and why it is important to tell the truth. Telling the truth demonstrates respect for the other person and allows individuals to make decisions with accurate information. If we found while exploring the "liar's" action that he or she was completely unaware that lying was wrong or bad we might excuse the person from moral wrongdoing because he or she did not know any better. When a person is unaware of the rightness or wrongness of actions, we consider him or her *amoral*.

Although it is difficult to believe that individuals would be unaware of the moral rules of the society in which they live, there are those who because of age or mental defect do not understand the moral implications of their actions. Persons who normally fall into this category are children, the mentally ill, or persons with severe cognitive disabilities. On the other hand, persons who know the difference between right and wrong conduct and yet choose to do the wrong thing are considered *immoral* and accountable for their actions.

Values

In the brief discussion of morality, it is clear that values are an important part of ethics. Values are the internal motivators for our actions. When individuals value something, they invest themselves psychologically and spiritually. They also attach emotions (positive or negative) and importance to persons, places, objects, actions, ideals, or goals that seem to be most relevant to or intimate with the self. Basic values and a value system are developed during childhood. Of course, early established values can be changed under great spiritual or emotional distress.

Values can also be changed when it becomes apparent that an old value does not effectively resolve a present dilemma and a new, more attractive and applicable, value does. A conflict of values is often the genesis for an ethical problem in clinical practice. Regardless of the origin of a value, the resulting personal and professional values can profoundly affect the ethical decisions occupational therapists make. For example, a first-year occupational therapy student used to think elders over age 85 should not receive any type of splinting because it was too costly and life expectancy was probably minimal. However, after graduating from occupational therapy training and interacting with older adults in the clinical setting the new therapist now values the lives of elders and has resolved the bias against ageism.

Sources of Moral Guidance

The basic definitions of ethics, morality, and values set a foundation to help separate ethical concerns from other types of problems and issues an occupational therapist faces in clinical practice. Once it is clear that a situation or problem involves ethics, the next question is where you should look to determine what is right or morally correct. Are morals grounded in one's own opinion? Or that of significant others? In the law and regulations that govern professional practice? In the opinions of one's professional group or association? In the religious or philosophical beliefs of the individual or institution?

This section explores alternative sources of moral guidance. What is important is not so much to determine what the right thing to do is but to reflect on the various sources of moral authority that have particular impact on your professional practice and personal decision making. One should consider how these sources of authority shape one's behavior and character.

Family and Peers

One of the primary sources of support and guidance for moral decision making are peers and family members. In two separate national studies (one of registered nurses and the other of pharmacists) the majority of respondents stated that they would first turn to their spouse for moral advice or counsel, followed by a peer [Haddad 1988, 1991]. Seeking the advice of someone who is close and trusted is not too surprising, and it is likely that occupational therapists would respond in the same way their colleagues in nursing and pharmacy did.

Individuals who know us well and share the same perspectives and values are logically the first-line resource for most health professionals faced with a moral problem. However, even though it is understandable why an occupational therapist might turn to a peer for ethical advice there is no reason to believe that the peer will be able to provide justifiable resolutions to the problem. In other words, peers and significant others may be sympathetic but they are not necessarily in the best position to help sort through the complicated ethical issues encountered in clinical practice.

Furthermore, significant others and peers would probably not be considered the *source* of moral authority, even if they were skilled in analyzing ethical problems. We must look further than the individuals who make up our families and our colleagues for moral guidance. For example, a therapist is faced with an ethical decision: whether or not to fabricate splints for a person who was burned over 90% of her body. Instead of the therapist asking his wife about the decision, the therapist networks with professional peers who are members of the hospital's ethics committee.

Laws and Regulations

At times it is difficult to distinguish between the law and ethics. Former Chief Justice of the Supreme Court Earl Warren described the relationship between the law and ethics as follows.

In civilized life, Law floats in a sea of Ethics. Each is indispensable to civilization. Without Law, we should be at the mercy of the least scrupulous; without Ethics, Law could not exist. Without ethical consciousness in most people, lawlessness would be rampant. Yet, without Law, civilization could not exist, for there are always people who, in the conflict of human interest, ignore their responsibility to their fellowman [Warren 1962].

Thus, there is a delicate and changeable relationship between ethics and law. Laws and specific regulations that govern health care practice order our professional and institutional relationships. In an ideal world, the law would embody our ethical commitments. Yet, sometimes the law and ethics diverge.

It is possible that an occupational therapist could conclude that he or she should engage in civil disobedience to violate the law or public policy to do what is ethical. Of course, this sort of decision to disobey a law or regulation should not be taken lightly. If ethics sometimes requires civil disobedience, it implies that what is ethical is not determined solely by public policy or law. Therefore, this reasoning argues, the law is not a sufficient source of authority for determining proper ethical conduct for an occupational therapist.

Professional Codes of Ethics

Health professionals recognize that the question of what is moral has to do with professional ethics. Occupational therapists might turn to a professional code of ethics as a source of moral guidance. For American occupational therapists, this would be the current Occupational Therapy Code of Ethics of the American Occupational Therapy Association [AOTA 2005].

An occupational therapist faced with an ethical problem could turn to the Occupational Therapy Code of Ethics to see what guidance it offers regarding the specific issues at stake. Often the Code will provide direction and assistance. "Health care professionals typically specify and enforce obligations for their members, thereby seeking to ensure that persons who enter into relationships with these professionals will find them competent and trustworthy" [Beauchamp and Childress 2001, p. 6]. Most health care professions codify these rules of conduct into a formal code of ethics.

The purpose of professional codes is to set minimal expectations of those who practice within their respective profession. Professional codes can also be aspirational in nature in that they set more than minimal expectations for members of the profession. The AOTA Code of Ethics states that the code "is an aspirational guide to professional conduct when ethical issues surface." One limitation of codes is that they tend to oversimplify moral responsibilities.

The occupational therapist is obligated to abide by the tenets of the Code of Ethics. It is possible that occupational therapists may believe that if they fulfill the requirements of the Code of Ethics they have done all they have to do, morally speaking. However, would an occupational therapist's conduct be always correct just because it conforms to the Code of Ethics of the AOTA?

Another limitation of codes of ethics is that the perspectives of the recipients of health care may be absent. What might the public proclaim as the fundamental obligations of occupational therapists if given the chance?

Finally, how do we account for changes in professional codes? Although the first version of the AOTA Code of Ethics was approved in 1977, it has already undergone several revisions. Each time the Occupational Therapy Code of Ethics changed, did the ethically correct behavior for occupational therapists really change—or only what AOTA members believed was the correct behavior? It seems that the foundation for ethics in occupational therapy is something more basic than current professional agreement based on these changes in the Code of Ethics.

Religion

If an occupational therapist worked in a hospital or ambulatory care center sponsored by a religious organization, the institution's ethical code may be derived from religious beliefs and ethical commitments of the sponsoring group. For example, if the institution were Catholic and located in the United States it would have to abide by the Ethical and Religious Directives for Catholic Health Care Services [U.S. Conference of Catholic Bishops 2001]. In addition, the occupational therapist may personally believe and hold to the beliefs and moral guidance of a religious tradition.

Should a religious tradition be considered a voice of moral authority? Religious traditions are a salient source of moral guidance on all-important matters of human life. Believers in a faith hold that a decision is right or morally correct because of divine authority. Thus, being a believer commits one to the ethical teachings of one's faith. Some argue that religion alone is the sufficient and ultimate justification for moral guidance. However, there is often plurality of beliefs regarding what is moral and good within a single faith tradition.

What if the religious beliefs of the institution and the occupational therapist differ? If there are differences in religious beliefs, whose beliefs should take precedence? For example, a female therapist receives an order to splint a male Hasidic Jew. The therapist recalls some information about the Hasidic Jewish culture. She thinks it may be inappropriate for her to touch this man's hand. The therapist is unsure what to do. She knows that this client needs her services and she is the only therapist in the clinic, but she also wishes to be culturally and religiously sensitive.

Because the moral authority for religious beliefs is by its very nature mutually exclusive, there would be no common language or set of ethical principles from which to engage in discussion. There is no common language because different people hold different religious beliefs. We would have to look for a view of ethics that is respectful and cognizant of religious beliefs but that exists outside individual belief systems in order to meet on common ground. In a pluralistic society, such as that encountered in the United States, secular ethical principles have great appeal because they are grounded on reason. Moreover, there is striking similarity among basic ethical principles and constructs held across diverse religious beliefs. This indicates that there is perhaps another, more basic source, of moral guidance. We now turn to three of these traditional approaches to secular ethics that allow us to talk across various faith traditions, cultures, and disciplines.

Classic Approaches to Ethics

One way of discussing morality is to observe that it involves obligations. The principles approach to ethics recognizes these obligations or duties and the universal nature of their application to moral decisions. Another way of viewing the moral life is through a more subjective lens, with a concern for actual persons and their needs and relationships. Care-based ethics attempts to focus on the specific ethical issues that arise within the web of human relationships that nurture and sustain us as human beings.

Finally, we can view the moral life outside the moral problems encountered in clinical practice and instead focus on the character of the occupational therapist. When decisions have to be made in occupational therapy practice it is often in a climate of stress and perhaps urgency. The best tools an occupational therapist can have for dealing with situations such as this are not those provided by principles or care-based reasoning but by a fixed habit of character or virtue. This provides a generally reliable response to ethical challenges. Virtue ethics takes the view that a person with a developed moral character knows when and what type of a decision needs to be made *and* has the perseverance to follow through. A brief description of each of these traditional approaches to ethics follows.

Principles Approach

Beauchamp and Childress [2001] are the architects of the *four principles approach* to ethics. Although there are more than the four ethical principles selected by Beauchamp and Childress, these four principles do provide a comprehensive framework for ethical analysis. The four principles are as follows:

- Respect for autonomy (respecting the decision-making capacity of autonomous persons)
- Nonmaleficence (the duty not to harm)
- Beneficence (the duty to do good)
- Justice (a group of norms or rules that assist in the fair distribution of burdens and benefits)

Each of these principles has played a central role in health care. Respect for autonomy requires that we not only respect other human beings but that we have a regard for their self-determination. Autonomous adults have the right to make decisions about their lives without undue interference or coercion from others. Therapists must be aware of the autonomy of their clients. For example, a therapist may want to provide a splint for an elder to retard deformity. The elder may explicitly state that he or she does not wish to have the splint made.

Nonmaleficence is sometimes referred to as the most basic of all ethical principles in health care. Nonmaleficence is a perfect duty because it is always binding and forbids harm to others. For example, a physician may write a prescription for a splint that you know will cause a client harm. The therapist's duty of nonmaleficence guides the therapist to handle the situation for a different outcome.

Beneficence is an imperfect duty and one that is sometimes binding. Beneficence asserts that we should promote and do good for others. All of the occupational therapist's efforts are directed to the patient's good in the sense that treatment and therapy are directed to improving function and well-being. The very act of splinting is a beneficent act because it is for the patient's welfare whether in the long or short term. In the relationship between health professionals and clients, the imperfect duty of beneficence takes on more weight and approximates the perfect duty of nonmaleficence.

Justice mediates the claims of self-interested individuals within communities. Distributive justice is of particular interest in health care because often there is not enough of a valuable resource for all those who need or want it, and decisions must be made about the fair distribution of such a resource. For example, a therapist knows that a client will benefit from a splint that is not covered by insurance. The therapist wishes to do good and refers the client to a pro bono clinic.

Generally speaking, principles are action guides to moral behavior. The principles approach responds most appropriately to the question of what is the morally correct thing to do. The principles are universally applicable (i.e., they apply to all people in all situations and provide a degree of impartiality to the decision-making process). Beauchamp and Childress emphasize that their four principles do not constitute a general ethical theory but provide a framework for identifying and reflecting on ethical problems [2001].

Principles must be specified to be of assistance in practical circumstances, especially when there is conflict between ethical principles. For example, a therapist is treating a client who is severely depressed and needs a splint to improve function. The client does not want the splint. The therapist must wrestle with the client's need for autonomy and the principles of beneficence and nonmaleficence. After specifying what autonomy, goods, and harms mean in the context of this case, the therapist could then turn to a more sophisticated level of reasoning to a moral decision; that is, ethical theory that prioritizes or balances the demands of the principles in conflict.

Care-Based Approach

Care-based reasoning emphasizes the particular and unique features of a situation. Care-based reasoning also emphasizes the moral relevance of such features as context, relationships, and power hidden in the more objective, universal view of the principles approach. A care-based approach to ethics recognizes that all persons are not situated so as to be independent decision makers of equal status. Many individuals (particularly clients) are disadvantaged, dependent, sometimes exploited, and often responsible for the care of others. All of these factors limit their ability to assert their rights in competition with the claims of others.

A care-based approach draws our attention to the actual persons involved in a case, and their needs, particular history, and connections. In addition, care-based theorists claim that a caring relationship is characterized by mutuality (recognition of the self in others) and transformation; that is, the relationship transforms or changes not only the recipient of care but the caregiver as well [Mayerhoff 1971, Gadow 1980]. The recognition and protection of relationships are of prime importance to care-based ethics.

The following example demonstrates the ethical dilemma arising from a situation in which relationships, context, and power are intertwined. A therapist may wish to honor a child's goal to independently hold a crayon. To accomplish this goal, the therapist must provide the child with a splint. The child's parents are adamantly opposed to the child's wearing the splint because they wish to preserve the child's "normalcy" and do not want equipment that calls attention to the disability.

Virtue-Based Approach

Virtue is a morally good habit of one's nature. Virtue makes work, interactions, and all types of human exchanges good and makes individuals good. The distinction between a habit and action is important if one is to understand virtue, as human beings are constantly required to make choices between good and bad alternatives and to discern the right and reject the wrong. We need a constancy of mind or will to adhere to right principles. All of this calls for a foundation of solid virtues. Thus, we do the right thing or are inclined to do good as a matter of habit or character. Goodness is a part of who we are and is evident in how we act. An occupational therapist must have the virtues of compassion, wisdom, justice, temperance, and fortitude—to name a few essential virtues—to be deemed a *good* occupational therapist.

According to Aristotle, virtue means doing the right thing in relation to the right person, at the right time, and in the right manner. In other words, we should strive for moderation in all things, not going to excess or falling short of the mark. For example, it is one thing to be courageous and another to take courage to the point of foolhardiness. If we exercise too little courage, we might be considered cowardly. Thus, to find the right balance is life's greatest good or *summum bonum* of the moral life. Virtue holds us fast to the right course. For example, a therapist's client tells her that her husband is abusing her and she is frightened to go home. The virtuous therapist makes the time to help this client and risk being reprimanded for low productivity units.

Application to Complex Cases

The three approaches to ethics provide different methods of analysis that highlight certain aspects of a case and minimize others. Each approach is applied to a different case dealing with occupational therapists involved in some aspect of splinting. The first case highlights the ethical principles of nonmaleficence and beneficence and an additional principle, proportionality, that helps balance the two.

Case One: Harms and Benefits of Splinting

Delaney, OTR/L, was somewhat surprised when she received an order for splinting for a client from the oncology service in the large medical center in which she worked. The occupational therapy department did not receive many referrals from oncology. Delaney was concerned that the order might be inappropriate when she noted the age and primary diagnosis of the client, Anne, who was dying of metastatic cancer of the breast. Anne is 82 years old and is no longer a viable candidate for any type of treatment for cancer. She had undergone surgery several years before. Surgery was followed by radiation and chemotherapy. However, the cancer had returned and metastasized to her bones.

Anne's husband died of cancer, and thus Anne had firsthand knowledge of what dying could be like. She told her physician, "I saw how Frank died surrounded by tubes and equipment. That's not for me. I don't want to die in the hospital. I want my family and friends with me, and I don't want to be in pain." Recently, Anne returned to the hospital for surgery to excise a tumor on her arm. Unfortunately, the tumor caused radial nerve compression that was not resolved by the surgery. The order Delaney received today was for a dynamic extension splint.

After Delaney finished reviewing the medical record, she walked down the hall to assess Anne's condition. Anne had fallen asleep in the chair in her room. As Delaney stood in the doorway and watched the slow rise and fall of Anne's thin chest, she wondered if splinting made any sense in this case. What did Anne stand to gain from the splinting procedure? The dynamic extension splint could cause discomfort. It did not seem right to inflict discomfort on Anne in addition to what she was already experiencing. How should Delaney weigh the potential benefit to be gained from splinting against Anne's overall prognosis?

There are at least two ethical questions raised by this case. The first is substantive: Is it ever appropriate to deliver care that offers little hope of benefit or is unduly burdensome to the client? The second is more procedural: What role should Delaney play in providing care to Anne? Clearly, the two are linked but separate issues.

Delaney is obligated by the principles of nonmaleficence and beneficence to avoid harm and to provide good. This statement appears fairly straightforward. Yet, we know that certain clinical procedures (splinting included) do cause harm in the form of inconvenience and discomfort. We justify this harm because of the potential benefit that will be realized through the present discomfort. It is worthwhile, in other words, to suffer some inconvenience and discomfort in the present for greater function from stretching of soft tissue in the long term.

The principle of proportionality recognizes the need to balance the goods and harms of all types of clinical care. The risks of harm must be constantly weighed against possible benefit. We not only have a duty to avoid harm and do good but to weigh and balance possible benefits against possible harms in order to maximize benefits and minimize harms. Normally, the provision of a dynamic extension splint would be considered a moral good. If the splint does its job, the client will have greater flexibility and use of the wrist and hand, adding to the overall quality of life.

In this case, however, Anne is already burdened with the pain and suffering of a terminal illness. It is unlikely that she will gain much benefit from the splint because there is little hope for an extended life span. In addition, the stretching provided by the splint will likely cause discomfort. Under other circumstances, the discomfort of the splint might be well worthwhile because of the benefits that would be gained in the long run. Anne made it clear that she did not want to be in pain while she was dying. Is the discomfort that will be caused by the splint the type of pain she meant?

Competent clients have the right, according to autonomy, to make decisions about the benefit and burdens of treatment. This is especially important when a client nears the end of life. A death with dignity is sometimes defined as a death that is not "unduly burdened" by the clinical environment and medical technology to prolong life [Catholic Health Association 1993]. The treatment or technology in this case is not "life-sustaining" (e.g., a ventilator or artificial nutrition and hydration). However, it does have an impact on the quality of life Anne will have until her death from other causes.

Clients are not obligated to undergo treatment that offers little hope of benefit or that involves excessive pain, expense, or other inconvenience. If the goals of treatment are not attainable (i.e., the use of particular therapy cannot or will not improve prognosis and recovery), the treatment need not be initiated or continued. The moral focus in this case is not on the type of disease or illness the client has, the state of medical science, or the type of treatment. In addition, questions of whether the treatment is customary, simple, inexpensive, or noninvasive are not the relevant ethical considerations.

The true moral focus regarding any treatment, splinting included, is the proportion between the benefit to the client and the burden involved. Furthermore, health care professionals are not mandated by law or morally obligated to render treatment that is deemed useless.

Delaney must first decide whether she considers the splint as plausible treatment. If the treatment is at least plausible, she has a duty to give Anne the relevant information about the splint and its possible benefits and burdens. This should be done in a manner that Anne can understand so that she can make a decision about the treatment that is in keeping with her values and previously expressed wishes. If Anne decides that the burdens of the treatment are disproportionate to the benefits, she is not obligated to undergo the splinting procedure; nor is Delaney morally obligated to provide treatment that Anne deems overly burdensome.

It should be noted that the physician has ordered a specific splint for Anne and Delaney cannot ignore this additional obligation to a professional colleague. The physician has a right to expect that his orders will be carried out unless there is a good reason they should not be. Delaney should explain the outcome of her interaction with Anne to the physician and work toward a mutually agreeable solution. Delaney could also offer other methods of support to Anne such as stretching exercises to improve the quality of her life for whatever time she has left.

The next case involves a situation in which the therapist is advised to deceive both the client and the third-party payer. The act of deception runs counter to the principle of respect for autonomy, and therefore requires justification. Another way to sort through the ethical issues and decide what ought to be done in this particular situation is through a care-based approach.

Case Two: Providing Less-Than-Optimal Services

The number of clients referred to the out-client rehabilitation clinic of Centerview Medical Center seemed to increase every week. Mark Petty, OTR/L, enjoyed the busy pace and the variety of clients he saw in the clinic. Mark was assigned a new client, Tung, a 28-year-old automobile manufacturing worker who had sustained a severe crush injury of his hand on the job. Mark noted that there were orders to evaluate and begin treatment. As Mark read further in Tung's medical record, he saw that the physician specifically requested a certified hand therapist's (CHT's) services. Mark was not a certified hand therapist, so he approached his supervisor, Vivian, to discuss the problem. Mark explained that the physician's orders specified a CHT.

"How soon can Tung see the CHT?" Mark asked Vivian. "She's just too busy to take any new clients," Vivian responded. "I'll tell you what to do. I would hate to lose this case. It looks like it will take at least a year of service to rehabilitate Tung. Why don't you just go ahead and provide services to him and have the CHT sign the notes? Who will know the difference?" Vivian then walked away.

Mark was left standing in the middle of the hallway with Tung's chart in his hand and a perplexed look on his face. Provide services to a client and have someone else sign off on them? On the face of it, that seemed very wrong to Mark. Yet he, too, would hate to lose this interesting case. He had briefly met Tung and instantly liked him. Would anyone really know the difference if he provided care to Tung or if the CHT did? Mark wondered what the right thing to do was. The application of a care-based approach includes the following [Fry et al. 1996]:

- Identifying the moral conflict within the specific context, considering the others who are involved in the conflict and how they are interrelated
- Feeling concern for relationships and individuals, and identifying oneself in relation to the individuals and problems involved

Generally speaking, if Mark were to take a care-based approach to resolving the ethical issues in the case he would have to ask himself what it means to be "caring" within the context of this situation and its specific responsibilities. The moral conflict involves whether or not to provide services that are less-than-optimal to Tung, in that Mark is not a CHT. Could this be considered a "caring" action? The context of this case is a busy outpatient setting, perhaps too busy to handle the volume of clients and maintain quality. Because the physician specifically ordered that a CHT provide the care the first logical alternative for Mark is to transfer Tung's care to a CHT. This is what Mark attempted to do and was told that the CHT caseload was backlogged.

If the beleaguered CHT at the Centerview Medical Center cannot see all of the clients who need her level of expertise, the clinic is obligated to either hire another CHT or to help support and prepare another therapist who is already a member of the staff (such as Mark). This would allow Mark to become eligible to take the certification examination to become a CHT. Both of these options are caring in several regards in that the special needs of all parties, including the overworked CHT, are considered.

The CHT would receive some assistance so that her work is more manageable, and probably less stressful, and clients would receive the level of care they deserve for their complex problems. However, these solutions are long term in nature and not immediately helpful to Mark. A caring, short-term solution could be to refer Tung to a CHT at another clinic or hospital. Alternatively, Mark could "trade" a patient with the CHT. In addition, Mark could work with the physician to see whether there is any room for negotiation about the requirement for the CHT. The latter option would be considered caring only if Mark truly believed he could deliver a quality of care approximating that of a CHT, perhaps under the indirect supervision of a CHT.

Vivian did not offer any of these alternative solutions to Mark's problem but suggested that Mark lie. Could a lie ever be considered a caring action? Perhaps, but in this situation we have to ask who the lie benefits? It appears that the clinic benefits because they won't lose reimbursement for a year's worth of billable service. Mark might also benefit to a limited extent because he would get to work with a client he likes and would learn from the experience of treating him.

Those who would be harmed are the physician and Tung. If either the physician or Tung found out that they had been deceived, how might they react? If Tung's care was insufficient, his function could be compromised. Of course, there are legal implications in the case, in that what Vivian has suggested is fraud. However, there are moral implications as well.

Care-based ethics also focuses on the relationship of the individuals involved. Lies have a way of eroding relationships because they damage trust. If Mark chose to follow Vivian's recommendation, the entire time he was treating Tung he would be doing so in a deceptive manner. It is important to understand that deception includes withholding information as well as outright falsehoods. In addition, Mark now knows that Vivian condones deception and this knowledge can hurt their relationship. Vivian did not demonstrate caring behavior to one of her subordinates but chose to place him in a moral dilemma in which he will be forced to oppose her recommendation in order to do the right thing.

Finally, because Mark "likes" Tung he may be more inclined to resist actions that are deceitful. Affection for clients makes it easier for us to recognize that they are fellow participants in life, facing the human condition. Another of the characteristics of care-based reasoning, as you recall, is mutuality; that is, empathizing with the other's position. If Mark were the client and had an injury similar to that suffered by Tung what sort of treatment would he want? As a client, would he accept the reasons for the deception Vivian has proposed? It is unlikely that any client would accept less than optimal care just so that the clinic could make a profit.

In the next case, an occupational therapist wrestles with the conflicting obligations often encountered in clinical settings between clients and colleagues. Everyone makes a mistake at one time or another, but what if the mistake of a colleague has serious implications for a client's well-being? Should the therapist's primary loyalty always lie with the client?

Case Three: Covering for a Colleague

Douglas, OTR/L, was filling in for a colleague and friend (Melody) who was absent from work with a bad case of the flu. Douglas and Melody attended the same occupational therapy program, and after graduation both ended up working for the same health system in a large urban setting. Douglas made it a habit to review the medical records, treatment plans, and progress reports of the clients he treated, even if he worked with them for only a day. He believed it was important to be familiar with their care and present status.

The first client on the schedule, Ben, was recovering from a flexor tendon injury, status post two weeks. The chart review indicated that Ben was a cooperative client. Douglas began with an assessment of Ben's condition before proceeding with therapy. Douglas immediately noticed that the tendon repair appeared to be ruptured. Douglas began to question Ben about his activities. Ben reported that Melody had removed the splint the previous day and engaged him in aggressive gripping exercises. "You know, I knew something was wrong right away with my hand last night when I was doing those gripping exercises on my own. Should the therapist have told me to do that?" Ben asked.

It appeared that Melody had not followed the protocol for flexor tendon injuries. Because she had given him a home exercise program with gripping exercises and put Ben through an inappropriate hand exercise regimen, the surgical repair was ruptured. Melody was responsible for the injury and the future pain and inconvenience Ben would have to undergo having surgical repair of the injury a second time. Ben's question hung in the air as Douglas thought about his obligations to a friend and colleague in contrast to his obligations to the client. This case raises numerous questions.

- Is this therapist simply inexperienced?
- How does one gauge the competence of a peer?
- How far does loyalty to peers extend?
- Is competency a matter of aesthetics?
- Are there sufficient safeguards in place to protect the public from incompetent providers?
- What are occupational therapy's obligations to society regarding the competence of its own practitioners and those in other fields?
- What does the public need to know?

It would be important to determine whether this was an isolated incident or a pattern in Melody's behavior. Overall competence is related to client good. Regardless of the reason for this particular act of incompetence, to remedy the incompetent behavior Douglas must access the systems in place in the organization (such as Melody's supervisor or the risk management department). To report a friend and colleague, Douglas must have the virtues of courage and perseverance. Douglas's first obligation as a health care professional is to the best interests of clients.

Douglas must also have the virtue of honesty. He has made an implied promise to clients to serve their best interests. In this case, that involves supplying information about what Douglas suspects is the cause of Ben's injury. It is possible that Ben injured his hand himself, although he denies it. However, even if that is so Melody should not have engaged him in inappropriate active hand exercises.

Douglas also has a general moral obligation to tell the truth. He should not lie. Before Douglas reveals the information about the ruptured tendon repair to Ben and the surgeon, who will also need to know, he would first want to speak to Melody and confirm what actually happened.

The morally virtuous occupational therapist is straightforward, thoughtful, and well-meaning. Given all of these virtues, Douglas must make a decision (and quickly) as to how he will respond to Ben about his injury. He can be loyal to his peer and friend and still do the right thing, but he will need a strong moral character in order to act.

The Occupational Therapy Code of Ethics would support actions that maintain high-quality standards of care. In addition, balanced with this mandate of client benefit is Principle 7, which states, "Occupational therapy personnel shall treat colleagues and other professionals with respect, fairness, discretion, and integrity." Douglas must make certain that Ben's welfare is protected, but he should do so in a way that minimizes harms to Melody.

Contribution of Ethics to Clinical Practice

In addition to the resources already enumerated to assist occupational therapists when making ethical decisions, there are also resources within organizations or institutions. For example, policies and guidelines provide excellent support when they are thoughtfully written in keeping with the ethical norms provided herein and the values of the organization as a whole. Policies or guidelines should be available for commonly encountered ethical issues, such as informed consent, determination of decision-making ability, confidentiality, futility decisions, fair and safe distribution of staff and workload, and the role of surrogate decision makers.

Furthermore, personnel in specific areas of care (such as hand rehabilitation or burn care) could work together to establish mutually held values about the complex issues that comprise daily clinical experience. For example, what are the values regarding conflicts between religious values and those held by the institution regarding end-of-life treatment and pain management? Unless dedicated time is spent reflecting on issues such as these, it is likely that decisions will be made during highly emotional and urgent circumstances with less than satisfactory results.

Finally, another resource that is becoming more common is the institutional ethics committee. Occupational therapists should not only seek out the advice and support of ethics committees when problems seem beyond resolution; they should also offer to serve on such committees, as their expertise and perspective are often missing from the committee's membership. Ethics committees offer the opportunity to discuss issues in a nonthreatening environment in a multidisciplinary manner. Although ethics committees do not make the decision for the individuals involved in an ethical problem, they do offer guidelines and affirm the values of the organization that form the parameters for decisions.

CASE STUDY 19-1*

Read the following scenario and answer the questions based on information in this chapter.

Mercedes, OTR/L, is the clinical therapy manager at Francis Medical Center in a moderate-sized city with many referrals from the surrounding rural community. She spends approximately 25% of her time treating clients, on both an inpatient and outpatient basis. The rest of her time is spent dealing with administrative responsibilities and management of the physical, occupational, and speech therapy staff and services.

Mercedes has recently hired Collin, a new occupational therapy graduate, who is planning to take his certification examination in 4 months. Until Collin can take and pass his examination, Mercedes decided she would review and co-sign Collin's documentation. Last week, Mercedes was reviewing Collin's treatment plan and documentation for several outpatients with complex upper extremity injuries. One client with a chronic radial nerve injury was being seen too many times and had no splint provision to prevent contractures or to position for function. As a result, Mercedes is concerned that Collin did not follow the usual diagnostic protocol to splint and monitor every other week. She realizes that Collin needs more supervision and networking to improve his services for efficiency and efficacy.

Mercedes knows that she does not have the flexibility or the time in her schedule to provide the mentoring Collin needs. There are no other qualified occupational therapists on staff, as one recently retired and the other is on maternity leave. Although recruitment is in progress, no one has been hired to take the retired therapist's place. Thus, Mercedes does not have another therapist to supervise and mentor Collin. What should Mercedes do? Should she limit the type of client Collin sees so that he does not treat clients with complex injuries? However, how will Collin gain the experience he needs to adequately manage complex clients if he is not allowed to treat them? What are Collin's responsibilities in this case?

1. Is there an ethical issue in the case? If so, list three questions pertinent to this position.

____

____

____

____

2. What is (are) the ethical problem(s) in the case? You may name them in terms of conflicts between principles or via a care-based or virtue approach.

____

____

____

____

3. Briefly describe four alternative actions Mercedes could take to resolve the ethical problem(s) in the case. For each alternative, name the ethical principle that is upheld or threatened by the alternative.

____

____

____

____

4. Use the Occupational Therapy Code of Ethics [2005] to determine what principle(s) of the Code would be helpful to Mercedes as she makes her decision. List the principle(s) and explain how it would be helpful.

____

____

____

____

*See Appendix A for the answer key.

SELF-QUIZ 19-1*

In regard to the following questions, circle either true (T) or false (F).

1. T F By looking at the virtues of individuals, we are able to gauge their character.
2. T F Moral principles serve as action guides as we make ethical decisions.
3. T F Beneficence is a perfect duty.
4. T F Respect for autonomy obligates us to do good for others.
5. T F The principle of nonmaleficence requires that we avoid harming others at all times.
6. T F Care-based reasoning is concerned with the universal abstract aspects of the moral life.
7. T F Although not legally binding, professional codes of ethics set forth the highest standards of professions.
8. T F Ethics is an attempt to state what we should do, be, or care about to attain the most of what is best in human life.
9. T F Justice is concerned with the fair distribution of burdens and benefits in a community.
10. T F Proportionality requires that we balance the harms and goods in a situation and work to maximize the good.

*See Appendix A for the answer key.

REVIEW QUESTIONS

1. How does one know if a situation involves ethics?
2. What is the difference among moral, amoral, and immoral behavior?
3. What are the basic differences between the three traditional approaches to ethics: principles, care-based, and virtue?
4. What are the four ethical principles that underlie the majority of interactions in health care?
5. What question does the principle approach to ethics best answer?
6. What does the principle of proportionality require us to do?
7. Can virtues be learned, practiced, and cultivated?
8. How does care-based ethics view the moral life?
9. How does virtue provide us with immediate responses to ethical challenges?
10. What are some of the limitations of professional codes of ethics?

References

American Occupational Therapy Association (2005). Occupational therapy code of ethics. American Journal of Occupational Therapy 59:639-642. Code available at *http://www.aota.org/general/coe.asp*.

Beauchamp T, Childress J (2001). *Principles of Biomedical Ethics, Fifth Edition*. New York: Oxford University Press.

Catholic Health Association (1993). *Caring for Persons at the End of Life*. St. Louis: Catholic Health Association.

Chater R, Dockter D, Haddad A, Rupp MT, Vivian JC, Weinstein B (1993). Ethical decision making in pharmacy. American Pharmacy NS33(4):73.

Fry ST, Killen AR, Robinson EM (1996). Care-based reasoning, caring, and the ethic of care: A need for clarity. Journal of Clinical Ethics 7(1):41-47.

Gadow S (1980). Body and self: A dialectic. The Journal of Medicine and Philosophy 5(3):172-184.

Haddad AM (1988). Ethical problems in nursing. In [editor], *Dissertation Abstracts International* #AAG8818621, Lincoln, NE: University of Nebraska at Lincoln.

Haddad AM (1991). Ethical problems in pharmacy practice: A survey of difficulty and incidence. American Journal of Pharmaceutical Education 55:1-6.

Jonsen AR (1998). *The Birth of Bioethics*. New York: Oxford University Press.

Mayerhoff M (1971). *On Caring*. New York: Harper & Row.

Solomon WD (1995). Normative ethical theories. In W Reich (ed.), *The Encyclopedia of Bioethics, Second Edition*. New York: Macmillan, p. 736.

United States Conference of Catholic Bishops (2001). *Ethical and Religious Directives for Catholic Health Care Services, Fourth Edition*. Washington, D.C.: U.S. Conference of Catholic Bishops. Text also available at *http://www.usccb.org/bishops/directives.htm*.

Warren E (1962). Special address to the Lewis Marshall Award Dinner of the Jewish Theological Seminary of America, New York. Quote appears in the *New York Times*, November 12, 1962, pp. 1-2, in an article by Milton Bracker, "Warren Favors Profession to Give Advice on Ethics."

Glossary

American occupational therapy code of ethics The professional code of ethics established by the American Occupational Therapy Association. This code sets forth the minimal expectations for occupational therapists.

Antideformity position A position that includes the wrist in 30 to 40 degrees of extension, the thumb in 40 to 45 degrees of palmar abduction, the thumb IP joint in full extension, the MCPs at 70 to 90 degrees of flexion, and the PIPs and DIPs in full extension.

Aponeurosis A strong sheet of fibrous connective tissue that serves as a tendon to attach muscles to bone or as a fascia to bind muscles together.

Arteriovenous anastomosis A blood vessel that connects directly to a venule without capillary intervention.

Assessment of Motor and Process Skills (AMPS) A functional assessment that requires the client to perform an IADL and assesses motor and process skills.

Autonomy The capability of an adult to make decisions for himself or herself.

Axonotmesis An interruption of the axon with subsequent degeneration of the distal nerve segment.

Basic biomechanical principles Principles that include assessment of normal and pathologic gait patterns in a clinically observable evaluation.

Beneficence The duty to do good.

Biofeedback machine Equipment used to identify muscle signals and sites.

Body powered Prosthesis activated and operated by body movements.

Boutonniere deformity A finger that postures with PIP flexion and DIP hyperextension.

Buddy straps Soft straps used to promote motion and support an injured digit to an adjacent digit.

Canadian Occupational Performance Measure (COPM) A client-centered outcome measure used to assess self-care, productivity, and leisure.

Care-based ethics Focuses on the specific ethical issues that arise within the web of human relationships that nurture and sustain us as human beings.

Carpal tunnel syndrome A common painful disorder of the wrist and hand induced by compression on the median nerve between the inelastic carpal ligament and other structures in the carpal tunnel.

Central extensor tendon This structure crosses the PIP joint dorsally and is part of the PIP joint dorsal capsule.

Circumferential A splint that fits around the circumference of an extremity.

Client-centered treatment Treatment that focuses on meeting client goals as opposed to therapist-designed or protocol-driven goals.

Collateral ligaments Ligaments on each side of the joint that provide joint stability and restraint against deviation forces. The radial collateral ligament protects against ulnar deviation forces, and the ulnar collateral ligament protects against radial deviation forces.

Complex regional pain syndrome A chronic pain condition thought to be a result of impairment in the central or peripheral nerve systems.

Componentry The compilation of components toward assembling a prosthesis.

Compression socks Socks used to reduce swelling formatation at an amputation site.

Conduction Transfers heat from one object to another. Heat is conducted from the higher-temperature object to the lower-temperature material.

Context A variety of interrelated conditions within and surrounding the client that influence performance, including cultural, physical, social, personal, spiritual, temporal, and virtual aspects.

Contracture An abnormal, usually permanent, condition of a joint characterized by flexion and fixation and caused by atrophy and shortening of muscle fibers or by loss of the normal elasticity of the skin such as that from the formation of extensive scar tissue over a joint.

Contralateral limb Limb on the opposite side to the referent.

Convection Transfers heat between a surface and a moving medium or agent.
Cubital tunnel syndrome The second most common site of nerve compression in the upper extremity following carpal tunnel. Injury to the nerve may occur as a result of trauma or prolonged or sustained motion that compresses the nerve over time.
Cumulative trauma disorders Musculoskeletal disorders resulting from repetitive motions (usually occupation) that develop over time. Symptoms include pain, inflammation, and function impairment.
Degrees of freedom The number of planes in which a joint axis(es) can move.
de Quervain's tenosynovitis The most commonly diagnosed wrist tendonitis that may be recognized by pain over the radial styloid, edema in the first dorsal compartment, and positive results from the Finkelstein's test.
Dorsal Pertaining to the back or posterior.
Double crush Nerves that are compressed at more than one site.
Dual site The use of an externally powered prosthesis from two muscle sites.
Dupuytren's contracture A contracture characterized by the formation of finger flexion contractures with a thickened band of palmar fascia.
Duty An obligatory task, conduct, or function that arises from one's position.
Ecchymosis A subcutaneous hemorrhage marked by purple discoloration of the skin.
Elbow arthroplasty The resurfacing or replacement of the elbow joint.
Elbow instability Injury that results from a dislocation of the ulnohumeral joint and injury to the varus and valgus stabilizers of the elbow and to the radial head.
Electrodes Round or square metal used to read or "pick up" muscle signals.
End feel Assessed by passively moving a joint to its maximal end range.
Ethics The exploration of moral duty, principles, human character or virtue, and human relationships involving the study of right and wrong, good and evil, moral conduct on an individual and societal basis, rules, promises, principles, and obligations.
Evidence-based practice The process of reviewing a body of literature in order to select the most appropriate assessment or treatment for an individual client.
Extensor lag The joint can be passively extended but cannot be fully actively extended by the client.
Externally powered Prosthesis operated by batteries.
Finger loops A method of applying dynamic force to a joint.
Finger sprain Stress or ligamentous injury to a joint. Occurs in varying grades of severity.
Flexion contracture A joint that cannot be passively extended to neutral.
Forearm trough A component of the wrist immobilization splint that rests proximal to the wrist on one or more surfaces of the forearm. It provides counterforce leverage to support the weight of the forearm.
Functional envelope Area of work in front and around a person's hands.
Functional position A position that includes the wrist in 20 to 30 degrees of extension, the thumb in 45 degrees of palmar abduction, the MCP joints in 35 to 45 degrees of flexion, and all PIP and DIP joints in slight flexion.
Fusiform swelling Fullness at the PIP joint and tapering proximally and distally. Often seen following finger PIP joint sprains.
Grasp The result of holding an object against the rigid portion of the hand that the second and third digits provide. The flattening and cupping motions of the palm allow the hand to pick up and handle objects of various sizes.
Grip force The amount of force given to a hand or a hook.
Handling characteristics The properties of thermoplastic material when heated and softened.
Harness Strap system to suspend or hold a prosthesis.
Heat gun An instrument used to make adjustments to thermoplastic materials.
Hook rubbers Rubber bands used for hooks used to increase hook grip.
Hypothenar bar A component of the wrist immobilization splint that palmarly supports the ulnar aspect of the transverse metacarpal arch.
Immobilization Splints designed to immobilize primary or secondary joints.
Integumentary system A system encompassing the integument (skin) and its derivatives.
Justice A group of norms or rules that assists in the fair distribution of burdens and benefits.
Lamination Hard, permanent finish of prosthetic socket.
Lateral bands Contributions from the intrinsic muscles that join dorsal to the PIP joint axis. They displace volarly in a boutonniere deformity and dorsally in a swan-neck deformity.
Lateral epicondyle The tissue at the lower end of the humerus at the elbow joint.
Mallet finger A finger that postures with DIP flexion.
McKie thumb splint A prefabricated neoprene splint designed to position the thumb in opposition and in which a supinator strap may be added. The primary function is to provide biomechanically sound weight bearing, grasp, and manipulation of objects.
Mechanical advantage The ratio of the output force developed by the muscles to the input force applied to the body structures the muscles move, especially the ratio of these forces associated with the body structures that act as levers.

Mechanoreceptors Sensory nerve endings that respond to mechanical stimuli such as touch, pressure, sound, and muscular contractions.

Medial epicondyle The part of the humerus that gives attachment to the ulnar collateral ligament of the elbow joint, to the pronator teres, and to a common tendon of origin (the common flexor tendon) of some of the flexor muscles of the forearm.

Median nerve One of the terminal branches of the brachial plexus, which extends along the radial parts of the forearm and the hand and supplies various muscles and the skin of these parts.

Memory The ability of thermoplastic material to return to its preheated (original) shape and size when reheated.

Metacarpal bar A component of the wrist immobilization splint that supports the transverse metacarpal arch dorsally or palmarly.

Mobilization Splints designed to move or mobilize primary or secondary joints.

Morality Concerned with human behavior or actions that are judged as either good or evil.

Myoelectrics The use of electronics to signal a muscle's electrical input.

Neoprene A soft splinting material consisting of rubber with nylon lining on one side and pile material on the other, thus making the Velcro hook attachment quick. Neoprene retains warmth, has some degree of elasticity, and has contour for a snug fit.

Neurapraxia A condition in which a nerve remains in place after a severe injury, although it no longer transmits impulses.

Neurotmesis A peripheral nerve injury in which laceration or traction completely disrupts the nerve.

Nonmaleficence The duty not to harm.

Oblique retinacular ligament Also called the ligament of Landsmeer, this structure is determined to be tight if there is limitation of passive DIP flexion while the PIP joint is extended.

Occupational deprivation A state wherein clients are unable to engage in chosen meaningful life occupations due to factors outside their control.

Occupational disruption A temporary and less severe condition than occupational deprivation that is also caused by an unexpected change in the ability to engage in meaningful activities.

Occupational profile The phase of the evaluation process that involves learning about a client from a contextual and performance viewpoint.

Occupation-based splinting A treatment approach that supports the goals of the treatment plan to promote the ability of clients to engage in meaningful and relevant life endeavors.

Olecranon process A proximal projection of the ulna that forms the tip of the elbow and fits into the oecranon fossa of the humerus when the forearm is extended at the proximal extremity of the ulna.

Orthosis A permanent device to replace or substitute for loss of muscle function.

Orthotic design principles Principles that consider the interaction of anatomic and mechanical structures as well as functional considerations of orthotic components and materials.

Orthotic terminology Terminology derived from the anatomic area affected by the orthosis.

Orthotic treatment objectives Objectives that establish short- and long-term goals that enhance functional level with minimal orthotic intervention.

Osteoarthritis The most common form of arthritis, in which one or many joints undergo degenerative changes—including loss of articular cartilage and proliferation of bone spurs.

Outrigger A projection from the splint base the therapist uses to position a mobilizing force.

Overuse syndrome Repetitive movements causing pain (usually contralateral limb).

Performance characteristics The properties of thermoplastic material after the material has cooled and hardened.

Phantom pain Burning, stabbing pain at the distal end of amputation.

Phantom sensation The feeling of presence of the nonexistent limb.

Physical agent modalities Modalities that produce a biophysiologic response through the use of light, water, temperature, sound, electricity, or mechanical devices.

Plasticity The quality of being plastic or formative.

Posterior elbow immobilization splint A custom-molded thermoplastic splint positioned in 80 to 90 degrees of flexion.

Posterior interosseous nerve syndrome A condition that includes weakness or paralysis of any muscles innervated by the posterior interosseous nerve and does not involve sensory loss.

Preformed splints Factory-produced splints premolded to a specific design.

Prehension The use of the hands and fingers to grasp or pick up objects.

Pressure Total force divided by the area of application.

Principles The universal nature of obligations and duties and their application to moral decisions.

Pronator tunnel syndrome The compression of the median nerve in the forearm between the two heads of the pronator teres muscle.

Protocols Written plans specifying the procedures for giving an examination, conducting research, or providing care for a particular condition.

Radial Pertaining to the radius or radial side of the forearm or hand.

Radial head The disc-shaped portion of the radius closest to the elbow.

Radial nerve The largest branch of the brachial plexus, supplying the skin of the arm and forearm and their extensor muscles.
Radial nerve injuries Injuries commonly occurring from fractures of the humeral shaft, fractures and dislocation of the elbow, or compressions of the nerve.
Radial tunnel syndrome A condition in which a nerve in the forearm is compressed, causing elbow pain and weakness of the wrist or hand but without causing a loss of sensation.
Reliability The consistency of an assessment.
Residual limb The distal end portion of an amputation.
Responsiveness An assessment's sensitivity to measure differences in status.
Rheumatoid arthritis A chronic systemic disease that can affect the lungs, cardiovascular system, and eyes. Joint involvement resulting from inflammatory disease of the synovium is the primary clinical feature. The disease may range from mild to severe and can result in joint deformity and destruction of varying degrees.
Scaphoid fracture A break in the boat-shaped bone of the hand.
Self-determination The ability of the individual to freely choose his or her own actions.
Sensory system modulation The brain's ability to regulate and balance excitation and inhibition of sensory input.
Single site The use of an externally powered prosthesis from one muscle site.
Socket A hard material (resin and plastic) used to make temporary or permanent prostheses.
Soft splints Prefabricated or custom splints made from various soft materials.
Spasticity A form of muscular hypertonicity with increased resistance to stretch.
Splint A temporary device that is part of a treatment program.
Static progressive tension A splint that uses nonelastic tension to provide a constant force.
Stress Any emotional, physical, social, economic, or other factor that requires a response or change.
Superficial agents Heating agents or thermotherapy agents that penetrate the skin to a depth of 1 to 2 cm. They include moist hot packs, fluidotherapy, paraffin wax therapy, and cryotherapy.
Suspension systems Straps used to suspend or hold a prosthesis.
Swan-neck deformity A finger that postures with PIP hyperextension and DIP flexion.
Tendonitis An inflammatory condition of a tendon, usually resulting from strain.
Tenosynovitis Inflammation of a tendon sheath caused by calcium deposits, repeated strain or trauma, high levels of blood cholesterol, rheumatoid arthritis, gout, or gonorrhea.
Terminal device Hand, hook, or tool used at the end of a prosthesis.
Terminal extensor tendon This delicate structure is formed by the uniting of the lateral bands and provides DIP extension.
Thermoplastic material Material that softens under heat and is capable of being molded into shape with pressure and then hardens upon cooling without undergoing a chemical change.
Three-point pressure A system consisting of three individual linear forces in which the middle force is directed in opposite direction to the other two forces.
Torque The effect a force has on rotational movement of a point. It can be calculated by multiplying the force by the length of the movement arm.
Torque transmission Splints that create motion of primary joints situated beyond the boundaries of the splint itself or that harness secondary "driver" joint(s) to create motion of primary joints that may be situated longitudinally or transversely to the driver joint(s).
Transhumeral amputation Amputation across the humerus bone.
Transradial amputation Amputation across the radius and ulna bones.
Transverse retinacular ligament This ligament helps prevent lateral band dorsal displacement and thereby contributes to the delicate balance of the extensor mechanism at the PIP joint.
Treatment protocol Written plan specifying the procedures for treatment.
Ulnar Pertaining to the long medial bone of the forearm or ulnar side of the forearm or hand.
Ulnar collateral ligament injury A common injury that can occur at the MCP joint of the thumb. This is also known as gamekeeper's thumb.
Ulnar nerve One of the termanl branches of the brachial plexus that supplies the muscles and skin on the ulnar side of the forearm and hand.
Validity The extent to which an assessment measures what it is intended to measure.
Values The internal motivators for an individual's actions.
Verbal Analog Scale A scale used to determine a person's perception of pain intensity. The person is asked to rate pain on a scale from 0 to 10 (0 refers to no pain and 10 refers to the worst pain ever experienced).
Virtue A morally good habit of one's nature.
Viscoelasticity The skin's degree of viscosity and elasticity, which enables the skin to resist stress.
Visual Analog Scale A scale used to determine a person's perception of pain intensity. The person is asked to look at a 10-cm horizontal line. The left side of the line represents "no pain" and the right side represents "pain as bad as it could be." The person indicates pain level by marking a slash on the line, which represents the pain experienced.

Volar Also called palmar, this term pertains to the palm of the hand or the sole of the foot.
Volar plate A fibrocartilaginous structure that prevents hyperextension of a joint.
Wallerian degeneration When a nerve is completely severed or the axon and myelin sheath are damaged, the segment of axon and the motor and sensory end receptors distal to the lesion suffer ischemia and begin to degenerate 3 to 5 days after the injury.
Wartenberg's neuropathy Compression of the superficial radial nerve that usually includes numbness, tingling, and pain of the dorsoradial aspect of the forearm, wrist, and hand.
Wearing schedules Planned schedules for donning and doffing splints.
Working memory The short-term storage of information in the brain.
Zones of the hand The division of the hand into distinct areas for ease of understanding literature, conversing with other health providers, and documenting pertinent information.

APPENDIX A

Answers to Quizzes, Laboratory Exercises, and Case Studies

Chapter 1

Self-Quiz 1–1 Answers

1. B
2. C
3. A

Case Study 1–1 Answers

1. B
2. C
3. A

Chapter 2

Self-Quiz 2–1 Answers

1. The therapist should seek to learn about the culture of the client, either through personal interview with the individual or family or through reading. If the client speaks a language that you do not speak, ensure that a translator is present so that information is accurately transmitted between you and the client. Different cultures may have views about illness and disability that are different from yours. They may also be of a different faith or have family obligations and responsibilities different from those you are accustomed to. Wearing a splint during certain ceremonies or religious events may not be acceptable to your client. Discuss the splint plan and appropriately explain the importance of compliance. If you learn that cultural difference may be a barrier to compliance, work with the client in an attempt to arrive at a workable solution.
2. The performance areas of play and education as well as developmentally appropriate activities of daily living (ADL) and instrumental activities of daily living (IADL) skills should be considered. Personal context factors such as age and gender will enter into color selection and the level of independence the child may have with splint donning/doffing and care. A younger child may need to have additional straps applied to prevent unwanted splint removal or shifting. An older child may be able to independently monitor a splinting schedule.

Case Study 2–1 Answers

1. Henry's wife, who is his primary caretaker, has accompanied him to the treatment sessions. As an important part of his social context, she is able to assist Henry with accurate completion of the intake interview. To ensure Henry's role, including competence as the husband and head of household within this traditional family, the therapist should first address questions to Henry and verify responses with his wife only if needed.
2. Splint care sheet should be written in large bolded font. Instructions should be written in simple phrases and line drawings used as appropriate to illustrate splint and strap placement. Black-and-white or photocopied photos should be avoided because they may not provide high contrast. High-contrast color photos taken of the splint on Henry's hand may assist with accurate placement. Splint care instructions must be reviewed with Henry and his wife using the splint care sheet prior to issuing the device. Henry should be asked to repeat instructions and precautions back to therapist with the assistance of his wife.
3. As with the splint care sheet, large font and line drawings can be used to assist with low vision. Instructions should be phrased simply and the order of the exercises should be clearly indicated. Line drawings

can be effective, as can color photographs of Henry's hand. Exercise instructions must be reviewed with Henry and his wife using the handout. Henry should be asked to demonstrate the exercises and verbalize repetitions and frequency with the assistance of his wife prior to leaving the clinic.

Case Study 2–2 Answers

1. Malcolm indicated that he is not satisfied with his handwriting, typing, or meat cutting abilities. All of these areas scored poor in performance and satisfaction. Despite these issues being caused by limited hand function, they should be addressed during the first treatment sessions in order to enhance the quality of life for Malcolm. Although these functions should return eventually as hand function improves, waiting for eventual hand movement, strength, and coordination will create an unnecessary lack of ability to complete meaningful life tasks. Handwriting and meat cutting are reported to be the most difficult and least satisfactory areas for Malcolm.
2. A client-centered treatment model and a rehabilitative approach will expedite Malcolm's return to function. The client-centered model focuses attention on his immediate concerns (handwriting, typing, meat cutting). The rehabilitative approach uses adaptations and modifications as treatment methods to enhance function.
3. The Canadian Occupational Performance Measure (COPM) was used to investigate the functional capabilities of the client within all areas of daily functioning. Issues were discovered within the patient's social, personal, and virtual contexts.

Chapter 4

Self-Quiz 4–1 Answers

Part I Answers

1. D
2. A
3. B
4. A
5. C

Part II Answers

1. distal palmar crease
2. proximal palmar crease
3. thenar crease
4. distal wrist crease
5. proximal wrist crease

Part III Answers

1. longitudinal arch
2. distal transverse arch
3. proximal transverse arch

Self-Quiz 4–2 Answers

1. F
2. F
3. T
4. T
5. F
6. T
7. F
8. T
9. T
10. F

Chapter 5

Self-Quiz 5–1 Answers

1. F
2. T
3. T
4. F
5. F
6. T
7. F
8. T
9. F
10. F
11. T
12. F
13. T
14. F

Chapter 6

Self-Quiz 6–1 Answers

1. F
2. T
3. T
4. T
5. F
6. T
7. F
8. F
9. F
10. T
11. T
12. F
13. F

Case Study 6–1 Answers

1. Randy has a radial nerve injury, which he sustained from falling asleep with his arm positioned over the top of a chair.
2. Never hesitate to call the physician's office. If the physician is not available, leave your question with the nurse.

3. The therapist should suggest a splint for radial nerve and research splints for that condition. He or she should review both textbooks and evidence-based practice articles, time permitting.
4. Randy should be educated about splint precautions, such as monitoring the splint for pressure sores, and about a splint-wearing schedule including removal for hygiene and exercise.
5. As discussed, compliance can be a tricky issue because so many factors need to be considered for why a person is noncompliant. Is Randy's noncompliance related to a self-image problem with the splint or for some other reason that he has not stated? Refer to Box 6–3 for ideas of factors contributing to noncompliance. The therapist should provide open-ended questions to get Randy's perception about his noncompliance and what it would take for him to become compliant with splint wear. More specific education, including sharing of research evidence about the importance of splint wear with a radial nerve injury for regaining function, would be helpful. This education would also help Randy understand the slow process of nerve regeneration. Due to Randy's history of alcohol abuse leading to the development of the condition, he may need psychosocial support beyond the therapy clinic. Psychosocial support can be tactfully suggested by the therapist and Randy can request a referral from his primary physician for intervention.

Case Study 6–2 Answers

1. Many areas were missing from the charting. Charting initially did not specify the extremity. It did not include client history of having de Quervain's tenosynovitis, or prior level of function. It did not mention prior treatment of receiving a prefabricated splint and did not specify where the reddened area was on the thumb. It provided an opinionated comment about client compliance. It would have been better to have provided factual information, such as a direct quote from Marie. The inclusion of normal measurements for range-of-motion, grip, and pinch strengths would make it easier for the reader to have a better understanding of deficits. It did not address the impact of the condition on doing work and home occupations. It did not address Marie's current level of pain. It should include the type of splint, position, and location. It should include a statement on fit, comfort, and function of the fabricated thumb immobilization splint. Goals are vague and not related to function. It would have been helpful to involve Marie with the goal setting, perhaps through administering the COPM.
2. In every situation, questions using the interactive clinical reasoning approach will be different. The following are a few of many suggested questions.
   - What questions do you have about wearing this fabricated splint? (This question may open up discussion, considering that Marie did not continue to wear the prefabricated splint due to developing some chafing on the volar surface of the thumb IP joint.)
   - How will you go about following a splint schedule based on the home and work demands in your life? (This question may be helpful, considering Marie's history of noncompliance with the first splint.)
   - What type of support do you need to help you with your splint and hand injury? (This question may help you better understand how Marie is coping with her condition.)
3. For this discussion, respect Marie's confidentiality by moving to a private area if in a large therapy room. You might assume that one reason Marie was noncompliant with the prefabricated splint was because it caused a reddened area on the thumb IP joint due to fitting improperly. However, you should tactfully question Marie for her reasons for noncompliance, which might be different from your assumption. Refer to Box 6–3 for ideas of factors that contribute to noncompliance and to Box 6–4 for ideas for open-ended questions to ask Marie. In any case, you should fabricate a well-fitted comfortable splint and monitor the fit carefully for potential pressure sores. Clear education about the reason for splint wear along with any evidence from research may help Marie's compliance. It will be important to check with Marie regularly about follow-through with the splint-wearing program. Consider making a phone call or e-mailing Marie to check on her level of compliance and to answer any questions.
4. Marie likely has worker's compensation insurance.

Chapter 7

Self-Quiz 7–1 Answers

1. T
2. T
3. F
4. T
5. T
6. F
7. F
8. T
9. F
10. F
11. F

Laboratory Exercise 7–2 Answers

Splint A

1. The wrist is positioned in extreme ulnar deviation. The wrist strap is placed incorrectly.
2. This extreme position stresses the wrist joint and possibly contributes to the development of other problems, such as wrist pain, pressure areas, and de Quervain's tenosynovitis.

Splint B

1. The wrist is positioned in flexion instead of a functional hand position of extension. Positioning in wrist extension helps with digital flexion. If the wrist is flexed, the client loses functional grasp. The wrist strap is placed incorrectly.

Splint C

1. MCP flexion is inhibited because the splint metacarpal bar is too high. The wrist appears to be radially deviated. The wrist strap is placed incorrectly.
2. Potential development of skin irritation or pressure areas exists with digital flexion, and the person does not have a full functional grasp.

Case Study 7–1 Answers

1. (1) The prefabricated splint was not the best choice because it migrated up the forearm and did not fit properly, limiting finger and thumb motions. (2) The splint was in the incorrect position of 20 degrees wrist extension and had not been readjusted to the correct position of neutral.
2. Wrist positioned as close to neutral as possible.
3. There are a variety of options for a splint-wearing schedule, but based on one recent study (Walker et al. 2000) the person should wear the splint all the time with removal for exercise and hygiene.
4. The therapist should observe areas such as the ulnar styloid, the first web space, and the volar and dorsal aspects of the hand over the metacarpal bones for skin irritation. Mrs. B. should notify the therapist immediately if irritation occurs. In addition, Mrs. B. should be educated to not perform full finger flexion in the splint due to that motion causing increased pressure on the carpal tunnel.
5. In this case, trust was violated because Mrs. B. dutifully followed a wearing regimen for a splint that did not correctly fit and was exacerbating her condition. As McClure [2003] suggests, providing research evidence specific to her situation might help her better understand the rationale for a custom-fabricated splint in a neutral position. Conservative management with splinting may help because the condition was caught early [Gerritsen et al. 2003] and because after giving birth carpal tunnel syndrome (CTS) symptoms may dissipate due to less fluid retention in the body and the client regaining hormonal balance.

Case Study 7–2 Answers

1. The therapist should splint Mrs. P's wrist in neutral to provide a low-load stretch.
2. The therapist should continue to serially splint the wrist to get Mrs. P's wrist into a functional wrist extension position.
3. This decision is made in collaboration with Mrs. P's physician based on her progress. Discontinuation of splinting could occur when Mrs. P. obtains more functional wrist extension because wearing the splint too long will result in muscle weakness and/or joint stiffness. Once the splint is removed, the therapist will continue to work on obtaining increased active wrist extension and normal wrist motions for function.

Chapter 8

Self-Quiz 8–1 Answers

1. T
2. F
3. T
4. F
5. T
6. T
7. F
8. F

Laboratory Exercise 8–1 Answers

1. thumb post
2. metacarpal (palmar) bar
3. forearm trough

Laboratory Exercise 8–3 Answers

1. The two problems are the following: (1) the metacarpal bar is too high to allow full finger MCP flexion and (2) the thumb IP joint flexion is limited because the material around the thumb extends too far distal.
2. An irritation might develop at the thumb IP joint (where the thumb opening is too high) and at the base of the index finger, where the metacarpal bar is too high. The splint limits full finger flexion.

Case Study 8–1 Answers

1. The hand is splinted in a hand-based thumb immobilization splint (MP radial and ulnar deviation

restriction splint) with the CMC joint in 40 degrees of palmar abduction and the MCP joint in neutral to slight flexion and ulnar deviation.
2. To provide rest and protection during healing.
3. The splint is worn continuously for 4 to 5 weeks, with removal for hygiene checks.
4. An option as suggested by Ford et al. [2004] is to fabricate a hybrid splint with a circumferential thermoplastic mold around the thumb covered by a neoprene wrap. This splint will provide stability to the MCP joint and allow for functional movements during skiing.

Case Study 8–2 Answers

1. Based on SY's symptoms, the therapists should fabricate a hand-based splint. Because only the CMC joint is involved, the splint designed by Colditz [2000]—which only immobilizes the CMC joint—would be appropriate.
2. To provide stability, and to control subluxation and pain.
3. Based on Colditz's [2000] recommendations, SY should wear the splint continuously for 2 to 3 weeks (with removal for hygiene). After that time period, she should wear the splint during times when the thumb is irritated by activities.
4. Because of the wrist and thumb involvement, the therapist would consider fabricating a forearm-based thumb splint.
5. The therapist should position the thumb MCP joint in 30 degrees flexion and in palmar abduction as tolerated.

Chapter 9

Laboratory Exercise 9–2 Answers

1. Thumb IP joint is flexed rather than extended; incorrect strap placement at distal forearm trough.
2. Radial deviation at the wrist; incorrect strap placement at distal forearm trough.
3. Poor wrist support; incorrect placement of straps at distal forearm trough.

Case Study 9–1 Answers

1. B
2. C
3. B
4. B
5. B

Case Study 9–2 Answers

1. Diabetes mellitus is associated with Dupuytren's disease.
2. Either a resting hand splint or a dorsal forearm-based static extension splint is appropriate to use after a Dupuytren's contracture release.
3. The therapeutic position includes wrist in neutral or slight extension and metacarpophalangeals (MCP), proximal interphalangeals (PIP), and distal interphalangeals (DIP) in full extension. The thumb does not need to be included in the splint.
4. Shelly should wear her splint well after the wounds have completely healed. After healing, she should wear the splint several weeks or months thereafter during the nighttime to provide stress and tension to counteract the scar contraction. (She may discontinue her resting hand splint in favor of individual finger splints.) The splint can be removed for hygiene, exercise, and ADLs.
5. To accommodate for bandage thickness, the design of the splint should be wider. As bandage bulk is reduced, the splint should be modified to maintain as close to an ideal position as possible. Therefore, thermoplastic material that has memory will assist with the modification process. In addition, because this is a fairly long splint a material with rigidity is helpful to adequately support the weight of the forearm, wrist, and hand.
6. Assuming no major complications in Shelly's rehabilitation, she may require outpatient therapy. At a minimum, Shelly should be seen for a home program and monitored until the wound heals. The therapy may entail a minimum of one visit per week.
7. Shelly may require assistance for any wound care and dressing changes initially. In addition, if she has difficulty with any one-handed techniques she may require some assistance with ADLs or instrumental ADLs (particularly writing). Temporary accommodations may be required at work or when driving if the automobile has a manual transmission.

Chapter 10

Self-Quiz 10–1 Answers

1. T
2. F
3. F
4. T
5. F
6. F
7. T
8. T
9. F
10. F

Case Study 10–1 Answers

1. Posterior elbow immobilization splint: elbow in 120 degrees of flexion, forearm in neutral, and wrist in 15 degrees of extension.

2. Supine on a plinth, with the shoulder in 90 degrees of forward flexion, elbow in 120 degrees of flexion, forearm in neutral rotation, and wrist in neutral extension of 15 degrees.
3. Protect the olecranon, medial and lateral epicondyles, radial and ulnar heads, by padding the bony prominences and molding the splint over the padding.
4. Splint is worn at all times, and removed for protected range-of-motion exercises only in a protected environment.

Case Study 10–2 Answers

1. A commercial brace that can be blocked at 90 degrees of flexion and allow for active flexion from 90-degree position as tolerated.
2. To wear the brace at all times, and to perform the exercises within the brace. The brace will be adjusted in therapy every week to increase the flexion angle by 10 to 15 degrees.

Chapter 11

Self-Quiz 11–1 Answers

1. T
2. T
3. F
4. F
5. T
6. T

Case Study 11–1 Answers

1. D
2. C
3. B
4. A
5. B

Chapter 12

Laboratory Exercise 12–1 Answers

1. It blocks the PIP joint.
2. It blocks the DIP joint.
3. It does not prevent the PIP from hyperextending, allowing the finger to still posture in a swan-neck deformity.

Self-Quiz 12–1 Answers

1. T
2. F
3. F
4. F
5. T

Case Study 12–1 Answers

1. The DIP joint of the right long finger.
2. All of the time except for skin care, during which time the joint needs to be supported in extension.
3. DIP gutter splint, dorsal-volar DIP splint, or stack splint.
4. Six to 8 weeks.

Case Study 12–2 Answers

1. Dorsal PIP splint because the injury involved the volar plate.
2. PIP joint in 20 to 30 degrees of flexion to protect the injured volar plate.
3. The index and long fingers should be buddy taped to support the injured long finger and maintain alignment. With injury to the radial collateral ligament, the middle phalanx would have a tendency to ulnarly deviate and the buddy strap helps correct this tendency.
4. Teach DS how to use self-adherent compressive wrap to treat the edema. Consider building up the girth of her tennis racquet handle to minimize stress on her injured joint.

Case Study 12–3 Answers

1. Yes, to improve her active PIP flexion.
2. Fabricate trial thermoplastic splints for a few fingers and assess if they help.
3. Important client factors are AW's job dealing with the public and what she finds to be most cosmetically appealing. Splints will be needed for multiple fingers and will be used long term, and thus streamlined fit and durability are desired qualities. Splint adjustability may also be beneficial because PIP size may fluctuate from swelling related to her arthritis.
4. During the daytime only because these are functional splints.

Chapter 13

Laboratory Exercise 13–1 Answers

S: "My pain has decreased."

O: Pt. reports that pain has decreased with resisted pronation from a score of 5 out of 10 to 2 out of 10. Manual muscle testing for the the pronator quadratus, pronator teres, flexor carpi radialis, palmaris longus and flexor digitum superficialis, flexor pollicis longus, and flexor digitorium profundus to index and long fingers were all 4 (good). The long-arm splint was discontinued on (date) with physician order.

A: PT was receptive to continue doing ADL and home program. PT plans to modify work and home activities to decrease repetitive pronation and supination. PT has been instructed in a light strengthening program.

P: OT will continue to monitor home program.

Self-Quiz 13–1 Answers

1. T
2. T
3. F
4. F
5. F
6. T
7. T
8. F
9. F
10. T
11. T
12. F

Case Study 13–1 Answers

1. Activities that require grasp and pinch.
2. An elbow splint. Due to interosseous weakness, the hand should be monitored for a possible hand-based splint for ulnar nerve.
3. The elbow is flexed 30 to 45 degrees and the wrist is in neutral to 20 degrees of extension.
4. There are a couple of options the therapist may consider. The first option is lining the splint to make it more comfortable. Another option would be to consider the comfort benefits of a prefabricated elbow splint. Care must be taken, however, that the prefabricated splint correctly position his elbow in the appropriate amount of flexion.
5. Because symptoms are continuous, the therapist should suggest that Mark wear the splint all of the time.
6. Mark must become aware of activities that irritate his condition, such as positioning his arm on the window frame.

Case Study 13–2 Answers

1. B
2. A
3. B
4. B
5. B
6. B

Chapter 14

Case Study 14–1 Answers

1. B. Because limited pain-free passive range of motion (PROM) is available at wrist and fingers, providing comfort offered by submaximum positioning and gentle stretch furnished by dynamic resistance is important. The hard-cone design allows orthotic management to begin even though the fingers are flexed. Because wrist and finger PROM are affected, orthotic design should span all affected joints.
2. Because the soft device has increased flexion tightness, the nursing staff should review the literature that addresses this dilemma. After discussion of other options, the staff members should be more open to attempt alternative splints.
3. E. Wrist and finger motions, though weak, are now adequate for light functional tasks. The present thumb web space tightness position remains the greatest threat to advanced prehension patterns.
4. With the thumb positioned in opposition, the client may be involved in some self-care activities such as grasping a napkin, assisting in combing hair, and arranging a bed sheet.

Chapter 15

Self-Quiz 15–1 Answers

1. T
2. F
3. F
4. T
5. F
6. T
7. F
8. F
9. T
10. F
11. T
12. T
13. T
14. T

Self-Quiz 15–2 Answers

1. A material that has high drapability and moldability is not a good choice for antigravity splinting. A material that has resistance to drape and memory is suitable. A slightly tacky splinting material that lightly adheres to underlying stockinette may be helpful. Preshaping techniques assist in molding.
2. A positioning soft splint such as soft roll or palm protector places the involved joints in submaximum extension. This position permits adequate skin hygiene.
3. A splint should not limit the use of uninvolved joints. An arthritis mitt splint immobilizes only the affected joints and positions the thumb in a resting position. The client can still use the fingers for functional activities at night.
4. Pad the outside of the splint.
5. The straps should be soft, wide foam straps that are cut a little long to adjust for edema. The splint design should be made wide enough to accommodate the edema.

Laboratory Exercise 15–1 Answers

1. The splint blocks the wrist and thumb IP joint.
2. The figure-of-eight is not properly positioned to effectively prevent hyperextension of the thumb IP joint. The figure-of-eight splint should be rotated and placed on the finger to prevent IP hyperextension

Case Study 15–1 Answers

1. B and C
2. A and C
3. B, C, and D
4. D

Case Study 15–2 Answers

1. A and D
2. D
3. A
4. D
5. C

Chapter 16

Laboratory Exercise 16–1 Answer

Two fabrication problems are present in this splint. First, the C bar does not fit into the web space of the thumb and provides inadequate positioning of the thumb between radial and palmar abduction. Second, the sides of the forearm trough are too high—resulting in bridging of the straps.

Laboratory Exercise 16–2 Answer

The straps are not keeping the wrist positioned in the splint. The distal forearm strap should be placed just proximal to the ulnar styloid, and a second strap should be added just distal to the ulnar styloid—preventing the flexor action of the wrist from lifting the wrist away from the splint's surface. The splint does not fit snugly into the thumb web space.

Laboratory Exercise 16–3 Answer

The splint does not fit snugly into the web space. In addition, the thumb trough is slightly too long and does not allow tactile contact of the tip of the thumb with an object being grasped.

Case Study 16–1 Answers

Option A would probably not be adequate to address concerns of losing range of motion of the wrist and fingers. Once range is lost, it can be difficult (if not impossible) to regain. Therefore prevention is paramount. Relying on passive range of motion may be disruptive to other activities and occupations during the day. The constant effects of moderately to severely increased tone will be difficult to overcome with activities alone. The thumb splints alone would not be adequate to address concerns with the wrist and finger flexors.

Option B would probably best meet Aaron's needs at this time. Prolonged stretch to the wrist and finger flexors could occur at night. Active functional movement during play, self-care, communication, and school activities could be emphasized during his waking hours. Because the left upper extremity is tighter and less functional, it would also be prudent to wear the left resting splint on this hand periodically during the day. A thermoplastic thumb splint for the right hand would control some of the increased tone in the hand but leave the wrist and fingers free for active and functional movement. Range-of-motion measurements would be required to determine optimal wearing schedules.

You will contact Aaron's parents to discuss your splinting recommendations and the purpose of the splints and to get their input. Assuming they are in agreement, you arrange a meeting with his parents prior to the splints' going home. At this time, you will review the purpose of the splints, demonstrate how to apply the splints, and provide an opportunity for the parents to practice donning and doffing the splints. You will also give the parents written instructions, precautions, and your phone number. Photographs of the splints on Aaron's hands will be included if needed.

Option C would be excessive use of resting hand splints at the present time. Aaron should continue to experience active movement and sensory feedback as much as possible during the day, especially with the right hand.

Option D would unnecessarily restrict active use of the hands during the day while leaving the wrist and finger flexors shortened during the night and on weekends. This family is involved in Aaron's programming, and you will address the issue of correct application at home by meeting with the parents as described under option B. If you have questions regarding follow-through at home, you should obtain more information about the family's strengths and limitations, the parent's understanding of intervention, and family routines. You should then individualize your style of collaboration and provide instruction for that family.

Case Study 16–2 Answers

Option A, resting hand splint, would not be appropriate because Maria has full passive range of motion in the left wrist and hand. Elongation of wrist and finger flexors is desirable but could be accomplished through weight-bearing activities.

Option B, a standard wrist cock-up (immobilization) splint, would not adequately address the problem of thumb adduction into the palm. It is likely that positioning the thumb in opposition will have an inhibitory effect on the wrist and hand. If the wrist flexion continues to be a problem after the thumb is addressed, other splinting or treatment options could be considered.

Option C, using a neoprene thumb splint as part of an overall intervention plan, is the correct answer. The thumb can serve as a key point of control for the hand, and once positioned may have an overall inhibitory affect. Tone is probably not severe enough to start with a thermoplastic thumb splint, but Maria might need additional assistance in the form of an added C bar attached to the neoprene thumb splint. If neoprene does not adequately limit thumb adduction, a thermoplastic thumb splint could be considered.

Chapter 17

Case Study 17–1 Answers

1. C
2. A.B.'s history of falls necessitates use of an orthosis. If strength and endurance improve, the device may be discontinued. Remind A.B. that falls result in fractured hips that often require placement in long-term care facilities.
3. A
4. D
5. Encourage A.B. to continue his walking program indoors at a local mall or health club. Inspect shoes to ensure that soles are not worn and that a non-skid surface is adequate for inclement conditions such as snow and ice.

Case Study 17–2 Answers

1. *Case A:* M.H. may be attempting to wear the orthosis over pants because it is easier to don and doff the device in this manner. If the device was donned under the pants with ample leg room, the device would be undetectable to others.
2. *Case B:* A video of T.F. walking with an ankle-foot orthosis (AFO) and without an AFO might illustrate that the AFO provides a more "normal" gait pattern. It would also be appropriate to discuss the effects of overstretching soft structures.
3. *Case C:* D.F.'s condition necessitates gentle prolonged stretch of the plantar surface structures. She may benefit from wearing specialty AFOs at night to increase stretching time and reduce overall pain.

Chapter 18

Self-Quiz 18–1 Answers

1. T
2. T
3. F
4. F
5. B
6. B
7. C
8. D
9. B
10. A
11. B
12. A

Chapter 19

Self-Quiz 19–1 Answers

1. T
2. T
3. F
4. F
5. T
6. F
7. F
8. T
9. T
10. T

Case Study 19–1 Answers

1. The guide to determining whether a situation involves ethics includes answering the following three questions: (1) Is there more than one morally plausible resolution?, (2) Is there no clearcut best resolution?, and (3) Is there direct reference to the welfare or dignity of others? In this case, because Collin is inexperienced one could expect that he would need supervision as he gains mastery over the techniques necessary to treat clients. Mercedes has already noted that Collin needs more supervision. Thus, the welfare of clients is affected. Mercedes realizes that the ideal solution would be for her to spend more time supervising Collin, but she does not believe this is possible because of her administrative duties. There is more than one morally plausible option in the case. Because the answer to two of the three criteria is "yes," the case does involve an ethical issue.
2. Clearly, the ethical principles of nonmaleficence and beneficence are involved. Mercedes and Collin have an obligation to protect all clients from unnecessary harm and to do good for them within the constraints of available resources. There are not enough qualified staff members to supervise Collin. The lack of senior staff members could be considered a problem of justice. There is not enough of Mercedes to go around. She is not capable of completing all of the tasks assigned to her, and thus she must make decisions about what takes priority.

A fair and equitable work setting should have adequate personnel to do the job safely and effectively. The current shortage of staff could be due to chance (i.e., the unfortunate coincidence of a retirement and maternity leave). However, both of these events are predictable. Thus, as the manager Mercedes should have foreseen that there would be a problem and have made advance plans for it. If Mercedes is making a good-faith effort to recruit replacement staff, we would not hold her accountable for sustaining a work environment that is unsafe and short staffed. We could, however, hold her accountable for poor planning and the impact this has had on Collin's orientation and client care.

According to care-based reasoning, Mercedes should consider what a caring work environment would look like for new employees and clients. It is true that novices do not become expert without experience, but how we provide experience makes a great deal of difference.

Finally, virtues that are required in this situation could include perseverance, compassion, courage, justice, and integrity. One of the alternatives available to Mercedes is to reassign her administrative and management responsibilities to someone else, in that there is no one else in her institution who is an occupational therapist and can supervise direct client care. It would take courage to delegate administrative authority, because it would require relinquishing power. However, if client care holds a central position in the values of the organization this is a plausible option.

3a. Mercedes could limit the type of clients Collin treats, selecting only those he can treat safely with minimal supervision. The principles that support this action are nonmaleficence and beneficence, in that clients would be protected. Collin would not receive the type of experience he would like, which might interfere with his autonomy but client welfare would not be in jeopardy.

3b. Mercedes could maintain the status quo and continue with things the way they are, with minimal supervision. The principles of nonmaleficence and beneficence are threatened. It is possible that Collin would not commit any serious mistakes, but because of his inexperience it is clear that clients would not be getting the quality of care they need or deserve.

3c. Mercedes could ask for release time from her administrative duties so that she could be free for direct client care. The principles of nonmaleficence, beneficence, and justice are supported by this action—in that client welfare is protected and Collin receives the type of supervision he should have to become a competent clinician.

3d. Hire on a temporary basis an occupational therapist for specific supervision of Collin and complex cases. This action may require greater expense, but it would allow Mercedes to continue with her administrative duties (if those duties contribute to the benefit of clients) and Collin would receive the supervision he needs. Clients would be protected from harm and would benefit from the expertise of an experienced therapist.

4. The principles in the Code of Ethics that are helpful in this case include principle 4, which demands the maintenance of high standards of competence. There is a clear responsibility for all occupational therapists to maintain their own level of competence and to monitor that of peers. Depending on the reason for incompetence, various methods can be taken to resolve the problem—such as further education, increased staffing, workshops, drug and alcohol treatment programs, and so on. In this case, Collin is incompetent because he is inexperienced and needs more supervision. This is a state that is temporary and could be resolved with adequate supervision. Second, principle 1C strictly enjoins protecting clients from harm. Mercedes should be guided by this principle above all others as she attempts to resolve the problem.

APPENDIX B

Forms

FORM 2-1 Occupation-based Splinting Checklist (OBS)

1. ______ Splint meets requirements of protocol for specific pathology; ensuring attention to bodily functions and structures.
2. ______ If indicated, splint design is approved with referring physician.
3. ______ Splint allows client to engage in all desired occupation-based tasks through support of activity demands.
4. ______ Splint supports client habits, roles, and routines.
5. ______ Splint design fits client's cultural needs.
6. ______ Splint design fits with temporal needs, including season, age of client, and duration of use.
7. ______ Splint design takes into consideration the client's physical environment.
8. ______ Splint design supports the client's social pursuits.
9. ______ Client's personal needs are addressed through splint design.
10. ______ Client is able to engage in the virtual world (e.g., cellular phone, PDA, computer use).
11. ______ Splint is comfortable.
12. ______ Client verbalizes understanding of splint use, care, precautions, and rationale for use.
13. ______ Client demonstrates the ability to don and doff splint.
14. ______ Adaptations to the physical environment are made to ensure function in desired occupations.
15. ______ Client indicates satisfaction with splint design and functionality within splint.

FORM 3-1 Hints for Drawing and Fitting a Splint Pattern

- ❍ Explain the pattern-making process to the person.
- ❍ Ask or assist the person to remove any jewelry from the area to be splinted.
- ❍ Wash the area to be splinted if it is dirty.
- ❍ If splinting over bandages or foam, cover the extremity with stockinette or a moist paper towel to prevent the plastic from sticking to the bandages.
- ❍ Position the affected extremity on a paper towel in a flat, natural resting position. The wrist should be in a neutral position with a slight ulnar deviation. The fingers should be extended and slightly abducted.
- ❍ To trace the outline of the person's extremity, keep the pencil at a 90-degree angle to the paper.
- ❍ Mark the landmarks needed to draw the pattern *before* the person removes the extremity from the paper.
- ❍ For a more accurate pattern, the paper towel can be wet and placed on the area for evaluation of the pattern, or aluminum foil can be used.
- ❍ Folding the paper towel to mark adjustments in the pattern can help with evaluation of the pattern.
- ❍ When evaluating the pattern fit of a forearm-based splint on the person, look for the following:
    - Half the circumference of body parts for the width of troughs
    - Two-thirds the length of the forearm
    - The length and width of metacarpal or palmar bars
    - The correct use of hand creases for landmarks
    - The amount of support to the wrist, fingers, and thenar and hypothenar eminencies
- ❍ When tracing the pattern onto the thermoplastic material, do not use an ink pen because the ink may smear when the material is placed in the hot water to soften. Rather, use a pencil, grease pencil, or awl to mark the pattern outline on the material.

FORM 5-1 Hand Evaluation Check-off Sheet

Person's history: interviews, chart review, and reports:

- ❍ Age
- ❍ Vocation
- ❍ Date of injury and surgery
- ❍ Method of injury
- ❍ Hand dominance
- ❍ Treatment rendered to date (surgery, therapy, and so on)
- ❍ Medication
- ❍ Previous injury
- ❍ General health
- ❍ Avocational interests
- ❍ Family composition
- ❍ Subjective complaints
- ❍ Support systems
- ❍ Activities of daily living responsibilities before and after injury
- ❍ Impact of injury on family, economic status, and social well-being
- ❍ Reimbursement
- ❍ Motivation

Observation:

- ❍ Walking, posture
- ❍ Facial movements
- ❍ Speech patterns
- ❍ Affect
- ❍ Hand posture
- ❍ Cognition

Palpation:

- ❍ Muscle tone
- ❍ Muscle symmetry
- ❍ Scar density/excursion
- ❍ Tendon nodules
- ❍ Masses (ganglia, fistulas)

Assessments for:

- ❍ Pain
- ❍ Skin and allergies
- ❍ Wound healing/wound status
- ❍ Bone
- ❍ Joint and ligament
- ❍ Muscle and tendon
- ❍ Nerve/sensation
- ❍ Vascular status
- ❍ Skin turgor and trophic status
- ❍ Range of motion
- ❍ Strength
- ❍ Coordination and dexterity
- ❍ Function
- ❍ Reimbursement source
- ❍ Vocation

Follow-up considerations:

- ❍ Splint fit
- ❍ Compliance

FORM 5-2 Splint Precaution Check-off Sheet

❍ Account for bony prominences such as the following:
- Metacarpophalangeal (MCP), proximal interphalangeal (PIP), and distal interphalangeal (DIP) joints
- Pisiform bone
- Radial and ulnar styloids
- Lateral and medial epicondyles of the elbow

❍ Identify fragile skin and select the splinting material carefully. Monitor the temperature of the thermoplastic closely before applying the material to the fragile skin.

❍ Identify skin areas having impaired sensation. The splint design should not impinge on these sites.

❍ If fluctuating edema is a problem, consider pressure garment wear in conjunction with a splint.

❍ Do not compress the superficial branch of the radial nerve. If the radial edge of a forearm splint impinges beyond the middle of the forearm near the dorsal side of the thumb, the branch of the radial nerve may be compressed.

FORM 5-3 Hints for Splint Provision

- ❍ Give the person oral and written instructions regarding the following:
  - Wearing schedule
  - Care of splint
  - Purpose of splint
  - Responsibility in therapy program
  - Phone number of contact person if problems arise
  - Actions to take if skin reactions such as the following occur: rashes, numbness, reddened areas, pain increase because of splint application
- ❍ Evaluate the splint after the person wears it at least 20 to 30 minutes and make necessary adjustments.
- ❍ Position all joints incorporated into the splint at the correct therapeutic angle(s).
- ❍ Design the splint to account for bony prominences such as the following:
  - MCP, PIP, and DIP joints
  - Pisiform
  - Radial and ulnar styloids
  - Lateral and medial epicondyles of the elbow
- ❍ If fluctuating edema is a problem, make certain the splint design can accommodate the problem by using a wider design. Consider pressure garment to wear under splint.
- ❍ Make certain the splint design does not mobilize or immobilize unnecessary joint(s).
- ❍ Make certain the splint does not impede or restrict motions of joints adjacent to the splint.
- ❍ Make certain the splint supports the arches of the hand.
- ❍ Take into consideration the creases of the hand for allowing immobilization or mobilization, depending on the purpose of the splint.
- ❍ Make certain the splint does not restrict circulation.
- ❍ Make certain application and removal of the splint are easy.
- ❍ Secure the splint to the person's extremity using a well-designed strapping mechanism.
- ❍ Make certain the appropriate edges of the splint are flared or rolled.

FORM 7-1 Wrist Immobilization Splint

Name: ______________________

Date: ______________________

Type of wrist immobilization splint:

Volar ❍ Dorsal ❍

Wrist position: ______________________

After the person wears the splint for 30 minutes, answer the following questions. (Mark *NA* for nonapplicable situations.) Discuss possible splint adjustments or changes you should make based on the self-evaluation. (What would you do differently next time?)

____

____

____

____

Evaluation Areas				**Comments**
Design				
1. The wrist position is at the correct angle.	Yes ❍	No ❍	NA ❍	
2. The wrist has adequate support.	Yes ❍	No ❍	NA ❍	
3. The sides of the thenar and hypothenar eminences have support in the correct position.	Yes ❍	No ❍	NA ❍	
4. The thenar and hypothenar eminences are not restricted or flattened.	Yes ❍	No ❍	NA ❍	
5. The splint is two-thirds the length of the forearm.	Yes ❍	No ❍	NA ❍	
6. The splint is one-half the width of the forearm.	Yes ❍	No ❍	NA ❍	
Function				
1. The splint allows full thumb motions.	Yes ❍	No ❍	NA ❍	
2. The splint allows full MCP joint flexion of the fingers.	Yes ❍	No ❍	NA ❍	
3. The splint provides wrist support that allows functional activities.	Yes ❍	No ❍	NA ❍	
Straps				
1. The straps are secure and rounded.	Yes ❍	No ❍	NA ❍	
Comfort				
1. The splint edges are smooth with rounded corners.	Yes ❍	No ❍	NA ❍	
2. The proximal end is flared.	Yes ❍	No ❍	NA ❍	
3. The splint does not cause impingements or pressure sores.	Yes ❍	No ❍	NA ❍	
4. The splint does not irritate bony prominences.	Yes ❍	No ❍	NA ❍	
Cosmetic Appearance				
1. The splint is free of fingerprints, dirt, and pencil and pen marks.	Yes ❍	No ❍	NA ❍	
2. The splinting material is not buckled.	Yes ❍	No ❍	NA ❍	

Continued

FORM 7-1 Wrist Immobilization Splint—cont'd

Therapeutic Regimen

1. The person has been instructed in a wearing schedule.	Yes ❍	No ❍	NA ❍
2. The person has been provided splint precautions.	Yes ❍	No ❍	NA ❍
3. The person demonstrates understanding of the education.	Yes ❍	No ❍	NA ❍
4. Client/caregiver knows how to clean the splint.	Yes ❍	No ❍	NA ❍

FORM 8-1 Thumb Immobilization Splint

Name: ______________________________

Date: ______________________________

Type of thumb immobilization splint:

Volar ❍ Dorsal ❍ Radial gutter ❍ Hand based ❍

Thumb joint position:______________________________

After the person wears the splint for 30 minutes, answer the following questions. (Mark *NA* for nonapplicable situations.)

Evaluation Areas				**Comments**
Design				
1. The wrist position is at the correct angle.	Yes ❍	No ❍	NA ❍	
2. The thumb position is at the correct angle.	Yes ❍	No ❍	NA ❍	
3. The thenar eminence is not restricted or flattened.	Yes ❍	No ❍	NA ❍	
4. The thumb post provides adequate support and is not constrictive.	Yes ❍	No ❍	NA ❍	
5. The splint is two-thirds the length of the forearm.	Yes ❍	No ❍	NA ❍	
6. The splint is one-half the width of the forearm.	Yes ❍	No ❍	NA ❍	
Function				
1. The splint allows full thumb IP flexion.	Yes ❍	No ❍	NA ❍	
2. The splint allows full MCP joint flexion of the fingers.	Yes ❍	No ❍	NA ❍	
3. The splint provides wrist support that allows functional activities.	Yes ❍	No ❍	NA ❍	
Straps				
1. The straps avoid bony prominences.	Yes ❍	No ❍	NA ❍	
2. The straps are secure and rounded.	Yes ❍	No ❍	NA ❍	
Comfort				
1. The splint edges are smooth with rounded corners.	Yes ❍	No ❍	NA ❍	
2. The proximal end is flared.	Yes ❍	No ❍	NA ❍	
3. The splint does not cause impingements or pressure sores.	Yes ❍	No ❍	NA ❍	
Cosmetic Appearance				
1. The splint is free of fingerprints, dirt, and pencil and pen marks.	Yes ❍	No ❍	NA ❍	
2. The splint is smooth and free of buckles.	Yes ❍	No ❍	NA ❍	
Therapeutic Regimen				
1. The person has been instructed in a wearing schedule.	Yes ❍	No ❍	NA ❍	
2. The person has been provided splint precautions.	Yes ❍	No ❍	NA ❍	
3. The person demonstrates understanding of the education.	Yes ❍	No ❍	NA ❍	
4. Client or caregiver knows how to clean the splint.	Yes ❍	No ❍	NA ❍	

Continued

FORM 8-1 Thumb Immobilization Splint—cont'd

Discuss possible splint adjustments or changes you should make based on the self-evaluation. (What would you do differently next time?)

FORM 9-1 Resting Hand Splint

Name: ____________________

Date: ____________________

Position of resting hand splint:

Functional position ❍ (mid joint)   Antideformity position ❍ (intrinsic plus)

Answer the following questions after the person wears the splint for 30 minutes. (Mark *NA* for nonapplicable situations.)

Evaluation Areas				**Comments**
Design				
1. The wrist position is at the correct angle.	Yes ❍	No ❍	NA ❍	
2. The MCPs are at the correct angle.	Yes ❍	No ❍	NA ❍	
3. The thumb is in the correct position.	Yes ❍	No ❍	NA ❍	
4. The wrist has adequate support.	Yes ❍	No ❍	NA ❍	
5. The pan is wide enough for all the fingers.	Yes ❍	No ❍	NA ❍	
6. The length of the pan and thumb trough is adequate.	Yes ❍	No ❍	NA ❍	
7. The splint is two-thirds the length of the forearm.	Yes ❍	No ❍	NA ❍	
8. The splint is half the width of the forearm.	Yes ❍	No ❍	NA ❍	
9. Arches of the hand are supported and maintained.	Yes ❍	No ❍	NA ❍	
Function				
1. The splint completely immobilizes the wrist, fingers, and thumb.	Yes ❍	No ❍	NA ❍	
2. The splint is easy to apply and remove.	Yes ❍	No ❍	NA ❍	
Straps				
1. The straps are rounded.	Yes ❍	No ❍	NA ❍	
2. Straps are placed to adequately secure the hand/arm to splint.	Yes ❍	No ❍	NA ❍	
Comfort				
1. The edges are smooth with rounded corners.	Yes ❍	No ❍	NA ❍	
2. The proximal end is flared.	Yes ❍	No ❍	NA ❍	
3. The splint does not cause impingements or pressure areas.	Yes ❍	No ❍	NA ❍	
Cosmetic Appearance				
1. The splint is free of fingerprints, dirt, and pencil or pen marks.	Yes ❍	No ❍	NA ❍	
2. The splint is smooth and free of buckles.	Yes ❍	No ❍	NA ❍	
Therapeutic Regimen				
1. The person has been instructed in a wearing schedule.	Yes ❍	No ❍	NA ❍	
2. The person has been provided with splint precautions.	Yes ❍	No ❍	NA ❍	
3. The person demonstrates understanding of the education.	Yes ❍	No ❍	NA ❍	
4. Client/caregiver knows how to clean the splint.	Yes ❍	No ❍	NA ❍	

Continued

FORM 9-1 Resting Hand Splint—cont'd

Discuss adjustments or changes you would make based on the self-evaluation. What would you do differently next time?

FORM 10-1 Elbow Immobilization Splint

Name: ______________________________

Date: ______________________________

Type of elbow immobilization splint:

Posterior ❍ Anterior ❍

Elbow position: ______________________________

After the person wears the splint for 30 minutes, answer the following questions. (Mark *NA* for nonapplicable situations.)

Evaluation Areas				**Comments**
Design				
1. The elbow position is at the correct angle.	Yes ❍	No ❍	NA ❍	
2. The elbow has adequate medial and lateral support (two-thirds the circumference of the elbow).	Yes ❍	No ❍	NA ❍	
3. The splint supplies sufficient proximal/lateral support (1 inch proximal to axillary crease).	Yes ❍	No ❍	NA ❍	
4. The splint is two-thirds the circumference of the upper arm.	Yes ❍	No ❍	NA ❍	
5. Distally the splint extends to the distal palmar crease.	Yes ❍	No ❍	NA ❍	
6. The splint is two-thirds the circumference of the forearm.	Yes ❍	No ❍	NA ❍	
Function				
1. The splint allows full thumb and digit motion.	Yes ❍	No ❍	NA ❍	
2. The splint allows full shoulder motion.	Yes ❍	No ❍	NA ❍	
3. The splint provides adequate elbow support to properly secure the elbow in the splint and prevent elbow motion.	Yes ❍	No ❍	NA ❍	
Straps				
1. The straps are secure and rounded.	Yes ❍	No ❍	NA ❍	
Comfort				
1. The splint edges are smooth with rounded corners.	Yes ❍	No ❍	NA ❍	
2. The proximal end is flared.	Yes ❍	No ❍	NA ❍	
3. The splint does not cause impingements or pressure sores.	Yes ❍	No ❍	NA ❍	
4. The splint does not irritate bony prominences.	Yes ❍	No ❍	NA ❍	
Cosmetic Appearance				
1. The splint is free of fingerprints, dirt, and pencil and pen marks.	Yes ❍	No ❍	NA ❍	
2. The splinting material is not buckled.	Yes ❍	No ❍	NA ❍	
Therapeutic Regimen				
1. The person has been instructed in a wearing schedule.	Yes ❍	No ❍	NA ❍	
2. The person has been provided splint precautions.	Yes ❍	No ❍	NA ❍	
3. The person demonstrates understanding of the education.	Yes ❍	No ❍	NA ❍	
4. Client/caregiver knows how to clean the splint.	Yes ❍	No ❍	NA ❍	

Continued

FORM 10-1 Elbow Immobilization Splint—cont'd

Discuss possible splint adjustments or changes you should make based on the self-evaluation. (What would you do differently next time?)

FORM 11-1 Radial Nerve Splint

Name: ______________________

Date: ______________________

Answer the following questions after the person wears the splint for 30 minutes. (Mark *NA* for nonapplicable situations.)

Evaluation Areas				**Comments**
Design				
1. The forearm trough is the proper length and width.	Yes ❍	No ❍	NA ❍	
2. The outrigger wire is at the appropriate angles and ½ inch wider than the MCPs at the level of the hand.	Yes ❍	No ❍	NA ❍	
3. The thermoplastic material on the MCP aspect of the outrigger is secure.	Yes ❍	No ❍	NA ❍	
4. The line to the outrigger is at a 90-degree angle from the long axis of the bone when the hand is at rest.	Yes ❍	No ❍	NA ❍	
5. The anchor hook is secure.	Yes ❍	No ❍	NA ❍	
6. The thermoplastic material patch adequately secures the outrigger.	Yes ❍	No ❍	NA ❍	
Function				
1. The wrist is maintained in neutral when the fingers are in extension.	Yes ❍	No ❍	NA ❍	
2. The outrigger or lines do not impede composite flexion of the fingers.	Yes ❍	No ❍	NA ❍	
3. The fit of the trough and straps prevents distal migration of the splint.	Yes ❍	No ❍	NA ❍	
4. The slings do not migrate distally with finger flexion and extension.	Yes ❍	No ❍	NA ❍	
Comfort				
1. Excessive pressure is not present on the radial or ulnar styloids.	Yes ❍	No ❍	NA ❍	
2. The edges are smooth with rounded corners.	Yes ❍	No ❍	NA ❍	
3. The proximal and distal ends are flared.	Yes ❍	No ❍	NA ❍	
4. Impingements or pressure areas are not present.	Yes ❍	No ❍	NA ❍	
5. Slings are durable enough to allow hand function over a long period of time.	Yes ❍	No ❍	NA ❍	
Therapeutic Regimen				
1. The person has been instructed in a wearing schedule.	Yes ❍	No ❍	NA ❍	
2. The person has been provided splint precautions.	Yes ❍	No ❍	NA ❍	
3. The person demonstrates understanding of the education.	Yes ❍	No ❍	NA ❍	
4. Client/caregiver knows how to clean the splint.	Yes ❍	No ❍	NA ❍	

FORM 12-1 Finger Splint

Name: ______________________________

Date: ______________________________

After the person wears the splint for 30 minutes, answer the following questions. (Mark *NA* for nonapplicable situations.)

Evaluation Areas				**Comments**
Design				
1. The PIP position is at the correct angle.	Yes ❍	No ❍	NA ❍	
2. The DIP position is at the correct angle.	Yes ❍	No ❍	NA ❍	
3. The splint provides adequate support and is not constrictive.	Yes ❍	No ❍	NA ❍	
4. The splint length is appropriate.	Yes ❍	No ❍	NA ❍	
5. The splint width is appropriate.	Yes ❍	No ❍	NA ❍	
6. The splint is snug enough to stay in place yet loose enough to apply and remove.	Yes ❍	No ❍	NA ❍	
Function				
1. The splint allows full MCP motion.	Yes ❍	No ❍	NA ❍	
2. The splint allows full PIP motion.	Yes ❍	No ❍	NA ❍	
3. The splint allows full DIP motion.	Yes ❍	No ❍	NA ❍	
4. The splint enables as much hand function as possible.	Yes ❍	No ❍	NA ❍	
Straps				
1. The straps are secure and the terminal edges are rounded.	Yes ❍	No ❍	NA ❍	
Comfort				
1. The splint edges are smooth, rounded, contoured, and flared.	Yes ❍	No ❍	NA ❍	
2. The splint does not cause pain or pressure areas.	Yes ❍	No ❍	NA ❍	
Cosmetic Appearance				
1. The splint is free of fingerprints, dirt, and pencil/pen marks.	Yes ❍	No ❍	NA ❍	
2. The splinting material is not buckled.	Yes ❍	No ❍	NA ❍	
Therapeutic Regimen				
1. The client or caregiver has been instructed in a wearing schedule.	Yes ❍	No ❍	NA ❍	
2. The client or caregiver has been provided splint precautions.	Yes ❍	No ❍	NA ❍	
3. The client or caregiver demonstrates understanding of the splint program.	Yes ❍	No ❍	NA ❍	
4. The client or caregiver demonstrates proper donning and doffing of splint.	Yes ❍	No ❍	NA ❍	
5. The client or caregiver knows how to clean the splint and straps.	Yes ❍	No ❍	NA ❍	

Continued

FORM 12-1 Finger Splint—cont'd

Discuss possible splint adjustments or changes you should make based on the self-evaluation. What would you do differently next time?

FORM 13-1: Anticlaw Splint

Name: ______________________________

Date: ______________________________

Answer the following questions after the splint has been worn for 30 minutes. (Mark NA for nonapplicable situations.)

Evaluation Areas				Comments
Design				
1. The splint prevents hyperextension of the MCP joints of the ring and little fingers.	Yes ❍	No ❍	NA ❍	
Function				
1. The splint allows full wrist motions.	Yes ❍	No ❍	NA ❍	
2. The splint allows full function of the middle and index fingers.	Yes ❍	No ❍	NA ❍	
Straps				
1. The straps avoid bony prominences.	Yes ❍	No ❍	NA ❍	
2. Straps are secure and rounded.	Yes ❍	No ❍	NA ❍	
Comfort				
1. The edges are smooth with rounded corners.	Yes ❍	No ❍	NA ❍	
2. The proximal end is flared.	Yes ❍	No ❍	NA ❍	
3. Impingements or pressure areas are not present.	Yes ❍	No ❍	NA ❍	
4. Splint pressure is well distributed over the proximal phalanx of the ring and little fingers.	Yes ❍	No ❍	NA ❍	
Cosmetic Appearance				
1. The splint is free of fingerprints, dirt, and pencil or pen marks.	Yes ❍	No ❍	NA ❍	
2. The splinting material is smooth and free of buckles.	Yes ❍	No ❍	NA ❍	
Therapeutic Regimen				
1. The person has been instructed in a wearing schedule.	Yes ❍	No ❍	NA ❍	
2. The person has been provided with splint precautions.	Yes ❍	No ❍	NA ❍	
3. The person demonstrates understanding of the education.	Yes ❍	No ❍	NA ❍	
4. Client/caregiver knows how to clean the splint.	Yes ❍	No ❍	NA ❍	

Discuss possible adjustments or changes you would make based on the self-evaluation.

____

____

____

____

____

____

____

FORM 14-1 Hard-Cone Wrist and Hand Splint

Name: ______________________

Date: ______________________

Type of cone wrist and hand splint:

Volar platform ❍ Dorsal platform ❍

Answer the following questions after the splint has been worn for 30 minutes. (Mark *NA* for nonapplicable situations.)

Evaluation Areas				**Comments**
Design				
1. The wrist position is at the correct angle.	Yes ❍	No ❍	NA ❍	
2. The correct cone-diameter size reflects the palm width and web-space size.	Yes ❍	No ❍	NA ❍	
3. The small end of the cone is placed radially and the large end is placed ulnarly.	Yes ❍	No ❍	NA ❍	
4. The thumb is positioned in palmar abduction with the web space preserved.	Yes ❍	No ❍	NA ❍	
5. The splint is two-thirds the length of the forearm.	Yes ❍	No ❍	NA ❍	
6. The splint is half the width of the forearm.	Yes ❍	No ❍	NA ❍	
Function				
1. The wrist is positioned in submaximal or maximal range.	Yes ❍	No ❍	NA ❍	
2. The fingers are positioned to provide firm pressure but not stretch the flexors.	Yes ❍	No ❍	NA ❍	
Straps				
1. The straps avoid bony prominences.	Yes ❍	No ❍	NA ❍	
2. The straps are secure and rounded.	Yes ❍	No ❍	NA ❍	
3. The active field materials are used over the extensor muscle bellies.	Yes ❍	No ❍	NA ❍	
4. The passive field materials are used over the flexor muscle bellies.	Yes ❍	No ❍	NA ❍	
Comfort				
1. The edges are smooth with rounded corners.	Yes ❍	No ❍	NA ❍	
2. The proximal end is flared.	Yes ❍	No ❍	NA ❍	
3. Impingements or pressure areas are not present. (The ulnar styloid is relieved.)	Yes ❍	No ❍	NA ❍	
Cosmetic Appearance				
1. The splint is free of fingerprints, dirt, and pencil or pen marks.	Yes ❍	No ❍	NA ❍	
2. The splinting material is not buckled.	Yes ❍	No ❍	NA ❍	

Continued

FORM 14-1 Hard-Cone Wrist and Hand Splint—cont'd

Therapeutic Regimen

1. The person/caregiver has been instructed in a wearing schedule.	Yes ❍	No ❍	NA ❍
2. The person/caregiver has been provided with splint precautions.	Yes ❍	No ❍	NA ❍
3. The person/caregiver demonstrates understanding of the education.	Yes ❍	No ❍	NA ❍
4. Person/caregiver knows how to clean the splint.	Yes ❍	No ❍	NA ❍

Discuss adjustments or changes you would make based on the self-evaluation.

____
____
____
____
____
____
____
____
____
____

APPENDIX C

Grading Sheets

GRADING SHEET 7-1 Wrist Immobilization Splint

Name: ______________________

Date: ______________________

Type of wrist immobilization splint:

Volar ❍ Dorsal ❍

Wrist position: ______________________

Grade: ________

1 = beyond improvement, not acceptable
2 = requires maximal improvement
3 = requires moderate improvement
4 = requires minimal improvement
5 = requires no improvement

Evaluation Areas						**Comments**
Design						
1. The wrist position is at the correct angle.	1	2	3	4	5	
2. The wrist has adequate support.	1	2	3	4	5	
3. The sides of the thenar and hypothenar eminences have support in the correct position.	1	2	3	4	5	
4. The splint is one-half the width of the forearm.	1	2	3	4	5	
5. The thenar and hypothenar eminences are not restricted or flattened.	1	2	3	4	5	
6. The splint is two-thirds the length of the forearm.	1	2	3	4	5	
Function						
1. The splint allows full thumb motion.	1	2	3	4	5	
2. The splint allows full MCP joint flexion of the fingers.	1	2	3	4	5	
3. The splint provides wrist support that allows functional activities.	1	2	3	4	5	
Straps						
1. The straps are secure and rounded.	1	2	3	4	5	

Continued

GRADING SHEET 7-1 Wrist Immobilization Splint—cont'd

Comfort					
1. The splint edges are smooth with rounded corners.	1	2	3	4	5
2. The proximal end is flared.	1	2	3	4	5
3. The splint does not cause impingements or pressure sores.	1	2	3	4	5
4. The splint does not irritate bony prominences.	1	2	3	4	5
Cosmetic Appearance					
1. The splint is free of fingerprints, dirt, and pencil and pen marks.	1	2	3	4	5
2. The splinting material is not buckled.	1	2	3	4	5

GRADING SHEET 8-1 Thumb Immobilization Splint

Name: ____________________

Date: ____________________

Type of thumb immobilization splint:

Volar ❍ Dorsal ❍ Radial gutter ❍ Hand based ❍

Thumb joint position: ____________________

Grade: ____________

1 = beyond improvement, not acceptable
2 = requires maximal improvement
3 = requires moderate improvement
4 = requires minimal improvement
5 = requires no improvement

Evaluation Areas						**Comments**
Design						
1. The wrist position is at the correct angle.	1	2	3	4	5	
2. The thumb position is at the correct angle.	1	2	3	4	5	
3. The thenar eminence is not restricted or flattened.	1	2	3	4	5	
4. The thumb post provides adequate support and is not constrictive.	1	2	3	4	5	
5. The splint is two-thirds the length of the forearm.	1	2	3	4	5	
6. The splint is one-half the width of the forearm.	1	2	3	4	5	
Function						
1. The splint allows full thumb IP flexion.	1	2	3	4	5	
2. The splint allows full MCP joint flexion of the fingers.	1	2	3	4	5	
3. The splint provides wrist support that allows functional activities.	1	2	3	4	5	
Straps						
1. The straps avoid bony prominences.	1	2	3	4	5	
2. The straps are secure and rounded.	1	2	3	4	5	
Comfort						
1. The splint edges are smooth with rounded corners.	1	2	3	4	5	
2. The proximal end is flared.	1	2	3	4	5	
3. The splint does not cause impingements or pressure sores.	1	2	3	4	5	
Cosmetic Appearance						
1. The splint is free of fingerprints, dirt, and pencil and pen marks.	1	2	3	4	5	
2. The splinting material is not buckled.	1	2	3	4	5	

Comments:

____

____

____

____

GRADING SHEET 9-1 Resting Hand Splint

Name: ______________________

Date: ______________________

Position of resting hand splint: ______________________

Functional position ❍ (mid joint) Antideformity position ❍ (intrinsic plus)

Grade: ______________

1 = beyond improvement, not acceptable
2 = requires maximal improvment
3 = requires moderate improvement
4 = requires minimal improvement
5 = requires no improvement

Evaluation Areas						**Comments**
Design						
1. The wrist position is at the correct angle.	1	2	3	4	5	
2. The MCPs are at the correct angle.	1	2	3	4	5	
3. The thumb is in the correct position.	1	2	3	4	5	
4. The wrist has adequate support.	1	2	3	4	5	
5. The pan is wide enough for all the fingers.	1	2	3	4	5	
6. The length of the pan and thumb trough is adequate.	1	2	3	4	5	
7. The splint is two-thirds the length of the forearm.	1	2	3	4	5	
8. The splint is half the width of the forearm.	1	2	3	4	5	
9. Arches of the hand are supported and maintained.	1	2	3	4	5	
Function						
1. The splint completely immobilizes the wrist, fingers, and thumb.	1	2	3	4	5	
2. The splint is easy to apply and remove.	1	2	3	4	5	
Straps						
1. The straps are rounded.	1	2	3	4	5	
2. Straps are placed to adequately secure the hand/arm to splint.	1	2	3	4	5	
Comfort						
1. The edges are smooth with rounded corners.	1	2	3	4	5	
2. The proximal end is flared.	1	2	3	4	5	
3. The splint does not cause impingements or pressure areas.	1	2	3	4	5	
Cosmetic Appearance						
1. The splint is free of fingerprints, dirt, and pencil or pen marks.	1	2	3	4	5	
2. The splinting material is not buckled.	1	2	3	4	5	

GRADING SHEET 10-1 Elbow Immobilization Splint

Name: ____________________

Date: ____________________

Type of elbow immobilization splint:

Posterior ❍ Anterior ❍

Elbow position: ____________________

Grade: ____________

1 = beyond improvement, not acceptable
2 = requires maximal improvement
3 = requires moderate improvement
4 = requires minimal improvement
5 = requires no improvement

Evaluation Areas						Comments
Design						
1. The elbow position is at the correct angle.	1	2	3	4	5	
2. The elbow has adequate medial and lateral support (two-thirds the circumference of the elbow).	1	2	3	4	5	
3. The splint supplies sufficient proximal/lateral support (1 inch proximal to axillary crease).	1	2	3	4	5	
4. The splint is two-thirds the circumference of the upper arm.	1	2	3	4	5	
5. Distally the splint extends to the distal palmar crease.	1	2	3	4	5	
6. The splint is two-thirds the circumference of the forearm.	1	2	3	4	5	
Function						
1. The splint allows full thumb and digit motion.	1	2	3	4	5	
2. The splint allows full shoulder motion.	1	2	3	4	5	
3. The splint provides adequate elbow support to properly secure the elbow in the splint and prevent elbow motion.	1	2	3	4	5	
Straps						
1. The straps are secure and rounded.	1	2	3	4	5	
Comfort						
1. The splint edges are smooth with rounded corners.	1	2	3	4	5	
2. The proximal end is flared.	1	2	3	4	5	
3. The splint does not cause impingements or pressure sores.	1	2	3	4	5	
4. The splint does not irritate bony prominences.	1	2	3	4	5	
Cosmetic Appearance						
1. The splint is free of fingerprints, dirt, and pencil and pen marks.	1	2	3	4	5	
2. The splinting material is not buckled.	1	2	3	4	5	

GRADING SHEET 11-1 Radial Nerve Splint

Name: ____________________

Date: ____________________

Wrist position at rest:

Grade: ___________

1 = beyond improvement, not acceptable
2 = requires maximal improvment
3 = requires moderate improvement
4 = requires minimal improvement
5 = requires no improvement

Evaluation Areas						Comments
Design						
1. The forearm trough is the proper length and width.	1	2	3	4	5	
2. The outrigger wire is at the appropriate angles and ½ inch wider than the MCPs at the level of the hand.	1	2	3	4	5	
3. The thermoplastic material on the MCP aspect of the outrigger is secure.	1	2	3	4	5	
4. The line to the outrigger is at a 90-degree angle from the long axis of the bone when the hand is at rest.	1	2	3	4	5	
5. The anchor hook is secure.	1	2	3	4	5	
6. The thermoplastic material patch adequately secures the outrigger.	1	2	3	4	5	
Function						
1. The wrist is maintained in neutral when the fingers are in extension.	1	2	3	4	5	
2. The outrigger or lines do not impede composite flexion of the fingers.	1	2	3	4	5	
3. The fit of the trough and straps prevents distal migration of the splint.	1	2	3	4	5	
4. The slings do not migrate distally with finger flexion and extension.	1	2	3	4	5	
Comfort						
1. Excessive pressure is not present on the radial or ulnar styloids.	1	2	3	4	5	
2. The edges are smooth with rounded corners.	1	2	3	4	5	
3. The proximal and distal ends are flared.	1	2	3	4	5	
4. Impingements or pressure areas are not present.	1	2	3	4	5	

Comments:

____

____

____

____

____

GRADING SHEET 12-1 Finger Splint

Name: ____________________

Date: ____________________

Type of finger splint:
Mallet finger ❍ PIP gutter ❍ PIP hyperextension block ❍ Other __________

Grade: __________

1 = beyond improvement, not acceptable
2 = requires maximal improvement
3 = requires moderate improvement
4 = requires minimal improvement
5 = requires no improvement

Evaluation Areas						**Comments**
Design						
1. The PIP position is at the correct angle.	1	2	3	4	5	
2. The DIP position is at the correct angle.	1	2	3	4	5	
3. The splint provides adequate support and is not constrictive.	1	2	3	4	5	
4. The splint length is appropriate.	1	2	3	4	5	
5. The splint width is appropriate.	1	2	3	4	5	
6. The splint is snug enough to stay in place yet loose enough to apply and remove.	1	2	3	4	5	
Function						
1. The splint allows full MCP motion.	1	2	3	4	5	
2. The splint allows full PIP motion.	1	2	3	4	5	
3. The splint allows full DIP motion.	1	2	3	4	5	
4. The splint enables as much hand function as possible.	1	2	3	4	5	
Straps						
1. The straps are secure and the terminal edges are rounded.	1	2	3	4	5	
Comfort						
1. The splint edges are smooth, rounded, contoured, and flared.	1	2	3	4	5	
2. The splint does not cause pain or pressure areas.	1	2	3	4	5	
Cosmetic Appearance						
1. The splint is free of fingerprints, dirt, and pencil/pen marks.	1	2	3	4	5	
2. The splinting material is not buckled.	1	2	3	4	5	

GRADING SHEET 13-1 Anticlaw Splint

Name: ______________________________

Date: ______________________________

Grade: ______________

1 = beyond improvement, not acceptable
2 = requires maximal improvement
3 = requires moderate improvement
4 = requires minimal improvement
5 = requires no improvement

Evaluation Areas						Comments
Design						
1. The splint prevents hyperextension of the MCP joints of the ring and little fingers.	1	2	3	4	5	
Function						
1. The splint allows full wrist motions.	1	2	3	4	5	
2. The splint allows full function of the middle and index fingers.	1	2	3	4	5	
Straps						
1. The straps avoid bony prominences.	1	2	3	4	5	
2. The straps are secure and rounded.	1	2	3	4	5	
Comfort						
1. The edges are smooth with rounded corners.	1	2	3	4	5	
2. The proximal end is flared.	1	2	3	4	5	
3. The splint is does not cause impingements or pressure areas.	1	2	3	4	5	
4. Splint pressure is well distributed over the proximal phalanx of the ring and little fingers.	1	2	3	4	5	
Cosmetic Appearance						
1. The splint is free of fingerprints, dirt, and pencil or pen marks.	1	2	3	4	5	
2. The splinting material is not buckled.	1	2	3	4	5	

Comments:

____

____

____

____

____

____

____

GRADING SHEET 14-1 Hard-Cone Wrist and Hand Splint

Name: ______________________

Date: ______________________

Type of cone wrist and hand splint:

Volar platform ❍ Dorsal platform ❍

Grade: ____________

1 = beyond improvement, not acceptable
2 = requires maximal improvement
3 = requires moderate improvement
4 = requires minimal improvement
5 = requires no improvement

Evaluation Areas						**Comments**
Design						
1. The wrist position is at the correct angle.	1	2	3	4	5	
2. The correct cone-diameter size reflects the palm width and web-space size.	1	2	3	4	5	
3. The small end of the cone is placed radially and the large end is placed ulnarly.	1	2	3	4	5	
4. The thumb is positioned in palmar abduction with the web space preserved.	1	2	3	4	5	
5. The splint is two-thirds the length of the forearm.	1	2	3	4	5	
6. The splint is half the width of the forearm.	1	2	3	4	5	
Function						
1. The wrist is positioned in submaximal or maximal range.	1	2	3	4	5	
2. The fingers are positioned to provide firm pressure but not stretch the flexors.	1	2	3	4	5	
Straps						
1. The straps avoid bony prominences.	1	2	3	4	5	
2. The straps are secure and rounded.	1	2	3	4	5	
3. The active field materials are used over the extensor muscle bellies.	1	2	3	4	5	
4. The passive field materials are used over the flexor muscle bellies.	1	2	3	4	5	
Comfort						
1. The edges are smooth with rounded corners.	1	2	3	4	5	
2. The proximal end is flared.	1	2	3	4	5	
3. Impingements or pressure areas are not present. (The ulnar styloid is relieved.)	1	2	3	4	5	
Cosmetic Appearance						
1. The splint is free of fingerprints, dirt, and pencil or pen marks.	1	2	3	4	5	
2. The splinting material is not buckled.	1	2	3	4	5	

APPENDIX D

Web Resources and Vendors

Societies, Organizations, Education

American Academy of Orthopaedic Surgeons
http://www.aaos.org/
American Hand Therapy Foundation
http://www.ahtf.org/
The American Occupational Therapy Association, Inc.
http://www.aota.org/
The American Occupational Therapy Foundation
http://www.aotf.org/
American Orthotic & Prosthetic Association
http://www.aopanet.org/
American Physical Therapy Association
http://www.apta.org//AM/Template.cfm?Section=Home
The American Society for Hand Surgery
http://www.handsurgery.org/
American Society of Hand Therapists
http://www.asht.org/
American Society for Surgery of the Hand
http://www.assh.org/AM/Template.cfm
Canadian Association of Occupational Therapists
http://www.otworks.com/otworks_page.asp?pageid=736
E-hand
http://www.eatonhand.com/
Exploring Hand Therapy
http://www.exploringhandtherapy.com/
Hand Rehabilitation Foundation
http://www.handrehabfoundation.org/
Handsights (special interest group of hand therapists attending the surgery meetings)
http://www.handsights.org/
Hand Therapy Certification Commission
http://www.htcc.org/
International Federation of Societies for Hand Therapy
http://www.ifsht.org/front.php
Journal of Hand Therapy
http://journals.elsevierhealth.com/periodicals/hanthe
World Federation of Occupational Therapists
http://www.wfot.org/

Splinting Materials and Accessories Suppliers

The following list is of course not exhaustive. Neither is the quality and/or service of products implied, and company contact information is subject to change.

AliMed 1-800-225-2610
http://www.alimed.com/
Bio Med Sciences, Inc. 1-800-25-SILON
http://www.silon.com/
Bioness, Inc.
http://www.bionessinc.com
Chesapeake Medical Products, Inc. 1-888-560-2674
http://www.chesapeakemedical.com/
DeRoyal 1-800-deroyal
http://www.deroyal.com/
Human Factors Engineering 928-684-9606
http://www.splinting.com/
Kinex Medical Company 1-800-845-6364
http://www.kinexmedical.com/
Larson Products, Inc. 614-235-9100
http://www.larsonmedical.com/
North Coast Medical 1-800-821-9319
http://www.ncmedical.com/main_index.asp?flash_enabled=N&sessionid={501D27F7-3D60-4350-844C-105D479D2A02}
Orfit Industries +32 (0) 3 326 20 26 (Belgium)
http://www.orfit.com/
Prostchotics, Functional Systems, LLC 1-877-675-2781
http://www.prosthotics.com
Sammons Preston Rolyan 1-800-323-5547 (to order catalog)
http://www.sammonspreston.com/
Silver Ring Splint Company 1-800-311-7028
http://www.silverringsplint.com/
UETECH 1-800-736-1894
http://www.uetech.com/
WFR Corporation 1-800-526-5247
http://www.reveals.com/

Index